Text Book
of
Pharmacognosy

Second Edition

Revised as per latest PCI syllabus

Text Book of Pharmacognosy

Second Edition

Revised as per latest PCI syllabus

Dr. Mohammed Ali

Faculty of Pharmacy
Jamia Hamdard (Hamdard University)
Hamdard Nagar, New Delhi - 110 062

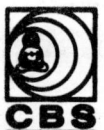

CBS Publishers & Distributors Pvt. Ltd.

New Delhi • Bengaluru • Chennai • Kochi • Kolkata • Mumbai
Bhubaneswar • Hyderabad • Jharkhand • Nagpur • Patna • Pune • Uttarakhand • Dhaka

Textbook of PHARMACOGNOSY

ISBN: 978-81-239-0278-4

Copyright © Author and Publisher

Second Edition: 2000
  Reprint: 2002, 2003, 2004, 2005, 2006, 2007, 2008, 2009, 2010, 2012, 2015, 2017, 2018, 2019, 2023

Published by Satish Kumar Jain and Produced by Varun Jain for

CBS Publishers & Distributors Pvt Ltd
4819/XI Prahlad Street, 24 Ansari Road, Daryaganj, New Delhi 110 002, India. 4819/XI Prahlad Street, 24 Ansari Road, Daryaganj, New Delhi 110 002, India.
Ph: 23289259, 23266861   Website: www.cbspd.com
                            e-mail: delhi@cbspd.com
Corporate Office: 204 FIE, Industrial Area, Patparganj, Delhi 110 092
Ph: 011-4934 4934 Fax: 011-4934 4935   e-mail: publishing@cbspd.com;
                            publicity@cbspd.com

Branches

- **Bengaluru:** Seema House 2975, 17th Cross, K.R. Road, Banasankari 2nd Stage, Bengaluru 560 070, Karnataka
  Ph: +91-80-26771678/79   Fax: +91-80-26771680   e-mail: bangalore@cbspd.com
- **Chennai:** 7, Subbaraya Street, Shenoy Nagar, Chennai 600 030, Tamil Nadu, India
  Ph: +91-44-26680620/26681266   Fax: +91-44-42032115   e-mail: chennai@cbspd.com
- **Kochi:** 42/1325, 1326, Power House Road, Opp KSEB, Power House, Ernakulam 682 018, Kochi, Kerala, India
  Ph: +91-484-4059061-65, 67   Fax: +91-484-4059065   e-mail: kochi@cbspd.com
- **Kolkata:** 147, Hind Ceramics Compound, 1st Floor, Nilgunj Road, Belghoria, Kolkata-700056, West Bengal, India
  Ph: +033-25633055, 033-25633056   e-mail: kolkata@cbspd.com
- **Lucknow:** Basement, Khushnuma Complex, 7 Meerabai Marg (Behind Jawahar Bhawan), Lucknow-226001, UP, India
  Ph: +91-522-4000032   e-mail: tiwari.lucknow@cbspd.com
- **Mumbai:** PWD Shed, Gala no 25/26, Ramchandra Bhatt Marg, Next to JJ Hospital Gate no. 2, Opp. Union Bank of India Noorbaug, Mumbai-400009, Maharashtra, India
  Ph: 022-66661880/89   e-mail: mumbai@cbspd.com

Representatives

• Hyderabad	0-9885175004	• Jharkhand	0-9811541605	• Nagpur	0-9421945513
• Patna	0-9334159340	• Pune	0-9923910676	• Uttarakhand	0-9716462459

Printed at Mudrak, Noida, UP

PREFACE TO THE SECOND EDITION

Every system of the world, including science, has developed through critical comments, discussion and suggestions. When the criticisms are abnormal and beyond limits, then there is a challenge. Popularity of the book among readers and their appreciation gave me enough courage to face such challenges.

When an edition of a book is revised, one tends to incorporate new advances into the overall structure of the first edition. In the present edition my emphasis is on providing a consistently readable format permitting clear understanding of up-to-date concise descriptions of various aspects of science of crude drugs. The traditional drugs are discussed to provide link between current findings. Recent informations concerning cultivation, chemical constituents and therapeutic efficacy of each drug have been included. The traditional medicinal systems in Chapter 1, drug constituents in Chapter 3 and pharmaceutical aids and technical products in Chapter 15 have been re-written. Microscopical aspects of the text have been revised thoroughly. Extensive tables summarizing drug informations may provide more knowledge of the subject. A new chapter entitled 'Variability in Drug Activity' is the additional attraction. Inclusion of questions at the end of each chapter will strengthen the interest of the readers. Every chapter has been carefully updated and revised. Most of the diagrams have been improved in their lay-out designs. The practical application of crude drugs is stressed throughout the book. Many of the simple illustrations have been re-drawn to improve accuracy and understanding.

I wish to thank my publisher, typists and artists for their untiring help. Many of my students and colleagues, present and past, have contributed useful suggestions and I am grateful to them. To our library staff thanks are due for their continued help in procuring much needed reference material. I express my deep gratitude to the authors of monographs of various pharmacopoeias, reports of the National Institute of Science Communication, New Delhi and of the Herbal Drugs and Phytopharmaceuticals from where I have gained knowledge for compiling the book.

I have made every effort to avoid printing errors. But ome of them may creep in present edition. I shall be bliged if the errors are brought to my notice. Constructive and helpful suggestions for improvement of the future editions of the book will be gratefully acknowledged.

—Mohammed Ali

CONTENTS

1

INTRODUCTION

Pharmacognosy is concerned with the study of crude drugs of vegetable and animal origins. The term materia medica is used to refer to all substances used in medicine such as pure chemical compounds, herbal drugs, mineral substances, and biological preparations like vaccines and sera. Pharmacognosy involved a comprehensive study of individual drugs and elucidation of general principles. The word "Pharmacognosy" was used by C.A. Seydler in 1815 (Greek : *Pharmakon* = drug; *Gnosy*=knowledge). The subject deals with biological, biochemical, therapeutic, and economic features of natural drugs and their chemical constituents. At present pharmacognosy involves the study of crude drugs and their natural derivatives. Thus, Digitalis and its isolated glycoside, digoxin; Datura and its isolated alkaloid, atropine; Opium and its purified compound morphine, all are treated as the subject of pharmacognosy. For studying a drug, the following points must be considered :

1. **Biological Source** : The biological source of a drug is mentioned in Latin language which also include the family to which it belongs. After the Latin name, the name of the botanist responsible for the classification is mentioned in abbreviated form. The plant family to which the drug belongs determines certain of its characters.

2. **Habitat** : The principal areas of collection and routes of transport are considered under this head.

3. **Plant Habit** : The general structure of the plant and morphology of crude drugs are studied.

4. **Cultivation, Collection and Preparation for Market**: These factors require particular attention when they affect the appearance or quality of the product.

5. **Morphology and Sensory Charactors** : A knowledge of the fine details of macroscopical sturcture is of vital importance in the examination of powdered drugs.

6. **Histology** : Microscopical characters such as cell structure and arrangement, starches, epidermal trichomes, calcium oxalate crystals and fibres are studied under this head.

7. **Commercial Varieties, Substitutes and Adulteration:** With a knowledge of the diagnostic characters of official drugs, a critical examination may be made of commercial samples to determine their quality, substances known to be potential substitutes or adulterations.

8. **Chemical Constituents** : The pharmacological active constituents, the percentage of the more potent components; constituents of affecting the mode of preparation, the identity and the class of such compounds are considered.

9. **Evaluation of Drugs** : The purity and quality of drugs are determined.

10. **Uses** : Various medicinal uses and toxic effects are studied.

PHARMACOGNOSY AND MODERN MEDICINE

Modern pharmacognosy has been developed rapidly due to the improvement made in the technology of isolation processes which include the development of techniques such as column, paper, thin layer, gas-liquid, high performance liquid and droplet counter current chromatographic procedures. These methods have allowed the rapid isolation of compounds previously difficult to obtain by classical procedures. The most important factor has been the development of new spectroscopic techniques which are used to identify structures of the isolated compounds.

Simultaneous advancement in the fields of chemistry, biochemistry, biosynthesis and pharmacology has developed pharmacognosy. Various active compounds have been isolated from plants which are used in modern medicine. With the advancement of synthetic organic chemistry most of the active constituents of plants used in medicine have been synthesized. However, in spite of phenomenal progress in the area of development of new drugs from synthetic sources and appearance of antibiotics as major therapeutic agents, plants continue to provide basic raw material for some of the most important drugs. Although more than 100 plants are used in modern medicine in various parts of the world, the list of most important ones along with their pharmacological properties is given in Table - 1.

Table 1. Important Active Constituents of Plants Used in Medicine.

Plants	Active Constituents	Pharmacological Activity
1. *Dioscorea* sp. *Agave* sp., *Solanum* sp.	Steroidal hormones	Anti-inflammatory, antiarthritic, hormonal
2. *Papaver somniferum*	Morphine, Codeine, Papaverine	Sedative, antitussive, smooth muscle relaxant
3. *Cinchona* sp.	Quinine Quinidine	Antimalarial, antiarrhythmic
4. *Datura* sp., *Hyoscyamus niger,* *Duboisia* sp.	Hyoscyamine Hyoscine Atropine	Parasympatholytic
5. *Digitalis lanata*	Digitoxin Digoxin Lanatosides	Cardiotonic
6. *Rauwolfia* sp.	Reserpine Rescinamine Deserpidine	Hypotensive Vasodialator
7. *Catharanthus roseus*	Ajmalicine	Vasodialator
8. *C. roseus*	Vincristine, Vinblastine	Anticancer
9. *Camellia sinensis* (Tea)	Caffeine	CNS stimulant

(Contd.)

Plants	Active Constituents	Pharmacological Activity
10. *Erythroxylum coca*	Cocaine	Anaesthetic
11. *Ephedra sp.*	Ephedrine	Sympathomimetic
12. *Pilocarpus jaborandi*	Pilocarpine	Parasympatho-mimetic
13. *Cephaelis acuminata, C. ipecacuanha*	Emetine	Antiamoebic
14. *Claviceps purpurea*	Ergometrine Ergotamine Ergotoxine	Oxytocic, Vascocontrictor, Vasodialator
15. *Plantago ovata*	Psyllium mucilage	Laxative
16. *Vinca minor, Voacanga africana*	Vincamine	Vasodialator
17. *Glycyrrhiza glabra*	Glycyrrhetic acid	Anti-inflammatory
18. *Cassia angustifolia, C. acutifolia*	Sennosides	Laxative
19. *Berberis sp.*	Berberine	Antidiarrhoreal
20. *Podophyllum peltatum*	Podophyllotoxin	Anticancer
21. *Colchicum autumnale*	Colchicine	Gout
22. *Theobroma cacao*	Theobromine	CNS stimulant, diuretic
23. *Coffea arabica*	Theophylline	CNS stimulant, diuretic

In addition to pure constituents the crude extracts of Belladonna, Ipecac, Opium, Henbane, Stramonium, Cascara sagrada, Glycyrrhiza, Rhubarb, Valerian, Podophyllum, Capsicum oleoresin, Digitalis and Aloe are used in modern medicine. Besides these, the essential oils of Japanese mint, Peppermint, Eucalyptus, Anise seed, Clove, Cinnamon leaf, Lemongrass and Camphor are also utilized in modern medicine.

Liver and stomach preparations of animals are used in therapy of pernicious anaemia. Bile secreted in liver is used in biliary secretion and parenterally as sodium salt to increase diuresis.

AYURVEDA AND DRUG DEVELOPMENT

Ayurveda is an ancient Indian system of health-care, both physical and mental, and literally means, science of life. Health in Ayurveda has been defined as a well balanced metabolism plus a happy state of being . Disease has been considered four fold,

1. body,
2. mind,
3. external factors and
4. natural intrinsic causes.

In Ayurveda treatment is done by a salubrious use of drugs, diets and practices.

Pharmaceutics occupies an important place in Ayurveda. Medicinal preparations are invariably complex mixtures, being derived from plant and animal products as well from minerals and metals.

Utilization of plants is mentioned in Rigveda and Atharvaveda. Charaka Samhita (900 B.C.) is the first recorded treatise on Ayurveda. It consists of eight sections divided into 150 chapters, and describes 341 plants used in medicine. The other treatise on Ayurveda is Sushruta samhita (600 B.C.) with special emphasis on surgery. It has six sections covering 186 chapters and describes 395 medicinal plants, 57 drugs of animal origin, and 64 minerals and metals as drugs. The next important authorty in Ayurveda was Vagabhatta of Sind, who practised during about 7th centrury A.D. His manuscript entitled 'Astanga Hridaya', is considered unrivalled for principles and practice of medicine. The manuscript is divided into six sections covering 120 chapters and contains 7444 verses. Madhava of Vijayanagar (12th century A.D.) comprised Madhava Nidana which consisted 69 chapters and 1552 verses. Sarangdhara (14th century), the author of Sarangdhara Samhita, systematized Ayurvedic Materia media. This book consists of three parts, 32 chapters, and 2500 verses. Bhava Mishra of Magadha wrote his treatise Bhava Prakashan in 1550 A.D. which contained 10,8 1 verses; nearly 470 medicinal plants are mentioned. In addition, about 70 pharmacy lexicons have been written. 'Raja Nighantu' by Narhari Pandita and 'Madanpala Nighantu' by Madanpala are considered as masterpieces on medicinal herbs.

Kashmir-born Dridhobala (9th century A.D.), a well known physician of India, re-constructed and re-edited the great Ayurvedic medical treatise *Charaka Samhita*. Another famous scholar of 9th century A.D. was Ugraditya Charya Jain, a native of Deccon, who wrote a treatise under the title *Kalyana Karaka*. He has described the use of mercury and many other compounds. Vrinda (1000 A.D.) composed a book of medicinal chemistry called *Siddhayoga*. The book describes methods for the preparation of various metallic drugs. Chakarapanidatta (1066 A.D.) wrote *Chikitsa Sarsamgraha* which described uses of more metals for curing diseases. A treatise called *Chikitsa Sarsamgraha* was written by Vangasena in 1200 A.D. The book describes uses of mica, iron, mercury, sulphur and copper.

CONTRIBUTION OF UNANI MEDICINAL SYSTEM TO PHARMACY

In the seventh and eighth centuries the Arabs conquered a great part of the ancient civilized world and extended their empire from Spain to India. Like the Romans, they respected the cultures of the conquered people. During the reign of Abbasid Caliph Harun al-Rashid (786-814 A.D.) Baghdad achieved fame as a city of learning. Some Indian physicians were invited to Baghdad, received the favours of the Caliph and settled there.

Juhanna ibn Masawaih (777-857 A.D.) translated the Greek manuscripts into Arabic and wrote a medical book. He modified the effects of certain remedies recommended as mixtures. The first London Pharmacopoeia was largely based on his formulae.

Manaka, a popular Indian physician at Baghdad, translated some books from Sanskrit into Arabic or Persian and composed *Kitab tafsir isma al-Aqaqir* which included a list of drugs and herbs of Indian origin.

The work of Persian born Abu Bekr Muhammad Ibn Zakaria or Rhaze (841 - 926) has been very much used in the European world. He wrote about one hundred medical books. His book, *Kitab al-Hawi*, has been used as a medical encyclopaedia. Abu'l Qasim al-Zahrawi or Albucasis, born in Spain in 936 A.D., practised as physician - pharmacist - surgeon and wrote on surgery and pharmaceutical subjects. Abu Mansur (C.970), a Persian pharmacologist, was the author of Arab Pharmacopoeia in which he described 466 vegetable drugs, 75 meneral drugs and 44 animal drugs. Al-Biruni (973-1050) of Khwarizm made great contribution towards the development of pharmacy. He defined pharmacognosy and pharmacology first of all, studied the natural products and their sources and mentioned 720 drugs in an alphabetical order in his book al - Saidana fil tibb.

Abu Ali al-Husain bin Abdallah or Avicenna (980 - 1037), born in Bukhara, was called as the "Prince of Physicians". His book, 'Qanun fil Tibb'. was used as a guide and authority up to 17th century. Ali ibn Abbas (994 A.D.), a persian medical author, wrote a medical encyclopaedia, Kitab al Maliki. Seville-born Abu Mervan or Ibn Zuhr or Avenzoar (1113-1199) was a medical botanist and pharmacist. His main work was on diet, which is incorporated in the book al-Aghdhiya. Abu'l-Walid Muhammad ibn Ahmad or Ibn Rushd, born in 1126 A.D. at Cardova in Spain, composed a medical book Kitab al-Kulliyat. Rabbi Moses (1135 - 1208) was a Jewish scholar and physician who wrote dietetic rules in a book. It describes diet and regimen including Rhubarb and tamarind pills. The publications of Spanish-born Ibn al-Baytar (1197-1248) gave the most comprehensive list of drugs. He mentioned detailed outlines for the preparation of rose water and recommended the use of Colocynth, Croton oil, Nutmeg and Pyrethrum. Ibn Serabi, an important pharmacist of the Muslim world, was famous for writing on medieval pharmacy. Abu'l Qasim-al-Iraqi (1300 A.D.) described the preparation and properties of an anaesthetic powder in his book Uyun al-Haqaiq.

The Arabs greatly improved pharmaceutical products and made them more elegant and palatable. Their pharmacy and Materia Medica were followed for a long time. The use of sugar is a chracteristic of Arab Pharmacy. Many drugs of India or of the East, such as Musk, Cloves, Cubebs, Dragon's blood, Galanga root, Betel nut, Sandalwood, Rhubarb, Nutmeg, Tamarind, Cassia bark, Croton oil, and Nux vomica were introduced by Arabs into Egypt. Alcohol, Jalap, Syrup, Aloe, Cinnamon, Camphor (Kafur), Anise, Zingiber, Myrrh, Styrax, Coffea, etc. are the Arabic names which are common in English. In the 7th century A.D. Arabs founded trading centres on the Malabar coast of South India. Through these centres they purchased spices, dyes, drugs and perfumes and introduced these articles in Iran, Turkey, Egypt and other countries.

It was in the 8th century that Arab Pharmacy and Medicine became two separate branches. This separation was made compulsory by law in 11th century and governmentally supervised stores were established in Baghdad. An inspector was appointed to check and ensure the supply of genuine herbs, and for inspecting the preparation of formulations for patients. There was deterrent punishment for adulteration of medicines and fake prescriptions. In Middle Ages schools of pharmacy were established for a regular pharmaceutical education. They discovered new and potent medicaments. If the new drugs proved bitter in taste, the ingenious Arab pharmacists devised chemical and mechanical methods to make them tolerable. The candy-coated pills were first employed by Avicenna who always tried to keep their patients cheerful. Arab pharmacists mixed rose-water and perfumes with medicines. They invented tinctures, confections, syrups, pomades, plasters, and ointments to ease the physicians task. The use of hashish and *bhang (Cannabis sativa)* and the behaviour of addicts of these drugs are described in the *Arabian Nights.* They invented the apothecary, which they called 'Saidala'. Ibn al-Attar, the son of a druggist, referred to the Sandalwood for therapeutic uses. In the reign of al-Mansur's son the drug shops were run by educated and morally responsible apothecaries.

Alchemy was developed along with medicine. The idea of "elixir of life", an "all-cure" was developed. The Arab pharmacists from the 9th century invented valuable techniques and apparatuses and included in their stock many of the commodities required in different branches of technology. Their pharmaceutical preparations consisted of powders, suspensions, syrups, electuaries, distilled medicinal waters and many other forms exceeding seventy in number. Some typical apparatuses were designed for manufacturing the medicines. Akbar the Great sent many Unani physicians all over India and paid attention to the profession of pharmacy. Most of the physicians were interested in medicinal plants and mentioned their preparations, properties, therapeutic effects, mode of administration and reactions in their books. Ilyas bin Shehab described many Indian drugs and herbs in his book *Rahat al - insan* during the rule of Firoz Shah Tughlaq (1351-1368 A.D.).

FUTURE OF HERBAL DRUGS

Plants are still a potent source of therapeutic agents. They are popularized due to their effectiveness, easy availability, low cost and comparatively being devoid of serious toxic effects. Some herbal drugs like *Achyranthes aspera* (diuretic), *Acorus calamus* (tranquilizer), *Artemisia vulgaris* (cardiac tonic), *Butea frondosa* (anthelmintic), *Bacopa monnieri* (memory), *Boerhaavia diffusa* (anti-inflammatory), *Cassia fistula* (cathartic), *Centella asiatica* (intelligence), *Curcuma longa* (anti-inflammatory), *Eugenia jambolana* (hypoglycemic), *Euphorbia thymifolia* (antiasthmatic) and *Sida rhombifolia* (anabolic) have been proven to exhibit the respective pharmacological actions. A derivative of artemisinin, prepared from *Atemisia annua*, is effective against resistant strains of *Plasmodium falciparum* where synthetic antimalarials fail to cure the disease. A derivative of podophyllotoxin obtained from *Podophyllum hexandrum* and *P. emodi* and taxol isolated from *Taxus baccata* have been approved as an anticancer agents in USA. A flavonoid, isolated from *Silybum marianum*, has been approved as drug against various liver disorders in Germany and other western countries. Iridoid glycosides, called valepotriates, obtained from *Valeriana* species, have been used as tranquilizer and sedative in Germany and other European countries. Total saponins from the Indian plant *Commiphora mukul*, often referred as guggulipid, have been approved as hypolipidaemic agent for lowering blood cholesterol.

AYURVEDIC MEDICINAL SYSTEM

Like all systems of Indian sciences, the origin of Ayurveda has been taken from the gods. Ayurveda was first perceived by Brahma, and he taught this science to Daksa - Prajapati, who taught it to the Aswni-Kumaras, and they taught it to Indra and so on. All the four Vedas are replete with references to various aspects of medicine. Many miraculous achievements in the field of medicine and surgery are mentioned in Vedas. The concept of digestion, metabolism, anatomical descriptions and discussion about several diseases are available. Different types of bacteria causing diseases are also described. The process of delivery, cauterization, toxins, control of evil sprites, rejuvenation therapies and aphrodisiacs have been mentioned. Medicinal plants, the different parts and their therapeutic effects are also described. Ayurveda believes in the existence of soul in the individual's body and in the unity of the body and the mind. Mental perversions affect the physical functions, and morbidity of the body affects the mental activities. Intellectual blasphemy, unwholesome conjunction of sense organs with their objects and vagaries of weather and time are causative factors of diseases. Forcible stimulation of natural strength, negligence in treatment, loss of good conduct, avoidance of health activities, malice, fear, anger, etc. are some examples of intellectual blasphemy. Unwholesome conjunction of sense organs include vision, sound, smell, taste and touch. Cold, heat and rain are characteristic features of seasonal diseases. *Rasa, rakta, mamsa, medas, asthi, majja* and *sukra* are the seven basic tissue elements. There are thirteen groups of enzymes which are responsible for digestion and metabolism in the body.

Principles of Ayurveda

Life in the purview of Ayurveda connotes a combination of body, sense organs, mind and soul. It is a system of health care which treats each person. The "TRIDOSHIC" concept is the fundamental principle in Ayurveda.

There are three basic constituents of the physiological systems according to this concept. These constituents are called "DOSHAS". They are the ultimate irreducible basic metabolic elements constituting the body and mind of the living organism. They are classified into VATA, PITTA and KAPHA. They correspond primarily to elements of air, fire and water. They determine the life processes of growth and decay.

Vata

The biological air humour is called "Vata" (air). It is primarily dry, cold and light. It is most important, or primary, of the three biological humours. It governs the other two and is responsible for all physical processes in general. It sustains effort, exhalation, movement and the discharge in impulses, the equilibrium of tissues and the coordination of senses. When aggravated, Vata (air) causes emaciation, debility, liking of warmth, tremors, distension, constipation, insomnia, sensory disorientation and incoherent speech. Vata is located in the colon, thighs, hips, ears, bones and organ of tough.

Pitta

The biological fire humour is called Pitta, sometimes also translated as bile. It is responsible for all chemical and metabolic transformation in the body. Pitta exists mainly in the acid form as fire and cannot exist directly in the body without destroying it. Pitta is primarily hot, moist and light. It governs digestion, heat, visual perception, hunger, thirst, lustre, complexion, understanding, intelligence, courage and softness of the body. Pitta in excess causes yellow colour of stool, urine, eyes and skin, hunger, thirst, burning sensation and difficulty in sleeping. High Pitta results in accumulation of internal heat or fever with inflammation and infections. Pitta is located in small intestine, stomach, sebacious glands, blood, lymph, organs and vision. Its primary site is in small intestine.

Kapha

The biological water humour is called Kapha, sometimes also translated as phlegm. Etymologically it means 'that which holds things together'. It provides substance and gives support and makes up the bulk of our bodily tissues. It also governs emotional traits as love, compassion, modesty, patience and forgiveness. Kapha is primarily cold, moist and heavy. It gives stability, lubrication, holding together of the joints and such qualities as patience. Kapha is the material substratum and support of the other two humours and also gives stability to the emotional nature. Excessive Kapha causes depression of the digestive fire, nausea, lethargy, heaviness, white colour, chills, looseness of the limbs, cough, difficult breathing and excessive sleeping. High Kapha results in the accumulation of weight and gravity in the body, inhibits normal function and causes hyroactivity through excessive tissue accumulation.

Treatment

Vata is treated by mild application of oils, mild sweating and purification methods. Pitta is treated with the ingestion of ghee (clarified butter), by purgation with sweet and cold herbs, by sweet, bitter and astringent foods and herbs, by applying cool, delightful and fragrant essential oils, by amounting the heat with Camphor, Sandalwood, Vetivert oils, etc. Kapha is treated by strong emetic and purgation methods according to the rules by all kinds of exercises, by smoking of herbs and by doing physical hard work.

Thus herbal medicine plays a major role in the treatment of Vata, Pitta and Kapha.

Ayurvedic Therapies

There are many different therapies applied in Ayurveda. They can all be defined in two groups viz :

(i) Tonification (supplementation-make heavy).

(ii) Reduction (elimination-to lighten)

Reduction therapies decrease body weight and are indicated for overweight accumulation of toxins and aggravated humours. It is indicated in acute stage of disease, when the attack is strong, and primarily for Kapha.

Tonification methods nourish deficiencies in body and are indicated in underweight, debility or tissue weakness. They are indicated in chronic diseases, in convalescence or after reduction methods have been used, and primarily for Vata. A mixed therapy is required for Pitta.

Ayurvedic methods of diagnosis are extremely simple. Stress is given on urine, stool, semen, flatus, vomiting, sneezing, eructation, yawning, hunger, thirst, tears, sleep and heavy breathing for diagnosis of a disease. Ayurveda also stresses upon the use of a wholesome diet along with the use of drugs for the successful treatment of diseases. Knowledge of the site of manifestation of the disease is essential for successful treatment. Pulse is examined in the early morning when the patient is in empty stomach. Pulse examination is carried out through the help of the radial artery.

In Ayurveda drugs are classified depending on their taste, attributes, potency, taste after digestion, and therapeutic effect. Four types of therapies - elimination therapy, alleviation therapy, psychic therapy and surgery, are used for the treatment of diseases. In addition to single drugs, compound formulations are generally used by Ayurvedic physicians in the form of pills, powders, decoctions, infusions, linctus, alcoholic preparations, medicated ghee, fractional distillation, collyrium, etc. Several pharmaceutical processes are followed for the preparation of medicines for easily administration; making the products delicious to the taste, easily digestable and assimilatable, therapeutically more efficacious, rendering them non-toxic and more tolerable and for preservation of medicines for a longer time. Ayruvedic drugs are administered both externally in the form of ointment, dusting powder, collyrium, ear drops and eye drops, and internally as tablets, pills, powder, syrups, etc. Along with medicines some regimens like sleep, walk, rest, physical exertion, etc. are also prescribed to the patients.

UNANI SYSTEM OF MEDICINE

Like Ayruveda, the Unani system of medicine is based on ancient principle. So there is a similarity between *Ayurveda* and *Tibb* regarding the contemplation of the same dogmatisms and traditionalism. The most important similarity is the principle of four elements which is identical to *Ayruveda's Panchbhuta* principle. According to four elemental principles of *Tibbi* discipline all the universal inanimate and animate things are produced from *Al-Nar* (Fire), *Al - hawa* (Air), *Al-ma* (Water) and *Al-ardh* (Earth). According to Ayruveda, all of the universal objects are made of *Panchbhuta* and body has its root and support of Doshas (*Tridosha* viz. *Vata, Pitta* and *Kapha),* Dhatus (seven metals : *Rasa, Rakta, Mansa, Meda, Asthi, Majja* and *Sukra)* and Mala (*Sweda, Mutra,* and *Purisha*). When these remain in the equilibrium and in normal functioning, then the health of an individual is maintained. In the same manner *Tibb* also maintains this view that the human body is composed of seven natural principles or components of the body known as *Al - umur Al - tabiyah.* The loss of the any one of these components may lead to diseases, or even death of the individual. These are as follows :

1. *Al - arkan* or *al - anasir* (Elements)
2. *Al - mizaj* (Temperament)
3. *Al - akhalt* (Humours - body fluids)
4. *Al a'za'* (Organs or members)
5. *Al - arwah* (Pneuma or vital spirit)
6. *Al - quwa* (Faculties or Powers)

7. Al - at'al (Functions)

In addition to these seven components, the essential causes influencing the human body are :
1. Atmospheric air
2. Foods and drinks
3. Physical or bodily movement and repose
4. Mental or Psychic movement and repose
5. Sleep and wakefulness
6. Evacuation and retention.

These factors essentially influence each and every body. Nobody could escape from these factors so long he is alive.

Some of the non essential causes are not concerned with every body and do not necessarily influence each and every human body. These are habit, habitat, profession, sex, temperament, other social factors, cosmic and terrestrial influences, etc. These factors influence to those only who come across them, therefore, they are considered non-essential. These are as :

1. Geographical conditions of the country and town and other related matters,
2. Residential conditions and related matters,
3. Occupation and related matters
4. Habits and related matters
5. Age and related matters
6. Sex and related matters
7. Any other factor antagonistic to nature and bodily health, e.g., micro-organisms, ionizing radiations, electricity and other natural forces.

The temperaments of persons are accordingly expressed by the words sanguine, phlegmatic, choleric and melancholic according to the preponderance in them of humours - blood, phlegm, yellow bile and black bile, respectively. The humors themselves are assigned temperaments - blood is hot and moist; phlegm cold and moist; yellow bile hot and dry; and black bile cold and dry.

Every person is supposed to have a unique humoral constitution which represents his healthy state. To maintain the correct humoral balance there is power of self preservation of adjustment called Quwwat-e-Mudabbira (Medicatrix naturae) in the body. If this power weakens imbalance in the humoral composition occurs, and this causes disease. In Unani medicine great reliance is placed on this power. The medicines used in this system, in fact, help the body to regain this power on the optimum level and thereby restore humoral balance, thus retaining health. The correct diet and digestion are also considered to maintain humoral balance.

Therapeutics

In Unani system of medicine various types of treatment are employed, such as Ilaj bit - Tadbeer (regimental therepy), Ilaj bil-Ghiza (dietotherapy), Ilaj bid-Dawa (pharmacotherapy) and jarahat (surgery).

The regimental therapy includes venesection, cupping, diaphoresis, diuresis, Turkish bath, massage, metastasis, cauterization, purging, emesis, exercise, leeching, etc. Dietotherapy aims at treating certain ailments by administration of specific diets or by regulating the quantity and quality of food, whereas pharmacotherapy deals with the use of naturally occurring drugs of herbal, animal and mineral origin. Similarly, surgery has also been in use in this system for quite long. The naturally occurring drugs used in this system are symbolic of life and are generally free from side-effect. If such drugs are toxic in crude form, then they are processed and purified in many ways before use. In Unani medicine although general preference is for a single drug, compound formulations are also employed in the treatment of various complex and chronic disorders. Since in this system, stress is laid on a particular temperament of an individual, the medicines administered are such as go well with the temperament of the patient, thus accelerating the process of recovery and also eliminating the risk of drug reaction.

Unani medicine aims of combating disease and preservation and promotion of health through curative, preventive, and promotive measures. For the treatment of various common and stubborn diseases, medicines obtained from natural sources e.g., plants, animals and minerals, are used in this sysem. Unani medicines are not only cheap and easily available, but are also effective and free from side effects.

Unani system of medicine has grown by experiences of

nations and countries like Egypt, Iraq, India, China, etc. Diagnosis of a disease is carried out by knowing past history of the patient and examination of pulse and other body organs. The Unani pharmaceutical preparations consist of powder, suspension, syrups, electuries, distilled medicinal waters and many other forms exceeding seventy in number.

HOMOEOPATHIC MEDICINAL SYSTEM

Homoeopathic medicinal system was started by the chemist, physician and pharmacist Samuel Hahnemann (1755-1843) of Germany who was dissatisfied with the side effects of the then current regimens of medication. He initiated the treatment of a disease with a low dose of those drugs which themselves produced similar symptoms of the disease in normal individuals. A medicine produces some symptoms in healthy state and if the identical symptoms are present in a sick person, then the patient will get relief with a minor dose of the medicine. According to Hahnemann, there is no any normal and natural method for diagnosis of a disease except its symptoms. This principle of the treatment of 'like with like' is quite the reverse of the allopathic system.

In any medicinal system there is no co-relation between the cause of the disease and human potency. According to homoeopathic medicinal system until the potency governing on the body of a human being is powerful and controls the functions of all organs, then the person will not be affected by a disease. A disease produced in the body and brain will effect on other body organs. The habits of telling lie, theft, deceit, evil, narcosis, under diet, anger, etc. are symptoms of mental diseases. After collecting the information about a disease, stress is given on mental disorders. Any symptom of a disease can not be complete without the governing power of the body.

Hahnemann's original observation involved Cinchona, which produced, in normal individuals, symptoms similar to those of malaria, for which the drug was used. In the same way, Belladonna on administration produced symptoms associated with Scarlet fever. If the symptoms of a disease are considered a manifestation of the body's own defence mechanism against the disease, then the homoeopathic treatment serves to stimulate such inherent defensive and curative processes. Hahnemann prepared a list of drugs with their effects on healthy individuals. A patient's symptoms could then be matched as closely as possible against the drug pictures and the appropriate treatment prescribed. In this way Nux vomica and Gelsemium root (yellow jasmine) became drugs for the treatment of influenza and the common cold.

Hahnemann observed that in the initial stages of treatment with the appropriate drugs at normal dosage rates, the illness appeared to be worsen in the beginning as the symptoms are inhanced by the drug. Therefore, subsequent doses are lowered. He observed that as the dose of a drug was reduced, its potency was enhanced. Thus, this process was no longer referred to as dilution but as potentiation. Thus, the homoeopathic treatment arrived at in conjunction with the patient's very detailed case history and constitutes the use of often very active drugs in extremely low doses. For the higher potencies of homoeopathic drugs the possibility of a current scientific explanation becomes non-existent, because individual doses at the dilution of the sixth or eight decimal may no longer contain a single molecule of the drug. Homoeopathic remedies have the distinct advantage that they are without side-effects.

Homoeopathic medicines are used in the form of mother tinctures, small pills, powder and distilled water. The patient should not take any kind of food or drink prior or after one hour of the dose.

For prescribing the medicine it is essential that information about characteristics of elements, mental symptoms and other symptoms should be collected. The medicine with more pronounced characters should be prescribed. If there is no relief then according to elements any medicine belonging to anti-soric, anti-cycotic and anti-syphilic category should be prescribed in one or two doses prior to the earlier medicine. Sora, syphilic and cycosis are related with the production of air, bile and cough as mentioned in Ayurveda. Diseases produced by air are identical to those which are produced by entering sora, e.g., mental exitement by bile and of syphilic and cycosis, respectively. These disorders are sometimes combined with each other. In some diseases the air and bile predominate and in others, cough and bile are in excess. In homoeopathy, diseases are not produced by the attack of microorganisms. Weak body potency is responsible for disease. This body potency becomes weak due to sora, syphilic and cycosis. Therefore, they are searched in the body.

Hahnemann's fundamental propositions peculiar to Homoeopathy may be said, as :

(a) that the action of drugs are demonstrable by observing the subjective symptoms, objective symptoms and pathological changes that occur when they are administered to healthy human subject.

(b) that the action of drugs so observed in a healthy human being constitutes their therapeutic potentiality with respect to the sick individual.

(c) that a similarity between disease processes in a particular individual and the known effects of a particular drug in healthy human being (known as drug proving of Homoeopathy) will lead to its successful application in the treatment of diseased individual (i.e. to bring a change in the altered dynamis).

(d) the conception of dynamis (vital force-active-driving force) is applicable in respect of health, disease and cure.

There are three essential processes involved in preparation of remedies : (a) Serial dilution (b) Succession (c) Trituration. Dilution is the meant by which we reduce the toxicity of the original crude drug. Serial dilution means that each dilution is prepared from the dilution that immediately proceeded it. Succession and trituration are the methods by which mechanical energy is delivered to our preparations in order to imprint the pharmacological message of the original drug upon the molecules of the diluent.

From the pharmaceutical point of view there are two main classes of original substance : (a) Soluble (b) Insoluble.

In the class of soluble substances mother tinctures (alcohol or water extraction) of the plant material are used. The symbol is used to denote the mother tincture of any soluble substance. For soluble substance alcohol and water are applied. At each stage rhythmical violent agitations are carried out, either by hand or machine, and this is known as "Succession". Insoluble natural substances are prepared in a different way. The diluent in one sense is lactose. The physical process applied at each stage is known as 'Trituration', it is a prolonged circular grinding with mortar and pestle. Once this trituration has obtained 6 x or 1/10, this be dispersed into alcohol water diluent. Thereafter, it is treated like a soluble substance.

These two major scales of preparing medicine are denoted as 'c' for centesimal scale and 'x' for decimal scale.

Centesimal scale involves a serial dilution 1/100, whereas decimal involves a serial trituration 1/10.

For the preparation of the homoeopathic potencies of a liquid drug substance three scales are in use, i.e. (a) Decimal (b) Centesimal and (c) Millesimal.

For the preparation of potencies from solid drug substances, (a) Decimal and (b) Centesimal scales are in use. When trituration attains the 6 x potency, then only it will be fit to be converted into liquid potency.

SIDDHA SYSTEM OF MEDICINE

Siddha is extensively practised in the southern parts of Tamil Nadu and in the neighbouring states.

Siddha is an ancient system of medicine. In treatment it uses minerals and metals mainly, but some products of vegetable and/or animal origin are also used. Work relative to Siddha contained atleast 3500 formulae written in Tamil initially on palm leaves.

Siddha medicine is essentially a psychosomatic system of medicine. Unlike Ayurveda importance is given more to minerals and metals rather than herbs in pharmaceutics. Herbs are used only to triturate and calcinate the metals into their basmam and sindooram.

As the world is made up of five elements or panchabutas, so also the human body. The human body is composed of earth and water, the soul is made up of air and ether and heat and fire combine them and make them to live together.

Hence, medicines for the human body are prepared based on the theory of panchabutas (metals of gold, lead, copper, iron and zinc). Gold and lead are used for the maintenance of the body. Iron, the only metal attracted by the electric power of magnet, and zinc, used for generating electricity, are employed in the medicine which are administered for the extension of life. Copper is used for the preservation of heat in the body. All the metals are used only after proper detoxification.

Siddha gives more attention to the disorders of the elements of the intrinsic factors of body than to the extrinsic ones.

The materia medica of Siddha science contains vegetables, minerals and marine elements and the three cordinal humours. All the drugs contain one or more of these humours.

The raw drugs are used either individually or in combination with other drugs. They are subjected to specific processes and the products are administered purification methods which include detoxification. A preparation contains several crude drugs.

SCOPE OF PHARMACOGNOSY AND PHYTOCHEMICAL INDUSTRY IN INDIA

Since indiscriminate use of synthetic drugs and antibiotics have resulted into serious symptoms all over the world, the demand of plant based raw materials for pharmaceuticals has increased enormously. Moreover, the synthetic drugs and intermediary chemicals are extremely expensive. The World Health Organization has emphasized the utilization of indigenous systems of medicines based on the locally available raw materials, i.e., medicinal plants. Furthermore, approximate one third of all drugs are plant-based and if bacteria and fungi are also included, nearly sixty per cent of pharmaceuticals are of plant origin. Our country is rich in large number of such plants that either be used directly or as the source of active principles in formulaion of drugs curing dreaded diseases. India as a whole is the richest source of medicinal plants which are distributed in almost all parts of the country. The herb collectors and small traders collect the drugs for the manufacturers of Ayurvedic and Unani medicines. But there is a shortage of these materials for maintaining the sustained supply to the plant based drug industries. It is also not proper under the present situation to be dependent only on natural resources to keep the wheel of the industries running all the time in view of the fast depleting natural wealth. This calls for the domestication and cultivation of these plants as well as increment of the drug production with uniformly high potency. At the same time increased demand of plant raw materials has led to over exploitation of wild plants resulting into serious hazard. This necessiates the urgent need of their systematic cultivation for constant supply to the user industries.

Domestication and cultivation of some of the important plants are necessary to cope up the demand of constant supply for the phytochemical industries. These plants include *Adhatoda vasica, Claviceps purpurea, Costus speciosus, Digitalis lanata, Dioscorea deltoidea, Hyoscyamus niger, Mentha piperita, Ruta graveolens, Santalum album, Solanum khasianum, S. lancinatum, Eucalyptus* species, etc.

There are many drugs which are imported to India. These include Balsam of Tolu, Peru Balsam, Benzoin, Storax, Copaiba, Asafoetida, Ipomoea, Colocynth, etc. If the cultivation of these drugs producing plants is carried out in India, sufficient foreign exchange can be saved.

As mentioned earlier, a derivative of artimisinin from *Artemisia annua*, podophyllotoxin obtained from *Podophyllum hexandrum* (*P. emodi*), silymarine flavanoid isolated from *Silybum marianum* seeds and total saponins from the Indian plant *Commiphora mukul* have been approved as drugs in various countries.

One of the new areas is medicine during the recent years has been the use of adaptogenic drugs from plants. Most of these drugs are used as general tonic and stimulants to improve the defence mechanism of the body and protect the body against stress and infection. These drugs also help the body to improve and tone up metabolism in old age and in persons weakened by serious diseases. These drugs, although not accepted in modern medicine, are now sold widely in Europe, USA and Asia mostly as health foods. Ginseng (*Panax* sp.), and Siberian Ginseng (*Eleutherococcus senticosus*), Korean ginseng (*Panax ginseng*), American Ginseng (*P. quinquefolium*), Ashwagandha (*Withania somnifera*), Brahmi (*Centella asiatica* and *Bacopa monnieri*) and Satwar (*Asparagus racemosus*) are used as adaptogenic drugs.

Inspite of the tremendous advance in medicine, there is a number of diseases for which modern medicine has no cure. In such cases it treats only symptoms to provide relief to patients. These include viral diseases, such as herpes (genitalis, simplex, zoster, etc.), muscular dystropy, parkinsonism, alcoholism, obesity, smoking, stress, genetic diseases, arthritic diseases, liver disorders, cancer, aids, etc. Recent trends have shown that plant drugs have the answer to such cases. Recently, a number of formulations based on Ayurvedic medicine have come to the market for control of liver disorders and some of these have been found effective against these diseases. There is a considerable scope to screen such plants for active constituents which may be used in future for treatment of such incurable diseases.

QUESTIONS

1. What is the importance of alternative systems of medicine in India ? Giving principles of Ayurveda, explain the role that modern pharmacognosy can play in proving effective drugs (Delhi University, 1988, Supple).

2. Giving historical background discuss the scope of pharmacognosy. What is its relevance in the modern drug scene (Delhi University, 1987) ?

3. Define Pharmacognosy and give its brief history and relationship with various allied sciences. (Jamia Hamdard, 1992).

4. Name the traditional systems of medicine practised in our country. Give the official source, chemical nature and uses of four traditional drugs which you have studied.

5. Discuss the development of Pharmacognosy giving the historical background. What are scopes of this discipline in providing authentic drugs ?

6. Discuss the basic principles of Ayurvedic and Unani systems of medicine. How is knowledge of pharmacognosy relevant to these medicines ?

7. What do you know about modern concept of pharmacognosy ?

2

CLASSIFICATION OF
CRUDE DRUGS

Higher plants, microbes and animals are the main sources of crude drugs. However, enzymes and antibiotics used in modern medicine are obtained from animals and microbes. For the study of crude drugs, they may be classified according to morphological, taxonomical, chemical and pharmacological characters. Each of these systems has its own merits and demerits. Morphological classification is more helpful to identify and detect adulteration. For studying evaluationary developments, the drugs are classified according to taxonomical classification. The activity of a drug is due to its chemical constituents and, therefore, the drugs are divided according to the presence of chemical components. Pharmacological classification of drugs is more relevant to study therapeutic utility of the drugs.

1. MORPHOLOGICAL CLASSIFICATION

Under morphological classification the drugs are arranged according to the part of the plant used such as leaves, stems, roots, barks, flowers, seeds, etc. The drugs obtained from the direct parts of the plants and containing cellular tissues are called as organized drugs, e.g. rhizomes, barks, leaves, fruits, entire plants, hair and fibres. The drugs which are prepared from plants by some intermediate physical processes such as incision, drying, or extraction with a solvent and not containing any cellular plant tissues are called as unorganized drugs, e.g. Aloe juice, Opium latex,

Agar, Gambier, Gelatin, Tragacanth, Benzoin, Honey, Beeswax, Lemongrass oil, etc. (Table 1).

The main drawback of morphological classification is that there is no co-relation of chemical constituents with the therapeutic actions. Usually this classification is adopted in the practical classes.

Table 1 : Gross Classification of Drugs on the Basis of Morphological Characters.

Plant Parts	Drugs
1. Organized Drugs	
Wood	Quassia, Sandalwood, Red Sandalwood.
Leaves	Digitalis, Eucalyptus, Gurmar, Pudina, Senna, Spearmint, Squill, Tulsi, Vasaka, Coca, Buchu, Hamamelis, Hyoscyamus, Belladonna, Tea.
Barks	Arjuna, Ashoka, Cascara, Cassia, Cinchona, Cinnamon, Kurchi, Quillaia, Wild Cherry.
Flowering Parts	Clove, Pyrethrum, Saffron, Santonica, Chamomile.
Fruits	Amla, Anise, Bael, Bahera, Bitter Orange peel, Capsicum, Caraway, Cardamom, Cassia, Colocynth, Coriander, Cumin, Dill, Fennel, Gokhru, Hirda, Lemon peel, Psoralea, Senna pod, Star anise, Tamarind, Vidang.
Seeds	Bitter Almond, Black Mustard, Cardamom, Colchicum, Ispaghula, Kaladana, Linseed, Neem, Nutmeg, Nux vomica, Physostigma, Psyllium, Strophanthus, White Mustard.
Roots and Rhizomes	Aconite, Ashwagandha, Calamus, Calumba, Colchicum corm, Dioscorea, Galanga, Garlic, Gentian, Ginger, Ginseng, Glycyrrhiza, Podophyllum, Ipecac, Ipomoea, Jalap, Jatamansi, Male fern, Picrorhiza, Piplamul, Rauwolfia.

Plant Parts	Drugs
	Rhubarb, Sassurea, Senega, Shatavari, Turmeric, Valerian, Squill, Serpentary, Indian Podophyllum, Krameria, Derris, Indian Valerian.
Plants and Herbs	Andrographis, Bacopa, Banafsha, Belladonna, Cannabis, Centella, Chirata, Chondrus, Datura, Ephedra, Ergot, Hyoscyamus, Kalmegh, Lobelia, Punarnava, Shankhpushpi, Stramonium, Vinca, Yeast.
Hair and Fibres	Cotton, Hemp, Jute, Silk, Flax.

2. Unorganized Drugs

Dried Latex	Opium, Papain.
Dried Juice	Aloe, Kino.
Dried Extracts	Agar, Alginate, Black Catechu. Pale Catechu, Pectin.
Gums	Acacia, Guar gum, Indian gum, Sterculia, Tragacanth.
Resins	Asafoetida, Benzoin, Colophony, Copaiba, Guaiacum, Guggal, Mastic, Myrrh, Peru Balsam, Sandarac, Storax, Tolu Balsam, Tar, Coal Tar.
Fixed Oils and Fats	Arachis, Castor, Chaulmoogra, Coconut, Cottonseed, Linseed, Olive, Sesame, Almond, Theobroma, Lard, Cod-liver, Halibut liver, Kokum butter.
Waxes	Beeswax, Spermaceti, Carnauba wax.
Volatile Oil	Turpentine, Anise, Coriander, Peppermint, Rosemary, Sandalwood, Cinnamon, Lemon, Caraway, Dill, Clove, Eucalyptus, Nutmeg, Camphor.
Animal Products	Beeswax, Cantharides, Cod liver oil, Gelatin, Halibut liver oil, Honey, Shark-liver oil, Shellac, Spermaceti wax, Wool fat, Musk, Mylabris, Lactose.
Fossil Organisms and Minerals	Bentonite, Kaolin, Kiesselguhr, Talc.

2. TAXONOMICAL CLASSIFICATION

Taxonomical classification is based on the principles of natural relationship and evolutionary development. They are grouped in phyllum order, family, genus and species. As all the entire plants are not used as drugs, therefore, it is of no significance of this division from identification point of view. This system also does not co-relate in between the chemical constituents and biological activity of the drugs. The taxonomical classification is summerized in Table 2.

Table 2. Taxonomical Classification of Drugs

Phyllum	Order	Family	Drugs
Angiosperms (Monocotyledons)	Liliflorae	Liliaceae	Scilla, Colchicum, Asparagus
		Dioscoreaceae	Dioscorea
	Microspermae	Orchidaceae	Vanilla
Angiosperms (Dicotyledons)	Papaverales,	Papaveraceae	Opium
	Rosales	Rosaceae	Almond, Quillaia, Rose oil
		Leguminosae	Balsam of Tolu, Glycyrrhiza, Senna
	Rutales	Rutaceae	Bael, Lemon, Orange peel
	Rhamnales	Rhamnaceae	Cascara bark
	Malvales	Malvaceae	Sida
	Umbelliflorae	Umbelliferae	Coriander, Caraway, Dill, Fennel
	Gentianales	Loganiaceae	Nux-vomica
		Gentianaceae	Chirata
		Apocyanaceae	Kurchi, Rauwolfia, Strophan-thus
	Tubiflorae	Convolvulaceae	Shankhpushpi
		Labiatae	Mentha, Ocimum

Phyllum	Order	Family	Drugs
		Solanaceae	Belladonna, Capsicum, Datura, Hyoscyamus
		Scrophulariaceae	Digitalis
	Plantaginales	Plantaginaceae	Plantago
	Dipsacales	Valerinanceae	Valerian
	Companulales	Lobeliaceae	Lobelia
		Compositae	Artemisia, Kuth
Bryophyta and Pteridophyta (Liverworts, Mosses and Ferns)	Filicales	Polypodiaceae	Male Fern
Gymnosperms	Genetales	Ephedraceae	Ephedra
	Coniferae	Pinaceae	Colophony
Thallophyta (Bacteria, Fungi, Lichens)			
Rhodophyta	Gelidiales	Gelidiaceae	Agar

3. CHEMICAL CLASSIFICATION

The biological activity of a drug is due to the presence of certain chemical constituents in the drug. Plants and animals synthesize chemical compounds such as fats, carbohydrates, proteins, volatile oils, alkaloids, resins, etc. and some of these are pharmacologically active constituents. A single active constituent may be isolated from the crude drug and used as a medicinal agent. More than 75 pure compounds derived from higher plants find their place in modern medicine. For example, the important traditional active plant principles are codeine, atropine, ψ-ephedrine, hyoscyamine, digoxin, hyoscine, digitoxin, pilocarpine, theobromine, theophylline, quinidine, quinine, emetine, caffeine, papaverine and colchicine. These active constituents are differentiated from the inert compounds like starch, cellulose, lignin, cutin, etc. The active constituent may be present in a very low concentration in the drug. The chemical classification of drugs is dependent upon the grouping of drugs with identical chemical constituents as shown in Table 3.

Table 3. Chemical Classification of Drugs

Chemical Constituents	Drugs
1. Carbohydrates	
Gum	Acacia, Tragacanth, Guargum, Sterculia
Mucilages	Plantago seed
Others	Starch, Honey, Agar, Pectin, Bael, Cotton
2. Glycosides	
Anthraquinone	Aloe, Cascara, Rhubarb, Senna,
Saponins	Quillaia, Arjuna, Glycyrrhiza, Dioscorea
Cyanophore	Wild Cherry bark,
Isothiocyanate	Mustard
Cardiac	Digitalis, Strophanthus,
(Steroidal)	Scilia
Bitter	Gentian, Calumba, Quassia, Chirata, Picrorhiza, Kalmegh
3. Tannins	Pale Catechu, Black Catechu, Ashoka bark, Galls, Myrobalan, Behera, Amla
4. Volatile oils	Cinnamon, Nutmeg, Fennel, Dill, Caraway, Coriander, Cardamom, Orange peel, Mint, Clove, Ginger, Valerian, Saffron, Banafsha, Tulsi, Anise, Lemongrass, Jatamansi, etc.
5. Lipids	
Fixed oils	Castor, Olive, Peanut, Cottonseed, Almond, Shark liver,
Fats	Theobroma, Lanolin
Waxes	Beeswax, Spermaceti
6. Resins	Colophony, Podophyllum, Jalap Cannabis, Capsicum, Turmeric, Ginger, Myrrh, Asafoetida, Storax, Balsam of Tolu, Balsam of Peru, Benzoin
7. Alkaloids	
Pyridine and Piperidine	Lobelia, Nicotiana, Areca nut
Tropane	Coca, Belladonna, Datura, Hyoscyamus, Stramonium, Henbane

(Contd.)

Chemical Constituents	Drugs
Quinoline	Cinchona,
Isoquinoline	Opium, Ipecac, Calumba
Indole	Ergot, Nux vomica, Rauwolfia, Catharanthus, Physostigma,
Amines	Ephedra
Steroidal	Kurchi, Veratrums
Purine	Tea, Coffee
Diterpene	Aconite
8. Proteins	Gelatin, Ficin, Papain
9. Vitamins	Yeast
10. Triterpenes	Rasna, Colocynth

4. PHARMACOLOGICAL CLASSIFICATION

In Pharmacological classification the drugs are grouped according to their therapeutic uses. Thus cardiotonic drugs include Digitalis, Squill and Strophanthus. Senna leaves and Castor oil are termed as purgative drugs. A particular drug containing known chemical constituents can be grouped according to its therapeutic use. The main drawback of this classification is that a drug can be placed in various classes according to its therapeutic use. Thus Cinchona can be grouped in antimalarial and antiarrhythmic catagories. The classification of drugs based on pharmacological action or therapeutic uses is given in Table 4.

Table 4 : Classification of Drugs Based on Pharmacological Action.

Pharmacological Action	Drugs
Anticancer	Vinca, Podophyllum, Taxus
Anti-inflammatory	Colchicum corm and seed, Turmeric
Antiamoebic	Ipecac root, Kurchi bark
Anthelmintic	Artemisia, Male Fern, Quassia wood, Vidang, Chenopodium oil
Antiasthmatic	Ephedra, Lobelia, Vasaka, Tylophora
Antispasmodic	Belladonna, Datura, Hyoscyamus
Astringent	Catechu, Tannic acid, Myrrh, Myrobalan, Ashoka bark

(Contd.)

Pharmacological Action	Drugs
Analgesic	Opium, Cannabis
Bitter tonics	Quassia wood, Nux-vomica, Gentian, Picrorhiza, Chirata, Kalmegh
Carminatives and	Cinnamon bark, Cardamom seed,
Flavours	Nutmeg fruit, Clove, Umbelliferous fruits, Peppermint, Saffron,
	Asafoetida, Oleo-gum resin, Mint, Tulsi, Ginger, Vanilla
Purgatives	Cascara bark, Senna, Rhubarb, Aloe, Castor oil, Plantago seed husk
Expectorant	Benzoin, Balsam of Tolu, Glycyrrhiza, Vasaka
Cardiotonic	Digitalis, Squill, Strophanthus
CNS Action	Ergot, Belladonna, Stramonium, Hyoscyamus, Ephedra, Physostigma
Hallucinogens	Cocaine, Cannabis
Tranquillizer	Rauwolfia roots.

QUESTIONS

1. Describe various systems of classification of crude drugs. Write their merits and demerits.
2. What are organized drugs ? Name five organized drugs containing glycosides as their main components. Give their biological sources and important diagnostic features.
3. What are the different systems of classifications of crude drugs ? Discuss the system based on the chemical constituents in detail.
4. Explain various classification of crude drugs. What are the advantage and disadvantage of morphological classification ?
5. Erumerate the different systems of classification of drugs. What is biochemical system of classification and what is its importance ?
6. Give the pharmacological classification of plant drugs.

3

DRUG CONSTITUENTS

The medicinal value of a crude drug depends on the presence of one or more chemical constituents of physiological importance. They may be glycosides, alkaloids, organized resins, enzymes, etc. A vegetable drug is composed of a number of tissues such as cells, fibres, vessels and other structures. The cell walls may consist of cellulose, lignins, tannins or cork cells. The cells of aromatic drugs like Cinnamon and Coriander contain volatile oils occurring in specialized cells or glands. The glycosides and alkaloids may occur in solution in the cell sap and deposit in the cells later on. The total contents of the cells are not used as physiological importance. For example, calcium oxalate occurs as a crystalline deposit and protein may occur as solid aleurone grains. Both these components are rejected in the preparation of a tincture or extract of the drug.

The unorganized drugs possess no cellular structure but consist of extracts, exudation, secretions and other products of the plants. The value of gums, gum-resins, oleo-resins, starch, fixed oils, catechu, and opium depends on the whole of the material present. The constituents of drugs of medicinal value generally belong to one of the following group: glycosides, enzymes, anthraquinone derivatives, alkaloids, tannins and other phenols, proteins, carbohydrates, gums, resins, fixed oils, fats, waxes and volatile oils.

CARBOHYDRATES

Carbohydrates are plant products which contain carbon,

hydrogen, and oxygen. The ratio of hydrogen and oxygen is the same as occurred in water, e.g. dextrose $C_6H_{12}O_6$ and sucrose $C_{12}H_{22}O_{11}$. Carbohydrates are widely distributed in plants; provide storage and transport of energy and are building blocks of the cell wall. They are classified as : mono- and oligosaccharides (True sugars); polysaccharides (Nonsugars), and the derived carbohydrates (gum, mucilage and pectin).

Polysaccharides consists of numerous units of monosaccharides. They are not sweet in taste. Starch, cellulose and dextrins are polysaccharides.

Gum, mucilage and pectin are derived carbohydrates which are composed of acid or ester forms. Gums are polyuronides formed due to combination of sugar and uronic acid units. Gums are used as emulsifier, suspending agents, tablet binders and thickeners.

Chemically, mucilages are similar to gums but differ in the nature of sugar and acid residue. They may contain sulphate groups or their salts. They form a clear colloidal solution and are used mainly as suspending agent. Mucilage is present in Agar, Plantago seeds and Linseed.

Pectins are consisted of methoxylated polygalacturonic acids. They are present in the inner portion of the rind of Citrus fruits and in apples. They swell in water and form stiff jellies.

GLYCOSIDES

Glycosides are compounds which upon hydrolysis give rise to one or more sugars (glycone) and a compound which is not a sugar (aglycone or genin). The aglycone is usually a compound containing one or more hydroxyl groups. The glycoside is formed by the elimination of a molecule of water between a hydroxyl group of the aglycone and a hydroxyl group of the sugar. The aglycone may be an alcohol (Salicin), anthraquinone derivative, phenol, aldehyde, acid, ester, or other compound.

The other important glycosides are anthraquinone glycosides, cardiac glycosides, cyanophore glycosides and isothiocyanate glycosides.

SAPONINS

Saponins are an important group of glycosides which are

widely distributed as plant constituents. The most important saponin-containing drugs are Quillaia and Senega. Most of the saponins are neutral and soluble in water. Like other glycosides, saponins are hydrolyzed to form a sugar (usually dextrose) and an aglycone, generally known as sapogenin. The sapogenins are insoluble in water, but soluble in weak alcohol. Their aqueous solutions form froths on shaking; produce stable emulsion on shaking with oils and fats; absorb and retain in solution a volume of gas (e.g., CO_2) several times greater than absorbed by an equal volume of water; an aqueous solution added to red blood corpuscles causes haemolysis, i.e., disintegration and solution of the corpuscles to form a clear red liquid.

ANTHRAQUINONE DERIVATIVES

The laxative action of certain drugs is attributed to derivatives of anthraquinones, $C_6H_4 (CO)_2 C_6H_4$. Various derivatives are obtained by replacing the hydrogen atoms by alkyl, hydroxyl and other groups. Many such derivatives occur in nature and often are combined with a sugar forming a glycoside. For example:

Chrysophanol : a dihydroxy methyl anthraquinone present in Rhubarb.

Emodin : a trihydroxy methyl derivative present in Cascara and Rhubarb.

Aloe-emodin : the primary alcohol derived from chrysophanol, present in Aloe, Rhubarb and Senna.

Rhein : the acid derived from aloe-emodin, present in Rhubarb and Senna.

The anthraquinone derivatives are often orange red coloured compounds. For their detection the filtrate is shaken with benzene or chloroform and set aside to form two layers. The organic layer is separated and shaken with an equal volume of solution of ammonia. A pink to reddish colour is developed.

LIPIDS-FIXED OILS, FATS AND WAXES

The term lipid is used for fixed oils, fats and waxes. Fixed oils are liquid at normal temperature while fats are solids or semi-solids at this temperature. Chemically, they are esters of glycerol with long chain fatty acids. These esters are termed as glycerides.

Fixed oils and fats are nonvolatile, insoluble in water and are lighter than it and form a permanent stain on a paper. They are sparingly soluble in cold alcohol (except Castor oil), but soluble in other organic solvents like petroleum ether, diethyl ether, chloroform, etc.

Waxes are esters of a higher alcohols (e.g. cetyl alcohol) with higher fatty acids. They are insoluble in water, soluble in many organic solvents and can be saponified by alcoholic alkali.

VOLATILE OILS

Volatile oils are flavouring constituents which evaporate on exposure at ordinary temperature. They are present in various plant parts such as flower petals (Saffron), fruits (Fennel), bark (Cinnamon), etc. They are secreted in particular secretory cells like glandular hairs, modified parenchyma cells, vittae or in lysigenous or schizogenous cavities.

Volatile oils are colourless liquids or crystalline or amorphous solids. They are slightly soluble in water, but highly soluble in ether, alcohol and other organic solvents. Like fixed oils they do not form permanent strains and cannot be saponified by alkalies.

Chemically, volatile oils are the mixture of monoterpenes and sesquiterpenes. They may be simple hydrocarbons, alcohols, ketones, aldehydes, phenols, ethers, oxides, esters, acids, aromatic or aliphatic compounds.

Phenolic volatile oils are present in drugs like Thyme, Clove, Creosote and Pine tar. They have antibacterial, antifungal and antiseptic properties.

RESINS, GUM-RESINS AND OLEO-RESINS

The resins are derived from living natural sources and most of them are plant products (except Shellac). The resinous exudation may consist almost entirely of resins (e.g. Benzoin), or it may be associated with volatile oil (e.g., Turpentine, Copaiba); or resin associated with gum(gum resin). If a considerable amount of volatile oil is present, the substance is called an oleo-gum-resin (e.g. Myrrh). The resins or oleo-resins, which contain benzoic or cinnamic acid either free or combined, are commonly called balsams (e.g. Benzoin, Balsam of Tolu, Balsam of Peru, Storax).

All resins are practically insoluble in water, soluble in organic solvents (e.g. alcohol) and terpentine oil.

A solution of a resin in a volatile solvent, on painting on a smooth surface, is dried rapidly and completely to form a hard transparent film. This film should not be darken with age or become impaired upon exposure to light or moisture.

Resins are not single chemical compounds, but are mixtures of various substances of complex chemical characters.

Resins are used. as purgative, cathartic, hydragogue, sedative, counter-irritant, anthelmintic, expectorant and laxative. Externally they are used as mild antiseptic in the form of cerates, ointments and plasters.

TANNINS AND OTHER PLANT PHENOLS

Tannins are complex phenolic compounds which are soluble in water and have an astringent and bitter taste. They are soluble in water; have an astringent taste; yield purple, violet, or black precipitates with iron compounds; are precipitated by a number of metallic salts like potassium dichromate, lead acetate and lead subacetate; combine with skin and hide to form leather and with gelatin and isinglass to form an insoluble compound; combine with alkaloids to form tannates, most of which are insoluble in water; and they yield a bulky precipitate with phenazone.

The tannin containing drugs are Cinchona, Clove, Catechu, Cinnamon, Hamamelis, Krameria, etc.

A considerable number of plant substances are phenolic compounds, e.g. the anthraquinone derivatives, morphine and the resinotannols. They form coloured compounds with ferric chloride. Certain plant pigments are also phenolic. For example,

1. *Hydroxy flavone glycosides* : They are derived from flavones or the related compound xanthones. These glycosides themselves are colourless, but form yellow salts. They occur in Clove, Hamamelis, Catechu, Buchu, Senega, Gentian, Digitalis and Stramonium. They yield a dull green or reddish-brown colour with ferric chloride.

2. *Anthocyanins* : They are phenolic plant pigments which may be red, blue, or purple. The exact colour depends upon the hydrogen ion concentration of the solution. For example, haematien is a reddish coloured anthocyanin of logwood which changes to blue upon addition of lime water.

Simple phenolic compounds are found in many plants and have different pharmaceutical uses. Vanillin is the aglycone of the glycosides of Vanilla pods and is used in confectionary and in perfumary. Similarly, eugenol (Clove), salicin, and arbutin are simple phenolic compounds.

ALKALOIDS

Alkaloids are complex substances, occurring in plants or animals, are basic or alkali-like and possess physiological activity. The term is usually restricted to compounds having one or more heterocyclic rings containing nitrogen. They are considered as derivatives of pyridine, quinoline or isoquinoline and contain carbon, hydrogen, oxygen, and nitrogen but a few are without oxygen. Mostly alkaloids are solid colourless crystalline products but few alkaloids, which generally do not possess oxygen, e.g., nicotine, coniine, spartein, are volatile colourless liquids. Some alkaloids are coloured, e.g. berberine (yellow) and sanguinarine (red).

Alkaloids combine with acids to give salts and are used in this form. A water-soluble alkaloidal salt or other compound is more useful than one insoluble in water. Alkaloids are fairly soluble in organic solvents, e.g. chloroform, ether, alcohol and benzene.

In plants alkaloids are found in various parts as in seeds (strychnine), in fruits (Piper), in leaves (Belladonna, Datura), in roots (Rauwolfia), in rhizomes and roots (Ipecac), in corm (Coichicum) and in bark (Kurchi, Cinchona).

ENZYMES AND OTHER PROTEINS

Enzymes are defined as organic catalysts produced by plants and animals with molecular weight from 13,000 to 8,40,000. At ordinary temperatures they bring about chemical changes, both synthetic and analytic. Most enzymes are insoluble in alcohol, ether, and other organic solvents, but are soluble in water. In some cases the enzymes are combined with the protoplasm which must be killed by an organic solvent (e.g., CHCl₃, toluene) or by mechanical means before extraction of the enzyme. Some enzymes do not pre-exist in the tissues, but are formed from substances termed 'zymogens'. In nature, decomposition of the zymogen is carried out by a complex substance, known as *kinase*, to form the enzyme when needed.

The term *substrate* is used to a substance which reacts with the enzyme. In nature, enzyme and substrate are sometimes present in the same cell and the reaction may take place continuously. In other cases, enzymes and substrate are found in different cells. The reaction starts on diffusion of one of the substance; the reaction is controlled by the plant. Some enzymes are combined with the protoplasm, and this represents one method of preventing diffusion.

The rate of chemical change brought about by enzyme is affected by certain factors. For examples, some substances, like *paralysers*, partially or entirely, inhibit the action of the enzymes. The substances, called *co-enzymes*, are required for the action. The · substances known as *accelerators* or *activators*, greatly accelerate the rate of reaction.

Temperature is another important factor in enzyme action. For each enzyme there is a particular temperature, called the optimum temperature and lies between 35°-45°C, at which reaction proceeds most rapidly. Most of the enzymatic reactions are inhibited below 10°C, and destroyed by heating to 100°C.

Enzymes are usually soluble in water. They are usually accompany with glycosides. Some drugs like Wild Cherry, Almonds, Mustard and Wintergreen, owe their value not to the glycoside present, but to its decomposition products by the enzymes.

Some important enzymes of medicinal importance are pancreatin of pancereas used to treat pancreatitis; trypsin of ox pancrease used to cure wounds, ulcers, abscesses and fistulas and as anti-inflammatory agent; chymotrypsin of pancreas of ox used identically as trypsin; fibrinolysin utilized to treat venous thrombosis and pulmonary embolism; pepsin of the gastric juice employed to treat achylia gastrica; hyaluronidase found in microorganisms, leaches, snake venom and mammalian testes, and used to facilitate the administration of fluids by hydronermolysis.

Papain is the dried and purified latex of the fruit of *Carica payaya* and used as a digestant. Chymopapain is a nonpyrogenic proteolytic enzyme obtained from the latex of *Carica payaya* and employed in the treatment of herniated lumbar intervertebral discs. Bromelains is a mixture of protein-digesting and milk-clotting enzymes obtained from the juice of the pineapple, *Ananas comosus*. It is used as adjunctive therapy to reduce inflammation and oedema and to reduce tissue repair.

Gelatin is obtained from animal collagen and is a pharmaceutical aid. Other protein based drugs are Absorbable Gelatin sponge and film, microfibrillar collagen surgical sutures, penicillamine, heparin sodium, heparin calcium, protamine sulphate and levodopa.

PEPTIDE HORMONES

Hormones are secreted by endocrine glands of animals. Thyroxine, conjugated oestrogens, insulin, epinephrine, oxytocin, vesopressin and gonadotropins are important mammalian hormones released directly into the blood. Thyroxin hormone of thyroid gland is used to treat thyroid insufficiency. Menopausal symptoms in females and dysmenorrhea are treated with conjugated oestrogens. Insulin, a polypeptide hormone secreted by the beta cells of the islets of Langerhans of pancrease gland, is employed to cure diabetes. Adrenal medulla of mammmals secretes the hormone epinephrine (adrenaline) which is utilized as vasoconstrictor to cure acute asthma. Oxytocin, a polypeptide hormone secreted by posterior pituitary gland, causes contraction of uterine muscles, stimulates the ejection of milk in lactating mothers, induce labour in pregnant women and stop haemorrhage after child birth. Another peptide hormone of the posterior lobe of pituitary gland, vasopressin, is used in the treatment of intestinal paralysis and diabetes. Gonadotropins are secreted by the interior lobe of the pituitary gland which control the production of sex hormones. They are employed to cure infertility and in cryptoichidism.

MICRO-ORGANISMS

Microorganisms (microbes) are the viruses, bacteria and rickettsiae which are sources of many biological substances of immunization importance. These drugs possess immunity against various infectious diseases. Immunity is acquired by administration of a vaccine, toxoid or antitoxin like diphtheria. Vaccines are suspended micro-organisms which may be obtained from viruses, bacteria and rickettsiae. On introduction into body, a vaccine stimulates the production of antibodies against pathogenic microbes. Viral vaccines are prophylactic agents used against polio, smallpox, rabies, influenza, measles and mumps. Rickettsial vaccine, prepared from gram-negative microorganisms, is the typhus vaccine which produces active immunity against typhus fever. Bacterial vaccine is the suspension of pathogenic bacteria in sodium chloride or other solvent. Bacteria vaccine includes Typhoid vaccine, Cholera vaccine, Plague vaccine, Pertussis vaccine (for whooping cough) and BCG vaccine (for tuberculosis).

The waste products of bacteria, called toxins, are dissolved in the surrounding culture medium after excretion. On treatment with formaldehyde their toxic properties are reduced but their antigenic property is not effected. These products are called fluid toxoids which are precipitated with alum, aluminium hydroxide or aluminium phosphate. The toxoids are used to induce artificial activity immunity in susceptible individual. For example, tetanus toxoid and diphtheria toxoid are the microbial products used to produce immunity in young children against diphtheria, tetanus and whooping cough.

MARINE PRODUCTS

Marine products are used a thickening, emulsifying and suspending agents. Carrageenan from *Chondrus crispus* (Irish Moss) and alginates from species of *Laminaria. Ascophyllum, Ecklonia, Nereocystis* and *Macrocystis* are used in adhesive formulations and as stabilizers, ingredients of ointment bases, suspending agent and tablet disintegrating agents. Agar, obtained from species of *Gelidium* and *Gracilaria,* is used as laxative, emulsifier, suspending agent and in the preparation of vaginal capsules, suppositories and nutrient media in bacteriological culture. Spermaceti, a solid waxy substance obtained from the oil of the sperm whale, *Physeter macrocephalus,* is used as a pharmaceutical aid for creams, ointments, cerates, soaps, cosmetics, etc. Shark liver oil, a fixed oil obtained from the liver of shark fish, *Hypoprion brevirostris*, is nutritive and used as a tonic and to treat xerophthalmia occurring due to deficiency of vitamin A. The marine fungus, *Cephalosporium acremonium*, produces the antibiotic cephalosporin C identical to penicillins. The strongly basic protein of low molecular weight, protamine, is obtained from the testes of the fish salmon. It is used as a heparin antagonist. Pralidoxine is produced from electric eel which acts as antidote for certain types of insecticide poisoning in humans. The Japanese drived red algae, *Digenea simplex*, contains the amino acid known as kainic acid from which an anthelmintic drug is prepared. Cod-liver oil is the source of vitamins A and D.

An anticoagulant agent has been isolated from the sea-anemone, *Rhodactis howesii.* Very potent anticancer agents, named dolastin 1-9, are present in Indian ocean sea-hare. The marine annelid, *Lumbriconeris heteropoda*, is toxic to some insects. The richest natural source of prostaglandin is the soft coral *Plexaura homomalla.* Many toxins occur throughout the complete range of marine life; they include irritants, CNS stimulants and depressants, haemolytic substances and protoplasmic poisons. Extracts of various marine algae contain vitamin C, folic acid, foilnic acid, niacin and vitamin B.

VITAMINS

Vitmains are organic compounds which are not synthesized within the body. They are essential in small amounts for the maintenance of normal health. The lack of specific vitamins causes diseases such as beriberi, rickets, scurvy and xerophthalmia. Vitamin B_2 (niacin) and pantothenic acid act as coenzymes. Vitamin B_{12} and folic acid take part in the biosynthetic transfer of 1-carbon unit. In the biosynthesis of hydroxyproline, vitamin C is required. Vitamin B_1 and B_6 are involved in the metabolism of carbohydrates. Many vitamins take part in metabolic oxidation-reduction reactions.

Vitamin A is obtained from animal products and it is involved in vision, growth and tissue differentiation. Vitamin B is a complex mixture of compounds. Liver and yeast are the main sources of the B vitamins. Vitamin C (ascorbic acid) prevents scurvy and is used as antioxidant. Good dietary sources of vitamin C are citrus fruits, tomatoes, strawberries, fresh fruits and vegetables. Vitamin D is essential for the absorption and utilization of calcium. It is obtained from fish liver oils, milk, cereals and synthesized in the body in sunshine. Vitmain E, a mixture of tocopherols, is widely distributed in plant oils, vegetables, grains, eggs and meats. Its deficiency causes muscular dystrophy, coronary disease and sterility. Vitamin K is widely distributed in diary products and many fruits and vegetables. It is necessary for normal clotting of blood.

ANTIBIOTICS

Antibiotics are the chemical substances produced by microorganisms and they have the capacity, in low concentration, to inhibit microorganisms through an antimetabolic mechanism. Penicillin G, obtained from a strain of *Penicillium chrysogenum*, is an agent acting against many pathogenic gram-positive bacteria and used to treat syphilis. Cloxacillin, dicloxacillin, methicillin, nafcillin and oxacillin are semisynthetic penicillins which are used for treatment of staphylococcal infections. Ampicillin has special clinical value for the treatment of infections caused by *Haemophilus influenza*, *Salmonella* species and *Shigella* species. Clavulanic acid is a fermentation product of *Streptomyces clavuligerus* and it controls many infectious diseases. Other antibiotics are cephalosporins (from *Cephalosporium acremonium)*, chloramphenicol (from *Streptomyces venezuelae)*, lincomycin (from *S. lincolnensis)*, cycloserine (from *S. orchidaceus)*, dactinomycin (from *S. parvullus)*, vidarabine (from *S. antibioticus)*, polymyxin B *(Bacillus polymyxa)*, colistin (*B. polymyxa)*, tyrothricin (*B. brevis)*, vancomycin (*S. orientalis)*, bleamycin (*S. verticillus)*, tetracyclines (*S. aureofaciens)*, mitomycin (*S. caespitosus)*, erythromycin (*S. erythreus)*, amphotericin B (*S. nodosus)*, navamycin (*S. natalensis)*, griseofulvin *(Pentcillium griseofulvum)*, rifampin (*S. mediterranei)*, novobiocin (*S. niveus and S. spheroides)*, stgreptomycin (*S. griseus)* neomycin, and paromomycin *(Streptomyces fradiae* and *S. rimosus* var, *paromomycinus)*, kanamycin (*S. kanamyceticus)*, gentamicin *(Micromonospora purpurea)*, tobramycin or nebramysin factor 6 or nebrarius), amikacin (semisynthetic antibiotic derived from kanamycin A by acylation), netilmicin *(Micromonospora inyoensis)* and spectinomycin *(Streptomyces spectablis* and *S. flavopersicus)*.

MISCELLANEOUS DRUGS

Ichthamol is a black tarry distillate obtained from bituminous schists containing fossil fish and possesses antiseptic and stimulant properties. Diatomaceous earth (siliceous earth, kieselguhr), made of shells of fossilized unicellular algae, is utilized in face powders, filtering aids, dentifrices and as chromatographic adsorbent.

Liver and stomach of healthy animals are converted into suitable preparations which are used as replacement therapy in pernicious anemia. Bile contains sodium salts of bile acids-dehydrocholic, taurocholic and deoxycholic acids. Bile acids, obtained from ox bile, are used in deficiency of biliary secretion and parenterally as sodium salts to increase diuresis. Carmine, a colouring principle obtained from cochineal insects, cantharidin, an irritant constituent of cantharidin insects, heparin, wool fat and lanolin are the other animal products which are used in some formulations and in cosmetics.

QUESTIONS

1. Give an account of the non-living cell content in plants with specific reference to the various microchemical tests for their identification.

2. Give a comparative account of chemical constituents present in crude drugs.

3. Describe biological sources and uses of the drugs in which the following chemical constituents are present: (a) Digitoxin (b) Atropin (c) Euginol (d) Curcumin.

4

DRUG ADULTERATION

An adulterated drug means one which does not conform to the official requirements. Adulteration involves incorporation of impurities. spoilage, deterioration, admixture, sophistication and substitution. The genuine drugs are substituted with spurious, inferior, defective or harmful substances. The spoiled or deteriorated drugs represent the greatest percentage of drug adulteration. In some cases the dealers substitute the drugs with cheap materials in case of scarcity or when the price of a drug is high. The adulteration may be due to faulty collection, imperfect perparation and incorrect storage as described hereunder :

FAULTY COLLECTION : In some cases the proportion of medicinally-active constituent reaches a maximum at a particular season, stage of development, or age. But collection of correct part of genuine plant without regard to time factors causes adulteration. The following are some examples:

(i) Season

Drug	Season of Maximum Activity
Solanaceous leaves	Flowering stage of the drug (Summer)
Wild Cherry bark	Autumn
Colchicum corm	Early summer
Male fern	Late autumn.

(ii) Stage of development and age

Drug	Stage and Age of Maximum Activity
Linseed	When fully ripe
Coriander	When fully grown and ripe
Wild Cherry bark	Bark of young stems
Belladonna root	Root of 3-4 years old.

Sometimes adulteration is done by collection of other less valuable part of a genuine plant. For example :

Drug	Official Part	Less Valuable Parts
Buchu	Leaves	Stems
Clove	Flower-buds	Flower-stalks
Senega	Root	Stems
Serpentary	Rhizome and roots	Sub-aerial stem

Ignorance or neglect on the part of collectors may lead to unintentional collection of drugs from the allied or foreign species. Such plants may bear a superficial resemblance to the genuine plant. In place of the genuine drugs, substituted products are available in the market. These substituents are identical in appearance. Some example are as :

Drug	Official Source	Source of Adulteration
Aconite	*Aconitum napellus*	*Aconitum deinorrhizum* and other species of *Aconitum*
Buchu	*Barosma betulina*	*Barosma crenulata, Barosma serratifolia*
Cascara sagrada	*Rhamnus purshiana*	*Rhamnus californica*
Myrrh	*Commiphora molmol*	*Commiphora erythaea* var. *brescens*
Belladonna leaf	*Atropa belladonna*	*Scopolia carniolica* *Phytolacca decandra* *Ailanthus glandulosa*
Indian *officinalis.* Belladonna	*Atropa* *acuminata*	Roots of *Althaea* leaves of *Phytolacca acinosa. Solanum nigrum*

(Contd.)

Drug	Official Source	Source of Adulteration
Pale Catechu	Uncaria gambier	and other species of Solanum and Datura Acacia catechu
Chamomile	Anthemis nobilis	Chrysanthemum parthenium
Digitalis	Digitalis purpurea	Verbascum thapsus; Symphytum officinale; Primula vulgaris; Digitalis thapsi
Tragacanth	Astragalus gummifer	Sterculia urens and other species of Sterculia.
Chirata	Swertia chirata	Swertia angustifolia S. alata, Rubia cordifolia and Andrographis paniculata
Cinnamon	Cinnamomum zeylanicum	Cinnamomum cassia
Balsam of Tolu	Myroxylon balsamum	Mixture of vanillin, Rosin, cinnamic and benzoic acids
Kalmegh	Andrographis paniculata	Chirata (Swertia chirata)
Ispaghula	Plantago psyllium	Salvia aegyptica, P. arenaria, P. lanceolate, P. major.
Linseed oil	Linum usitatissitmum	Vegetable oils of rape-seed, cottonseed, soya-bean, sunflower and saf-flower and rosin, mineral and fish oil.
Ipecac	Cephaelis ipecacuanha	Richardia scabra, Cryptocoryne spiralis, Psychotria emetica, Manettia ignita, Hybanthus ipecacuanha, Asclepias curassavica, Anodendron paniculatum. Calotropis gigantea, etc.

(Contd.)

Galanga	*Alpinia officinarum*	*Acorus calamus*

Drug	Official Source	Source of Adulteration
Saffron	*Crocus sativus*	Flower and floral parts of some *Compositae* family, e.g., *Calendula* species, *Carthamus tinctorius;* corn silk.
Saussurea oil	*Saussurea lappa*	Elecampane oil
Punarnava	*Boerhaavia diffusa*	*Trianthema portulacastrum*
Rauwolfia	*Rauwolfia serpentina*	*Rauwolfia beddomei, R. densiflora, R. micrantha, R. perakensis, R. nitida, R. tetraphylla; Ophiorrhiza mungos* and *Clerodendrum* species
Nux-vomica	*Strychnos nux-vomica*	*S. potatorum* and *S. nux-blanda*
Pyrethrum	*Chrysanthemum cinerariaefolium*	*C. leucanthemum*
Datura	*Datura stramonium*	*Xanthium strumarium, Carthamus helenioides, Chenopodium hybridum.*
Cardamom	*Elettaria cardamomum*	Orange seeds, Unroasted coffee grains
Calamus	*Acorus calamus*	*Alpinia galanga; Aconitum* species
Areca nut	*Areca catechu*	Sogo palm nuts (*Metroxylon* sps.), tapioca (*Manihot esculenta*), sweet potato (*Ipomoea batatas*), nuts of *Caryota urens.*
Liquorice	*Glycyrrhiza glabra*	*Abrus precatorius*
Ashoka bark	*Saraca indica*	*Trema orientalis* bark
Kurchi bark	*Holarrhena antidysenterica*	*Wrightia tinctoria* bark
Devadru bark	*Polyalthia longifolia*	*Saraca indica* bark

(Contd.)

| Hindisana leaves | *Cassia angustifolia* | *Cassia auriculata* leaves |

IMPERFECT PREPARATION : Collection of other and less valuable parts of the genuine plant may cause adulteration. For example, stems are collected with leaves. The adulteration done by non-removal of inert or undesirable parts of the drugs is illustrated by the following examples:

Drug	Official Composition	Inert and Undesirable Part
Ginger	Rhizome freed from cork	Cork
Male fern	Rhizome and leaf bases	Roots and dead portions
Orange and Lemon peels	Outer part of the pericarp	Inner white spongy part of pericarp
Ipecac	Roots or rhizomes	Aerial stem
Fennel	Fruit	Undeveloped or mould attack fruits
Saffron	Stigma and style-tops	Parts of corolla
Quillaia	Inner part of the bark	Rhytidome
Tamarind	Fruits freed from the brittle outer part	Outer part of pericarp
Pyrethrum	Flower heads	Stem and leaf

Neglect of proper conditions for drying leads adulteration in the following drugs :

Drug	Faulty Treatment
Colchicum corm	Drying at a temperature above 65°C which accelerates the rate of hydrolysis of colchicine.
Digitalis	Leaving in a wilted condition for long period, thereby providing suitable conditions for the decomposition of the glycosides by enzymes, or drying above

(Contd.)

60°C thereby promoting hydrolysis of the glycosides.

Drug	Faulty Treatment
Gentian	Allowing excessive fermentation before drying in which sugars are converted to alcohol and carbon dixoide and the proportion of water-soluble extract is reduced below the official minimum.
Cod-liver oil	Excessive heat used in separating the oil from the livers affect the proportion of vitamins, odour and colour.

INCORRECT STORAGE : Incorrect storage spoils many drugs. The quality, value or usefulness of the drug has been impaired or destroyed by the action of moisture, light, temperature and microorganisms (fungi and bacteria) and the article becomes unfit for human consumption. Many examples of spoilage are found in food industry. All drugs which are unfit for human or animal consumption are legally considered as adulterated. The impairment of the quality or value of an article by the abstraction or destruction of valuable constituents by distillation, extraction, aging, moisture, heat, fungi, insects or other means deteriorate the drugs considerably. A few examples are :

Drug	Storage Conditions
Cascara sagrada	To be collected at least one year before being used.
Male fern	To be used after the internal green colour is lost.
Digitalis, Belladonna leaf, Hyoscyamus and Stramonium	To be preserved in a dry place or a container which prevents excess of moisture to prevent enzymatic hydrolysis.
Cod-liver oil	Protected from light, which would decompose the vitamin A.
Volatile oil	Protected from light, and stored in well-closed containers in a cool place.
Lard	Protected from moisture.
Squill	Powdered squill hardens by absorption of moisture.
Coffee	Caffeine is lost by over-heating.
Ergot	Protected from molds.

DELIBERATE ADULTERATION

Substitution of exhausted drugs : Many drugs are extracted on a large scale for the isolation of an active constituent or volatile oil, or for the preparation of an extract. The exhausted material may be used entirely or in part as a substitute for the genuine drug. This extraction procedure does not bring any change in the morphology of the drug. Some example are :

Drug	Constituent Removed
Clove	Volatile oil
Umbelliferous fruits	Volatile oil
Indian hemp	Resin
Glycyrrhiza	Glycyrrhizin and other water-soluble matter
Jalap	Resin
Balsam of Tolu	Balsamic acid
Ginger	Gingerol, volatile oil and resin
Tea	Caffeine
Cardamom	Volatile oil
Saffron	Volatile oil
Cardamom powder	Hulls powder

Sometimes foreign matters are added which are cheap in comparison with the drug and are usually dense and inconspicuous upon cursory examination. Replacement wholly or in part by a fictitious mixture of similar composition is occasionally a cause of adulteration. Admixture with non-plant substances resembling to a particular drug is commonly practised. For example :

Drug	Foreign or Fictitious Matters
Cochineal	Barium sulphate, barium carbonate, lead carbonate and animal charcoal.
Myrrh	Quartz and other mineral matter
Resins and Copaiba	Colophony.
Black pepper	Seeds of papaya

(Contd.)

Drug	Foreign or Fictitious Matters
Saffron	Materials coloured with coal-tar dye, oil and glycerine
Papain	Arrowroot starch, dried milk of cactus, gutta-parcha, rice flour and pepsins.
Nux-vomica powder	Olive stone powder
Pyrethrum powder	Lead chromate, Turmeric, and fustic
Coca leaves	Novacaine, boric acid, sodium carbonate and bicarbonate, lime chalk, starch, lactose and quinine.
Honey	Cane sugar, corn syrup and artificial invert sugar.
Asafoetida	Gum arabic, gum-resins, rosin, gypsum, red clay, chalk, barley or wheat flour, slices of potato, etc.
Clove	Clay material
Caraway	Clay material
Lemon oil	An admixture of citral and other terpenes.
Balsam of Peru	An admixture of synthetic benzyl benzoate, Storax, Benzoin and Balsam of Tolu.
Nutmeg	Broken kernels moulded with clay; shaped pieces of wood.

CONFUSION OF COMMON VERNACULAR NOMENCLATURE

Common vernacular names of different plants in different regions of India cause this type of adulteration. In different regions the same plant is known by different names. Sometimes different drugs are known by the same name. For example, the drugs *Trianthema portulacastrum* and *Boerhaavia diffusa* are known by the common name "Punarnava". In most of the states "Brahmi" is obtained from the plant *Hydrocotyle asiatica* while in eastern parts of India the plant 'Herpestis monniera' is used as "Brahmi". The plants *Evolvulus alsinoides*, *Convolvulus microphyllus* and *Clitoria ternatea* are sold by the name "Shankhpushpi". Similarly for

"Boch" the rhizomes and roots of *Acorus calamus, Alpinia officinarum* and *Anacyclus pyrethrum* are available. Rasna is also a controversial drug and three different plants-*Pluchea lanceolata* (in north India), *Vanda roxburghii* (in Bihar and Bangal) and *Alpinia officinarum* (in south India) are sold as Rasna. Other examples are :

Agaru (*Aquilaria agallocha* in Sanskirt. and Bangali; *Commiphora roxburghii*, in Telgu and Sanskrit; *Excoecaria agallocha* in Sanskirt)

Akasbel (*Cassytha filiformis*, Mumbai; *Cuscuta reflexa* in Hindi).

Al (*Morinda umbellata*, Mumbai, *Morinda citrifolia*, M.P. and south Maharastra).

Babuna (*Matricaria chamomilla* in Punjabi and Mumbai; *Cotula anthemoides* in Hindi and Punjabi; *Corchorus depressus* in Punjabi).

Banda (*Viscum album* in Hindi; *Dendrophthoe falcata* in Hindi and Punjabi; *Hedera helix* in Punjabi).

Bhangra (*Indigofera linifolia* in Mumbai and Bengali; *Eclipta alba* in Hindi; *Wedelia calendulacea* in Hindi; *Sonchus arvensis* in Punjabi).

Chitra (*Plumbago indica* in Hindi and Mumbai; *Berberis asiatica* in Nepal; *Drosera lunata* in Punjabi).

Gaozaban (*Onosma bracteatum* in Bengal and Urdu; *Macrotomia benthami* in Punjab and Indian Market; *Anchusa strigosa* in Indian Market).

Hing (*Ferula narthex* in Hindi, Bengal and Mumbai; *F. foetida* in Hindi and Mumbai).

Kasni (*Cichorium endivia* in Hindi and Mumbai; *C. intybus* in Hindi, Bengali, Mumbai, Telgu).

Luban (*Boswellia serrata* in Hindi and Mumbai; *Styrax benzoin* in Hindi, Mumbai and Bengal).

QUESTIONS

1. Define adulteration. How will you evaluate a drug by chemical tools?

2. What do you mean by adulteration? Describe different means of adulteration in crude drugs. Support your answer with suitable examples.

3. What is adulteration? How are crude drugs adulterated by faulty collection and incorrect preparation.

5

EVALUATION OF DRUGS

Evaluation of drugs deals with the correct identification of the plant and determination of quality and purity of the crude drugs. Actual collection of the drug is done from the identified plant or animal. For this purpose research gardens have been maintained. The characters of an unknown sample are compared with the authentic monographs written in the pharmacopoeia. The high quality of the drug is maintained by collection of the drug from the correct natural source at proper time; preparation of samples of the collected drugs by proper cleaning, drying and to free from dirt, and proper preservation of the cleaned, dried and pure drug.

The evaluation of a drug is done by studying its organoleptic, microscopic, biological, chemical, and physical properties.

ORGANOLEPTIC EVALUATION

Organoleptic evaluation means study of a drug with the help of organs of sense which includes its external morphology, colour, odour, taste, sound of its fracture, etc.

Morphological Characters : To study morphology of a drug, its shape and size, colour and external markings, fracture and internal colour, odour and taste are examined. The organized drugs are classified into :

1. **Barks :** Which are tissues in a woody stem outside the inner fascicular cambium, e.g., Cinnamon, Cinchona, Quillaia, Ashoka and Kurchi.

2. **Underground Structures :** Which may be rhizomes, roots, bulbs, corm, and tubers; they are often swollen due to storage of carbohydrates and other chemicals, e.g., roots (Podophyllum, Liquorice, Jatamansi, Rauwolfia), rhizomes and stolons which are underground stems and have buds, scale leaves and scars, (Ginger, Turmeric, Dioscorea).

3. **Leaves :** These are photosynthetic organs arising from a node on a stem. The shape, margin, base, apex and venation of leaves help in the identification of the drugs. Senna, Tulsi, Vasaka and Digitalis leaves can be easily identified.

4. **Flowers :** These are reproductive organs of a plant and possess different shapes, size and colour, e.g., Saffron, Banafsha, Pyrethrum.

5. **Fruits :** Fruits arise from the ovary and contain seeds, e.g. Cardamom, Colocynth, Almond, Vidang, Bahera, Amla and Bael.

6. **Seeds :** Seeds are developed from the ovules in carpels of the flowers and characterized by the hilum, micropyle and sometimes raphe. The seed drugs are Ispaghula, Linseed, Nux-vomica, Psoralia.

7. **Herbs :** The whole aerial part is sometimes used as a drug, e.g. Brahmi, Chirata, Kalmegh, Pudina, Shankhpushpi, etc.

The shape of a drug may be cylindrical (Sarsaparilla), sub-cylindrical (Podophyllum), conical (Aconite); fusiform, ovoid or pyriform (Jalap), and terete or disk-shaped (Nux-vomica). The drug may be simple, branched, curved or twisted. The length, breadth and diameter are measured in millimeters or centimeters. In case of conical drugs the size of both parts is mentioned.

External markings are mentioned as :
1. furrows, ridges, etc.,
2. wrinkles,
3. annulations,
4. fissures, .
5. nodules,
6. projections,
7. scars of leaf, stem-base, root, bud, bud-scale, etc.

The fractures may be complete, incomplete, short, fibrous, splintery (breaking irregularly), brittle (easily broken), tough and weak.

Sensory Characters : Colour, texture, odour and taste are useful in the evaluation of drugs. This method is especially applicable to drugs containing volatile oils or pungent principles (e.g. Capsicum), and to the detection of the effects of inadequate drying or damp storage. The external colour varies from white to yellowish grey, brown, orange or brownish black. The colour of some drugs changes if they are dried in sunlight in place of shade.

The odour of a drug may be either distinct (characterisic) or indistinct. The terms used to define odour are aromatic, balsamic, spicy, alliaceous (garlic-like), camphoraceous (camphor-like), terebinthinate (turpentine-like) and others. Leaves of different species of *Mentha* can be distinguished by smell. Clove and exhausted clove are differentiated by odour. Deteriorated Cantharides have ammonical smell while spoiled Ergot has rancid and ammonical smell.

Taste is a particular sensation production by certain substances when these come into contact with taste buds present in epithelial layer of the mouth. The taste may be sour (acidic), salty (saline), sweet (saccharine), bitter, alkaline and metallic. Substances possessing no taste are mentioned as tasteless. The tastes due to a characteristic odour are grouped as aromatic, balsamic, spicy, alliaceous, camphoraceous and terebinthinate. The taste produced by distinctive sensations to the tongue are classified as mucilaginous, oily, astringent (producing a contraction of the tissues of the mouth), pungent (warm biting sensation), acrid (unpleasant, irritating sensation) and nauseous (causing vomiting).

The drugs like Ginger and Capsicum have pungent taste; Gentian, Chirata and Kalmegh have bitter taste; Glycyrrhiza and Honey are sweet in taste. Linseed and Isphagula are mucilaginous; fixed oils have bland taste; calcium oxide is astringent; Podophyllum, Kaladana, Jalap and Ipomoea are acrid; while Ipecac, Acorus, and *Tylophora indica* contain nauseous taste.

Glycyrrhiza has hard and fibrous fracture due to the presence of fibrous and woody tissues. Aconite has a horny fracture due to gelatinization of starch.

Colour of drugs are standardized and determined by the Inter-Society Colour Council-National Bureau of Standard method. For example, reserpine is described as a "white or pale buff to slightly yellowish, odourless crystalline powder".

MICROSCOPIC OR ANATOMICAL EVALUATION

Schleiden (1847) used microscope for the examination of drugs. Microscopic examination of section and powder drugs, aided by stains, helps in distinction of anatomy in adulterants. Further, microscopical examination of epidermal trichomes and calcium oxalate crystals is extremely valuable, especially in powdered drugs. In the powdered drugs the cells are mostly broken, except lignified cells. The cell contents such as starch, calcium oxalate crystals, aleurone, etc. are scattered in the powder. Some fragments are specific for each powder which may consist of parts of cells or groups of cells.

Plant parts are made up of specific arranged tissues, spores (Lycopodium) or hairs (Lupulin). Histological characters are studied from very thin transverse, or longitudinal sections properly mounted in suitable stains, reagents or mounting media.

The size, shape and relative positions of the different cells and tissues, chemical nature of the cell walls and of the cell contents are determined. The basic arrangement of tissues in each drug is fairly constant. Fibres, sclereids, tracheids, vessels and cork are least affected by drying. Starch, calcium oxalate, epidermal trichomes and lignin are examined carefully.

Microscope is also used for a quantitative evaluation of drugs and adulterated powders. This is done by counting a specific histological feature such as stomatal index, vein-islets and vein termination numbers, palisade ratio, etc. These features are compared with the standard samples.

Palisade Ratio : The average number of palisade cells beneath each epidermal cell is called as palisade ratio. It is determined from powdered drugs with the help of camera lucida.

Stomatal Number : The average number of stomata per square millimeter of the epidermis is known as stomatal number. The range and average value for each surface are recorded.

Stomatal Index : The percentage proportion of the number of stomata form to the total number of epidermal cells of a leaf is termed the stomatal index :

$$S.I. = S/E+S \times 100;$$ where S = number of stomata per unit area, E = number of ordinary epidermal cells in the same unit area.

Stomatal number varies considerably with the age of the leaf but the stomatal index is highly constant for a given species.

Vein-Islet Number : The word 'Vein-islet' is used for the minute area of photosynthetic tissue encircled by the ultimate divisions of the conducting strands. *Vein-islet number* is defined as the number of vein-islets per square mm calculated from four contiguous square mm in the central part of the lamina, midway between the midrib and the margin. The average range of vein-islet numbers for Senna are : *Cassia senna* (26), *C. angustifolia* (21); for Coca: *Erythroxylum coca* (11), *E. truxillense* (20); for Digitalis. *Digitalis purpurea* (3.5) *D. lanata* (2.7); *D. lutea* (4.4), *D. thapsi* (1.2).

Veinlet Termination Number : It is defined as the number of veinlet terminations per mm^2 of leaf surface. A vein termination is the ultimate free termination of a veinlet or branch of a veinlet. By this character different Coca leaves and Senna leaflets are differentiated.

LYCOPODIUM SPORE METHOD

Lycopodium (syn. Club-moss spores, Lycopodium seeds; vegetable sulphur) consists of the spores of the clubmoss, *Lycopodium clavatum* Linn. (Fam. Lycopodiaceae, Phyllum. Pteriodophyta); grows in the North America, Russia, Poland, India and Pakistan. The sporangial spikes are cut and dried and the spores are separated by shaking. Lycopodium is a light yellow, extremely mobile and flammable powder without odour or taste. It contains about 50% fixed oil, which consists mainly of glycosides of lycopodiumoleic acid; sugars (3%), phytosterin and alkaloids of the annotine type.

Lycopodium spores are exceptionally uniform in size (about 25 μm) and 1 mg of lycopodium contains an average of 94,000 spores. The number of spores per milligram is determined by direct counting and by calculation based on specific gravity and dimensions of the spores. It is possible to evaluate many powdered drugs if well-defined particles may be counted as in case of pollen grains or starch grains; or if single layered tissues or cells of the area of which may be traced at a definite magnification and the actual area calculated; or if characteristic particles of a uniform thickness, the length of which can be measured at a definite magnification and the actual length calculated. Mounts containing a definite proportion of the powder and lycopodium are used and the lycopodium spores counted in each of the fields in which the number or area of the particles in the powder is determined.

In this method the moisture content of the powdered material is determined. A mixture of weighed quantity of the powder and lycopodium spores is suspended in a suitable viscous liquid. A drop of this suspension is mounted and examined with a 4 mm objective. The number of lycopodium spores and the number of characteristic particles are counted in 25 various fields. The same experiment is repeated with a second similar suspension. From the mean of these results and a knowledge of the weights of lycopodium and powder in the mixture, the number of characteristic particles in 1 mg of the powder may be determined.

By employing lycopodium spore method the number of pollen grains in pyrethrum powder (1000-2000/mg), starch granules in wheat powder (400 granules/mg) and starch grain in Ginger (261400 grains/mg) have been determined.

Lycopodium spore method is also used to determine size of a particular type of particle in powders such as epidermal fragments of leaves, single layer of scalerenchyma, or isolated fibres. The procedure is almost the same as used for counting of particles. The particle size is traced with the help of camera lucida and the spores are counted. The tracings are cut out and weighed and their area calculated by weighing a sheet of known area of the paper used. This area divided by the magnification used $(420)^2$ gives the actual area of the particles in a certain weight of the powdered drug, which is calculated from the number of spores counted and the weight of spores and powder in the suspension. By this method epidermal area of Indian Senna stalk (100 cm^2), sclerenchyma layer in Linseed, fibres in the Cinnamon bark and number of beaker cells in testa of Cinnamon seed have been measured.

CHEMICAL EVALUATION

Chemical evaluation involves the determination of active constituents by a chemical process. Chemical tests are used to identify certain crude drugs to determine purity. Chemical tests for alkaloids, carbohydrates, steroids. phenolic compounds, saponins, proteins, amino acids, fixed oils and volatile oils are performed. Titrimetric assay, iodine value, saponification value, acid value, acetyl value, ester value, peroxide value, hydroxyl value and ash value are determined. Tropane alkaloids in Datura, Belladonna and Stramonium are determined by Vitali-Morin reaction. Potassium chlorate and hydrochloric acid are used to estimate emetine in Ipecac. Strychnine in Nux-vomica is detected with ammonium vanadate and sulphuric acid. Bornträger's test is useful for detecting anthraquinone glycosides, present in Senna, Rhubarb, Cascara and Aloe. Alkaloid contents can be evaluated by determining total alkaloidal contents by acid-base titration.

Preparation of an extract by an appropriate solvent is sometimes applied to determine the quality of drugs. The solvent may extract a single constituent, e.g. fixed oil from crushed Linseed. Further examples of the use of extractive tests are in cases of Gentian, Colocynth seeds, Indian hemp, Ginger, Calumba, Rhubarb, Glycyrrhiza and Myrrh.

Drugs containing volatile oils are examined for authenticity and quality by determining the percentage of volatile oil yielded by steam distillation in a suitable apparatus. Standards for content of volatile oil in drugs usually allow a somewhat smaller percentage from powdered drugs as compared with the whole drug due to inevitable loss on grinding, volatilization and decomposition.

On ignition of crude drugs a residue of mineral substances or ash remains, derived from the cell wall and cell contents. The ash value is useful in determining authenticity and purity of drugs. For a number of official drugs, a limit is placed on the yield of acid-insoluble ash, i.e. the ash remaining after extraction of the total ash with dilute acid. This residue consists chiefly of silica, partly derived from the constituents of the cells and their walls and partly from foreign mineral matters, mainly soil. Acid-insoluble ash limits are imposed especially in cases where foreign silica may be present or when the calcium oxalate contents of the drug is high. Pharmacopoeial limits for acid insoluble ash vary from 0.5 (Agar) to 12 percent (Hyoscyamus). Glandular trichomes present in Hyoscyamus have a capacity of retaining clay and thus the acid insoluble ash value is higher in such cases. In case of Glycyrrhiza the total ash figure is of importance which indicates the care taken in the preparation of the drug. For the determination of total ash values the carbon must be removed below 450°C, since alkali chlorides would be lost due to volatile at high temperature. The total ash usually consists of carbonates, phosphates, silicates and silica. In case of Ginger a minimum percentage of water-soluble ash is determined to detect the presence of exhausted ginger.

PHYSICAL EVALUATION

Physical constants such as elasticity in fibres, viscosity of drugs containing gums, swelling factor of mucilage containing materials, froth number of saponin drugs, congealing point of volatile and fixed oils, melting and boiling points and water contents (loss on drying at 110°C) are some important parameters used in the evaluation of drugs. Ultraviolet light is also used for determining the fluorescence of extracts of some drugs (Gambir, Senna) and colours of alkaloids as : aconite (light blue), berberine (yellow), emetine (orange) and quinine (dense fluorescence in dilute sulphuric acid). The florescence of Belladonna leaf and root, Wild Cherry bark and Jalap is due to the presence of a coumarin, β-methyl asculetin. Pale Catechu shows fluorescence in alkaline solution due to gambir-fluorescin. Aloe exhibits a green fluorescence in a solution containing borax. Many other drugs show a marked intensity of colour or a characteristic colour under UV light. Rhubarb is differentiated from Rhapontic, Chinese or Indian Rhubarb by its marked fluorescence in UV light.

Physical constants are extensively applied to the active principles of drugs, such as alkaloids, volatile oils, fixed oils, etc. Solubility expresses number of ml of solvent require to dissolve one gram of the drug. For example, 1 g of codeine sulphate is soluble in 30 ml of water, and in 1300 ml of alcohol, Alkaloids and other nitrogenous compounds are soluble in dilute hydrochloric acid. Melting points are recorded for solid fixed oils (fats) and alkaloids.

Most of the monoterpenes have asymmetric carbon.

Therefore, they are optical active. For example, Peppermint oil has optical rotation as $-18°$ to $-32°$. Specific gravity is important with nutgalls. The galls that will not sink in water are considered to be inferior quality. In Jalap, the specific gravity should be higher than water. This constant is also important for volatile oils and lipids. Refractive index is particularly important in volatile oils and fixed oils. It is in between 1.45-1.46 for Peppermint oil at 20 degree.

Spectrocopic analysis (UV, IR, NMR, Mass), and radioimmuno assays are applied more frequently to the active individual drugs components. Chromatographic techniques such as paper, column, thin-layer, gas-liquid (GLC) and high performance liquid chromatography (HPLC) provide information about the chemical constituents present in the drug.

The foreign organic (animal, animal excreta, insects, fungi, bacteria, or mould) and inorganic matters should be in pharmacoepeal limits. They are determined by sedimentation or floatation method. If the drug is not prepared properly, the total ash value will be more.

BIOLOGICAL EVALUATION

The drugs, which cannot be assayed satisfactorily by chemical or physical means, are evaluated by biological methods. Tests are carried out on intact animals, animal preparations, isolated living tissues or micro-organisms. Since living organisms are used, the assays are called 'biological assays'. Biological standardization procedures are generally less precise, more time consuming and more expensive to conduct than chemical assays. Therefore, they are generally used if the chemical identity of the active principle has not been fully elucidated; if, no adequate chemical assay has been derived for the active principle as in case of insulin; if the drug is composed of complex mixture and activity, e.g. Digitalis; if the purification of crude drug is not possible, e.g. separation of vitamin D from irridiated oils; and if the chemical assay is not a valid indication of biological activity.

A biological assay measures the actual biological activity of a given sample. In any one test the animals of only one strain are used. For some assays a specific sex must be used. The male rat has faster growth rate than the female. Therefore, use of both male and female in a growth test should be avoided. Bioassays are conducted by determining the amount of a solution of unknown potency required to produce a definite effect on suitable test animals or organs under standard conditions. To minimize the source of errors resulting from animal variation, standard reference preparations are used in certain bioassay procedures.

Bacteria such as a *Salmonella typhi* and *Staphylococcus aureus* are used to determine antiseptic value of certain drugs. In another microbiologic methods the living bacteria, yeast and molds are used for assaying vitamins and to determine the activity of antibiotic drugs. Mice are used to test Rabies vaccine, Diphtheria toxoid and other biologics. The 'rat line test' is utilized for the assay of vitamin D preparation. Guinea pigs are employed to test the toxicity and antigenicity of diagnostic Diphtheria toxin and tetanus toxoid. Oxytocic activity of vasopressin injection is also tested on guinea pigs. Oxytocic injection is assayed on young domestic chickens by injecting into an exposed crural or brachial vein and observing changes in blood pressure. Digitalis glycosides are assayed on pigeons by transfusing the drug through the alar vein into the blood stream and noting the lethal effects. Cats are utilized in tests for drugs with depressor activity and glucagon injection. Mydriatic drugs such as atropine are evaluated on cat's eye. Curare alkaloids, e.g. tubocurarine chloride, and pyrogens in antibiotic solutions are assayed on rabbits. Ophthalmic preparations are tested on rabbit eyes. Dogs are the test animals to determine pressor activity in drugs and to assay Veratrum viride preparations. Anthelmintic drugs (Male fern) are evaluated on earthworms. Evaluation of Ergot is carried out on cock's comb or rabbit intestine or its uterus. Human beings are also used to note the activity of drugs in clinical trial.

There are some disadvantages of bioassays. Quantitative accuracy is usually less than observed with most chemical analyses. Techniques and interpretations involved vary with different operators. The effect measured in the test animals is different from that observed in treating patients.

A simple bioassay utilizing brine shrimp *(Artemia salina)* is available for determining new biological activities in plant extracts. The eggs of this creature, which serve as food for tropical fish, are allowed to hatch in a brine solution. The shrimp are exposed to different concentrations of the test material and an LC_{50} (median lethan concentration) value in µg/ml is calculated. A broad range of compound show toxic effect to the shrimp. The procedure is rapid, reliable and cheap. Another procedure, called potato-disc assay, involved observation of the inhibition of crown gall tumors induced on potato discs by *Agrobacterium tumefaciens* by plant extracts or isolated compounds. This method is used for detecting in preliminary fashion anticancer activity.

QUESTIONS

1. (a) Describe the various non-living cell contents. How will you test them chemically or microscopically ?
   (b) What chemical tests will characterize (i) lignified cell wall and (ii) suberized and cutinized cell walls.

2. What do you understand by the term 'Evaluation of Drugs'? Discuss the usefulness of qualitative and quantitative microscopic evaluation giving suitable examples to illustrate your answer.

3. Explain palisade ratio, stomatal number, stomatal index, veinislet number, vein termination number and give suitable examples where these parameters have helped in the crude drug evaluation.

4. Give the importance of vein islet number, stomatadal index, palisade ratio and lycopodium spores in quantitative evaluation of pharmacognostic drugs. Give suitable examples to support the answer.

5. Give the importance of ash valve, calcium oxalate, trichomes and lycopodium spore method in adulteration. Support your answer with suitable examples.

6. Why is it necessary to evaluate the drugs ? What different methods will you use to evaluate crude drugs ?

7. Describe various organoleptic methods with suitable examples used for the evaluation of drugs.

8. Discuss morphological and chemical methods of evaluation of herbal drugs.

6

CARBOHYDRATES

The carbohydrates include simple sugars and polysaccharides. They are carbonyl alcohols containing the elements carbon, hydrogen and oxygen. The last two elements are usually present in the same proportions as in water. Carbohydrates are the primary products of photosynthesis and from them the plant synthesizes various chemical constituents by subsequent organic reactions. They are most abundant components of both plants (cellulose, starch, sugars) and animals (glycogen). Sugars are united with many compounds to form glycosides.

Generally carbohydrates are divided into two groups :

(1) monosaccharides or simple sugars, and

(2) polysaccharides.

Sugars are polyhydroxy-aldehydes or ketones and contain an unbroken chain of carbon atoms. Oligosaccharides are carbohydrates whose molecules consist of not more than a few monosaccharide units linked through oxygen. They are subdivided into disaccharides, trisaccharides, etc. They are hydrolyzed with water in the presence of catalysts or enzymes to produce monosaccharide molecules. On the basis of number of carbon atoms in the molecule monosaccharides are classified as trioses (with three carbon atoms), tetroses (four carbon atoms), pentoses (five carbon atoms), and hexoses (six carbon atoms). Sugars are soluble in water, crystalline compounds and sweet in taste. Monosaccharides like glucose possessing aldehydic group are called aldoses, ketone group containing sugars (fructose) are known as ketoses.

Polysaccharides are substances of very high molecular weight consisting of large number of monosaccharide units linked through oxygen. The hydrolysis of polysaccharide, by enzymes or reagents, yields in a succession of cleavage and the end products are monosaccharides. On the basis of these final products polysaccharides yielding hexose are called hexosans; starch yielding glucose is known as glucosan and inulin producing fructose is termed as fructosan. The fundamental unit of plants is made of a polysaccharide, cellulose, which consists of glucose units joined by β-1, 4-linkages. The other plant constituents of high molecular weight are hemicelluloses which are more soluble and more easily hydrolyzed. Gums and mucilages are related to hemicelluloses. Gums consist largely of pentose and hexose moeties and hydrolysis yields galactose and arabinose. Hemicellulose on hydrolysis produces another type of sugars like glucose, mannose and xylose. Gums are formed by decomposition of the cellulose or by injuring the plant and some of them constitute an important group of drugs as emulsifying agents, suspending agents for insoluble powders in mixtures, as adhesive in pills and tablets, and for the preparation of hand lotions and other cosmetic items. Pectins are also related to cellulose in structural skeleton. Polysaccharides are neither sweet nor crystallizable, insoluble in water and does not form colloidal solutions.

CHEMICAL TESTS

1. **Fehling's Solution Test :** The substance (0.5 g.) is heated with dilute hydrochloric acid to hydrolyse a polysaccharide. The reaction mixture is neutralized by addition of sodium hydroxide solution and then Fehling's solutions 1 and 2 are added. Red precipitate of cuprous oxide is produced on heating in case of reducing sugars (all monosaccharides, and many disaccharides like lactose, maltose, cellobiose and gentiobiose). Non-reducing sugars include some disaccharides (sucrose and trihalose) which on boiling with acids are converted into reducing sugars.

2. **Molisch Test :** A solution of carbohydrate is prepared in water containing α-naphthol. On addition of concentrated sulphuric acid along the side of test tube a purple ring is formed on the junction below aqueous layer. With insoluble carbohydrates (e.g. cellulose)

the colour will produce on shaking the reaction mixture.

3. **Osazone Formation** : A sugar on heating with phenylhydrazine hydrochloride, sodium acetate and acetic acid forms yellow crystals of osazone.

4. **Resorcinol Test for Ketoses (Selivanoff's Test)** : A crystal of resorcinol is added to the solution and heated with an equal volume of concentrated hydrochloric acid. Pink colour is produced in case of ketoses (e.g. fructose, honey or hydrolyzed inulin).

5. **Test for Pentoses** : A solution of the material is heated with equal volume of hydrochloric acid containing a little phloroglucinol. A red colour is formed in case of pentoses.

6. **Keller-Kiliani Test for Deoxysugars** : A deoxysugar (found in cardiac glycosides) is dissolved in acetic acid containing a trace of ferric chloride and transferred to the surface of concentrated H_2SO_4. A reddish-brown colour is formed at the junction which turns blue latter on.

7. **Furfural Test** : A carbohydrate sample is heated in a test tube with a drop of syrupy phosphoric acid to convert it into furfural. A disk of filter paper moistened with a drop of 10% solution of aniline in 10% acetic acid is placed over the mouth of the test tube. The bottom of the test tube is heated for 30-60 seconds. A pink or red stain appears on the reagent paper.

HONEY

Synonyms : Purified Honey, Mel, Clarified Honey, Strained Honey; Madhu (Hindi).

Biological Source : Honey is a sugary secretion deposited by the honeybees, *Apis mellifera* Linn. and other species of *Apis* in the honeycomb. It must be free from foreign substances such as parts of insects, leaves, etc., but may contain pollen grains.

Order : Hymenoptera.

Family : Apidae.

Habitat : Honey is produced mainly in England, West Indies, California, Canada, Chile and in some parts of Africa, Australia and New Zealand.

Collection : Honeybees live in swarms which are gathered into hives. A hive contains :

1. a single queen bee,
2. the males or drones, and
3. the worker bees which are undeveloped females.

The worker bees possess a long, hollow tube to insert into the nectaries of the flowers. The tube is formed from the maxillae and labium. They take nectar from the flowers and pass it through the oesophagus into the honey-sac or crop. The nectar, which is an aqueous solution of sucrose (25%), is mixed with salivary secretion containing the enzyme invertase and then is hydrolyzed into the invert sugar. On returning at the hive the worker bees deposit the contents of the honey sac in the previously prepared cell of the honeycomb. The filled cell is sealed by wax. For collecting the honey, the honeycomb is smoked to remove bees, the comb is cut and honey is collected either by drainage or by expression. The honey obtained by latter procedure is contaminated with the wax. For getting purified honey, it is heated at 80°C when the impurities float on the surface which are removed.

Characters : Honey is thick, syrupy, translucent liquid when fresh. The colour is pale yellow or reddish-brown and it possesses pleasant odour and sweet taste which are dependent upon the floral source of the product. The honey obtained form *Eucalyptus* and *Banksia* species has somewhat unpleasant odour and taste and the honey collected from *Datura stramonium* is poisonous. On storage it becomes opaque and granular due to the crystallization of dextrose.

Chemical Constituents : Honey consists chiefly of glucose (30-40%), fructose (40-50%) and small amounts of sucrose (0.1-10%), dextrin, formic acid, volatile oil and pollen grains. In addition to these, traces of enzymes, vitamins, proteins, maltose, melezitose, pentosans, gums, trace elements, amino acids and colouring matter are also present in honey.

Uses : Honey shows mild laxative, bactericidal, sedative, antiseptic and alkaline characters. It is used for cold, cough, fever, sore eye and throat, tongue and duodenal ulcers, liver disorders, constipation, diarrhoea, kidney and other urinary disorders, pulmonary tuberculosis, marasmus, rickets, scurvy and insomnia. It is applied as a remedy on open wounds after surgery. It prevents infection and promotes healing. Honey works quicker than many antibiotics because it is easily absorbed into the blood stream. It is also useful in healing of carbuncles, chaps, scalds, whitlows and skin inflammation; as vermicide; locally as an excipient, in the treatment of aphthae and other infection of the oral mucous membrane. It is recommended in the treatment of pre-operative cancer. Honey, mixed with onion juice, is a good remedy for arteriosclerosis in brain. Diet rich in honey is recommended for infants, convalescents, diabetic patients and invalids.

Honey is an important ingredient of certain lotions, cosmetics, soaps, creams, balms, toilet-waters and inhalations. It is used as a medium in preservation of cornea.

Adulterants : Honey is adulterated with cane sugar, corn syrup and artificial invert sugar which is obtained by acid hydrolysis of sucrose. The sugar contains furfural which gives red colour with resorcinol in the presence of hydrochloric acid. On prolonged heating or storage of the honey furfural may be formed in the genuine honey.

Chemical Tests : Adulteration in honey is determined by the following tests :

1. **Fiehe's Test for Artificial Invert Sugar :** Honey (10 ml) is shaken with petroleum or solvent ether (5 ml) for 5-10 minutes. The upper ethereal layer is separated and evaporated in a China dish. On addition of 1% solution of resorcinol in hydrochloric acid (1 ml) a transient red colour is formed in natural honey while in artificial honey the colour persists for sometime.

2. **Reduction of Fehling's Solution :** To an aqueous solution of honey (2 ml) Fehling's solutions 1 and 2 are added and the reaction mixture is heated on a steam bath for 5-10 minutes. A brick red colour is produced due to the presence of reducing sugars.

3. **Limit Tests :** The limit tests of chloride, sulphate and ash (0.5%) are compared with the pharmacopoeial specifications.

STARCH

Synonym : Amylum

Biological Source : Starch of pharmaceutical use consists of polysaccharide carbohydrate occurring as discrete granules in the mature grain of corn, *Zea mays* Linn. (Fam: Gramineae) or of wheat, *Triticum aestivum* Linn. (Gramineae), or tubers of potato, *Solanum tuberosum* Linn. (Solanaceae) or rice, *Oriza sativa* Linn. (Gramineae), or arrowroot, *Maranta arundinacea* Linn. (Marantaceae). Commercial starch is also obtained from tapioca or cassava starch, *Manihot utilissima* Pohl. (Fam : Euphorbiaceae).

Geographical Source : Commercially the starch is produced in U.S.A., Argentina, India, China, Japan and other tropical and sub-tropical countries.

Preparation : Various procedures are used to prepare a particular starch. In cereal grains starch is present in the endosperm along with cell debris, oil, soluble and insoluble proteins (gluten). These substances are removed during the preparation of starch.

1. Preparation of Maize Starch

The grains are softened by soaking in an aqueous solution of sulphurous acid (0.2%) at 50°C for 2-3 days to free the starch from fibres. The softened grain is crushed in rollers to separate embryo or germs. The germs are used to prepare germ oils (fixed oils) which are source of vitamins and contain unsaturated fatty acids like linoleic and linolenic acids. The milky liquid is filtered through sieves to remove cell-debris and some of gluten as it is lighter than starch. The remaining proteins may be separated by repeated tabling method in which the suspension is allowed to flow slowly through toughs about 40 m long and 0.7 m wide shallow tables when the heavier starch deposits first. In a modified procedure the total mixture of starch and proteins is fractionated into gluten and starch by the use of special starch purification centrifuges. Traces of proteins are separated by treating starch with dilute alkali to dissolve the former. Then the starch is dried by flash dryers or a moving-belt dryer.

2. Preparation of Rice Starch

Broken rice pieces are softened by macerating in aqueous sodium hydroxide solution (0.4%) and then crushed. The ground material is mixed with water and the starch is separated by standing or by means of a centrifuge. It is washed, dried at 50-60°C and powdered.

3. Preparation of Wheat Starch

To the wheat flour water is added to prepare dough and then kept for one hour to allow gluten to swell. The balls of dough are shaken with water on grooved rollers. Liquid containing starch falls below from which it is separated by centrifugation, washed and dried.

4. Preparation of Potato Starch

Potatoes are washed, crushed in a rasping machine and the cell-debris is removed from the pulp by rotary sieves after addition of water. The liquid contains starch, soluble proteins, salts and some cellular tissues. On standing, the starch separates more rapidly. It may be purified by centrifugation. The washed starch is dried and pulverized.

Characters : Starch occurs in irregular, angular powder or a white mass, insoluble in cold water and forms a colloidal solution on boiling. On cooling the solution forms a translucent jelly. It produces deep blue colour with iodine solution. Starch granules undergo gelatinization on heating or by treating with sodium hydroxide solution or concentrated solution of calcium or zinc chlorides or chloral hydrate. Maize starch is almost neutral, rice starch is slightly alkaline and potato starch is slightly acidic.

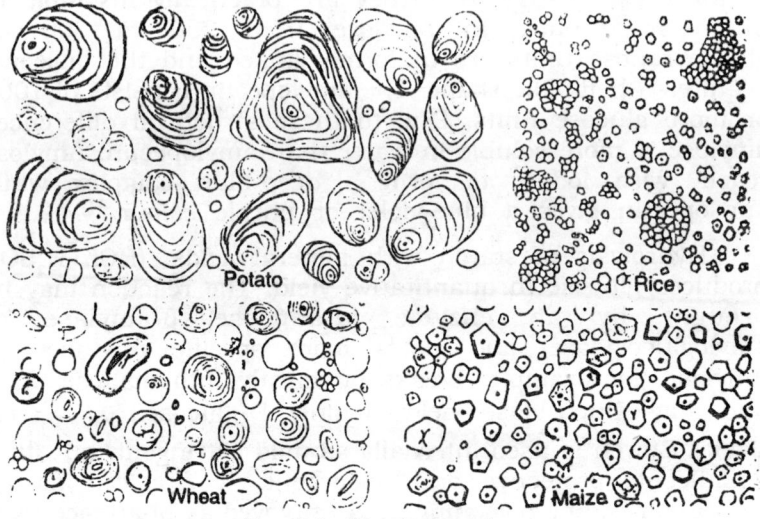

Fig. 6.1. Starch granules

Microscopically, starch granules contain central or eccentric hilum, concentric rings or striations and differ in size and aggregation. In maize starch granules are 10-35 μm in size, angular, polyhedral, hilum is central, distinct and contain a cavity or from 2 to 5 rayed cleft. The striations are absent. Rice starch is composed of 2-10 μm diameter compound and simple granules with an angular outline and aggregated from 2 to 150 components. The granules are polyhedral with sharp angles. Striations are absent and hilum is centric. Wheat starch contains larger granules lenticular, smaller ones globular, size is from 2 to 45 μm. Few compound granules are present. The hilum is central and unclaft. Concentratic and faint striations are observed. Potato starch contains most of simple granules, wedge or mussel-shaped. The diameter is from 2 to 110 μm. Hilum is in the form of α point, near the narrower point and eccentric. Concentric striations are well-marked. Few compound granules of 2 or 3 components are fused together.

Chemical Constituents : Starches are generally mixtures of two types of polymers :

(1) amylose, a linear (1-4)-α-D-glucan, and

(2) amylopectin, a branched D-glucan with mostly α-D (1-4) and aproximately 4% α-D (1-6) linkages.

The strach in corn contains approximately 27% amylose and 73% amylopectin. These two polymers are so associated in the crystal lattice that they are practically insoluble in water or alcohol. In amylose from 250 to 300 D-glucopyranose units are uniformly linked and the molecule acquires a helix-like shape. The amylopectin consists of 1000 or more glucose units. Due to these structural differences amylose is more soluble in water than amylopectin. Amylose reacts with iodine to form a deep-blue complex while amylopectin gives a blue-violet or purple colour.

Hydrolysis of starch with mineral acids, (HCl, H_2SO_4) produces glucose in quantitative yield. The reaction may be brought by an enzyme (α-amylase, β-amylase or amyloglucosidase) and yields more specific products. β-Amylase, for example, breaks off mostly into maltose units and amyloglucosidase yields mainly D-glucose.

Uses : Starch is used internally as mild astringent, nutritive, demulcent, protective and absorbent. It is given as an antidote in iodine poisoning. It is employed as pharmaceutical aid, as tablet disintegrant, filler and binder. Externally it is used as an absorbent, emollient, in dusting powders and in ointments. Starch is the starting material for the preparation of glucose, dextrose, and dextrin. Some official preparations of starch are Mucilage of Starch B.P.C., Zinc Starch Dusting powder B.P.C., and Zinc oxide paste, I.P.

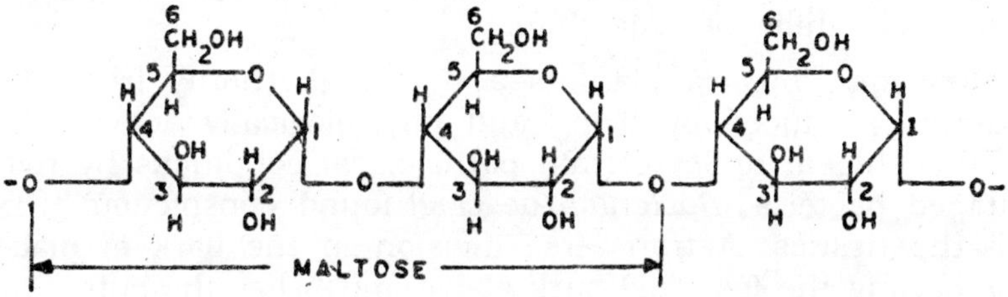

β-Amylose

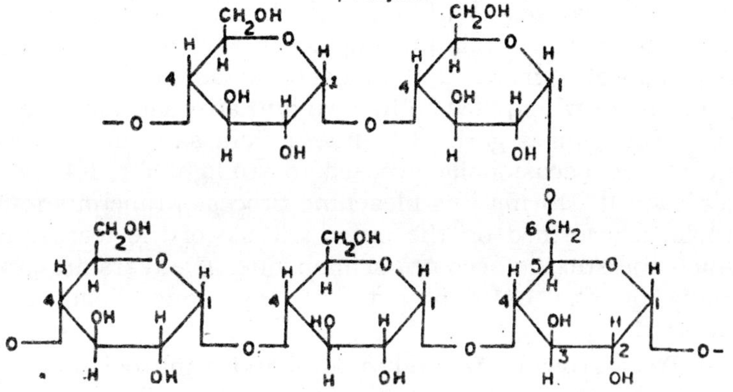

Amylopectin

Tests for Identification

1. Dissolve starch (1 g) in water (15 ml) by heating on a water bath. A viscous transluscent jelly is formed on cooling.
2. Fehling's solution test is positive.
3. It shows Molisch's test for carbohydrates.
4. Solution of starch (1 ml) forms a deep blue colour on addition of iodine solution (1 drop). On warming the colour disappears and re-appears on cooling.

ACACIA GUM

Synonyms : Acacia, Gum Acacia, Gum Arabic, Acaciae gummi.

Biological Source : Acacia gum is the dried gummy exudate obtained from the stem and branches of *Acacia senegal* Willd. and of some related species like *Acacia arabica* Linn.

Family : Leguminosae.

Habitat : *A. senegal* is found in Sudan, Central Africa, West Africa and north-western India particularly Haryana, Gujarat and rocky hills of Rajasthan.

Collection : Acacia plant is a 6 m high thorny tree. The gum is produced by living and physiologically active cells of the phloem under certain pathological conditions by rod-shaped bacteria *(Bacterium acaciae)* found conspicuously in all the tissues. A transverse incision in the bark is made for peeling the loosened bark above and below the cuts. The cambium measuring 0.5-1.0 m in length and 5-7.5 cm in breath is exposed. Within a month new phloem cells are produced in the cambium. The tears of gum are formed on this exposed surface due to bacterial action or the action of a ferment which flow on its own and are collected in leather bags. The gum is garbled to free it from sand and vegetable debris and occasionally exposed to sunlight for 3-4 months to bleach it. During this bleaching process numerous minute cracks are formed on the outer surface of the tears due to which the surface becomes semiopaque. The tears are graded finally on the basis of external appearance, packed and exported.

Trees growing in sandy plains and semi-rocky sites give higher gum-yield than those growing in rocky areas.

Characters : Acacia gum occurs in rounded or ovoid, irregular or broken tears, 1-3 cm in diameter. Outer surface contains numerous fine cracks. Colour is white or pale yellow. The gum is very brittle and the exposed surface is transparent and glassy. It is odourless and taste is bland and mucilaginous. It is freely soluble in equal weight of water to form a viscous and acidic solution. The gum is insoluble in alcohol and other organic solvents.

Chemical Constituents : Acacia gum contains chiefly arabin which is the mixture of calcium, magnesium and potassium salts of arabic acid. On hydrolysis arabic acid yields L-rhamnopyranose, galactopyranose, L-arabofuranose and the aldobionic acid 6-β-D-glucuronosido-D-galactose. Further hydrolysis yields L-arabinose, D-galactose, D-glucuronic acid and rhamnose. The gum also possesses enzymes like oxidases, peroxidases and pectinases.

Uses : Acacia gum is demulcent, emollient, and used as emulsifying and suspending agent for the administration of insoluble drugs. It is employed as an adhesive and binder in tablets especially in lozenges. Due to its demulcent properties it is used in various formulations for cough, diarrhoea and throat problems. Internally, Acacia gum is used in inflammation of intestinal mucosa. It is also used to cover inflamed surfaces such as burns, sore nipples, etc.

Purity Tests : 1. An aqueous solution of the Acacia gum (5 g) is prepared by dissolving in water (15 ml) to perform the following tests for identity :

1. The aqueous solution is slightly acidic and becomes more acidic on keeping.

2. On standing it does not form viscous gelly-like mass. No sediment should be deposited on standing in case of pure gums.

3. To the aqueous solution (5 ml) a few drops of dilute solution of lead acetate are added. No precipitate is formed due to absence of Tragacanth and Agar.

4. It does not form blue or brown colour with iodine solution due to absence of starch and dextrin.

5. With ferric chloride solution it does not produce any violet or green colour due to absence of tannins.

6. To the solution of gum acacia resorcinol (0.1 g) and hydrochloric acid (2 ml) are added and then heated on a water-bath. No yellow or pink colour is developed due to absence of sucrose or fructose.

7. Fine powder of the gum (5 g) is dissolved in distilled water (100 ml), dilute hydrochloric acid (10 ml) is added and the reaction mixture is boiled gently for 15 minutes. The hot solution is filtered by suction through a sintered glass crucible, washed thoroughly with hot water, dried at 105°C and weighed. The insoluble matter should not exceed 50 mg in case of pure gum.

Test for Identification

1. To the aqueous solution (5 ml) borax (0.1 g) is added. A stiff translucent mass is obtained.

2. To the dilute aqueous solution few drops of lead sub-acetate are added. A white, bulky precipitate is produced.

3. To the aqueous solution (5 ml) few drops of 1% alcohol

solution of benzidine are added along with 10% hydrogen peroxide (0.5 ml). On shaking blue colour is produced due to enzyme oxidase.

4. Gum acacia responds positively to Fehling's solution test of reducing sugars and Molisch's test of carbohydrates.

5. To the aqueous solution (5 ml), alcohol (10 ml) is added gradually by shaking. The cloudy liquid on addition of glacial acetic acid (0.5 ml) forms a white precipitate. It is filtered and to the clear filtrate ammonium oxalate solution (50 ml) is added. The filtrate becomes cloudy again.

Allied Drugs : Gatti gum (Indian gum) is obtained from *Anogeissus latifolia* Wallich (Fam. Combretaceae). Its tears are of different colour and the outer surface is dull. Some of tears are vermiform in shape and their surface shows fewer cracks than the natural acacia. Aqueous solution of this gum has the viscosity between those of Acacia and Sterculia gums. With lead subacetate solution it forms very slight precipitates.

Starch, Tragacanth, Talka gum, Dextrin and cheaper gums from Acacia species are other adulterants of Acacia gum.

TRAGACANTH

Synonyms : Gum tragacanth, Anjira (Hindi).

Biological Source : Tragacanth is the dried gummy exudation obtained by incision from the stems of *Astragalus gummifer* Labil. (White gavan) or other Asiatic species of *Astragalus* such as *A. kurdicus*, *A. adscendens* and *A. strobiliferus.*

Family : Leguminosae.

Harbitat : Tragacanth plant is most widely found in Iran, also in Asia Minor, Syria, Anatolia, Iraq, Turkish, Greece and Afghanistan.

Collection : The Tragacanth plants are 1 meter high thorny branching shrubs. The gum is produced physiologically in the plant cells. When a one-or two years old plant is injured, the cell wall of the pith and then of the medullary rays are gradually converted into gum. This change is called as "gummosis". The gum absorbs water and a considerable pressure is created within the stem which forces the gum to the surface through the incision in the form of soft, solid Tragacanth. In contact of the air it is hardened due to evaporation of water. The shape of the gum depends on the shape of the incision made. The gum is collected by the natives and packed.

Characters : Tragacanth occurs as thin, flattened, curved or ribbon-like flakes, length up to 2.5 cm, breadth 1.2 cm. Colour is white or pale yellow, translucent. The surface is marked with concentric ridges which indicates the successive exudation and solidification. Longitudinal striations caused by small irregularities in the incision are present on the surface. The fracture is short and horny. It is odourless and has a little insipid, mucilaginous taste. Tragacanth is entirely insoluble in alcohol and other organic solvents.

Chemical Constituents : Tragacanth consists of tragacanthin (water-soluble portion) and bassorin (water-insoluble protion). The insoluble portion swells to a gel and consists of 60-70% bassorin which is a complex of polymethoxylated acids. Tragacanthin is probably demethoxylated bassorin consisting of 30% of the gum. The gum is composed of sugar and uronic acid units. On hydrolysis of Tragacanth, galacturonic acid, D-galactopyranose, L-arabofuranose and D-xylopyranose are obtained. Starch and protein are also present in Tragacanth.

Uses : Tragacanth is used in pharmaceutical as compounding and dispensing agent, e.g. to suspend heavy insoluble powders, as an excipient for tablets and to impart consistency to touches; also in making emulsions and emulsifying agents for oils and resin; as stabilizer, thickener, and texturizer in food. As Tragacanth is resistant to acid hydrolysis, it is preferred for use in highly acidic conditions. It has demulcent and emollient properties and is used in various cosmetic formulations like hand lotions. It is also used in adhesives (mucilages, pastes); in textile sizing, textile printing and general printing inks, and in dyeing with insoluble colour lakes.

Allied Drugs : Tragacanth of lower grades, known as *hog gum* or *hog tragacanth*, is used in textile industry and pickle manufacture. The pieces are of different shape, yellow to black in colour and contaminated with earth. Their ashes give a strong reaction for iron. It is adulterated with *Chitral gum* obtained from *Astragalus strobiliferus,* Sterculia gum obtained from *Sterculia urens,* insoluble *Shiraz gum* of unknown origin imported from Iran and *Vermicelli tragacanth*

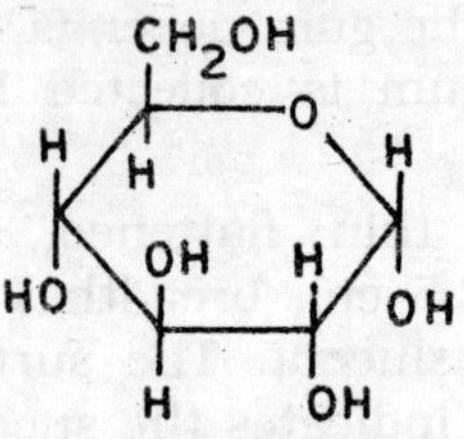

α-D-Glucose

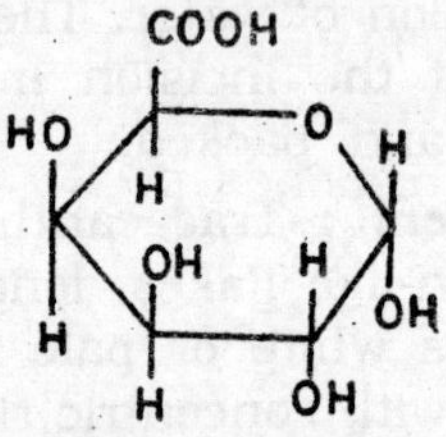

D-Galacturonic acid

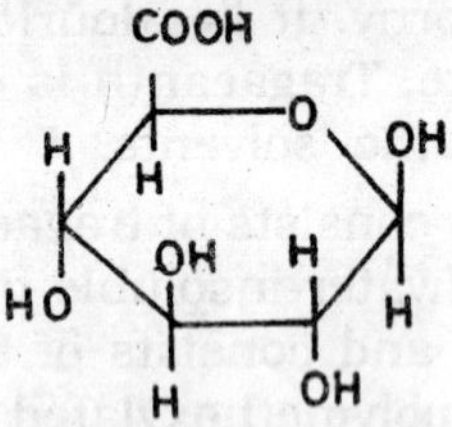

β-D-Glucuronic acid

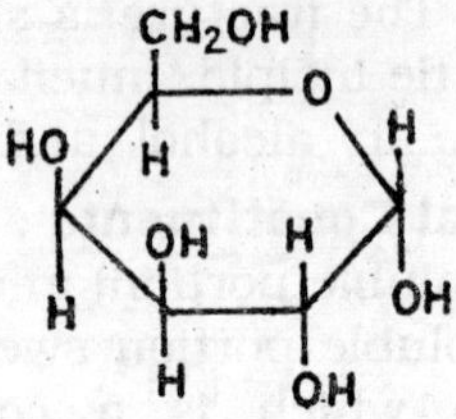

Galactose

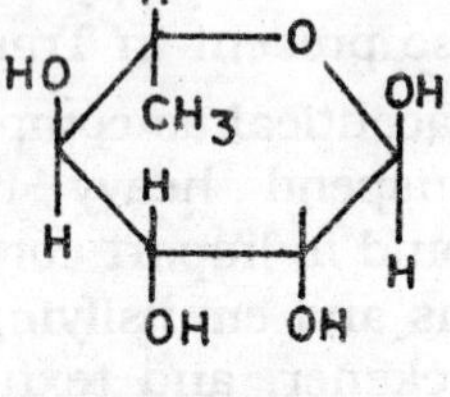

Rhamnose

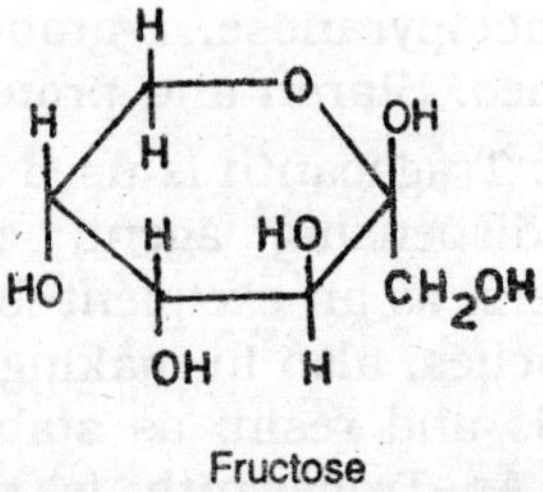

Fructose

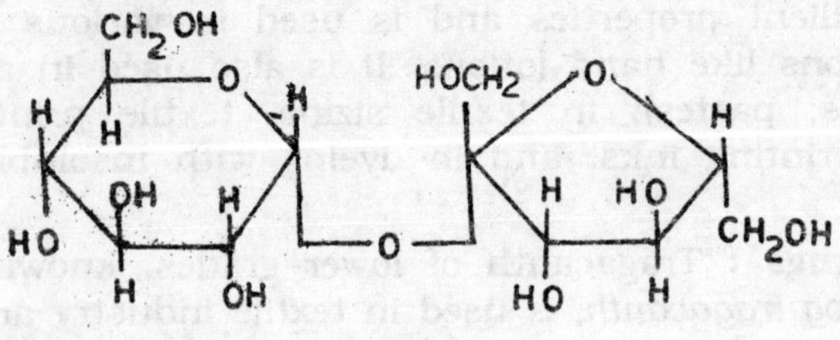

Sucrose

obtained from *Astragalus cylleneus.*, a species found in Greece.

Tests for Identity

1. Tragacanth contains about 30% of water soluble portion.
2. On boiling with sodium hydroxide solution a brown or yellow colour is formed.
3. It responds positively with Molisch's test and Fehling's solution test.
4. It swells and forms a smooth, nearly uniform stiff, opalescent mucilage free from cellular fragments.
5. Powdered material (0.5g) is dissolved in water (1 ml) to form a homogenous mucilage. The mucilage is diluted with water (5 ml) and barium hydroxide solution added. A slightly flocculent precipitate is formed. On heating for ten minutes, it gives an intense yellow colour.

STERCULIA GUM

Synonyms : Kadaya; Mucara; Kullo; Katilo; Kuteera, Gum Karaya, Karaya gum, Indian Tragacanth, Bassora Tragacanth.

Biological Source : Sterculia is the dried gummy exudate of the tree *Sterculia urens* Roxb., *S. villosa, S. tragacantha* or from *Cochlospermum gossypium* Decand. (Fam. Bixaceae).

Family : Sterculiaceae.

Habitat : The tree is found mainly in India (Gujarat, Maharastra, Madras, Rajasthan, M.P. and Chota Nagpur), Pakistan and to some extent in Africa.

Collection : The gum exudes naturally or from incisions made to the heartwood and is collected twice a year, before and after the monsoon season (April-June and September). The gum of first collection has the highest viscosity. The dried irregular masses of several kilograms in weight are picked up, bark pieces are removed, packed and exported.

Characters : Sterculia gum occurs in irregular, translucent striated mass. The pure gum is colourless, medium grade is pinkish tinge and lower grades are very dark. In water it is slightly soluble but swells to many times. It has a distinct odour of acetic acid.

Chemical Constituents : Sterculia gum consists of an acetylated, branched heteropolysaccharide with a high composition of D-galacturonic acid and D-glucuronic acid moieties.

Hydrolysis of the gum affords D-galactose, L-rhamnose, D-galacturonic acid, aldobiouronic acid, acetic acid and an acid trisaccharide. Uronic acid residues are present in 37% amount in the gum.

Uses : Sterculia gum is used as a bulk laxative, emulsifying and suspending agent and a dental adhesive. The powdered gum is used in lozenges, pastes and denture fixative powder. It is also employed in wave set solution, skin lotions, textile and printing industries and in the preparation of compositae building materials.

AGAR

Synonyms : Agar-agar, Gelose; Japan agar, Bengal isinglass; Ceylon isinglass, Chinese isinglass, Japanese isinglass; Vegetable Gelatin, Kanten.

Biological Source : Agar is the dried, hydrophilic, colloidal, polysaccharide complex extracted from the agarocytes of algae known as *Gelidium cartilagineum* (L.) Gaillon (Family Gelidiaceae), *Gracilaria confervoides* (L.) Grev. (Family Sphaerococcaceae) and some other speices of *Acanthopeltis*, *Ceramium*, and *Pterocladia*. (Family : Rhodophyceae). *Gelidium* Provides about 35% of the total agar source.

About 18 important species of marine red algae occur in Indian coasts. The seven species, viz *Gracilaria corticata*, *G. crassa*, *G. edulis*, *G. foliifora*, *G. verrucosa*, *Gelidiella acerosa* and *Pterocladia capillacea* are used to prepare Agar.

Habitat : Agar is prepared from Japan, Korea, South Africa, Mexico, Atlantic and Pacific coasts of U.S.A., Spain, and New Zea land.

Collection and Preparation : Algae are cultivated on the coast. The development of algae takes place on poles which are withdrawn from time to time to strip off the algae. The seaweed is washed for 24 hours in running water, beaten and shaken to remove sand and shells, extracted in steam heated digesters with dilute acids and then with water for 30 hours. The hot mucilaginous decoction is filtered through linen. On cooling a jelly is formed which is cut into bars. The bars are converted into strips by passing through wire netting. Water is removed by successively freezing, thawing and drying at about 35°C. The agar ice block weighing about 150 kg is crushed, melted, and filtered through a rotary vacuum pump. The moist agar flakes so obtained are dried by currents of dry air in tall cylinders.

Characters : Agar occurs in the form of a transparent or translucent, agglutinated, yellowish-white slender, lustrous, flattened strips or as fine or granulated powder. It is tough in damp, brittle in dried form, odourless or with a slight odour and taste is mucilaginous. Agar is insoluble in cold water and alcohol, slowly soluble in hot water to form a viscid solution and its 1% solution forms a stiff firm jelly on cooling.

Chemical Constituents : Agar is composed of the calcium salt of acidic polysaccharides. It can be separated into a natural gelling fraction, *agarose*, and a sulphated non-gelling fraction, *agaropectin*. The structure is believed to be a complex range of polysaccharide chains having alternating α-(1→3) and β-(1→4) linkages. On hydrolysis Agar yields galactose and sulphate ions. It is a hetrogeneous polysaccharide. Agarose, responsible for the gel strength, consists of alternate residue of 3,6-anhydro-L-galactose and D-galactose. The viscosity of agar solutions is due to the presence of agaropectin which is a sulphated polysaccharide in which galactose and uronic acid moieties are partly esterified with sulphuric acid.

Uses : Agar is used to treat chronic constipation, as a laxative, suspending agent, an emulsifier, a gelating agent for suppositories, as surgical lubricants, as a tablet excipient, disintegrant, in production medicinal encapsulations and ointments; as dental impression mold base. It is extensively used as a gel in nutrient media for bacterial cultures; as a substitute for gelatin, insiglass, etc., in making emulsions including photographic, gel in cosmetics, as thickening agent in food especially confectionaries and dairy products, in meat canning; sizing for silk and paper; in dyeing and printing of fabrics and textiles; in adhesive, etc.

Chemical Tests

1. Agar responds positively to Fehling's solution test.
2. Agar gives positive test with Molisch's reagent.
3. Aqueous solution of Agar (1%) is hydrolyzed with concentrated hydrochloric acid by heating for 5-10 minutes. On addition of barium chloride solution to the reaction mixture, a white precipitate of barium sulphate is formed due to the presence of sulphate ions. This test is absent in case of Starch, Acacia gum and Tragacanth.

4. To Agar powder a solution of ruthenium red is added. Red colour is formed indicating mucilage.

5. Agar is warmed in a solution of potassium hydroxide. A canary yellow colour is formed.

6. An aqueous solution of agar (1%) is prepared in boiling water. On cooling it sets into a jelly.

7. To agar solution an N/20 solution of iodine is added. A deep crimson to brown colour is obtained (distinction from Acacia gum and Tragacanth).

8. To a 0.2% solution of Agar an aqueous solution of tannic acid is added. No precipitate is formed indicating absence of Gelatin.

9. It does not gives any precipitate with Millon's reagent due to absence of Gelatin.

10. On heating Agar with soda lime no ammonia is evolved due to absence of Gelatin.

11. To the ash of Agar dilute hydrochloric acid is added and examined under microscope. Skeletons and fragments of diatoms and sponge spicules are observed.

ISPAGHULA (Plantago)

Synonyms : Psyllium seed; Flea seed; Plantain seed; Isabgol; Ishabgul; Spogel seed.

Biological Source : Ispaghula consists of cleaned, dried, ripe seed of *Plantago psyllium* Linn, or of *Plantago indica* Linn. (*P. arenaria* Wald.), known as Spanish or French Psyllium seed, or of *Plantago ovata* Fork, known as Blonde Psyllium or Indian Plantago.

Family : Plantaginaceae.

Habitat : *P. psyllium* Linn. is indigenous to the Mediterranean region and west Asia, presently cultivated in France, Spain and Cuba. *P. ovata* is found in Punjab hills and other parts of north-west India, Sind and Baluchistan and is cultivated in Bengal, Karnataka, Gujarat and Maharashtra.

Cultivation and Collection : The plant is a stemless or sub-caulescent soft, hairy annual herb. It is cultivated by spreading seeds in November in well drained loamy soil. To the fields ammonium sulphate fertilizer is added and they are irrigated at an interval of 8-10 days for about 8 times.

The crop is harvested in four months in March/April. The plants are cut just above the ground, dried and seeds are separated by thrashing.

Characters : The seeds of *P. ovata* are 2.0-3.3 mm in length, 1-16 mm in breadth; dull, pinkish grey-brown; long to elliptical in outline, boat shaped; the dorsal surface is convex with a small elliptical or elongated shining reddish brown spot while the ventral surface is concave with a deep furrow, not perfectly reaching to either end of the seeds. At the furrow a hilum is present which is covered by a thin membrane and appears as a red spot in the centre. The outer surface is smooth, hard and translucent. The seeds are odourless and taste is bland but mucilaginous.

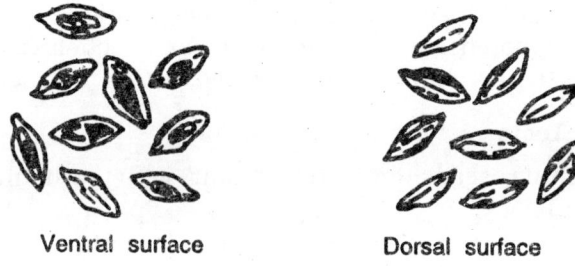

Ventral surface   Dorsal surface

Fig. 6.2. Ispaghula

Chemical Constituents : The seeds contain hydrocolloidal polysaccharide (mucilage) in the outer seed coat (20-30%), fixed oils, tannin, aucubin glycoside (iridoid), sugars, sterols and protein. The mucilage of Ispaghula is colloidal in nature and its composition varies with the conditions of preparation. It is mainly composed of xylose, arabinose and galacturonic acid; rhamnose and galactose have also been reported. Two polysaccharide fractions have been separated from the muscilage. One fraction is soluble in cold water and on hydrolysis yields xylose (46%), an aldobiouronic acid (40%), arabinose (7%) and insoluble residue. The other fraction in soluble in hot water forming a highly viscous solution which sets as a gel on cooling and yields on hydrolysis xylose (80%), arabinose (14%), aldobiouronic acid (0.3%) and trace of galactose. The fatty oil is composed of linolenic, linoleic, oleic, palmitic, stearic and lignoceric acids. *P. ovata* is a good source of linoleic acid. The amino acids reported in the seeds are valine, alanine, glycine, glutamic acid, cystine, lysine, leucine and tyrosine.

Uses : Seeds are demulcent, cooling, diuretic and used in inflammatory conditions of mucus membrane of gastrointestinal and genitourinary tracts. They are used to cure chronic dysentery, diarrhoea, duodenal ulcer, gonorrhoea, constipation and piles. Isabgol preparations are given after colostomy to assist the production of smooth solid faecal mass. The mucilage is not digested by enzymes and intestinal bacteria in the gut and comes out unchanged. Jelly-like mucilage absorbs irritating products and toxins of the gut and they are expelled from the body. The seeds are used in febrile conditons and the affections of kidneys, bladder and urethra. A decoction of seeds is prescribed in cough and cold, and the crushed seeds made into poultice are applied to rheumatic and glandular sweelings. Recently anticancer, antitoxic, antiatherosclerosis, hypocholesteremic, hypo-glycemic, hypotensive, cardiac depressant, cholinergic and cervical activities have been reported.

Chemical Tests

1. Ispaghula seeds form red colour with ruthenium red solution.

2. On adding water mucilage swells forming surrounding layer outside the seed.

3. **Determination of Swelling Factor :** The drug (1 g) is placed in a 25 ml graduated cylinder. Water is added up to 20 ml mark and left for 24 hours with occasional shaking. The seeds are allowed to settle for 1-2 hours and the total volume occupied by the swollen seeds is noted. The swelling factors for the seeds are as : 14 ml for *P. psyllium;* 10 ml for *P. ovata* and 8 ml for *P. indica.*

Adulterant and Substitute : *P. lanceolata* Linn., occurring wildly in India, is adulterated in Ispaghula. Its seeds are oblong elliptical in shape with yellowish brown colour. The seeds of *P. asiatica,* (syn. *P. major* L.), found in Andhra Pradesh and Tamil Nadu, are substituted to Ispaghula. It is also adulterated with the seeds of *P. arenaria.* The seeds of *Salvia aegyptica* are frequently mixed which also yield copious mucilage. The seeds of *P. media* L. have different colour and swell very little in water.

BAEL

Synonyms : Bel, Bengal quince; Fructus belae, Bael fruit.

Biological Source : Bael consists of the entire unripe fruit or its slices of *Aegle marmelos* Corr.

Family : Rutaceae.

Habitat : Bael plant is found all over India in sub-Himalayan forests, Bengal, central and south India and also in Burma and Sri Lanka.

Collection : Tree is slender, deciduous, nearly 12 m in height. Generally bael is propagated by seeds which are covered with earth and watered. The tree can be propagated by root-cuttings and layers. The unripe or half-ripe fruits are collected, epicarp is removed and cut into transverse slices or irregular pieces.

Morphology : The fruit is a woody, large berry with green colour when unripe and yellowish brown on maturing, diameter 10-20 cm. The fruit is sub-spherical in shape, epicarp is hard, woody, smooth, about 2 mm thick, slightly granular. A circular scar is left by the removal of the stalk. Internally it consists of reddish-brown pulpy endocarp; mesocarp consists of 10-15 capsules, each containing several hairy, oblong, multicellular seeds surrounded by reddish mucilage. Odour is faint and aromatic and taste is mucilaginous and sweet.

The peripheral part just within the rind is fleshy and thick and has a pleasant resinous odour. The walls separating the chambers are yellow. The chambers are full of amber-or honey-coloured, viscous, very sticky or glutinous, translucent pulp.

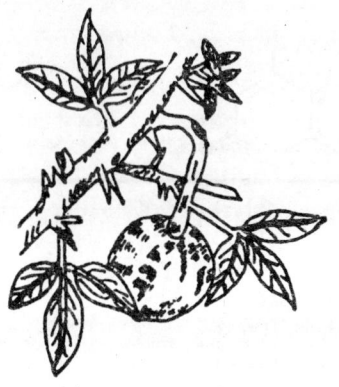

Fruit on a branch

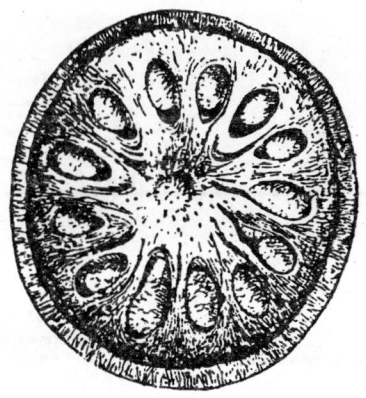

Transverse section of the fruit

Fig. 6.3. Bael fruit

Chemical Constituents : Fruit contains marmelosins (0.4%) which are the active constituents, in addition to carbohydrates (11-15%) including reducing sugars (3-4%), allo-imperatorin, β-sitosterol, tannins (20%), proteins (1%), vitamins A and C and volatile oil. Marmelosin is a furocoumarin which is identical with imperatorin. Fruits are also the source of alkaloids namely O-methylhalfordinol and isopentylhalfordinol. The furanocoumarin, alloimperatorin methyl ether, has also been isolated. It also contains marmelide (1,1-dimethyl allyl ether), psoralen, gum, etc. The fruit yields 2% water-soluble gum which on hydrolysis gives galactose, arabinose, D-galacturonic acid and rhamnose.

Uses : Unripe fruit is astringent, digestive, demulcent, stomachic, and used in diarrhoea and dysentery. Ripe fruit is sweet,aromatic, cooling, alterative and nutritive. When taken fresh, it is useful in habitual constipation, chronic dysentery and dyspepsia. Fresh juice is bitter and pungent. Root and stem barks are used as antipyretic. Aegelin, a sterol isolated from the leaves, has been tried to treat bronchial spasm. The cathartic action is caused by the swelling of the mucilaginous seed coat, therefore giving bulk and lubrication. The seeds should be taken with a considerable amount of water. In combination with powdered anhydrous dextrose, sodium bicarbonate, monobasic potassium phosphate, citric acid and others, plantago husk is used as remedy of constipation.

Marmelosin A : $R_1=R_2=H$
Marmelosin B : $R_1=H$; $R_2=Me$
Marmelosin C : $R_1=Me$; $R_2=H$

GUAR GUM

Synonyms : Guar flour; Decorpa; Jaguar; Jaguar gum; Guaran; Gum cyamopsis; Cyamopsis gum; Burtonite V-7-E.

Biological Source : Guar gum is the ground endosperms of *Cyamopsis tetragonolobus* (L.) Taub.

Family : Leguminosae.

Habitat : The plant is cultivated in dry climates in India (Maharastra, Gujarat, Karnataka and Rajasthan), Pakistan, and U.S.A. (Taxes).

It is robust erect annual, 1-3 in high plant, bearing cluster of thick and fleshy pods.

The plant is hardy and drought-resistant. It grows well on deep alluvial soils and sandy loams. It is cultivated usually as a mixed crop. The seeds are sown broadcast in northern India in May-June and harvested in September-October.

Characters : Guar gum is a pale-yellow free flowing powder; completely soluble in cold and hot water; practically insoluble in oils, greases, hydrocarbons, ketones and esters. Water solutions are tasteless, odourless, nontoxic and neutral. It is stable to heat. It has five to eight times the thickening power of starch. It forms thick colloidal solution in water and swells rapidly. The water soluble fraction (85%) is called guaran.

Chemical Constituents : Guar gum contains mainly of a high molecular weight hydrocolloidal |polysaccharide| which is a galactomannan. Guaran consists of linear chains of $(1\rightarrow4)$-β-D-mannopyranosyl units; 1,6-linked α-D-galactopyranosyl units are attached to alternate mannose units. Ratio of D-galactose to D-mannose is 1:2. On hydrolysis Guar gum yields galactose and mannose. It also contains small amount of proteins (5-7%).

Chemical Tests

1. Powdered Guar gum on treatment with ruthenium red does not form pink colour (difference from Sterculia and Agar).

2. Aqueous solution of Guar gum is converted to a gel by small amount of borax.

3. Aqueous solution of Guar gum is precipitated with 2% solution of lead acetate.

4. Aqueous solution of Guar gum does not produce any colour with iodine solution.

Uses : Guar gum is used as a thickening agent, as a tablet binder and disintegretor; as an emulsifying agent, as a protective colloid, stabilizer, thickening and film forming agent for cheese, salad dressings, ice creams, soups; in pharmaceutical jelly formulations; in suspensions, emulsions, lotions, creams, toothpastes; in the mining industry as a flocculent, as a filtering agent; and in water as a coagulant aid.

PECTIN

Biological Source : Pectin is a purified complex polysaccharide substance present in cell walls of all plant tissues which functions as an intercellular cementing material. It is a purified carbohydrate obtained from the dilute acid extract of inner portion of the peel of citrus fruits or from apple pomace. Lemon or orange rind is the richest source of pectin which contains about 30% of this polysaccharide. Other sources of pectin are papaya, guava, mangoes, and roots (beets and gentian).

Geographical Source : On commercial scale pectin is prepared in India, U.S.A., Switzerland and some other European countries.

Guaran

Preparation : Pectin occurs in the middle lamellae of cell walls, and in an insoluble form is called as protopectin. It is converted to the soluble form by treating the fruit pulp with a 20-times its weight of dilute acid at high temperature (90°C) for 30 minutes at pH 3.4-4. The aqueous solution is filtered, and alcohol is added to the filtrate to precipitate pectin. The precipitated pectin is separated and dried under reduced pressure.

Characters : Pectin occurs as a coarse or fine powder, yellowish-white in colour, practically odourless, and taste is mucilaginous. It is almost completely soluble in 20 parts of water, forming a viscous opalescent and colloidal solution containing negatively charged, very much hydrated particles. Aqueous solution is acidic to litmus. It is insoluble in alcohol and in other organic solvents. It dissolves more readily in water. It is stable under mildly acidic conditions. Depolymerization takes place in more strongly acidic or basic conditions.

Chemical Constituents : Pectin occurs naturally as partial methyl ester of α-$(1\rightarrow4)$ linked D-polygalacturonate sequences interrupted with $(1\rightarrow2)$-L-rhamnose residue. On hydrolysis it produces D-galactose, L-arabinose, D-xylose and L-fucose.

Chemical Tests

1. Pectin (1 g) is dissolved in water (10 ml). A stiff gel is produced.

2. To 1% aqueous solution of pectin add 2% aqueous solution of sodium hydroxide (5 ml). Within 20 minutes a transparent gel is produced. On shaking the gel with dilute hydrochloric acid gelatinous precipitates are formed which turn white on boiling.

Uses : Pectin is used in the treatment of diarrhoea due to property of colloidal absorption of toxins. It is also used as haemostatic for haemorrhage, as emulsifying agent, gelling agent, as a plasma substitute, for preparation of cosmetics, jellies and as a thickening agent in food industry for the sauces, jams and ketchup. As a colloidal solution, it has the property of conjugating toxins and enhancing the physiological action of the digestive tract through its physical and chemical properties. In the upper intestinal tract, pectin has a surface area composed of ultramicroscopical particles.

These particles, called micelles, have the property of colloidal absorption of toxins.

Pectic acid

ALGIN

Synonyms : Alginic acid sodium salt; Sodium alginate; Sodium polymannuronate; Kelgin; Minus; Protanal.

Biological Source : Algin is a gelling polysaccharide extracted with dilute alkali from giant brown seaweed, *Macrocystis pyrifera* (giant kelp), Family Lessoniaceae; or from *Laminaria digitata* (horsetail kelp), Family Laminariaceae, or from *Laminaria saccharina* (sugar kelp). Other sources are the species *Ascophyllum, Ecklonia* and *Nereocystis.*

Geographical Source : USA (California), Norway, Chile, China, Canada, Iris Republic, Australia, Iceland, UK (Scotland), and South Africa.

Preparation : The dried milled seaweed is macerated with dilute sodium carbonate solution. The resulting paste-like mass is diluted with soft water to separate the insoluble matter by modern super-decanters or continuous-setting devices. The resulting clear liquor contains most of the alginate orginally present in the algae. It is poured into dilute sulphuric acid or dilute calcium chloride solution, when the insoluble alginic acid or its salt, calcium alginate, is precipitated as a bulky, heavily hydrated gel from which liquor is separated by roller or expeller presses. Wood pulp-like product is obtained which is agitated aganist a stream of hydrochloric acid. Then calcium is removed and the highly swollen pulp of alginic acid is roller-pressed and then neutralized with sodium carbonate to give sodium alginate. In an another procedure the sodium alginate may be precipitated from the clear liquor by addition of ethyl alcohol directly or after partial evaporation.

Characters : Algin is a cream-coloured powder, soluble in water, forming a viscous and colloidal solution, insoluble in alcohol and in hydro-alcoholic solution in which the alcohol content is >30% v/v. It is insoluble in chloroform, ether and in aqueous acid solutions when the pH is below 3. It liberates carbon dioxide from carbonates. With compounds containing ions of alkali, metals, or ammomium or magnesium, it reacts to give salts (alginates) which are water soluble. The salts of most other metals are water-insoluble.

Chemical Constituents : Alginic acid is composed of residues of D-mannuronic and L-glucuronic acids; the chain length is long and varies with the method of isolation and the source of algae. The sugar units are joined by β-1, 4-glycosidic linkages. Its molecular weight varies from 220 to 860 units.

Algin

Uses : Alginates are used as stabilizing, thickening,emulsifying, deflocculating, gelling and film-and filament-forming agents in the rubber, paint, textile, food (including as stabilizing colloid), cosmetics and pharmaceutical industries. It is also used in drilling muds; in coatings, in the flocculation of solids in water treatment; as sizing agent, thickener, emulsion stabilizer, suspending agent in soft drinks and in dental impression preparations. Alginate fibres are used as absorable haemostatic dressings.

Algin is metabolized in the body. It has a caloric value of about 1.4 calories per gram. Alginic acid is relatively less soluble in water. It is used as a tablet binder and thickening agent. Gel-forming properties are associated with salts of different polyvalent cations and alginic acid. The propylene glycol ester of Algin has been prepared. It is useful in formulations that require greater acid stability than that of the parent hydrocolloid.

QUESTIONS

1. What are carbohydrates ? How are polysaccharides formed in the plants ? Enumerate the polysaccharides containing uronic acid or other units. Give some useful tests for sugars and other carbohydrates (Delhi University, 1988).

2. How will you differentiate the following pair of drugs: (a) Maize starch and Potato starch (b) Acacia and Gelatin (c) Agar and Starch (d) Sterculia gum and Acacia gum.

3. What are gums and mucilage ? Give official source, chemical constituents and uses of Ispaghula, Agar, Bael and Guar gum.

4. Give chemical constituents and chemical tests for the identification of the following drugs :
   (a) Tragacanth (b) Honey (c) Acacia gum (d) Algin.

5. Give the sources of starch that are commonly used in pharmaceutical practice. Discuss their microscopic characteristics and method of determining purity.

6. Give a pharmacognostic account of :
   (a) Guar gum (b) Starch (c) Acacia gum (d) Bael.

7. What are gums ? How are they formed in plants ? What is their usual composition ? Give a complete pharmacognostic account of one gum studied by you.

8. What is Agar ? How is it obtained ? Give important chemical test for identification of Agar.

9. Describe purity tests and uses of Honey, Acacia gum and Agar.

10. Discuss the biological sources, chemical constituents and uses of the carbohydrate drugs belonging to the following families : (a) Apidae (b) Sterculiaceae (c) Plantaginaceae (d) Rutaceae.

11. Give the source, methods of preparation, chemical constituents and uses of the following : (a) Sodium alginate (b) Pectin (c) Plantago.

7

GLYCOSIDES

Glycosides are compounds which upon hydrolysis give rise to one or more sugars (glycones) and a compound which is not a sugar (aglycone or genin).

In a glycosidic compound a sugar residue is linked to C-1 through oxygen (O-glucoside), nitrogen (N-glucoside) or sulphur (S-glucoside) moiety. β-D-Glucose is the most common sugar found in glycosides. The other sugars detected are rhamnose, digitoxose, and cymarose (deoxysugar). The glycosides from individual sugars are called glucoside, rhamnoside, galactoside, fructoside, etc.

In glycosides the hydroxyl of a sugar is condensed with the hydroxyl of the non-sugar component. The secondary hydroxyl within the sugar molecule is condensed to form an oxide ring. Thus, they may be considered as acetals or sugar ethers. By acid or base catalyzed or enzymic hydrolysis glycosides yield the parent sugar together with the non-sugar compound. The sugar component is known as the *glycone*; while the nonsugar residue is called as *aglycone*. The aglycone may be an alcohol, phenol, cyanohydrin or complex fused ring or heterocyclic hydroxy compounds. More than one molecule of sugars may be present in glycosides which are formed by either separate linkages or stepwise substituion of the sugars to the aglycone. In plants only β-forms of glycosides are formed, although the α-linkage is detected in nature in some carbohydrates such as sucrose, glycogen and starch. In α-strophanthoside, the outer glucose molecule occurs in α-linkages and the inner glucose possesses β-linkage.

Most of the glycosides are colourless, crystalline compounds. Anthracene glycosides are red or orange coloured compounds and flavone glycosides are yellowish in colour. They are soluble in water and alcohol, but insoluble in other organic solvents like petroleum ether, solvent ether, chloroform, carbon tetrachloride, etc. Glycosides are optically laevorotatory.

β-Form   α-Form

Classification

Various types of classifications of glycosides have been mentioned. On the basis of linkage of sugar molecule to aglycone, they are divided as follows :

1. **O-glycosides** : In these glycosides the sugar is combined with alcoholic or phenolic hydroxyl function of aglycone; e.g. digitoxin.

2. **N-glycosides** : In these glycosides nitrogen of amino group ($-NH_2/-NH-$) is condensed with a sugar, e.g., nucleoside.

3. **S-glycoside** : These glycosides contain a sugar moiety attached to a sulphur of the aglycone, e.g., isothiocyanate glycosides.

4. **C-glycosides** : Condensation of a sugar directly to a carbon atom gives rise to C-glycosides, e.g., aloin, and cascaroside. These glycosides are not hydrolyzed with acids, alkalies or enzymes.

On the basis of the chemical nature of aglycone the glycosides are classified as follows :

1. **Steroidal Glycosides** : These glycosides contain a sterol as an aglycone, e.g. diosgenin.

2. **Flavonoid Glycosides** : A flavonoid aglycone is present in these glycosides, e.g. rutin.

3. **Anthracene Glycosides** : In these glycosides, sugar moiety is attached to an anthracene aglycone, e.g. frangulin, barbaloin.

4. **Cyanophoric Glycosides** : Cyanogen is the aglycone part. They yield hydrocyanic acid on hydrolysis, e.g. amygdalin, prunasin.

5. **Triterpenic Glycosides** : A triterpene molecule is condensed with a sugar component, e.g., glycyrrhizin.

6. **Alcohol Glycosides** : e.g. Salicin.

7. **Lactone Glycosides** : e.g. Hydroxycoumarin glycosides.

8. **Isothiocyanate Glucosides** : e.g. Sinigrin, sinalbin.

9. **Saponin Glycosides** : e.g. Dioscin.

On the basis of nature of sugars the glycosides are called as glucosides, fructosides, rhamnosides, ribosides, etc.

Pharmacological classification of glycosides is dependent on their activities. For example, cardiac glycosides exhibit their action on heart. Glycosides possessing bitter taste are called bitter glycosides, e.g. glycosides of Gentianceae.

Glycosides are used for the treatment of various illness. Digitalis and Strophanthus contain cardiac glycosides and are used as cardiac stimulant drugs. Anthraquinone glycosides, present in Senna, Cascara, Rhubarb and Aloe, are used as laxative. Picrorhiza roots and rhizomes possess picroside glycosides and are utilized as bitter tonic and to protect damaged liver. Wild Cherry bark and Scilla glycosides have expectorant properties. Dioscin is a saponin glycoside found in the tubers of *Dioscorea* species and its hydrolysis furnishes diosgenin aglycone. Various steroidal drugs have been synthesized from diosgenin. Some glycosides are less effective in original form, but produce active compounds on hydrolysis. For example, sinigrin, a glycoside of black mustard, is non-irritating in its natural form, but on hydrolysis a powerful irritating substance, allylisothiocyanate, is formed.

SAPONIN GLYCOSIDES

Saponins are highly complex glycosides which are widely distributed in the higher plants. The drugs like Quillaia,

Sarsaparilla and Senega have their medicinal properties due to the saponins they contain. Saponins form colloidal solution in water which give a soap-like froth on shaking. They have the property of causing haemolysis of red blood corpuscles, even at great dilution. Most of the saponins are highly toxic when injected into the body, much less so when taken orally. They are very toxic to fish. On hydrolysis they yield an aglycone known as 'sapogenin' which may be a steroid or a triterpene and the sugar moiety may be glucose, galactose, a pentose or a methylpentose. Saponins have a high molecular weight and they are purified with difficulty.

Steroidal saponins are less common than the pentacyclic triterpenoid type in plants. They are related with compounds such as sex hormones, cortisone, diuretic steroids, vitamin D, withanolides and cardiac glycosides. Natural sapogenins differ only in their configuration at carbon atoms 3, 5 and 25.

Cardiac Glycosides : These are steroidal glycosides and show highly specific and powerful action upon the cardiac muscles. The sugar part is attached at C-3 position of the steroidal nucleus. The steroid aglycone or genins are of two types :

(i) Cardenolides which are C_{23} steroids having an α, β-unsaturated five - membered lactone ring attached at 17β position. These compounds are present in Digitalis, Strophanthus, Oleander, Calotropis and Convallaria.

(ii) Bufadienolides which are C_{24} steroids having double unsaturated six-membered lactone ring at the 17α position. The name bufadienolides has been derived from the generic name for the toad, *Bufo*, since the compound bufalin was isolated from the skin of toads.

Cardenolides are distributed in excess amount in nature. For maximum cardiac activity the aglycone should possess an α, β-unsaturated lactone ring attached β-position at 17-carbon of the steroid nucleus and the A/B and C/D ring junctions should have the cis-configuration. The sugar portion of the glycoside helps in its absorption and distribution in the body. Oxygen substitution on the steroid nucleus also affects the distribution and metabolism of the glycosides. When number of hydroxyl groups is increased on the molecule, the more rapid is the action in the body.

Cardiac glycosides increase the force of systolic contraction and decrease the heart rate.

The sugar units, attached at C-3 of the steroid, are composed of up to three sugar molecules. Glucose, rhamnose, digitoxose and cymarose are the sugars usually attached to the aglycone. Cardiac glycosides containing cyclic sugars have been isolated from *Calotropis* species.

DIGITALIS

Synonyms : Foxglove; Purple foxglove; Fairy gloves; Digifortis; Digitora; Neodigitalis; Pil-digis, Folia digitalis; Digitalis folium.

Biological Source : Digitalis consists of dried leaves of *Digitalis purpurea* Linn. possessing not less than 0.3 per cent of total cardenolides calculated as digitoxin. The collected leaves are immediately dried at a temperature below 60° and stored in a water proof container. The moisture should not be less than 5 per cent. (Family : Scrophulariaceae).

Habitat : Southern and Central European countries, England, Germany, Holland, France, Northern U.S.A. and in Kashmir. In India it is cultivated in Kashmir at Tangmarg and Kishtwar at 2000-2300 m; Darjeeling district and the Nilgiris.

Cultivation and Collection : Digitalis is a biennial herb occurring wildly. For its cultivation especially stained seeds are sown in a soil consisting of equal parts of clean sand, garden soil, manure and leaf mould in March. After about two months the seedlings are transferred in fields. The leaves are collected in the early afternoon from September to November by hand. Leaves of the first year crop contain maximum amount of active constituents. The leaves are dried immediately after collection below 60°C. If drying is rapidly, then characteristic green colour remains as such. Dried leaves are packed in air-tight containers. Usually a desiccating substance like silica gel or calcium oxide is placed in the container to absorb moisture. Some plants are allowed to grow for the next year during flowering and seeds are developed which are used for cultivation of the next crop.

Characters : The leaves are linear or oblong-lanceolate, with obtuse or rounded apex, size 10-10 cm long and 4-8 cm wide. The margin is crenate to dentate with water pores on many teeth. Lamina is decussate at the tapering base. Upper surface is pubescent, dark green and little wrinkled and veins are depressed. The lower surface is greyish-green and veins are more prominent. Both the surfaces are hairy, but the lower surface is more hairy in comparison to upper one. Venation is pinnate, all types of veins are less prominent on the upper surface; lateral veins leave the mid-rub at an acute angle and anastomose on the margin. Petiole is winged, 2.5-10 cm in length. Odour is distinct and taste is bitter.

Chemical Constituents : Digitalis contains about 35 glycosides and some of these glycosides are summarized in Table 1. The most important compounds of medicinal importance are digitoxin, gitoxin, and gitaloxin which are secondary glycosides. These glycosides possess a linear chain of three deoxy sugars at C-3 of the aglycone and not the terminal glucose as in purpurea glycosides A and B. These two glycosides are the prominent active components of the fresh leaves. When the drug is dried, enzymatic degradation takes place resulting the removal of terminal glucose to give digitoxin, gitoxin and gitaloxin.

Purpurea glycosides A and B and glucogitaloxin are the primary glycosides which contain a linear chain of three digitoxose sugar moieties terminated by the fourth sugar glucose at C-3 of the aglycone residue.

In addition to cardiac glycosides the presence of tannins, inositol, luteolin, acids, fatty matters, antirhinic acid, digitalosmin, digitoflavone and pectin have been reported in the drug. It also contains anthraquinone derivatives such as 1-methoxy-2-methylanthraquinone, 3-methoxy-2-methylanthraquinone, digitolutein (3-methylalizarin-1-methyl ether), 3-methylalizarin and 1,4,8-trihydroxy-2-methylanthraquinone.

Uses : Digitalis is used as a cardiac stimulant and tonic. The drug stimulates cardiac muscles, increases the systole of heart ventricle and normalizes the heart frequency. In this way the drug is useful in congestive heart failure, atrial flutter and atrial fibrillation.

Chemical Tests

Digitalis glycosides respond to the following tests due to five-membered lactone ring present at C-17.

    1. **Keller-Kiliani Test :** To an extract of the drug in

glacial acetic acid few drops of ferric chloride and concentrated H_2SO_4 are added. A reddish-brown colour is formed at the junction of two layers and the upper layer turns bluish green. This test indicates the presence of digitoxose.

2. **Legal Test** : To a solution of glycoside in pyridine sodium nitroprusside solution and sodium hydroxide solution are added. A pink to red colour is formed.

3. **Baljet Test**.: To a leaf lamina sodium picrate reagent is added. A yellow or orange colour is formed in the presence of glycosides.

Table 1. Some Cardioactive Glycosides of *Digitalis purpurea*.

	Glycoside	Aglycone	Sugar moieties
1.	Purpurea glycoside A	Digitoxigenin	(Digitoxose)$_3$-glucose-
2.	Digitoxin.	Digitoxigenin	(Digitoxose)$_3$-
3.	Glucodigitoxigenin-digitoxoside	Digitoxigenin	(Digitoxose)$_2$-glucose-
4.	Gluco-evatromonoside	Digitoxigenin	Digitoxose-glucose-
5.	Purpurea glycoside B	Gitoxigenin	(Digitoxose)$_3$-glucose-
6.	Gitoxin	Gitoxigenin	(Digitoxose)$_3$-
7.	Glucogitoroside	Gitoxigenin	Digitoxose-glucose-
8.	Digitalinum verum	Gitoxigenin	Digitalose-glucose-
9.	Stropeside	Gitoxigenin	Digitalose-
10.	Glucogitaloxin	Gitaloxigenin	(Digitoxose)$_3$-glucose
11.	Gitaloxin	Gitaloxigenin	(Digitoxose)$_3$-
12.	Glucogitaloxigenin-bis-digitoxoside	Gitaloxigenin	(Digitoxose)$_2$-glucose-
13.	Gluco-lanadoxin	Gitaloxigenin	Digitoxose-glucose
14.	Gluco-verodoxin	Gitaloxigenin	Digitalose-glucose
15.	Verodoxin	Gitaloxigenin	Digitalose-

ALLIED DRUGS

Digitalis lanata : (Grecian Foxglove, Wooly foxglove). The leaves of *Digitalis lanata* Ehrh. (Fam. Scrophulariaceae)

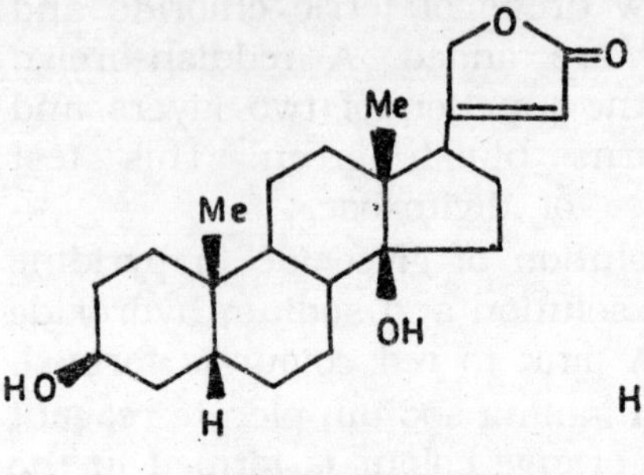

Digitoxigenin

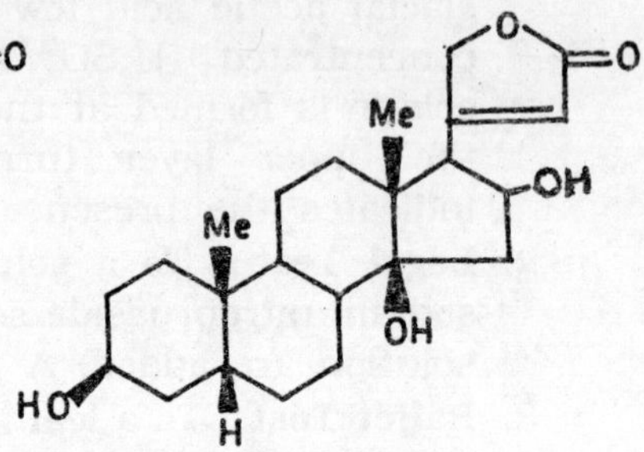

Gitoxigenin

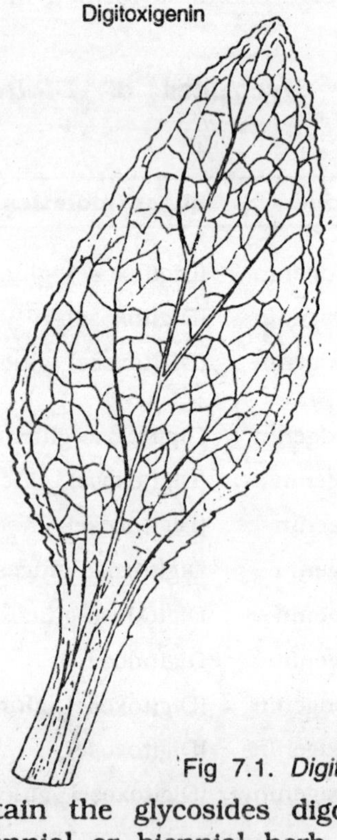

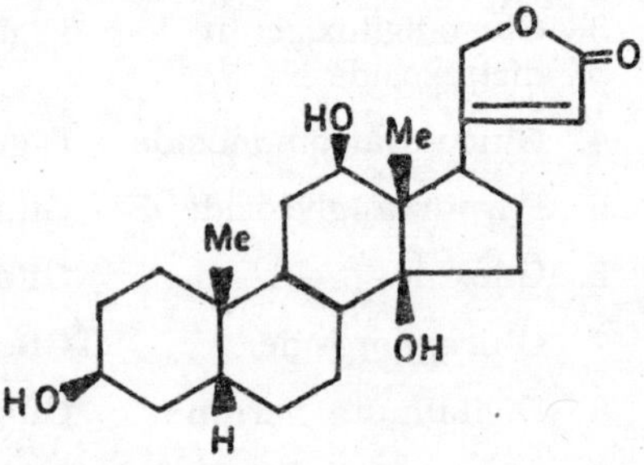

Digoxigenin

Fig 7.1. *Digitalis purpurea* leaf

contain the glycosides digoxin and lanatoside C. It is a perennial or biennial herb, nearly 1m in height, found in Europe, Holland, Ecuador and in Kashmir at Tangmarg and Baramulla. The leaves are sessile, oblong, up to 30 cm in length and 4 cm broad. The margin is entire and acuminate apex. The veins are joined to the midrib at a very acute angle.

D. *lanata* contains lanatosides A, B, C, D and E, acetyldigitoxin, digitoxin, glucogitoroside, digitalinum verum, deacetyl-lanatoside C, digoxin, glucolanadoxin, and glucoverodoxin. The aglycone parts of lanatosides A-E are given in Table-2. Some flavone derivatives, e.g., scutellarein, luteolin and dinatin have also been reported from *D. lanata*.

D. lanata leaves are used for the preparation of lanatosides and digoxin.

In addition to *D. lanata* the leaves of *D. thapsi*, found in Spain and Italy, *D. lutea*, and *D. ferruginia* are used as allied drugs.

Tabel 2 : Some Cardioactive Glycosides of *D. lanata* Leaves

Glycoside	Aglycone	Sugar Moieties
Lanatoside A	Digitoxigenin	Glycose-acetyldigitoxose-(digitoxose)$_2$-
Lanatoside B	Gitoxigenin	Glucose-acetyldigitoxose-(digitoxose)$_2$-
Lanatoside C	Digoxigenin	Glucose-acetyldigitoxose-(digitoxose)$_2$-
Lanatoside D	Diginatigenin	Glucose-acetyldigitoxose-(digitoxose)$_2$-
Lanatoside E	Gitaloxigenin	Glucose-acetyldigitoxose-(digitoxose)$_2$-
Digitoxin	Digitoxigenin	(Digitoxose)$_3$-
Glucoevatromonoside	Digitoxigenin	Glucose-digitoxose-
Digitalinum verum	Gitoxigenin	Glucose-digitalose-
Glucolanadoxin	Gitaloxigenin	Glucose-digitoxose-
Glucoverodoxin	Gitaloxigenin	glucose-digitalose-
Acetyldigitoxin	Digitoxigenin	Acetyldigitoxose-(digitoxose)$_2$-
Acetyldigoxin	Digoxigenin	Acetyldigitoxose-(digitoxose)$_2$-
Deacetyl-lanatoside C	Digoxigenin	Glucose-(digitoxose)$_2$-

Adulterants : Digitalis is adulterated with the leaves of mullein (*Verbascum thapsus* Linn.), comfrey (*Symphytum officinale* Linn.), primrose (*Primula vulgaris* Huds.), elecampane (*Inula helenium* Linn.), ploughman's spikenard (*Inula conyza* DC) and nettle (*Urtica dioica*).

STROPHANTHUS

Synonyms : Strophanthus seeds; Semina strophanthi.

Biological Source : Strophanthus is the ripe seeds of *Strophanthus kombe* Olive, or *S. hispidus* DC.

Family : Apocynaceae.

Habitat : East and central Africa.

Collection : Seeds are collected usually from wild plants. The plants are large climbers. Fruits are many-seeded, dehiscent and consist of two divergent follicles. Mature fruits are collected in June-July, epicarp and mesocarp are separated and seeds are removed. The seeds are washed and dried.

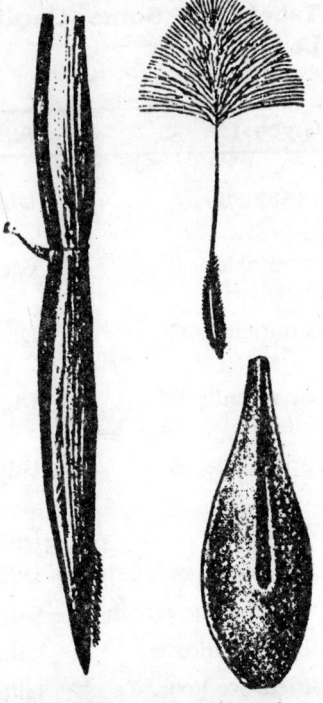

Chemical Constituents : Strophanthus contains a cardiac glycoside strophanthin-K (2-5%), kombic acid, choline, trigonelline, fixed oil (30%), resin and mucilage. Strophanthin-K, is a mixture of K-strophanthoside, K-strophanthin-β and cymarin and the genin part of all these glycosides is strophanthidin. The genin strophanthidin is coupled to a trisaccharide consisting of cymarose, β-glucose and α-glucose.

The enzyme α-glucosidase removes the terminal α-glucose to yield K-strophanthin-β and the enzyme, strophenthobiase, present in seeds, converts this to cymarin and glucose.

Fig. 7.2. Seed of Strophanthus

Uses : Strophanthus is used as cardiac tonic, diuretic and arrow poison.

Allied Drugs : *Strophanthus gratus* contain 4-8% of ouabain (G-strophanthin). Ouabain has also been reported in the wood of African *Acokanthera ouabaio*.

Seeds of *S. sarmentosus* contain a number of glycosides with sarmentogenin as the aglycone.

Strophanthidin

Ouabagenin

Choline $(CH_3)_3 \overset{+}{N} CH_2 \overset{+}{C}H_2 OH] Cl^-$

Sarmentogenin

Trigonelline

Cymarose

SQUILL

Synonyms : Sea onion; Bulbus Scillae; Meerzwiebel, Scilla bulb; White Squill; European Scilla; Radix scillae.

Biological Source : Squill consists of the dried sliced scales of the fleshy inner bulb of the white variety of *Urginea maritima* (L.) Baker *(Scilla maritima* L.). The central part of the bulb is removed during its preparation.

Family : Liliaceae.

Habitat : Mediterranean seacoasts of Spain, France, Italy, Greece, Algeria, Morocco; Algiers and Cyprus.

Collection : The bulbs grow half immersed in the sandy soil. It is collected in August during flowering stage. Outer membraneous scales, fibrous roots and central portion are removed. Then the bulbs are cut transversely into thin slices, dried in the sun or stove heated and packed in bags or in barrels. On drying about 80% weight is lost.

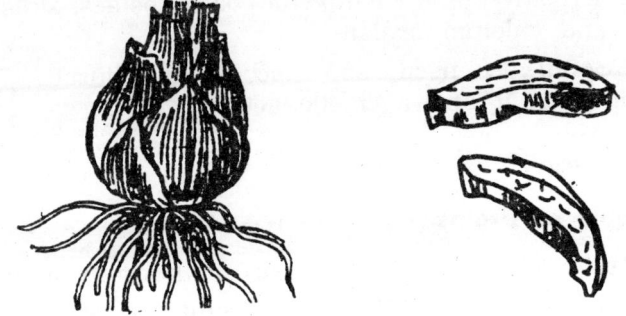

Fig. 7.3. Squill

Morphology : Squill bulbs are pear-shaped, tapering at both ends, diameter 15-30 cm. Surface contains longitudinal furrow. Colour is yellow, fracture is short and brittle. The slices of the drug are nearly 0.5-5 cm long, tapering at both ends. The odour is slight and taste is bitter, mucilaginous and acrid. The drug is hygroscopic and should be stored carefully in air-tight containers.

Chemical Constituents : The drug contains about a dozen of cardioactive glycosides scillaren A, scillaren B, glucoscillaren A, proscillaridin A, scillaridin A, scilliglaucoside, scillipheoside, glucoscillipheoside, scillicyanoside, scillicoeloside, scilliazuroside and scillicryptoside.

Scillaren A.   Scilliroside

Two-third amount of the total glycosides is of scillaren A. On hydrolysis it forms the aglycone scillarenin (bufadienolide), rhamnose and glucose. In addition to glycosides the drug also contains various flavonoids, like quercetin derivatives and kaempferol polyglycosides; sinistrin, mucilage and calcium oxalate.

Uses : Squill is used as expectorant, diuretic, and cardiotonic, but it shows emetic action.

ALLIED DRUGS

Indian Squill or Urginea

It consists of dried longitudinal slices of the bulb of *Drimia indica* (syn. *Urginea indica* Kunth) (Family Liliaceae). The drug is found in western Himalaya, Bihar, Chota Nagpur, Konkan and Coromandel Coast. It is a small glabrous herb, bulb diameter is about 1.5 cm or more, flowers appearing before the leaves drooping or spreading. Surface of the bulb is fleshy and longitudinally ribbed, fracture is brittle, yellowish colour, odour is slight and taste is bitter and acrid.

It is also cultivated is sandy soils near the sea-shore in south India. The bulb prefers a sandy soil and average temperature of 15°C. The plants are grown from seeds and in 5-6 years the bulbs develop. Bulbs are also raised from the bulblets. Planting is generally done in rows. The bulbs are collected in the early autumn when the leaves wither after flowering. The bulbs are cleaned of the soil, the dry outer scales separated and cut into four parts. The core is cut out and the quarters are finally sliced. The slices are dried in the sun, or on slow fire to lose 80% of their weight and packed in bags or barrels.

Indian Squill occurs in the form of curved or irregularly shaped strips, 3-6 cm long, 3-8 mm broad and 1-3 mm thick. They are thickened in the middle, but tapering towards the ends, translucent or yellowish white, and slightly darker in colour than the European Squill. They are brittle when dried, but become tough when moistened; fracture is brittle. It is odourless and has a slight bitter, mucilaginous and acrid taste.

In large doses it is emetic and cathartic and may cause cardiac depression. It is used to treat cough, dropsy, rheumatism, skin troubles; to remove warts and corns; as cardiac tonic, expectorant and diuretic.

Indian Squill contains scillarens A and B and mucilage is consisted of mannose, glucose and xylose. Scillaren A yields on hydrolysis proscillaredin A and than scillaredin A. With iodine water a reddish purple colour is formed and this test is negative with European Squill.

Red Squill : Red Squill is a variety of *Urginea maritima* (Fam. Liliaceae). It contains cardiac glycosides and glycosides scilliroside and scillirubroside. Red Squill is used as a rodenticide to kill rodents. When taken by rodents, convulsions, respiratory failure and death occur. It contains cardic glycoside scillaren A and enzyme scillarenase composed of proscillaridin and glucose.

ANTHRAQUINONE GLYCOSIDES

Anthraquinone glycosides possess anthracene or their derivatives as aglycone. Hydrolysis of these glycosides yields aglycones which are di-, tri- or tetrahydroxyanthraquinones.

The glycosides are found in the drugs like Senna, Aloe, Rhubarb, Cascara, Cochineal, etc. In addition of hydroxy groups, some other groups have been detected, for example, methyl in chrysophanol, hydroxymethyl in aloe-emodin and carboxyl in rhein.

Anthraquinone derivatives are usually orange-red compounds, soluble in water or dilute alcohol. When the alcoholic or ethereal extract of powdered drug is treated with ammonia or caustic soda solution, a pink, red or violet colour is formed.

Anthranols and anthrones are the reduced anthraquinone derivatives found in free or combined state as glycosides. They are converted to other compounds in solution. They are pale yellow, non-fluorescent substances, and insoluble in alkali. They contain significant therapeutic action of the crude drugs.

Oxanthrones are intermediate products between anthraquinones and anthranols. They are present in Cascara bark and produce anthraquinone on oxidation.

In dianthrones two anthrone molecules are combined at C-10 which may be identical or different. These compounds are found in species of *Cassia, Rheum* and *Rhamnus*. Sennosides are the glycosides belonging to dianthrone group.

Aloin-type or C-glycosides are obtained from *Aloe* species. They are resistant to normal acid hydrolysis.

The anthraquinone aglycones in free state exhibit little therapeutic activity. The anthraquinone and related glycosides act as stimulant cathartics and increase the tone of the smooth muscle in the wall of large intestine. Glycosides of anthranols and anthrones exhibit more drastic action than the related anthraquinone glycosides.

SENNA

Synonyms : Alexandrian Senna (Egyptian Senna); Tinnevelly Senna (Indian Senna); Senna Leaves; Folia sennal.

Biological Source : Senna consists of dried leaflets of *Cassia acutifolia* Delile (*C. senna* L.) known as Alexandrian Senna, and of *C. angustifolia* vahl, known as Tinnevelly Senna. It contains about 2.5% of hydroxyanthracene glycosides, calculated as sennoside B.

Family : Leguminosae.

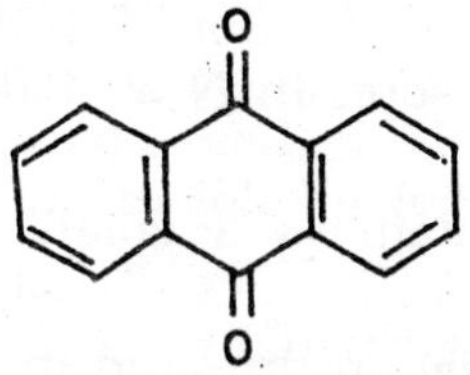

Anthraquinone

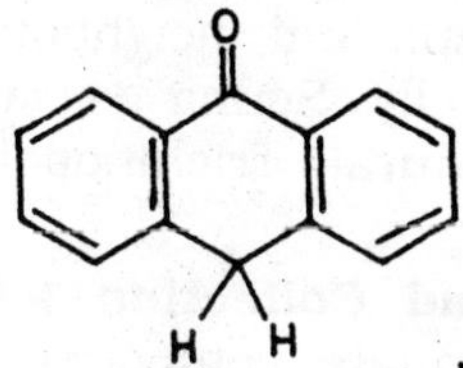

Anthrone

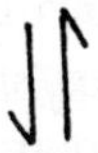

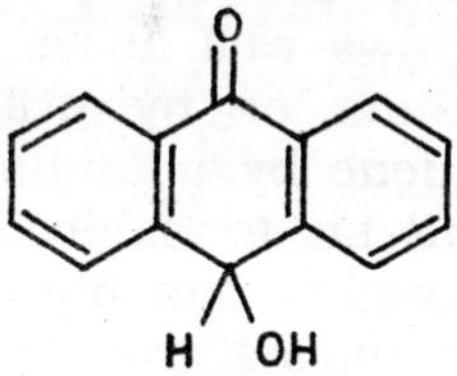

Oxanthrone

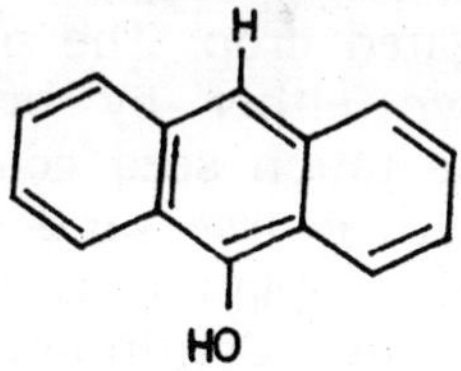

Anthranol

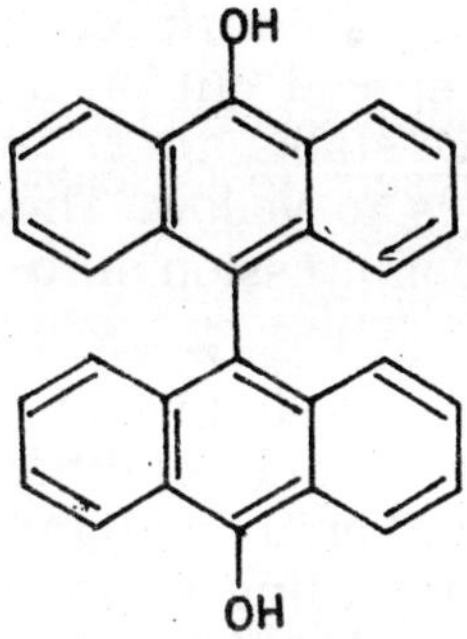

Dianthranol

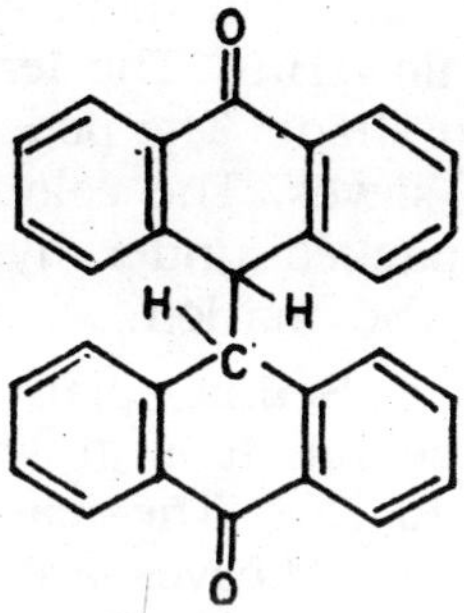

Dianthrone

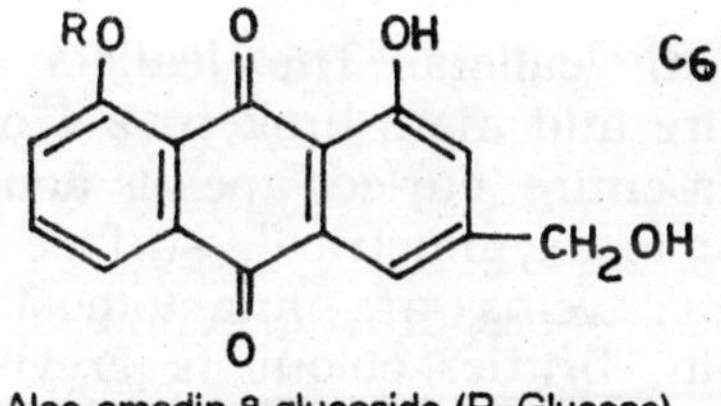

Aloe-emodin-8-glucoside (R=Glucose)
Aloe-emodin (R=H)

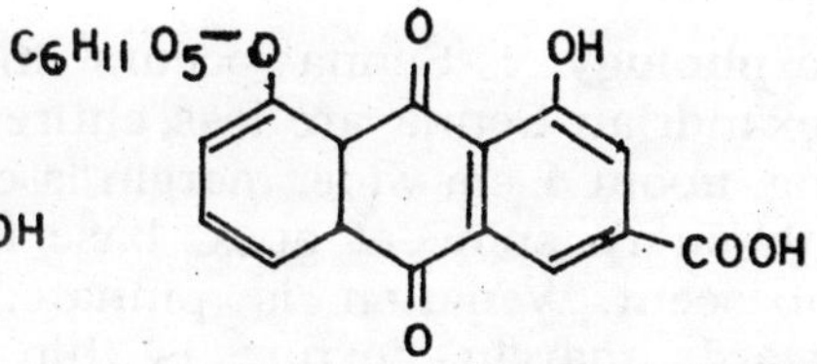

Rhein-8-glucoside

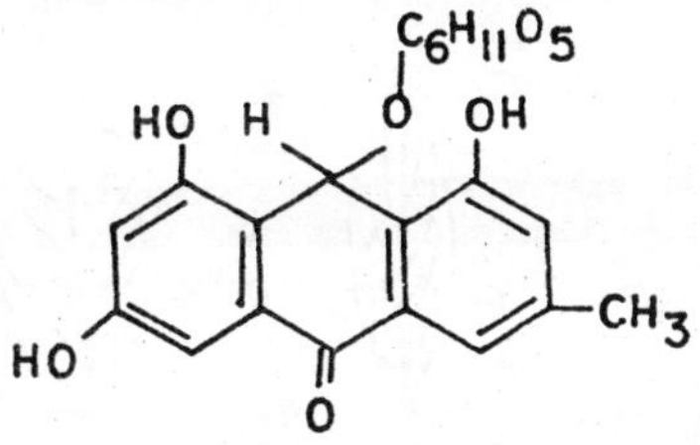

Emodin-oxanthrone glucoside

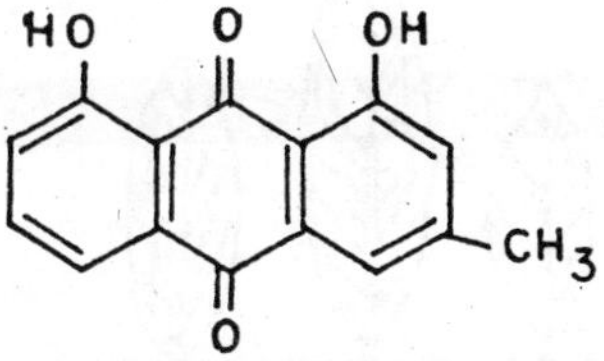

Chrysophanic acid

Habitat : Egypt and neighbouring region for Alexandrian Senna; Tinnevelly Senna is cultivated in South India in Tinnevelly, Madurai, Trichinopoly, Mysore; in N.W. Pakistan and Jammu.

Cultivation and Collection : The plant is a small shrub bearing paripinnate compound leaves.

C. *angustifolia* is cultivated usually on dry land in south India. It is grown on rice land immediately after the rice crop is harvested. It may be given a light irrigation and grown as a semi-irrigated crop. The plant grows well above 10°C. Seeds are sown either by broadcasting or by dribbing. Abrading of the tough seed coats is done by pounding the seeds lightly with coarse sand in a mortar to induce quick germination. The plants require bright sunshine and occasional drizziling. Continuous rains during growth spoils the quality of the leaves. When the leaves are fully grown and are thick and bluish in colour, they are stripped off by hand before flowering. The leaves are spread out on a hard floor to dry in shade. The pods and large stalks are separated by means of sieves. The colour changes to yellow. They are graded and packed under hydraulic compression into balls and sent to the market.

Tinnevelly Senna plants are more luxuriant than Alexandrian senna. It is grown on dry or wet conditions as a successor to rice. The leaves are gathered by hand and dried in the sun. Leaves are graded according to their size and colour of the leaflets, compressed into bales and exported.

Morphology : Senna occurs in leaflets. The leaflets of Alexandrian Senna are less entire and more broken, 2-4 cm long, about 1 cm wide; margin is entire, curled, apex is acute with sharp spine at apex, base is asymmetrical, surface is pubescent, venation is pinnate, veins are anastomosing towards margin, texture is thin, brittle; colour is greyish green, odour is faint, taste is mucilaginous and slightly bitter.

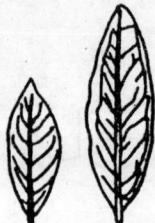 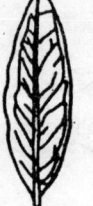 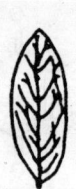 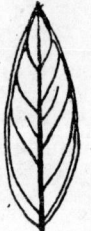 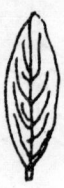 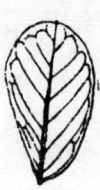

Indian Senna   Alexandrian Senna   Palthe Senna   Dog Senna

Fig. 7.4. Senna leaves

Tinnevelley Senna differs slightly from the Egyptian Senna. Its leaflets are 2.4-6 cm long, shape is lanceolate and colour is yellowish green.

Epidermal trichomes are present on the leaflets which are unicellular, conical, thick-walled and with a warty cuticle. Lamina is isobilateral.

Chemical Constituents : Senna contains dianthrone glycosides, the sennosides A, B, C and D, aloe-emodin-dianthrone-diglycoside, rhein-anthrone-8-glycoside, rhein-8-diglycoside; aloe-emodin-8-glucoside and aloe-emodin-anthrone diglucoside. In addition to these two naphthalene glycosides, viz. 6-hydroxymusizin glycoside and tinnevellin glycoside have been isolated. Senna also contains flavonoids like kaempferol, its glucosides (kaempferin), isorhamnetin; a sterol and its glucoside, mucilage, calcium oxalate, resin and free anthraquinones.

Chemical Test

1. **Bornträger Test for Anthraquinones** : Senna leaves are boiled with dilute H_2SO_4, filtered, the filtrate is extracted with chloroform or ether. On addition of ammonia to the extract in organic phase pink to red colour is formed due to the presence of anthraquinone compounds.

2. A little drug extract is treated with 5 N sodium hydroxide and sodium hyposulphite. On heating red colour appears.

Uses : Senna is used as purgative and cathartic. It is stimulant laxative. The drug is used in acute constipation and in all cases in which defaecation with a soft stool is required; e.g. with haemorrhoids, after anal-rectal operations, before and after abdominal operations, with anal fissures, for the evacuation of X-ray contrast media from intestines, etc. The sennosides are first hydrolyzed by the intestinal bacteria and then reduced to anthrone stage, the actual active form.

There may be reddening of urine (harmless) and passage of some of the anthracene derivatives into mother's milk which may cause diarrhoea in infants. Overdose may lead to colicky abdominal pains and the formation of thin, water stools.

Allied Drugs : *Bombay, Mecca* and *Arabian Sennas* are the leaves of *Cassia angustifolia* found in Arabia and used as a substituent.

Dog Senna is obtained from the leaves of *Cassia obovata*. The leaves are ovate and it contains about 1% anthraquinone derivative.

Palthe senna is obtained from *Cassia auriculata*. This adulterant does not contain any sennosides. It can be examined by with a hand lens by the dense pubescence on the lower surface of the leaf, and by the trichomes, which are very long, slightly wirty, and more sharply covered towards the tips. With 80% sulphuric acid, palthe senna gives a carmine-red colour due to conversion of leuco-anthocycinidin to the oxonium salt. In addition to these, leaves of other senna are substituted.

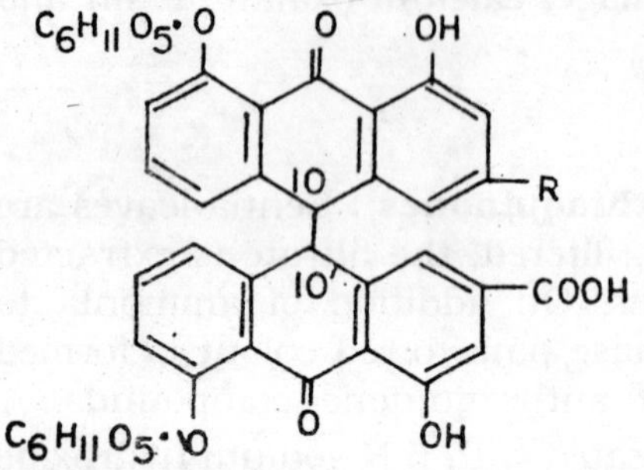

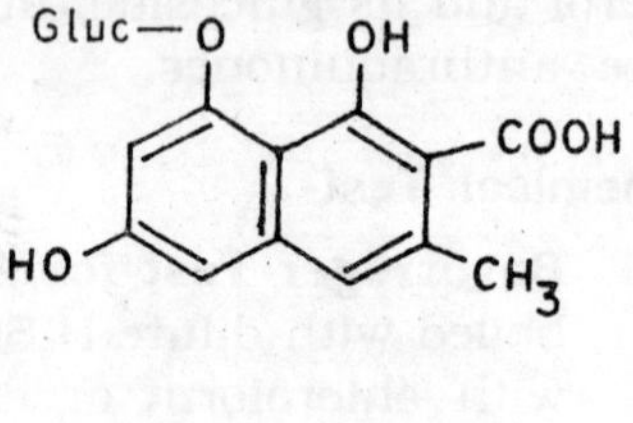

6-Hydroxymusizin glycoside

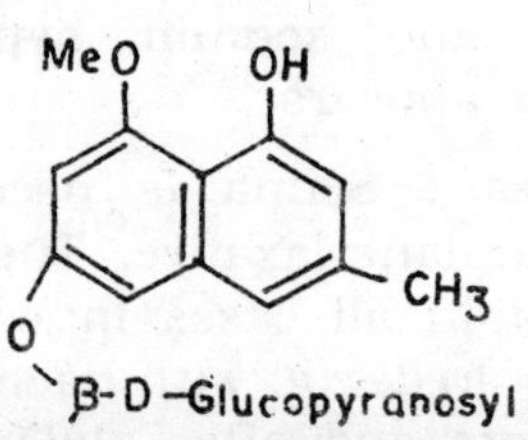

	R	10-10¹
Sennoside A	COOH	trans
Sennoside B	COOH	meso
Sennoside C	CH₂OH	trans
Sennoside D	CH₂OH	meso

Tinnevellin glycosede

RHUBARB

Synonyms : Rheum, Rhizome Rhei, Rhei Radix, Revandchini (Hindi); Rhubarb rhizome; Turkey Rhubarb, Radix rhei.

Biological Source : Rhubarb is the dried rhizome and roots of *Rheum officinale* Baill, *R. palmatum* L. or other species of *Rheum* (excepting *R. rhaponticum* L.), deprived of most of its bark. It contains about 2.5% of hydroxyanthracene derivatives, calculated as rhein.

Family : Polygonaceae.

Habitat : China, Tibet, Nepal, Central Asia; cultivated in Europe, southern Siberia, and North America.

Collection : Rhubarb grows at a high altitude of 3000 m. The plant is perennial bearing large and vertical rhizome and thick-branched roots.

The drug is collected in autumn or spring from 6-10 years old plants by digging out. Roots are cut and outer bark is separated by peeling. The big rhizomes are cut longitudinally into small pieces, dried and exported.

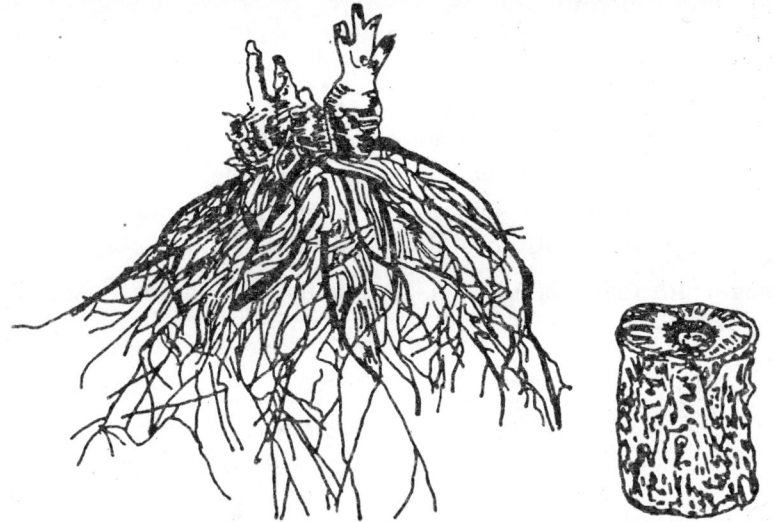

A. Rhizome with small roots   B. Rhizome piece

Fig. 7.5. Rhubarb

Morphology : The drug occurs as round or flat pieces, 5-15 cm long, diameter is 3-8 cm; shape is cylindrical ; surface is smooth, firm, non-shrunken and bright yellow showing white reticulations due to fusiform or lozenge-shaped cut ends. Fracture is irregular and granular. Odour is characteristic and aromatic; taste is bitter and astringent. Holes in pieces of the drug may be caused by insect attack or made for hanging the drug up to dry.

Chemical Constituents : Rhubarb contains free anthraquinones and their glycosides (3-12%) such as chrysophanol, aloe-emodin, emodin, physcion and rhein. Anthrones or dianthrones of chrysophanol, emodin, aloe-emodin, or physion are reported. The dianthrone glucosides of rhein (sennosides A and B) and the oxalates of these (sennosides E and F) are isolated. Heterodianthrones are derived from two different anthrone molecules; for example, palmidin A (aloe-emodin anthrone and emodin anthrone); palmidin B (aloe-emodin anthrone and chrysophanol anthrone), palmidin C (emodin anthrone and chrysophanol anthrone), sennidin C, rheidin B and rheidin C.

Besides these, Rhubarb contains glucogallin, free gallic acid, (-)-epicatechin gallate, catechin, rheotannic acid, erythroretin, methylchrysophanic acid, rhubarberon, cinnamic acid and calcium oxalate.

Chemical Tests

1. Bornträger's test described under Senna is positive due to anthraquinone derivatives.
2. It gives pink colour with ammonia.
3. A blood red colour is formed on treating Rhubarb powder with 5% KOH solution.

Uses : Rhubarb is used as a laxative; in larger doses as a purgative.

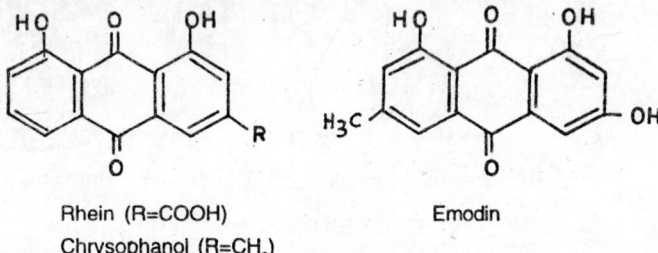

Rhein (R=COOH)
Chrysophanol (R=CH₃)

Emodin

OTHER RHUBARBS

Indian Rhubarb : It consists of the dried rhizomes and roots of *R. emodi* and *R. webbianum*. *R. emodi* is a stout herb, 1.5-3.0 m in height, distributed in the Himalayas from Kashmir to Sikkim at altitudes of 3,300-5,200 m. It is also cultivated in Assam for its leaves consumed as vegetable. Roots are very stout.

The drug is collected from the wild plant, found in the hills of Kangra, Kulu, Kumaun, Nepal and Sikkim. The herb is drought resistant, and can be propagated either through rhizome-cuttings or seeds. The plant requires deep, rich soil, mixed with well-rotten manure. The cuttings are planted in early spring at a spacing of 1.2 - 1.5 m beneath the surface. Aerial portions wither away during winter and die, but the rhizomes regenerate during the ensuring spring. Rhizomes and roots are dug up in September from 3 to 10 years old plants. They are washed and cut into pieces of proper size, kiln- or sun-dried, and stored in air-tight containers and protected from sunlight.

Indian rhubarb contains a number of anthraquinone derivatives based on emodin, emodin-3-monomethyl ether (physcion), chrysophanol, aloe-emodin and rhein. These occur free and as quinone, anthrone or dianthrone glycoside. The astringent principle consists of gallic acid, present as glucogallin, along with tannin and catechin. The drug also contains cinnamic and rheinolic acids, volatile oil, starch and calcium oxalate. Free chrysophanic acid, sennoside A and sennoside B are also present. The characteristic odour of the essential oil is due to presence of eugenol.

Indian rhubarb is used as a purgative and astringent tonic, in atonic dyspepsia, and for cleaning teeth. Powdered roots are sprinkled over ulcers for quick healing.

Chinese Rhapontic (Rhapontic rhubarb) : It is obtained from *Rheum rhaponticum.* Its odour is sweet. It contains anthracene derivatives and a stilbene derivative, rhaponticin. Its alcoholic extract on filter paper shows a distinct blue fluorescence in U.V. light due to rhaponticin.

Japanese Rhubarb : It is a hybrid of *R. coreanum* and *R. palmatum* and contains anthraquinone derivatives, naphthalene glycosides, stilbene glycosides and *d*- catechin.

ALOE

Synonyms : Aloes; Ghrit kumari (Sansk)

Biological Source : Aloe is dried juice of the leaves of *Aloe barbadensis* Mill. (*A. vera* L.), *A. ferox* Mill and *A. africana* Mill. or their hybrids. It contains about 28% of hydroxyanthracene derivatives, calculated as anhydrous barbaloin.

The liquid is obtained from the transversely cut leaves which is concentrated by boiling and solidifies on cooling.

Family : Liliaceae.

Habitat : There are about 180 species of Aloe and most of them are found in South Africa and West Indies. *A.*

barbadensis is a native of Northern Africa but it is planted in Indian gardens and many other tropical countries. Aloe plant is a typical xerophyte with thick, fleshy, strongly cuticularized spiny margined leaves arranged in rosette formation. Erect unbranched flower rises after rainy season in winter. It fluorishes on poorest soil and can be propagated easily by means of a sucker.

Commercial Varieties of Aloe

1. *Aloe barbadensis* (Syn. *A. vulgaris, A. officianalis*) : This is known as Curacao Aloe or Barbados Aloe. It is native of northern Africa. At present it is cultivated in Aruba, Bonaire and Curacao islands near West Indies. It is coarse - looking perennial plant with a short stem found in semi-wild parts; leaves 30-60 cm, erect, crowded in basal rosette, full of juice, glaucous - green, narrow-lanceolate, long-acuminate, smooth; flowers yellow, in dense racemes terminating the scapes. The juice of the Aloe is collected in a tin vessel. It is packed in gourds. The Aloe is also known as Hepatic Aloe or Liver Aloe. The plant of *A. barbadensis* is of herbaceous type.

2. *Aloe ferox* and its hybrids : This drug is called as Cape Aloe and occurs wildly on the Islands of Socotra, South Africa, Kenya and neighbouring mainland of East Africa. The juice of the plant is collected in canvas or goat skin. Cape Aloe is exported from the Republic of South Africa and largely used in veterinary practice. The plant of *A. ferox* is of the arborescent type.

3. *Aloe perryi* : This Aloe is known as Socotrine and Zangibar Aloes. This is cultivated in Socotra and Zangibar Islands. It has simple stem, 2.5 cm in diameter, scarcely rising above the ground, and crowded leaves much shorter than those of *A. succotrina*. The plant is suitable to grow in the limestone-tract and can be cultivated in the driest situation and poorest soil. Zangibar Aloe is packed in skins of carnivorous animals. This Aloe is also called as Monkey skin Aloe. The juice of Socotrine Aloe is collected in goat or sheep skin.

Collection : The Aloe leaves contain spines at the margins. For collection of juice of *A. barbadensis*, (Curacao Aloe) the leaves are cut in March-April in V-shaped and a vessel is kept under the incision. The juice is evaporated in copper vessel on open fire, poured into cans or tins, allowed to solidify and exported. The methods of preparation of aloes from different varieties are varied slightly. The juice of *Aloe perryi* (Scotorine Aloe) is collected in goat's or sheep's skin container which is evaporated itself without applying heat. The latex of leaves of *Aloe ferox* (Cape Aloe) is boiled in a drum for about 4-5 hours on an open fire. It is then cooled quickly for getting vitreous or shiny aloe.

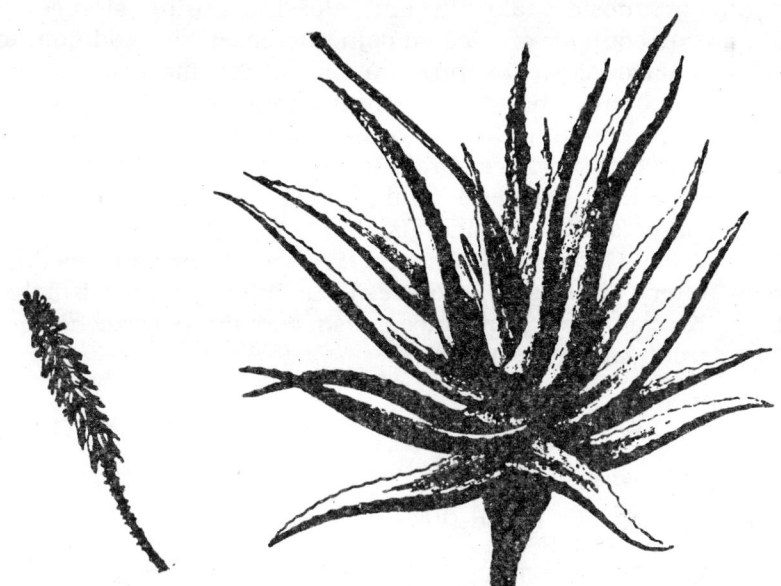

Fig. 7.6. Aloe vera

Characters : Aloe is available as opaque masses, colour ranges from reddish black to brownish black, fracture is waxy. Cape Aloe is glassy mass having characteristic, sour odour, taste is nauseous and bitter. Curacao Aloe is yellowish brown to chocolate brown in colour, opaque, breaks with a waxy fracture, nauseous and bitter taste and iodoform-like odour.

Chemical Constituents : Aloe contains a mixture of crystalline glycosides known as 'aloin' (4-5% in Cape Aloe; 18-25% in Curacao Aloe), resin (16-63%), emodin and volatile oil. It also possesses the anthraquinone glycosides like barbaloin (aloe-emodin anthrone C-10 glucoside); chrysophanic acid, β-barbaloin, and iso-barbaloin. Barbaloin is a C-glycoside and it can not be hydrolyzed easily. The

O-glycosides present in the Aloe are aloe-emodin-8-glucoside and emodin oxanthrone glucoside. Aloe resin is the ester of p-coumaric acid or p-hydroxycinnamic acid with aloe resinotannol.

The principal constituents of aloin are barbaloin, isobarbaloin, β-barbaloin, aloe-emodin and resins. Phenolic glucosides identified are isoeleutheraol, β-D-glucopyranoside, aloesaponol III-8-0-β-D-glucopyranoside, aloesaponol II-6-0-d-glucopyranoside, aloenin and aloesin. During storage of aloin the content of aloe-emodin increases. In addition to these, flavonoids, oxanthraquinones, coumarins, amino acids, monosaccharides, polysaccharides, oils, sterols, triterpenes, vitamin C and group B vitamins, citric, L-malic and formic acids are present in all aloes. Cholesterol, compesterol, β-sitosterol and lupeol are found in lipid fraction. Presence of minerals B, P, Al, Mg, Cu, Ni, Ca, K, Si, Fe, Pb, Cr, Ba, Ag, Zn and Sr have been confirmed. A new bitter C-glucoside, aloe resin D, has also been isolated from Kenya aloe. Some aloes also contain polysaccharides "aloeferon" and "aloeulcin".

Aloin (R = H)
Barbaloin (R = OH)

Aloesin

Chemical Tests : Aqueous solution of Aloe is used to perform the following tests :

1. **Schonteten's Test :** To a solution (5 ml) borax (0.2g) is added and it is heated to dissolve completely. Few drops of the liquid are poured in a test-tube filled with water. A green fluorescence is produced.

2. **Bromine Test :** A pale yellow precipitate of tetrabromaloin is formed on addition of bromine.

3. **Nitric Acid Test :** On addition of nitric acid (2 ml) to a solution of Aloe (5ml), Cape aloe forms a brown colour which changed rapidly to green; Curacao gives a deep brownish-red; Socotrine a pale brownish-yellow; Zanzibar a yellow-brown colour.

4. **Nitrous Acid Test :** To an aqueous solution of Aloe a small amount of sodium nitrite and few ml of acetic acid

are added. Pink colour is developed.

5. **Klunge's Isobarbaloin Test** : To an aqueous solution (20 ml) copper sulphate solution (1drop) is added followed by sodium chloride (1 g) and 90% alcohol (10 ml). A purple colour is formed due to the presence of isobarbaloin. This test is sensitive in case of Curacao Aloe.

6. **Modified Bornträger's Test** : Aloe (0.1 g) is boiled with dil. HCl (5 ml) and 5% solution of $FeCl_3$ (5 ml) for 5 minutes. The solution is cooled, filtered and the filtrate is shaken with benzene. The benzene layer is separated, ammonia solution is added to this when a pink colour is formed.

Uses : Aloe is used as purgative and given in constipation. It is one of the ingredient of Compound Benzoin Tincture, Ointment of aloe-gel is used to cure burns caused by heat, sun or radiation and skin irritations. The plant is valued to cure many skin diseases, ulcerative skin conditions, wounds, burns, snake bite, as hair tonic, to treat enlarged spleen; tonic for stomach and brain, as a febrifuge and emmenagogue to relieve buring sensation.

Allied Drug

Indian Aloe : It is obtained from *Aloe vera* Var. *Officinalis.* It is found on the coasts of Bombay, Gujarat and Madras.The colour of the aloe is dark. It contains aloin but *iso*-barbaloin is almost absent. It is widely used in cosmetic products.

Aloe is substituted by Socotrine and Zangibar varieties from *Aloe perryi* and Natal Aloe *(A. candelabrum).* Socotrine Aloe occurs as yellowish-brown to blackish brown, opaque masses and breaks with a porous fracture. Zanzibar in identical but has a waxy fracture. Natal Aloe grows near Pietermaritzburg. It contains nataloin, homonataloin, and a resin consisting of nataloresinotannol and paracoumaric acid. Mocha Aloe is imported from Bombay. It is black, brittle, glassy aloe with strong odour and is of inferior quality. Jafferabad Aloe in nearly black.

CASCARA BARK

Synonyms : Sacred bark; Chittem bark; Chittim bark; Purshiana bark; Persian bark; Bearberry bark; Bearwood; Cascara sagrada; Rhamnus purshiana; Cortex rhamni.

Biological Source : Cascara is the dried bark of *Rhamnus purshiana* DC usually collected one year before its use.

Family : Rhamnaceae.

Habitat : Cascara is grown on the Pacific coast of North America, British Columbia, Oregon, Washington, California and Kenya.

Collection : The bark is collected during April-August from 6-12 meters high tree.The bark is removed from the tree by making longitudinal incisions. The trees are often felled and the bark is separated from larger branches. It is dried in the shade or in sun by keeping cork upper side. The bark is stored by protecting from rain and damp. The dried bark is cut into small pieces.

The bark occurs in quills, channelled or flat pieces, length up to 20 cm, thickness 1-4 mm with short fracture Odour is slight and distinct; taste is bitter.

Chemical Constituents : Cascara contains anthracene derivatives which are normal O-glucosides (10-20%) and C-glucosides (80-90%) and free anthraquinones. Cascarosides A, B, C and D contain both O- and C- glucosidic linkages.

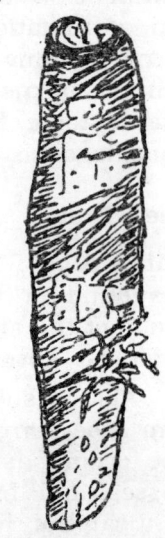

Two aloins, namely barbaloin derived from the aloe-emodin anthrone and chrysaloin derived from chrysophanol anthrone, are the C-glycosides. Cascara possesses O-glycosides derived from emodin, emodin oxanthrone, aloe-emodin and chrysophanol. Various dianthrones such as those of emodin, aloe-emodin and chrysophanol and the heterodianthrones palmidins A, B and C have been reported in Cascara bark. It also contains aloe-emodin, chrysophanol and emodin in the free state.

Fig. 7.7. Bark of Cascara sagrada

Chrysaloin

Cascaroside A = 10β, R=OH
Cascaroside C = 10β, R=H;

Cascaroside B = 10α, R=OH
Cascaroside D = 10α, R=H

Uses : Cascara is purgative and generally used in the form of liquid extract, elixir or tablets prepared from a dry extract.

DIOSCOREA

Synonyms : Wild yam; Colic root; Rhematism root.

Biological Source : Dioscorea is the dried rhizome of several species of *Dioscorea* like *D. villosa, D. prazeri* Prain & Burk; *D. composita* and *D. spiculiflora; D. deltoidea* and *D. floribunda.*

Family : Dioscoreaceae.

Habitat : North America and Mexico. In India the plants grow wildly in Western Himalayas up to an altitude of 3000 m.

Dioscorea plants are climbing; roots tuberous; tubers large; stem leafy.

Dioscorea species are distributed throughout India except in the dry north-western region. These plants are cultivated mostly as garden crops or subordinate crops with ginger, turmeric, brinjal, sweet potato or maize. They thrive best in deep sandy loams with adequate moisture and good drainage. The field should be well prepared by digging to considerable depth and manuring liberally. Farmyard manure is usually applied. Both tuber tops and aerial tubers borne on the stems are used for propagation. The planting period is generally April-June after the onset of the monsoon, but it may vary according to local condition and the species. Vines are allowed to trail on ground or are trailed over stakes or trees near by. The crop is ready after 5-8 months of planting. During this period, the field is hoed and weeded and earthed up round the stems.

Tubers are variable in shape and size. Some species produce large cylindrical tubers penetrating deep into the ground while others produce globose tubers, close to the soil surface. Tubers are either solitary-one from each plant - or several of them are clustered together at the base of the plant. The yield ranges from 2 to 14 tons per acre dipending upon the variety cultivated, the soil and the cultural treatment. Discoreas are stored in cool sheds under dry earth or sand for about 6 months.

The yams of several species are soft, fleshy and edible.

Chemical Constituents : Dioscorea is a source of saponin glycoside diosgenin. Botagenin and diosgenin are obtained from the root of *Dioscorea spiculiflora*. Diosgenin is obtained by hydrolysis of dioscin. Dioscorea also contains small quantities of hecogenin having keto group at 12 position of diosgenin; and an acrid resin. Dioscin on acidic hydrolysis yields diosgenin, rhamnose and glucose.

Diosgenin   Hecogenin

The alkaloid, dioscorine, and the saponin, dioscin, occur in varying quantities in different species. American species contain the steroidal sapogenins, diosgenin, yamogenin, kryptogenin, etc. Botogenin, obtained from *D. mexicana*, is a starting material for the synthesis of cortisone, used in the treatment of rheumatoid arthritis and rheumatic fever.

Uses : Diosgenin is used for the production of various steroidal drugs like progesterone, and as a cheap source of carbohydrate food. Some species, e.g. *D. alata*, are used for the extraction of starch. Some of them are rich in vitamins B_1, B_2 and B_6.

Allied Species : *D. alata*, a native of south east Asia, is the most important cultivated species throughout the tropics. They are starchy and used as vegetable, anthelmintic, in leprosy, piles and gonorrhoea.

D. bulbifera is a large unarmed climber with stems twining to the left. The tubers are used mostly as famine food, to prepare starch, for washing wool and as fish bait in Kashmir, applied for ulcers, in piles, dysentery and syphilis.

D. deltoidea is an extensive climber with unarmed stem twining to the left. The tubers are rich in saponin and are used for washing silk, wood and hair, and in dyeing. They kill lice.

D. esculenta is a prickly climber; tubers 4 to many stalked, produced in branches close to the surface of the ground. The tubers are starchy and free from dioscorine. They have a sweetish taste; in flavour and mealiness, closely resemble potatoes. The Tubers are applied for swelling.

D. glabra is a climber with stems twining to the right. This species occurs in Assam, Bengal, Bihar, Orissa, Andaman and Nicobar Islands. The tubers are used as food edible.

D. hamiltonii is a climber with angled glabrous stem twining to the right. *D. hispida* is a climber with prickly stem twining to the left. The tubers are large, contain high amount of starch and used as famine food. The toxic principle is dioscorine which is distributed throughout the plant. The milky juice of tubers with the juice of *Antiaris toxicaria* is used as arrow poison.

D. oppositifolia is a climber with glabrous or finely pubescent stem. The tuber is usually single with few rootlets; skin reddish; flesh white, soft and edible. The tubers are used externally to reduce swellings.

D. pentaphylla is a tall, slender, prickly climber. Tubers are almost invariably single; texture and shape variable, skin brown, yellow or purplish. They are used to disperse swellings and as tonic.

D. prazeri is a climber with smooth or slightly ridged, unarmed stem. The tubers contain saponin and used for hair wash for killing lice and as fish poison.

D. puber is a large unarmed climber. The tubers are edible.

GLYCYRRHIZA

Synonyms : Liquorice; Licorice; Liquorice root; Mulethi (Hindi), Sweetwood; Radix glycyrrhizae.

Biological Source : Glycyrrhiza consists of the dried unpeeled roots and rhizome of *Glycyrrhiza glabra* L. var. *typica* or of *G. glabra* var. *glandulifera* or of other varieties of *G. glabra* yielding a yellow and sweet wood. It contains not less than 4% of glycyrrhizinic acid.

Family : Leguminosae.

Habitat : The drug is found from southern Europe to central Asia in Iran, Iraq, Russia, Arabia, Afghanistan, Turkestan, Asia Miror, Greece and Siberia. The plant is cultivated in Punjab, sub-Himalayan tracts from Chenab eastwards, Sind, Peshawar valley, to Burma and in Andaman Islands.

Cultivation and Collection : The plant is a 1 m high perennial herb. It is cultivated by planting rhizome or stolon cuttings in well moist sandy soil in March. It grows better near the banks of river in sunny climate. Manure is added for favourable growth. Drug is collected from 3-4 years old plants during autumn. Roots and rhizomes are dug out, rootlets and buds are removed, washed in water and cut into small pieces.

Morphology : The drug occurs in peeled or unpeeled stolons and roots, length 5-30 cm, diameter 1-2 cm, cylindrical, branched or unbranched. Unpeeled drug is longitudinally wrinkled; contains dark, reddish-brown bark. The peeled drug has yellow colour. Fracture is fibrous; odour faint and typical; taste, sweet.

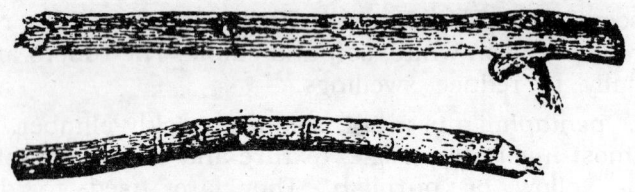

Fig. 7.8. Glycyrrhiza

Chemical Constituents : Glycyrrhiza contains 6-14% of glycyrrhizin (the glucoside of glycyrrhetic acid), sugars and resin. The saponin like glycoside, glycyrrhizin, is 150 times as sweet as sugar. On hydrolysis the glycoside is converted into the aglycone glycyrrhetic acid and two moles of glucuronic acid. Glycyrrhetic acid is a pentacyclic triterpene of β-amyrin series. Other hydroxy-and deoxytriterpenoid acids related to glycyrrhetic acid and 20-epimer of glycyrrhetic acid (liquiritic acid) have been reported in the drug. The yellow colour of Glycyrrhiza is due to the presence of more than 30 flavonoids like isoliquiritin (a chalcone), liquiritin, liquiritigenin, isoliquiritigenin, rhamnoliquiritin and various 2-methylisoflavones. The other constituents are a coumarin named as liqcoumarin (6-acetyl-5-hydroxy-4-methylcoumarin), 5-15 per cent of sugars (glucose, mannitol, sucrose), asparagine (1-2%), β-sitosterol, starch (20%), protein, bitter principles (glycyramarin), umbelliferone (coumarin), 22, 23-dihydrostigmasterol, malic acid and resin. Liquiritin on hydrolysis affords liquiritigenin and glucose.

Uses : Glycyrrhiza possesses tonic, laxative, demulcent, diuretic, emmenagogue and emollient properties and used in genito-urinary diseases, coughs, sore throat, in scorpion-biting, as demulcent, in inflammatory affections or irritable conditions of the bronchial tubes, bowels and catarrh; and to relieve peptic ulcer pain. Glycyrrhiza is added to chewing gums, chocolate candy, cigarettes, smoking mixtures, snuff and chewing tobacco. Glycyrrhetinic acid is used to cure rheumatoid arthritis, Addison's disease and various inflammatory conditons.

Substituents and Adulterants : *Glycyrrhiza uralensis* is a source of Manchurian Liquorice. It resembles Russian Liquorice in appearance. The bark is pale chocolate-brown in colour and exfoliates readily. It contains only a small percentage of sugar and gives a pungent extract. *G. glabra* var. *typica* is the source of Spanish Liquorice collected chiefly in Sicily and Spain. The drug consists of pieces of underground roots. Unpeeled pieces are dark reddish or purplish brown in colour and longitudinally wrinkled. The fracture is fibrous in the bark and splintery in the wood. Peeled pieces are smooth and yellow. The drug has a faint characteristic odour and a sweet taste free from bitterness.

Russian Liquorice is derived from *G. glabra* var. *glandulifera.* It is collected in southern Russia chiefly from wild plants. It consists mainly of roots and some pieces of rootstock. Bigger pieces are longitudinally split. Unpeeled pieces are purplish; taste is sweet accompanied by a perceptible, bitterness and acridity. It is usually exported in peeled form.

Persian Liquorice is derived from *G. glabra var. violacea* and is collected chiefly from the Tagris and Euphrates valley in Iraq. It is usually thicker than other varieties and is marketed in an unpeeled state.

Roots and rhizomes of some related plant genera are also used as substituents and adulterants of Liquorice. The roots of *Abrus precatorius* are used as adulterant in the trade as Indian Liquorice.

QUILLAIA BARK

Synonums : Quillaja; Soap bark, Quillary bark, Panama bark; China bark, Murillo bark, Panama wood; Cortex quillaiae.

Biological Source : Quillaia bark is the inner dried bark of *Quillaia saponaria* Molina and other species of *Quillaia.*

Family : Rosaceae.

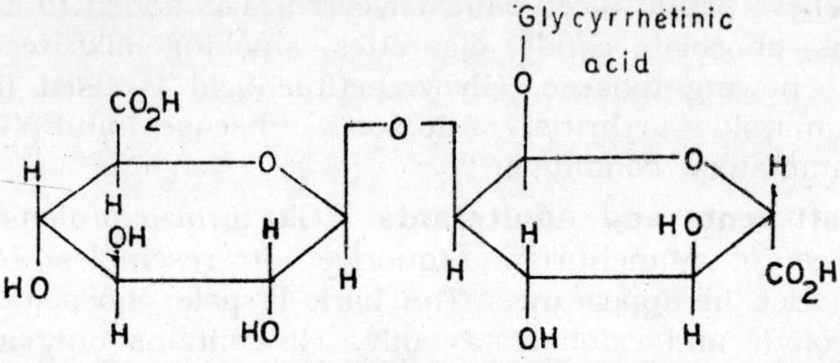

Glycyrrhetinic acid

Glycyrrhizic acid

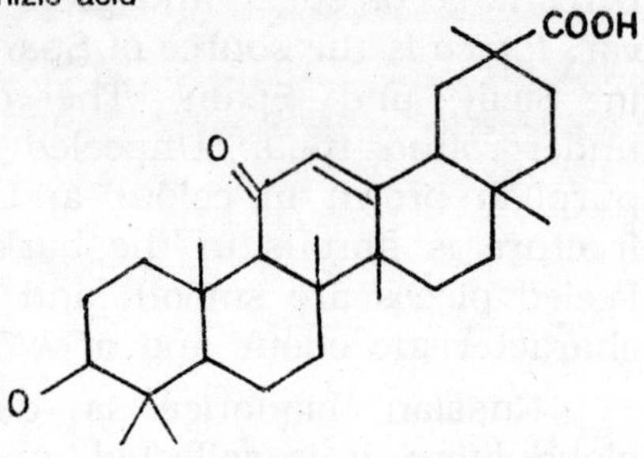

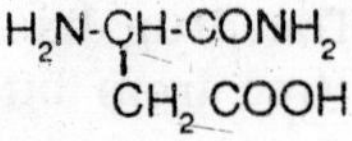

$H_2N-CH-CONH_2$
$\quad CH_2 COOH$
Asparagine

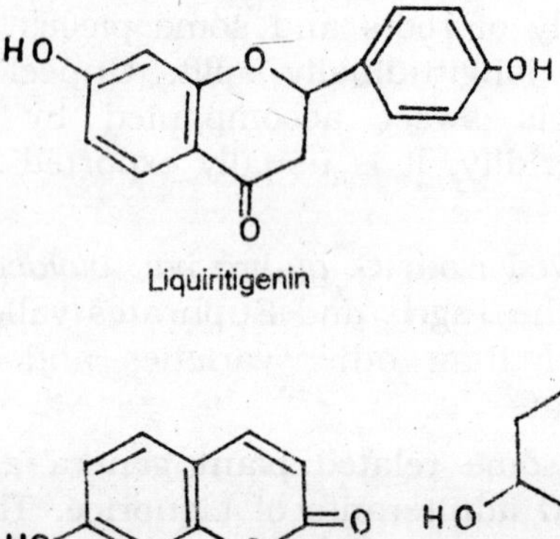

Glycyrrhetinic acid

Liquiritigenin

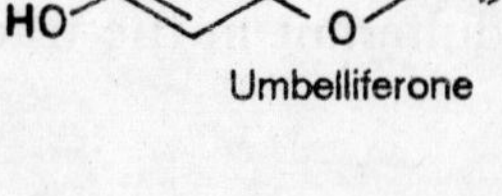

Umbelliferone

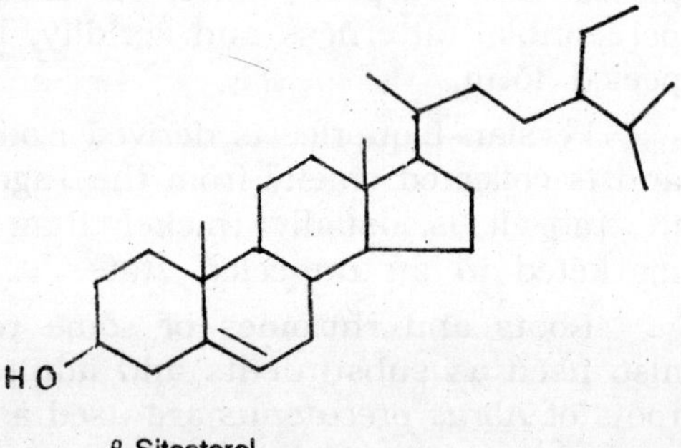

β-Sitosterol

Habitat : *Q. saponaria* is about 18 m high evergreen, graceful tree found in Peru, Chile, Bolivia, South America, California and India.

The bark is collected from the stem; outer, dark-coloured rhytidome is removed, dried and graded. It consists mainly of saponaceous inner bark (phloem).

Morphology : Quillaia bark occurs in flat pieces, about 1 m long, 20 cm wide, and 3-10 cm thick. Outer surface is brownish-white, smooth and contains reddish- or blackish-brown patches of rhytidome adhere to the outer surface. The rhytidome is made of dead secondary phloem. The inner surface is yellowish-white and smooth. Fracture is splintery. Large crystals of calcium oxalate are present. Odour is sternutatory and taste is acidic and astringent.

Chemical Constituents : Quillaia bark contains saponins (10%), quillaic acid, calcium oxalate, starch, sucrose and tannin. Quillaia saponin on hydrolysis forms pentacyclic triterpenoid, quillaic acid (Quillaja sapogenin), and a sugar glucuronic acid.

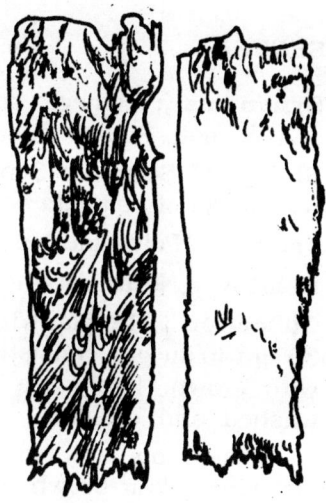

Chemical Tests

1. Powdered drug on shaking with water produces soap like froth which persists for some time.

2. On addition of a small portion of drug or its alcoholic extract in a drop of blood on a microscopic slide, a haemolytic zone surrounding the drug is formed.

Outer surface Inner surface
Fig. 7.9. Quillaia bark

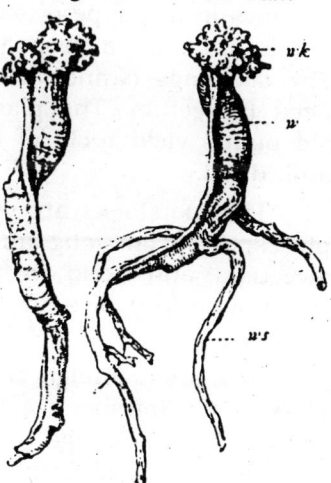

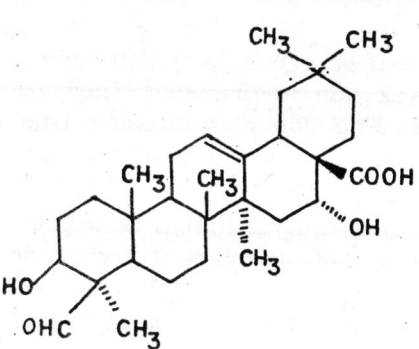

Quillaic acid

Fig. 7.10. Roots of *Polygala senega* (Senega root)

Uses : Quillaia bark is used as an emulsifying agent, for coal tar emulsion, cleaning industrial equipments, washing delicate fabrics, to prepare tooth powders, tooth pastes, hair shampoos, hair tonics, tar solutions and metal polishes. The drug is highly irritating and causes nausea and is expectorant on internal consumption. It is diuretic and a cutaneous stimulant.

SENEGA

Synonyms : Senega snakeroot; Seneca snakeroot; Rattle snake root; Radix senegae.

Biological Source : Senega consists of the dried roots and rootstocks of *Polygala senega* Linn. or *P. senega* var. *latifolia*.

Family : Polygalaceae.

Habitat : North America, Canada, Japan.

Collection : The plant is a pluricaulous perennial herb, 20—30 cm in height consisting of yellow twisted, branched roots with crown. Roots are dug out, aerial parts are removed, washed and dried.

The roots are twisted, curved, tapering, longitudinally striated, colour-brown, odour is methyl salicylate-like, taste is first sweet and then acrid.

Senega thrives in the open and also in partial shade. It grows in any type of soil, containing a fair amount of leaf-mould. It can be propagated either by seed or rootstocks. The seedlings cannot withstand frost in the first year and need protection. The plants grow slowly and nearly 4-year old plants yield roots of the required size. They are cleaned and dried.

The rootstocks are yellowish orange to brownish conical pieces, 5-20 cm long and 2-12 mm in diameter. They are sweetish, and acrid in taste. The odour is characteristic, resembling that of methyl salicylate. Powered Senega causes sneezing.

In market foreign Senega *(P. senega)*, Indian Senega *(P. chinensis)*, Nowshera or Pakistan Senega (roots of *Andrachne aspera*), Delhi Senega, Kulu Senega, Tuticorin yellow *(Glinus oppositifolius)* and Tuticorin Brownish green are available.

Chemical Constituents : Senega contains a mixture of saponins A, B, C and D (8-10%), polygallic acid (senegenic acid), polygalitol (1, 5-anhydro-sorbitol), anhydride of the hexahydric sugar alcohol sorbitol, sucrose, fat, sterols, methyl salicylate, volatile oil and fixed oil. Hydrolysis of the crude saponin (senegin) yields glucose, presenegenin, senegenin, senegenic acid, polygallic acid and hydroxysenegin. Senegenin is a chlorinated triterpenoid. The roots also contain 2, 3, 27-trihydroxy-12-oleanene-23, 28-dioic acid, α-spinasterol and free fatty acids.

Uses : Senega is used as a stimulant, expectorant in chronic bronchitis, and as emetic.

Side effects include nausea, diarrhoea, stomach upsets and dizziness.

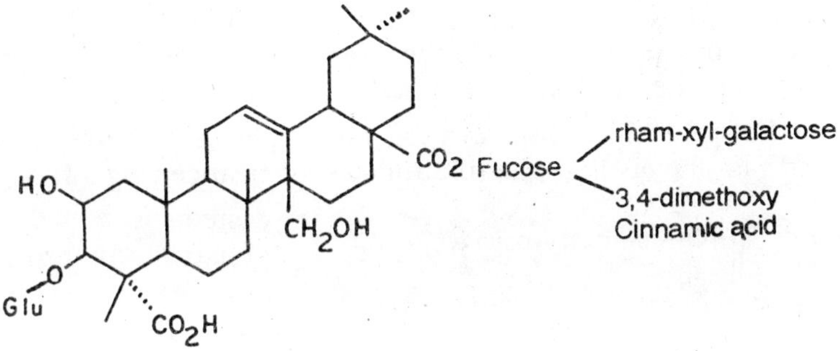

Senegin II

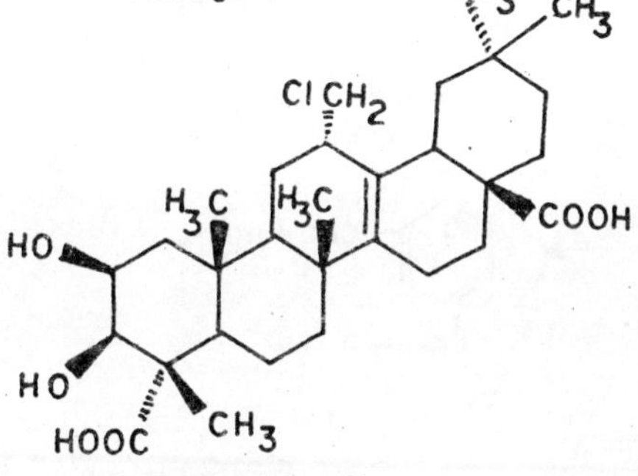

Senegenin

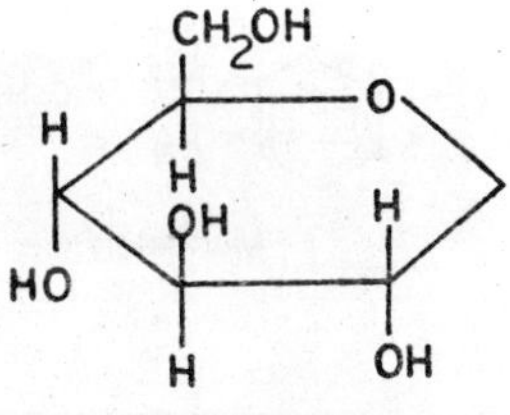

Polygalitol

CYANOGENETIC OR CYANOPHORE GLYCOSIDES

Cyanogenetic glycosides on hydrolysis yield hydrocyanic acid as one of the products. The glycoside amygdalin is most widely distributed in nature. Usually these glycosides are derived from the nitrile of mandelic acid. This group is represented by amygdalin which is the major component of bitter almonds and in kernels of apricots, cherries, peaches, plums and many other seeds of the Rosaceae. Prunasin is found in *Prunus padus* and yields d-mandelonitrile on hydrolysis as the aglycone. Other cyanogenetic aglycosides are prulaurasin from cherry laurel leaves and sambunigrin from *Sambucus nigra.*

Cyanogenetic glycosides contain nitrogen, but the sugar moiety is attached to oxygen and not to nitrogen. The sugar residue of the molecule may be a monosaccharide or a disaccharide as gentiobiose or vicianose. Amygdalin on hydrolysis yields two molecules of glucose. The enzyme emulsin, found in almond kernels, consists of two enzymes, amygdalase and prunase. The first enzyme breaks the molecule to liberate one of mandelonitrile glucoside. The latter enzyme liberates the remaining glucose forming benzaldehyde-cyanohydrin known as mandelonitrile.

Drugs containing cyanogenetic glycosides are widely used as flavouring agents and as anticancer agents.

Chemical Tests

Sodium Picrate Test : A strip of filter paper is dipped in 10% aqueous solution of picric acid. It is drained and re-dipped in 10% sodium carbonate solution and drained again. To powdered drug in a flask, water is added to moisten it. Sodium picrate paper is kept on the mouth of flask with cork. Hydrocyanic acid vapours turn the paper brick red or maroon-coloured.

BITTER ALMOND

Synonyms : Badam (Hindi); Amygdala amara.

Biological Source : Bitter almond is the dried ripe seeds of *Prunus amygdalus* Batsch var. *amara* or *P. amygdalus* var. *dulcis.*

Family : Rosaceae.

Habitat : Italy, Spain, southern France, North America, and in Kashmir.

Cultivation : The almond requires a cold and dry climate, but a fairly warm weather during its ripening period. The trees are raised from seeds which are sown in nurseries and seedlings transplanted after one year. The trees are planted 6-8 m apart in circular pits. The trees tend to grow large with long branches. The fruit is borne largely on short-spurs. The almond crop comes to harvest from July to September. Almonds are graded into several classes to meet the demand for specific purposes. Unshelled almonds are stored in a cool, dry and well-ventilated place.

Characters : Almond tree is about 5 m in height. The bitter almond is 1.5-2 cm long, rounded at one end and pointed at the other. Cinnamon-brown coloured testa is present which is removed by soaking in hot water. The oil kernel consists of two large, oily planoconvex cotyledons. A small plumule and radicle are present. Some almonds possess cotyledons of unequal sizes. The presence of bitter almonds in sweet almonds can be detected by the sodium picrate test for cyanogenetic glycosides.

Chemical Constituents : Bitter and sweet almonds contain fixed oil (40-55%), proteins (20%), mucilage and emulsin. The bitter almonds contain a colourless, crystalline, cyanogenetic glycoside amygdalin (about 3%). In the presence of water the enzyme emulsin acts upon amygdalin and decomposes it into

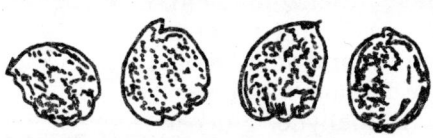

Fig. 7.11. Bitter Almond Fruits.

a volatile oil which is a mixture of benzaldehyde and hydrocyanic acid. A casein like protein, amandin, is also present in bitter almond.

Uses : Bitter Almond seeds have demulcent, mild laxative, stimulant and nervine tonic properties. Almond oil is used as a flavouring agent in the preparation of toilet articles, as a vehicle for oily injections and in manufacturing of liquors. Due to the presence of hydrocyanic acid in the volatile oil, it gives relief in bronchitis and cough.

WILD CHERRY BARK

Synonyms : Wild black cherry, Cherry bark; Virginian Prune Bark; Prune bark, Cortex Pruni Virginianae; Prunus Virginiana; Prunus serotina.

Biological Source : Wild Cherry bark is the dried stem bark of *Prunus serotina* Ehrh.

Family : Rosaceae.

Habitat : United States and Canada.

Collection : Wild Cherry plant is a tree, 30 m high or more. The bark is collected in autumn from young branches and stem, cork and cortex are removed by peeling to get 'rossed bark', dried and preserved in containers.

Morphology : The drug occurs in curved or channelled pieces, length up to 10 cm, width 5 cm, thckness 0.3-1.4 mm. Outer surface of unpeeled bark (unrossed bark) is reddish-brown, covered with thin papery, glossy, exfoliating cork cells and bears very conspicuous whitish lenticles. The outer surface of the bark is rough with pale buff-coloured lenticels. Inner surface is reddish-brown with striated and reticulately furrowed appearance. Patches of wood adhering to the inner surface are sometimes present. The fracture is granular and short. Slightly moist drug contains benzadehydic odour. Taste is bitter and astringent.

Chemical Constituents : Wild Cherry bark contains a cyanogenic glycoside, prunasin (d-mandelonitrile glucoside), the enzyme prunase, benzoic acid, trimethylgallic acid, p-coumaric acid, starch, tannin and volatile oil.

The enzyme emulsin hydrolyzes prunasin to benzaldehyde, glucose and hydrocyanic acid. The bark

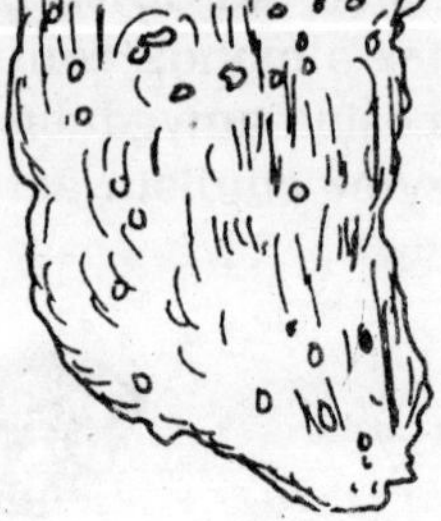

Fig. 7.12. Wild Cherry bark

possesses resin which yields the fluorescent compounds, e.g. scopoletin, on hydrolysis.

Uses : Wild Cherry is used in cough preparations as sedative expectorant and as flavouring agent.

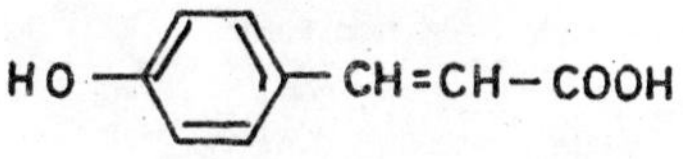

p-Coumaric acid

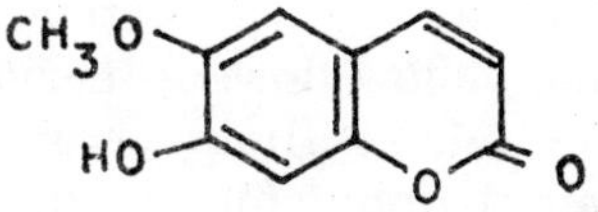

Scopoletin

ISOTHIOCYANATE GLYCOSIDES

Isothiocyanate glycosides contain sulphur and present in many Cruciferous plants. On hydrolysis they produce isothiocyanate aglycones which may be aliphatic or aromatic. Sinigrin from Black Mustard, sinalbin from White Mustard and gluconapin from Rapeseed are isothiocyanate glycosides. Sinigrin on hydrolysis in the presence of the enzyme, myrosin, yields allyl isothiocyanate, glucose and potassium acid sulphate. The activity of the fixed oil content of these seeds is due to allyl isothiocyanate. These glycosides are irritant and employed as counter-irritant externally in neuralgia and rheumatism.

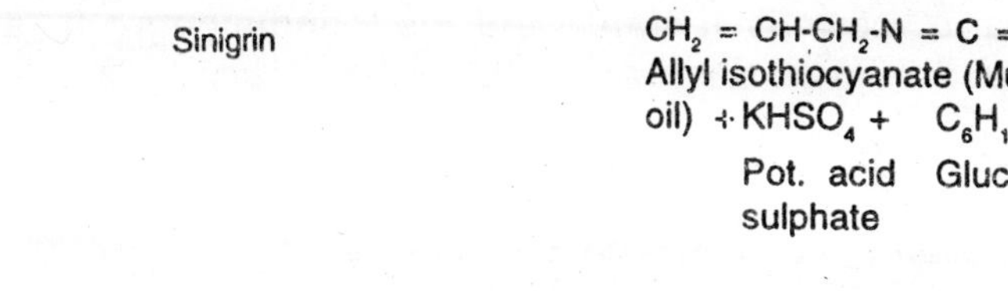

Sinigrin

Myrosin

$CH_2 = CH\text{-}CH_2\text{-}N = C = S$
Allyl isothiocyanate (Mustard oil) $+ KHSO_4 + C_6H_{12}O_6$
Pot. acid   Glucose
sulphate

MUSTARD

Synonyms : Black Mustard, Brown Mustard, Red Mustard, Sinapis Nigra; Semina Sinapsis Nigrae.

Biological Source : Mustard is the dried ripe seed of *Brassica* *nigra* (L.) Koch. or of *B. juncea* (L.) Czern. & Coss. or of these varieties.

Family : Cruciferae.

Habitat : Europe, U.S.A., southwestern Asia, India. *B. juncea* is abundantly cultivated in upper Indian region.

Collection : The plant is an annual herb with erect slender stems, yellow flowers. Leaves large, pinnatifid, without basal lobes, terminal lobe much larger. The aerial parts of the plant are cut after maturation. Seeds are removed by thrashing or beating of the dried parts and then sieving.

Characters : Seeds are small, brown to red colour, globular in shape, testa is minutely pitted, embryo is oily, yellow in colour, consisting of two cotyledons.

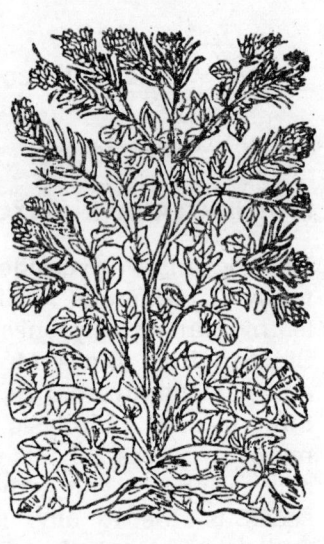

Fig. 7.13. Brassica nigra

Chemical Constituents : Mustard contains fixed oil (30-35%), proteins (20%), sinigrin (potassium myronate), myrosin, sinapine sulphocyanate, erucic acid, behenic acid and sinapolic acid. Sinigrin is the active constituent of the drug and its amount varies from 0.7 to 1.3%. In the adjacent cell of sinigrin an enzyme, myrosin, is present. In the presence of water myrosin activates the hydrolysis of sinigrin and yields allyl isothiocyanate, potassium hydrogen sulphate and glucose.

Uses : Mustard is used in the form of plasters, as rubefacient, vesicant, counter-irritant and as condiments. It acts as emetic in large doses.

Sinalbin

Erucic acid
$$CH_3(CH_2)_7 CH=CH(CH_2)_{11}COOH$$

Sinapine

Allied Drugs : White Mustard or Sinapsis alba Bois. is the dried ripe seed of *Brassica alba* Bois. (Fam. Cruciferae). The seeds are globular in shape, 1.5-2.5 mm in diameter. It contains the glucoside sinalbin and myrosin. In the presence of moisture, sinalbin is hydrolyzed into sinapin hydrogen sulphate, acrinylisothiocyanate and glucose. The isothiocynate is an oily liquid with pungent taste. Sinapine hydrogen sulphate is the salt of an unstable alkaloid. The seeds also contain fixed oil (30%), protein (20-25%) and mucilage.

White Mustard is used as counter-irritant, emetic and carminative.

OTHER GLYCOSIDES

Flavonol glycosides or flavonoids are widely distributed in nature. Rutin, quercitrin, and Citrus biflavonoids are the examples of flavonoid constituents. The phenolic glycoside salicin is found in several species of *Salix* and *Populus*. Salinigrin, isolated from *Salix discolour*, is formed by combination of glucose with m-hydroxybenzaldehyde. Several glycosides of hydroxylated coumarin derivatives are found in plant kingdom. Bitter glycosides are found in Gentianaceae species which are used as stomachic, febrifuge, bitter tonic and in digestive disturbances.

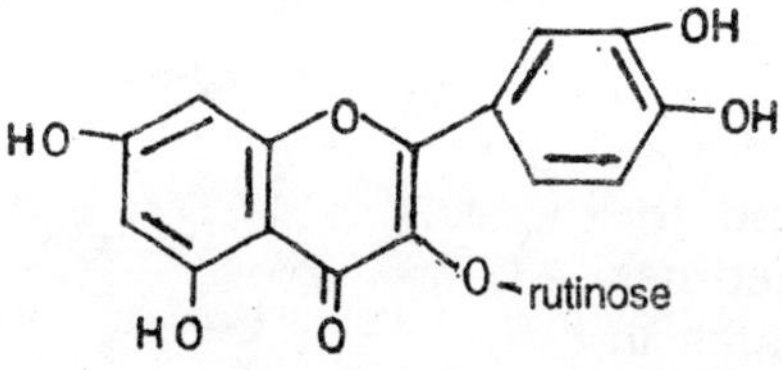

Rutin

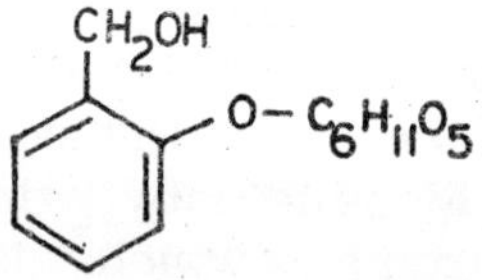

Salicin

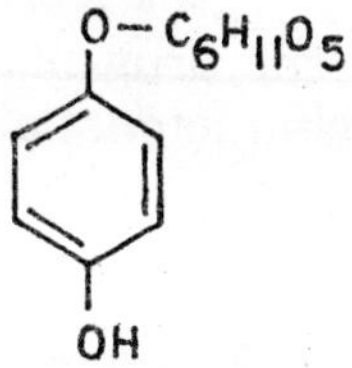

Arbutin

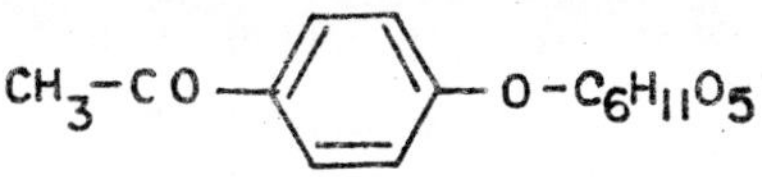

Picroside (Salinigrin)

GENTIAN

Synonyms : Yellow Gentian, Pale Gentian, Gentian root, Bitter root; Radix Gentianae.

Biological Source : Gentian is the dried rhizome and roots of *Gentiana lutea* Linn. It contains about 33% of water-soluble extractives.

Family : Gentianaceae.

Habitat : Central and southern Europe, Asia Minor, Pyrenees.

G. *lutea* requires a moist situation, good drainage and a suitable soil consisting of loam, peat and grit. Seeds are slow to germination, seedlings frequently taking several years to appear. The roots and rhizomes are collected from the 2-5 years old plants during May-October and allowed to ferment in heaps. They are then washed, dried in the open and cut into variable length.

Collection : The plant is a large perennial herb. The drug is collected from a 2-5 years old plant in the autumn. Turf is stripped and the rhizomes are dug up. It is cut into pieces of different length and dried quickly first in air and then in sheds.

Morphology : Gentian consists of brownish, subcylindrical, entire or longitudinally split pieces of rhizomes and roots, 15-20 cm or more in length and 2.5 to 8 cm in thickness at the crown. The root is longitudinally wrinkled and the rhizome, which is sometimes branched, frequently terminates in one or more buds and bears numerous encircling leafscars,

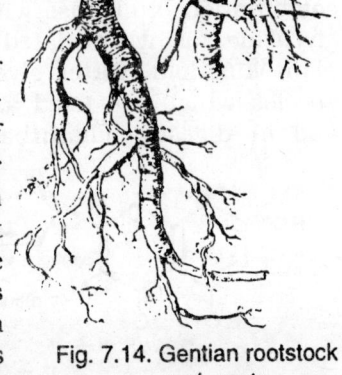

Fig. 7.14. Gentian rootstock and roots

which appear as transverse annulations. The drug in brittle and breaks with a short fracture. It has a characteristic odour and the taste is sweet at first and intensely bitter afterwards.

Chemical Constituents : Gentian contains the bitter glycoside gentiopicrin (~2%) as a principal active constituent. On hydrolysis it yields the aglycone mesogentiogenin and glucose. Gentiopicrin is a secoiridoid, gentiopicroside, and it is decomposed on fermentation and drying of the drug. Other bitter compounds are gentisin, gentiopicroside, amaropanin, amarogentin and amaroswerin. Gentian also centains abundant of starch, trisaccharide gentianose, disaccharide gentiobiose, sucrose, alkaloid gentianine, yellow xanthone pigments gentisin (or gentianin), isogentisin, and its glycoside gentioside, gentiin, gentiamarin, gentisic acid, tannins, pectin and calcium oxalate.

Uses : Gentian is used as a bitter tonic and stomachic for increasing appetite and to cure debility.

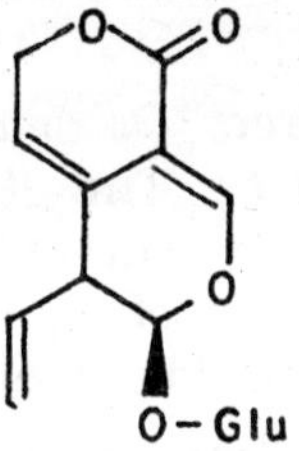

Gentiopicroside (Seco-iridoid)

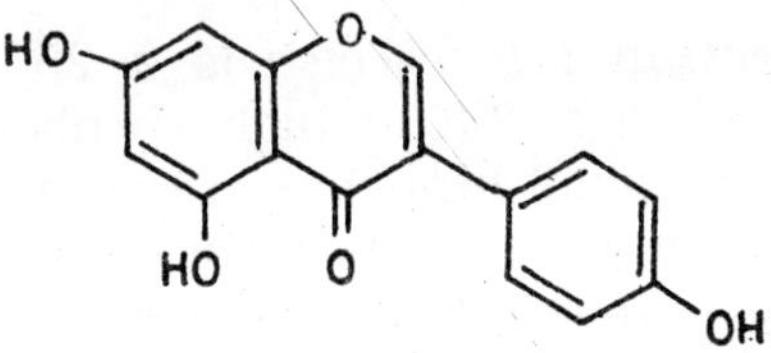

Genistein

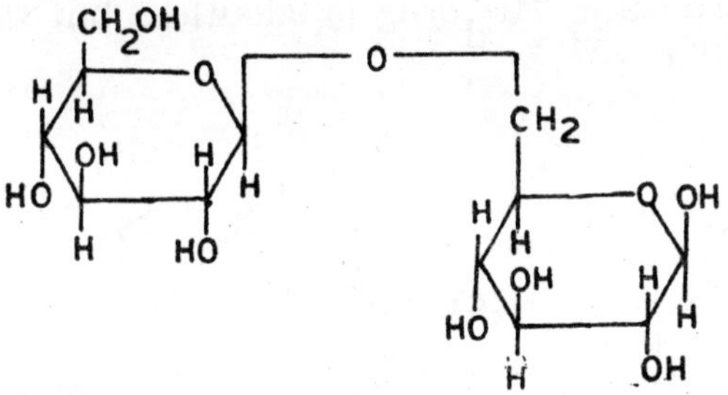

Gentiobiose

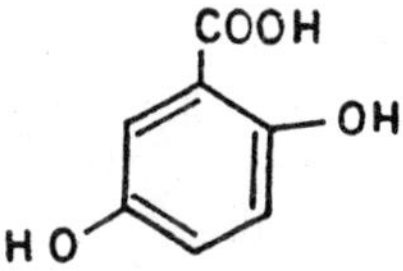

Gentisic acid

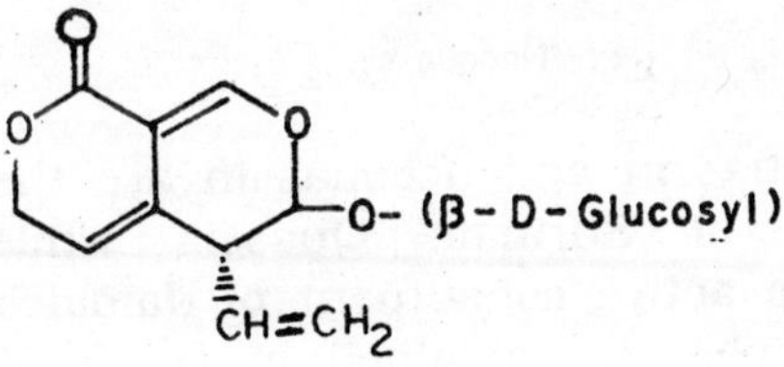

Gentiopicrin

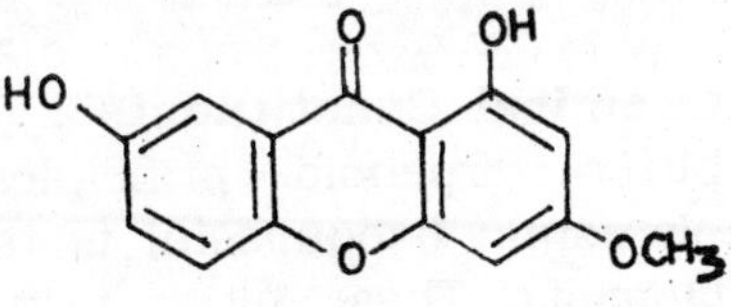

Gentisin

QUASSIA

Synonyms : Bitter wood, Bitter ash; Quassia wood; Lignum quassiae.

Biological Source : Quassia is the dried stem wood of *Picrasma excelsa* (Swartz) Planchon (syn. *Picroena excelsa* or *Aeschrion excelsa)* which is known in commerce as Jamica

Quassia, or of *Quassia amara* Linn. which is known in commerce as Surinam Quassia.

The plant is propagated by seeds, cuttings or layers.

Family : Simarubaceae.

Habitat : *P. excelsa* inhabits in West Indies, Jamaica and the Caribbean Islands. *Quassia amara* Linn. is a native of Brazil and Guiana and is cultivated in Colombia, Panama and the West Indies.

Collection : *P. excelsa* is a 25 m high tree; *Q. amara* is a branching, 2-3 m high shrub or small tree. The stem is cut and small branches are separated. Bark is removed from the stem and big branches are cut into logs of up to 30 cm length or chips and dried to check mould's growth.

Morphology : Quassia is found in logs, chips or rasping. The logs are up to 30 cm in length, covered with a dark grey cork. The colour of wood is white in beginning and becomes yellow on exposure. The drug is odourless but the taste is intensely bitter.

Quassin   Neoquassin

Chemical Constituents : Quassin and neoquassin are the bitter terpenoid principles of Surinam Quassia while picrasmin (isoquassin) is the active constituent of Jamaica Quassia. These bitter principles are obtained in 0.1-0.2% yields and appear commercially under the name of quassin. Other compounds reported from Quassia are 18-hydroxyquassin, scopoletin (coumarin) and cathine-6-one (alkaloid).

Uses : Quassia is used as a bitter tonic, as an insecticide in the form of fly poison on fly-paper, and as an enema for the expulsion of thread worms.

FLAVONOL GLYCOSIDES

The flavonol glycosides and their aglycons are called flavonoids. A large number of different flavonoids are found in nature. These are yellow pigments of higher plants. The important flavonoids are rutin, quercitrin, hesperidine, hesperetin, diosmin and naringen. Rutin and hesperidine are known as vitamin P or permeability factors. They are used in the treatment of different disorders such as capillary bleeding and increased capillary fragility. Bioflavonoids are reported to treat symptoms of the common cold.

ALCOHOL GLYCOSIDES

Salicin is an alcoholic glycoside obtained from several species of *Salix* and *Populus*. The important sources are *Salix purpurea* and *S. fragilis*. Salicin is hydrolyzed into D-glucose and saligenin by emulsin. Salicin has antirheumatic properties. Its actions are similar to that of salicylic acid.

ALDEHYDE GLYCOSIDES

Vanilla contains an aldehydic aglycone, vanillin. Vanilla is the cure, full grown unripe fruit of *Vanilla planifolia* or of *V. tahitensis* (Family Orchidaceae). The plants are perennial, climbing, dioecious epiphytes attached to the trunks of trees and found in eastern Maxico. The plant is propagated from cuttings. The fruits are collected, cured by dipping in worm water and repeated sweating between woolen blankets in the sun for two months. Green Vanilla contains two glycosides, glucovanillin and glucovanillic alcohol. Vanilla is used as flavouring agent and as a pharmaceutical aid. It is a source of vanillin.

QUESTIONS

1. What are bitters, saponins, thiocyanate glycosides and cardiac glycosides ? Give official source and uses of Senna, Aloe, Rhubarb and Strophanthus.

2. (a) What are cardiac glycosides ? Write official source and chemical constituents of Digitalis.

(b) What are bitter glycosides ? Give official source and chemical constituents of Black Mustard.

(c) What are saponin glycosides ? Write a short note on Dioscorea.

3. (a) Name two different cyanogenetic types of principles present in drugs. Mention the drugs in which they are present.

(b) Differentiate between hydragogus and irritant purgatives.

(c) Explain the Keller-Kiliani test.

(d) Why chrysarobin is not used internally as purgative. What is its actual use ?

4. Draw the labelled diagrams of the following drugs and mention their uses :

(a) Digitalis (b) Strophanthus (c) Wild Cherry bark (d) Rhubarb (e) Aloe.

5. Give the important diagnostic features of

(a) Dioscorea (b) Digitalis (c) Rhubarb

(d) Quillaia bark. What are their uses ?

6. What are glycosides ? Classify drugs containing glycosides. Give important substitutes and adulterants of Digitalis.

7. Describe 'Indian Senna' under a suitable pharmacognostic scheme.

8. What are saponin glycosides ? Discuss their occurrence, properties and pharmaceutical significance. Write a note on diosgenin.

9. Give distinguishing features of the following :

(a) *Urgenia scilla* and *Urginia indica;*

(b) *Rheum palmatum* and *Rheum emodi.*

(c) Glycyrrhizine and Glycyrrhetinic acid.

10. Enumerate method of extraction, separation and isolation of diosgenin from Dioscorea tubers.

11. Discuss the biosynthesis of cardiac glycosides and their distribution is nature. Give a comparative account of glycosides of Digitalis, Strophanthus and Scilla.

12. What are glycosides ? How are they classified ? Describe different steps involved in the biosynthesis of digitoxin.

8

TANNINS

Tannins are complex organic, non-nitrogenous derivatives of polyhydroxy benzoic acids which are widely distributed in the vegetable kingdom. They are the active constituents of materials like oak bark, which are used in the tanning of skins. They are present in aerial parts, e.g. leaves, fruits, barks or stem; generally occur in immature fruits, but disappears during ripening process. New leaves of deciduous plants contain high concentration of tannins. Tannins occur in many crude drugs. They probably serve as a protective to the plant during growth and are destroyed or deposited as end products of metabolism in some dead tissues of the mature plant, i.e., outer cork, heartwood, galls, etc. Some phenolic substances, such as gallic acid, catechins and chlorogenic acid often occur with tannins and are called as 'pseudotannins'. Most of the true tannins have the molecular weight in between 1000 to 5000.

Most tannins are very complex substances which can only be isolated in the pure state with the greatest difficulty. Many of them are glycosidal in nature (e.g. glucogallin). The gallotannins on hydrolysis yield a sugar and gallic acid. Tannins are non-crystalline substances, occur as mixtures of polyphenols and form colloidal solutions with water. Their aqueous solutions are acidic in nature and possess sharp 'puckering' taste. They are precipitated with solutions of gelatin and alkaloids. They produce greenish black or blue colour with ferric chloride and deep red colour with potassium ferricyanide and ammonia. They form precipitate with salts of copper, lead, and tin and by strong aqueous potassium dichromate or 1% chromic acid.

Tannins precepitate and combine with proteins. The protein tannin complex is resistant to proteolytic enzymes. This property is known as astringent action and many tannin- containing drugs are used in medicine as astringent. During healing process of burns, the proteins of the exposed tissues are precipitated producing a mildly antiseptic, protective layer under which the new tissues are regenerated. Tannins are used in the tanning process of animal hides to convert them into leather. Aqueous solutions of tannins are used to precipitate gelatin, proteins and alkaloids in the laboratory. They are used as healing agents in inflammation, leucorrhoea, gonorrhoea, burns, piles, diarrhoea and as antidote in the treatment of alkaloidal poisoning. Their deep red coloured complexes with iron salts are used to manufacture inks.

Tannins are classified as :
1. Hydrolysable tannins
2. Condensed tannins and
3. Pseudotannins.

1. **Hydrolysable Tannins** : These tannins are esters of a sugar, usually glucose with one or more trihydroxybenzene carboxylic acids. They are hydrolyzed by acids or enzymes to yield several molecules of phenolic acids such as gallic and ellagic acids. The phenolic acids are combined to a central glucose residue by ester linkages. The tannins derived from gallic acid are known as gallitannins and from that of ellagic acid as ellagitannins. Gallitannins occur in Rhubarb, Cloves, Chestnut, Rose petals, Bearbery leaves, Chinese leaves, Turkish galls, Maple and Chestnut. The sources of ellagitannins are Myrobalans, Pomegranate bark and rind, Eucalyptus leaves, Chestnut, Oak bark, etc. These tannins form blue or black colour with ferric chloride, and pyrogallol on heating. They do not give blue colour with bromine solutions.

2. **Condensed Tannins (Proanthocyanidins)** : Condensed tannins are resistant to hydrolysis and they are derived from the flavanols, catechins and flavan-3, 4-diols. On treatment with acids or enzymes they are decomposed into phlobaphenes. On dry distillation condensed tannins produce catechol. Therefore, these tannins are

called as catechol tannins. Condensed tannins are found in bark (Cinnamon, Cinchona, Wild Cherry, Willow, Acacia, Oak and Hamamelis), roots and rhizomes (Krameria and Male fern), seeds (Cacoa, Kola, Areca and Guarana), leaves (Hamamelis and Tea) and extracts (Catechu, Acacia, Butea gum, etc.). These tannins give green colour with ferric chloride solution, produce catechol on heating, yield phloroglucinol with conc. HCl or vanillin-HCl and phlobaphene on oxidation.

3. **Pseudotannins** : Pseudotannins are phenolic compounds of lower molecular weight and they do not show the goldbeater's skin test. They occur as gallic acid (in Rhubarb), catechins (in Catechu, Acacia, Cutch, Kinos, Cacoa, Guarana), chlorogenic acid (in Mate, Coffee and Nux vomica) and ipecacuanhic acid in Ipecacuanha.

Solubility : Tannins are freely soluble in water, alcohol, glycerol, acetone and dilute alkalies. They are sparingly soluble in chloroform, ethyl acetate and some other organic solvents.

Phlobaphenes are soluble in alcohol but practically insoluble in water. Phlobaphenes result from phlobatannins in many ways. They are slowly deposited from a cold aqueous solution of a phlobatannin, and rapidly if the solution is subjected to prolonged boiling, or if boiled with sulphuric acid. Glycerine appears to minimize conversion of phlobatannins to phlobaphenes.

Chemical Tests

1. **Goldbeaters Skin Test** : A small piece of goldbeater's skin (a membrane prepared from the intestine of an ox) is soaked in 2% hydrochloric acid, rinsed with distilled water and placed in a solution of tannin for 5 minutes. The skin piece is washed with distilled water and kept in a solution of ferrous sulphate. A brown or black colour is produced on the skin due to the presence of tannins.

2. **Gelatin Test** : To a solution of tannin (0.5-1%) aqueous solutions of gelatin (1%) and sodium chloride (10%) are added. A white buff-coloured precipitate is formed.

3. **Phenazone Test** : A mixture of aqueous extract (5 ml) of a drug and sodium acid phosphate (0.5g) is heated,

cooled and filtered. A solution of phenazone (2%) is added to the filtrate. A bulky coloured precipitate is formed.

4. **Catechin Test (Matchstick Test)** : A matchstick is dipped in aqueous plant extract, dried near burner and moistened with concentrated hydrochloric acid. On warming near a flame the matchstick wood turns pink or red due to formation of phloroglucinol.

5. **Chlorogenic Acid Test** : An extract of chlorogenic acid containing drug is treated with aqueous ammonia. A green colour is formed on exposure to air.

6. **Vanillin-Hydrochloric Acid Test** : (Vanillin 1 g, alcohol 10 ml, concentrated hydrochloric acid 10 ml). When a drug is treated with vanillin-hydrochloric acid reagent, pink or red colour is formed due to formation of phloroglucinol.

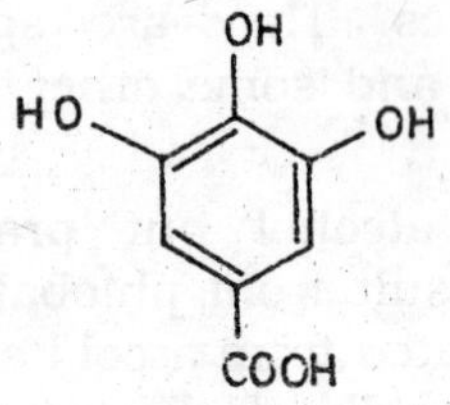

Gallic acid

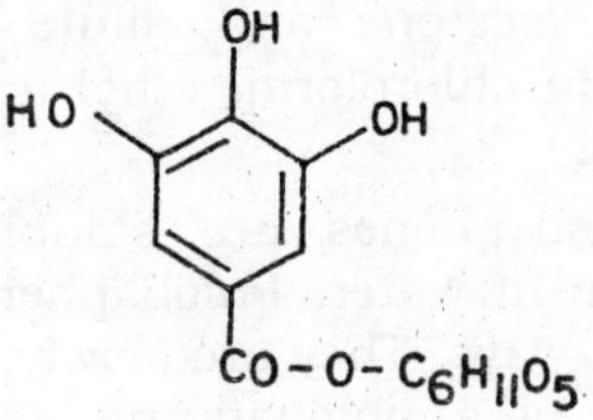

Glucogallin

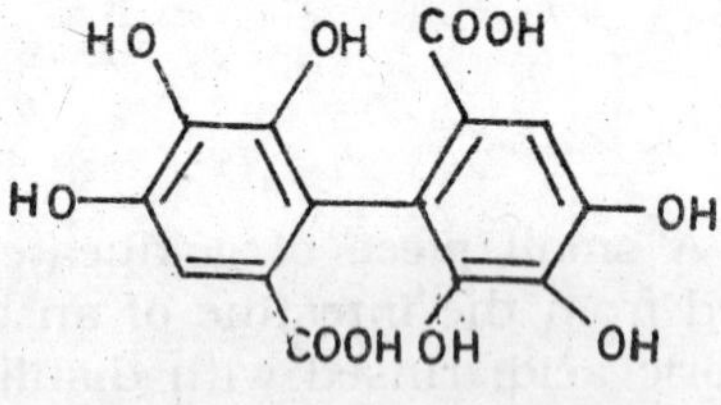

Hexahydroxydiphenic acid

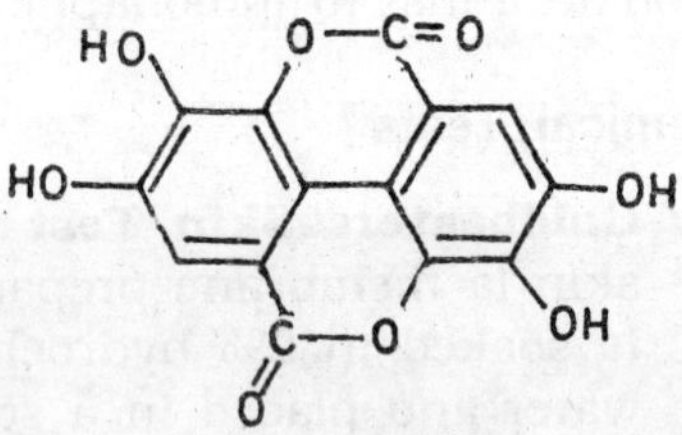

Ellagic acid

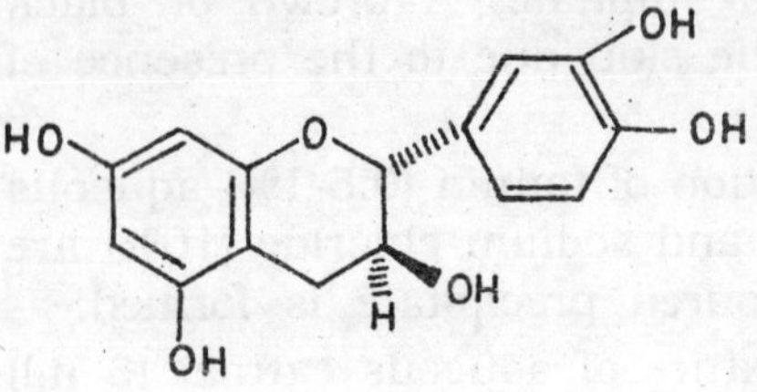

(+)-Catechin

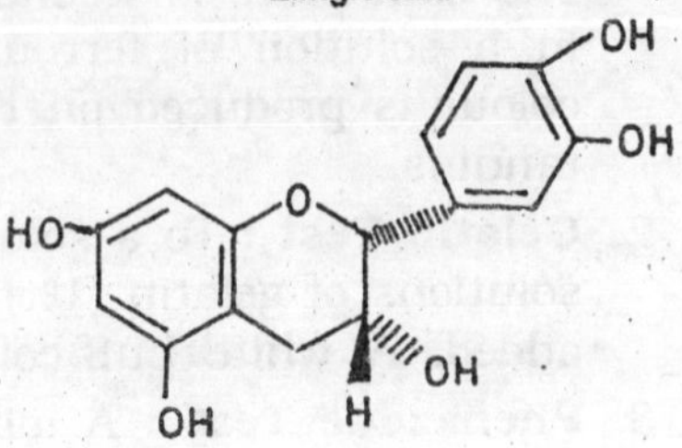

(+)-Epicatechin

PALE CATECHU

Synonyms : Gambier; Catechu; Gambier Catechu; Terra japonica.

Biological Source : Pale Catechu is the dried aqueous extract of leaves and twigs of *Uncaria gambier* (Hunter) Roxb. (syn. *Ourouparia gambier)*.

Family : Rubiaceae.

Habitat : The plant is indigenous to Malaya and cultivated in Indonesia, Malaya and Borneo.

Preparation : Plant is a climbing shrub and grown from seeds. The leafy twigs up to 50 cm in length are cut at an interval of 4-6 months from 2 to 10 years old plant. The leaves and twigs are boiled with water for 3 hours in a large pan. The leaves and twigs are removed and the extract is concentrated to form a yellowish green pasty mass. It is cooled in shallow wood tube, put into trays or tin containers and cut into cubes of uniform size. The cubes are dried in sun, packed and exported. Sometimes semisolid mass is packed into bales. It contains more water, less tannins and is of inferior quality.

Characters : Pale catechu occurs as cubes of 2.5 cm length and breadth. Sometimes cubes are broken and adhere to each other. Colour is dark reddish-brown, internal surface is pale brown and dull. Cubes break easily and are friable. The fractured surface appears porous internally. The drug is odourless and taste is astringent followed by bitterness in the beginning and sweetish afterwards.

Chemical Tests

1. **Gambir-Fluorescin Test** : A mixture of alcoholic extract of Pale Catechu (1 g), sodium hydroxide solution (5 ml), and petroleum ether (5 ml) is shaken and kept for sometimes. The petroleum ether layer shows green fluorescence.

2. Catechin or matchstick test is positive in Pale Catechu.

3. Vanillin-hydrochloric acid test is positive in Pale Catechu.

4. **Chlorophyll Test** : powdered drug (0.5 g) is heated with chloroform (5 ml) on a water bath for 1-2 minutes. The organic layer is filtered in a white China dish and

evaporated on the water. A greenish residue is remained due to the presence of chlorophyll.

Chemical Constituents : Pale Catechu contains catechins (7-33%), catechutannic acid (22-50%), catechu red, quercetin, pyrogallol, Gambir fluorescein, fixed oil and wax. It contains not less than 70% water-soluble substance and not less than 60% alcoholic soluble portion.

Quercetin (R = H)
Quercitrin (R = Rhamnose)

Catechin is crystallized into white, accicular crystals which are water soluble. Removal of one mole of water from catechin gives catechutannic acid which is an amorphous phlobatannin.

Uses : Pale Catechu has astringent action and is used in diarrhoea, in lozenges, for tanning and dyeing fabrics brown or black.

BLACK CATECHU

Synonyms : Cutch, Catechu; Cachou: Peru Catechu; Cashoo; Catechu nigrum; Kattha (Hindi).

Biological Source : Black Catechu is a dried aqueous extract prepared from the heartwood of *Acacia catechu* Willd.

Family : Leguminosae.

Habitat : The tree is a native of India and found in Burma.

Preparation : The tree is felled and bark as well as sapwood are removed, cut into small pieces and boiled with water in earthenware or stainless steel vessels. The decoction is filtered and concentrated to get a viscous mass. The thick syrup is poured into wooden frames on papers, cooled and the solidified product is cut into small pieces.

Characters : Black Catechu occurs in black, irregular mass. Outer surface is rough and dull and rarely glossy. Fracture is hard and brittle and the broken surface is dark brown with a dull gloss and porous. It is partially soluble in cold water and alcohol and completely soluble in hot water. The drug is odourless and taste in bitter in the beginning and astringent afterwards.

Chemical Constituents : Black Catechu contains a mixture of catechin isomers, acacatechin (2-12%), catechutannic acid or phlobatannin (25-35%), gum (20-30%), quercitrin, quercetin, catechu red and water. Acacatechin contains (-)-epicatechin which is the *trans-* form of acacatechin. During the extraction of heartwood chips with boiling water epicatechin undergoes epimerization and recemization to dl-acacatechin. Isomers of acacatechin present in Black Catechu are l-acacatechin (m.p. 230°) and d-iso-acacatechin (m.p. 226-228°).

Acacatechin is insoluble in cold water but soluble in hot water. It undergoes oxidation to catechutannic acid in the presence of water.

Uses : Black Catechu possesses cooling and digestive properties. It is used in relaxed condition of throat, mouth and gums and in cough and diarrhoea. Externally as an astringent medicament it is applied to ulcers, boils, and skin eruptions and in a number of medicinal preparations.

Black Catechu is mainly used as an ingredient of betal leaf (Paan) and *Paan masala.*

Chemical Tests

1. Catechin (match-stick) test is positive.
2. Vanillin-hydrochloric acid test is positive.
3. Gambir-fluorescin test is negative distinguishing it from Pale Catechu.
4. Chlorophyll test is also negative distinguishing Black Catechu from Pale Catechu.
5. Add a few drops of a fresh aqueous extract to lime water (10 ml); a brown colour is produced and on standing for three minutes a red precipitate is formed.
6. To an aqueous solution (2%), add solution of ferric ammonium sulphate; a dark green colour is formed. Add sodium hydroxide solution, the colour changes to purple.

GALLS

Synonyms : Turkey galls, Galla, Nutgall, Aleppo galls, Blue galls, Gallae ceruleae.

Biological Source : Galls are vegetable outgrowths formed on the twigs of dyer's oak. *Quercus infectoria* (Fam. Fagaceae) due to deposition of eggs of the gall-wasp *Adleria gallaetinctoriae* Olivier (Fam. (Cynipidae).

Habitat : The plant is found in Turkey, Syria, Persia, Cyprus and Greece.

Preparation : The plant is a 2 m high small tree or shrub. The gall-wesp lays eggs on the twigs in early summer. Larvae come out from the eggs and enter into the soft epidermis near the growing point of the twigs. The larvae secrete an enzyme from its mandible which stimulates abnormal development of vegetable tissues around the larvae. During this process their is rapid conversion of starch in the surrounding tissues into sugars which stimulates cell division. Shrinkage of tissue takes place due to disappearing of starch and a central cavity is formed in which development of larvae and pupae takes place. The larva remains in the galls for 5 to 6 months. The mature insect bores the covering of the galls and escapes. The colour of galls changes from bluish-grey to white during this process. The galls are collected before escaping the insect.

Characters : Galls are globular or subspherical in shape, 1-2.5 cm in diameter with short basal stalk. Numerous rounded projections are present on the outer surface. 'White galls', from which the insects have emerged, contain circular holes, 2-3 mm in diameter, on the lower part on one side. Colour is grey or white and the projections are dark brown in colour. White galls are brownish or yellowish-brown. Gall are hard and heavy and shrink in water. Taste is very astringent.

Chemical Constituents : Galls contain tannin known as gallotannic acid (50-70%), gallic acid (2-4%), ellagic acid, β-sitosterol, methyl betulate, methyl oleanolate, starch, calcium oxalate, nyctanthic acid, roburic acid and syringic acid.

Uses : Galls are used as astringent, for tanning and dyeing, and in the manufacture of inks and tannic acid.

Allied Drugs

Chinese and Japanese Galls : They are produced on the petioles of the leaves of *Rhus chinensis* (Anacardiaceae) by an aphis, *Schlechtendalia chinensis*. The galls on breaking show a large, irregular cavity and contain tannin (57-77%). They are used as astringent and to treat haemorrhoids.

Crowned Aleppo Galls : They are about globular, 0.5 cm in diameter, stalked and contained a crown of projections near the apex. They are produced by an insect, *Cynips polycera.*

Hungarian Galls : They are formed on a tree, *Quercus robur*, growing in Yungoslavia, by an insect *Cynip lignicola.* They are used in tanning.

English Oak Galls : They are produced by *Adleria kollari* on *Quercus robur* and contain tannins (15-20%).

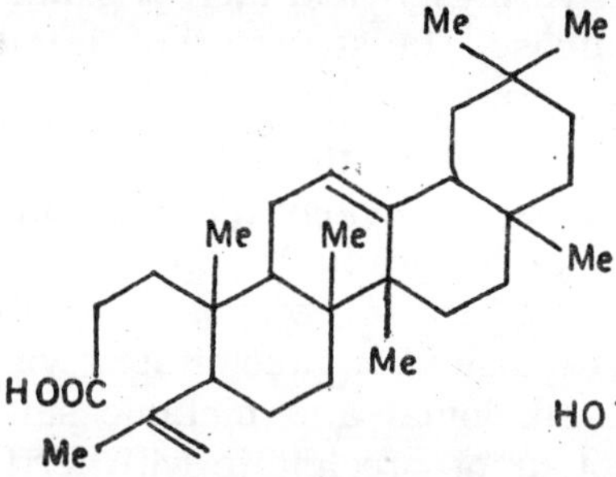

Nyctanthic acid

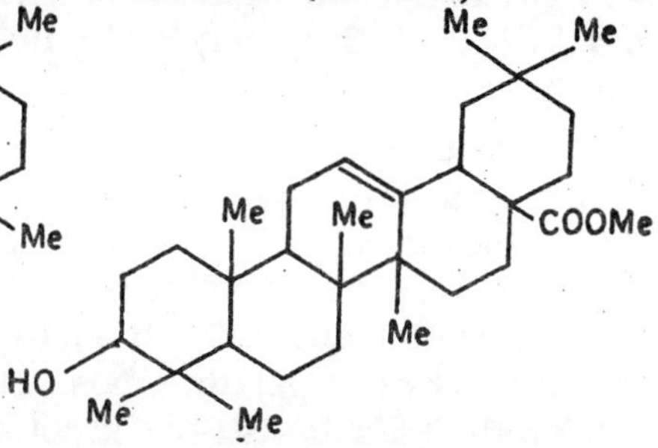

Methyl oleanolate

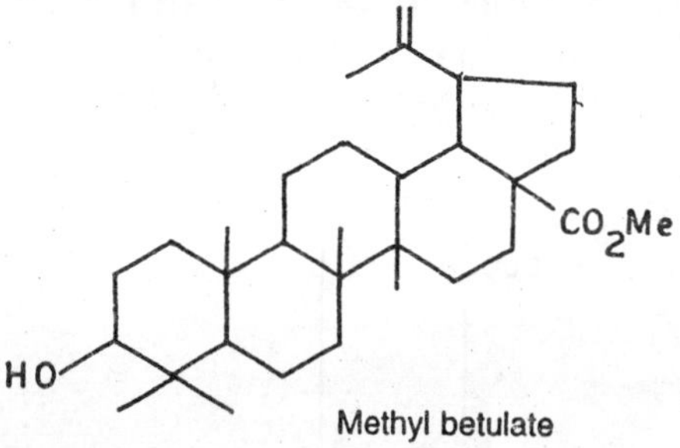

Methyl betulate

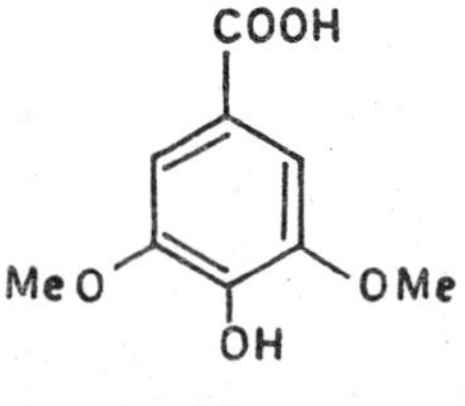

Syringic acid

TANNIC ACID

Synonyms : Tannin, Gallotannin, Gallotannic acid.

Biological Source : Tannic acid occurs in nutgalls of *Quercus infectoria* Oliv, bark of the oak species, in Sumac and Myrobalan. It is produced from Turkish or Chinese nutgalls, the former containing, 50-60%, the latter about 70%. Galls are produced by an aphis, *Schlerchtendalia chinensis*, on the petioles of the leaves of *Rhus chinensis* (Fam. Anacardiaceae).

Preparation : Tannic acid is obtained by extracting powdered galls with a mixture of ether, alcohol and water. Two layers are formed; the aqueous layer contain gallotannin and the free gallic acid is present in the ethereal layer which is evaporated to get the gallic acid. Tannic acid is purified by various procedures.

Previous to extraction the galls are exposed to a moist atmosphere for some time, during which fermentative changes occur and the yield is increased.

Chemical Composition : The chemistry of the tannic acid is most complex and non-uniform. Tannic acid is not a single homogenous compound but a mixture of esters of gallic acid with glucose. Chinese Galls on hydrolysis yield methyl gallate and 1, 2, 3, 4, 6-pentagalloyl glucose. The structure of tannic acid named corilagin is given hereunder.

Tannic acid is yellowish white to light brown, amorphous, bulky powder or flakes, or spongy masses; faint characteristic odour, astringent taste, gradually darkens on exposure to air and light, mp 210-215°, decomposes mostly into pyrogallol and CO_2. It gives insoluble precipitates with albumin, starch, gelatin, most alkaloidal and metallic salts and produces a bluish-black colour or precipitate with ferric salts. One gram of tannic acid is dissolved in 0.35 ml water, 1 ml warm glycerol; very soluble in alcohol and acetone, practically insoluble in benzene, chloroform, ether, petroleum ether, carbon disulphide and carbon tetrachloride.

Corilagin

Uses : Tannic acid is astringent and is used as hemostatic, in solution for burns and as a heavy metal antidote and in case of alkaloidal poisoning. It is also used as mordant in dyeing, manufacturing ink; sizing paper and silk; printing fabrics, with gelatin and albumin for manufacturing of imitation horn and tortoise shell, tanning, clarifying beer or wine, in photography, as coagulant in rubber manufacturing, for commericial preparation of gallic acid and pyrogallol and as a reagent in analytical chemistry.

Utilization of certain tannin-rich plant materials for long time may be harmful due to their carcinogenic activity. The habitual chewing of betal nut (Areca catechu) produces oral and esophageal cancer. The drug contains piperidine-type alkaloids like arecoline, arecaidine, guvacine and guvacoline and is also rich in condensed tannins. Utilization of ordinary tea (leaves of Camellia sinensis) without milk causes esophageal obstruction. Milk binds tannins of the tea and it becomes less harmful.

The property of precipitation of proteins by tannins is also utilized in the process of vegetable tanning. It converts animal hides to leather. The tannin affects the pliancy and toughness of the leather and acts as a preservative due to its antiseptic action. Different types of tannins produce a variety of leather. Certain hydrolyzable tannins form a bloom leather whereas the nonhydrolyzable tannins give the tanner's red leather. Solutions of tannins are used in the laboratory as reagents for the detection of gelatin, proteins and alkaloids due to their precipitating properties.

QUESTIONS

1. Enlist four plant drugs containing tannins and give their exact botanical source, chemical constituents and therapeutic uses

2. What are tannins? Name the drugs which contain tannins . and give their official source, chemical constituents and uses

3. Describe tannins. Discuss official sources, chemical constituents and uses of tannin containing drugs.

4. How is Black Catechu differentiated from Pale Catechu? Describe biological source, chemical constituents, preparation and uses of Black and Pale catechues.

9

FATS, OILS AND WAXES

Fixed oils and fats are esters of glycerol with higher long-chain fatty acids such as palmitic, stearic, oleic, and linoleic acids. Fats are solid or semi-solid at 15.5-16.5°C while oils occur as liquid at this temperature. These compounds are obtained from plants (Arachis oil, Castor oil) or animals (Lard, Cod liver oil). There is no chemical difference in fats and oils. The fatty acids may be saturated (e.g., palmitic acid, stearic acid) or unsaturated (e.g. oleic acid), but usually they contain unbranched carbon chains and have an even number of carbon atoms.

Most of the saturated glycerides are solid at ordinary temperature, but most unsaturated glycerides are oily liquids. Therefore, vegetable oils contain larger proportions of unsaturated glycerides than the solid animal fats. The identity, quality and purity of fatty substances are determined by finding out their acid value, saponification value, Reichert-Meissl number, iodine number, melting point, specific gravity and refractive index.

If the fatty acid present in a glyceryl ester is the same, then it is known as 'simple' glyceride. For example, tripalmitin, tristearin, and triolein are simple glycerides. If different fatty acids are present in a glyceride, then it is called as mixed glyceride, e.g., 2-oleodipalmitin and 1-oleo-2-palmitostearin. In mixed glycerides two or sometimes three different acid groupings are present. Animal fats, such as Lard and Suet, and 'fixed' or fatty vegetable oils, such as Olive oil, Almond oil, and Theobroma oil, are mixtures of glycerides. On hydrolysis they yield both saturated and unsaturated acids. In addition to glycerides, the oils and fats contain other substances like phosphatides, phytosterols, stigmasterol, hydrocarbons, fat-soluble vitamins A, D and E and some volatile substances.

Seeds are the principal source of fats and oils. The oil containing seeds are Sesame seed, Coconut, Arachis, Castor, etc. The compounds are also present in Olive fruits, Cod liver, Shark, etc. The fats and oils are important products used as pharmaceutically, industrially and as articles of food.

Fixed oils and fats are separated from plant parts by hot or cold expression in hydraulic press or by extraction with an organic solvent. Animal fats are isolated by heating the animal tissues with steam. The fat melts which floats on the top and is separated by decantation.

Fats and oils have certain common characteristics. They are greasy subtances and are lighter than water. They are insoluble in water, sparingly soluble in alcohol, and freely soluble in solvent like petroleum ether, chloroform and benzene. Their specific gravity is always less than water and, therefore, they float on the aqueous surface. When a drop of fats or oils is placed on a paper, they form a permanent translucent stain on it. Due to this property they are called as fixed oils. They cannot be distilled and on heating they are decomposed producing an odour of scorched fat due to formation of acraldehyde ($CH_2=CH\text{-}CHO$). Many fats and oils become rancid on long exposure to air, give acidic reactions and develop very disagreeable odour. In moist conditions the hydrolysis of fats is affected with lipase enzyme and free fatty acids are formed. In the presence of light and micorganisms keto-, keto acid-, oxide- and peroxide-derivatives of fatty acids are produced and all these substances are responsible for rancidity of fats.

The oil obtained by expression contains water, mucilaginous matter, and ground seed tissues in suspension. It may also have a strong odour and a dark colour. The presence of a very small proportion of fatty acid affects the taste and flavour of oils. The oils is purified and refined by removing free fatty acids, decolourization, deodourization and demargination. Free fatty acids are removed by adding sodium hydroxide solution and the resulting sodium salts are separated by suitable means. For decolourizing, the oil is heated to about 200°C for about 30 minutes with 2-4% fuller's earth and 0.2-1.0% of animal charcoal, followed by filtration. For deodourization, the oil is placed in an autoclave, vacuum is created in the apparatus and then superheated for a very short time. In demargination process, the solid glycerides are removed at room temperature. Cod-liver oil is to be demarginated and this is accomplished by cooling it to about 0°C; at which tempearture a portion solidifies and is separated by filtration, the filtrate constituting non-freezing Cod Liver oil.

Catalytic reduction of unsaturated fatty acids in the presence of hydrogen and a catalyst (e.g., Raney Nickel or Pd-C) yields saturated compounds which are solid at normal temperature. Vegetable ghee is prepared by hydrogenation of oils.

A thin layer of Linseed oil is dried and forms a hard transparent film. This oil is, therefore, called as drying oil and used in paints and varnishes. Cottonseed oil resinifies and dries without forming a thin film. Such oils are called semi-drying oils. Some Oils, like Olive oil, neither dry nor form a thin layer. Such oils are called as non-drying oils.

Fatty acids are used to treat skin lesions (linolenic and linoleic acids), wounds, burns, sunburns, eczema and dandruff; as emollient, laxative (Castor oil), in the preparation of ointments, liniments and suppositories, as a source of vitamins A, D and E; as cholesterol suppressant, antifungal agent, and in the manufacture of soaps, glycerine, paints, varnishes and lubricants.. Chaulmoogra oil is utilized to cure leprosy.

Saturated Fatty Acids Detected in Oils and Fats

Butyric	$CH_3 (CH_2)_2 COOH$
Isovaleric	$(CH_3)_2 CHCH_2 COOH$
Caproic	$CH_3 (CH_2)_4 COOH$
Caprylic	$CH_3 (CH_2)_6 COOH$
Capric	$CH_3 (CH_2)_8 COOH$
Lauric	$CH_3 (CH_2)_{10} COOH$
Myristic	$CH_3 (CH_2)_{12} COOH$
Palmitic	$CH_3 (CH_2)_{14} COOH$
Stearic	$CH_3 (CH_2)_{16} COOH$
Arachidic	$CH_3 (CH_2)_{18} COOH$
Behenic	$CH_3 (CH_2)_{20} COOH$
Lignoceric	$CH_3 (CH_2)_{22} COOH$
Cerotic	$CH_3 (CH_2)_{24} COOH$

Unsaturated Fatty Acids Detected in Oils and Fats

Palmitoleic	$CH_3 (CH_3)_5 CH=CH (CH_2)_7 COOH$
Oleic	$CH_3 (CH_2)_7 CH=CH (CH_2)_7 COOH$
Ricinoleic	$CH_3 (CH_2)_5 CHOH-CH_2 CH=CH (CH_2)_7 COOH$
Linoleic	$CH_3 (CH_2)_4 CH=CHCH_2 CH=CH (CH_2)_7 COOH$
Linolenic	$CH_3 CH_2 CH=CHCH_2 CH=CHCH_2 CH=CH- (CH_2)_7 COOH$
Eleostearic	$CH_3 (CH_2)_3 (CH=CH)_3 (CH_2)_7 COOH$
Licanic	$CH_3 (CH_2)_3 (CH=CH)_3 (CH_2)_4 CO(CH_2)_2 COOH$
Parinaric	$CH_3 CH_2 (CH=CH)_4 (CH_2)_7 COOH$
Tariric	$CH_3 (CH_2)_7C\equiv C (CH_2)_7 COOH$
Gadoleic	$CH_3 (CH_2)_9 CH=CH (CH_2)_7 COOH$
Arachidonic	$CH_3 (CH_2)_4 (CH=CHCH_2)_4 (CH_2)_2 COOH$
Cetoleic	$CH_3 (CH_2)_9 CH=CH (CH_2)_9 COOH$
Erucic	$CH_3 (CH_2)_7 CH=CH (CH_2)_{11} COOH$
Selacholeic or nervonic	$CH_3 (CH_2)_7 CH=CH (CH_2)_{13} COOH$

CASTOR OIL

Synonyms : Castor bean oil; Castor oil seed; Ricinus oil; Oil of Palma Christi; Tangantangan oil; Neoloid; *Oleum Ricini,* Cold-drawn Castor oil.

Biological Source : Castor oil is a fixed oil obtained by cold-expression from the seeds of *Ricinus communis* Linn.

Family : Euphorbiaceae.

Habitat : The plant is extensively cultivated in temperate climate such as India, South America, African countries, Brazil, China, East and West Indies and Thailand. The plant is an annual soft-wooden 15 meters high tree.The fruit is a three-celled spiny capsule, each cell has an ovoid albuminous seed.

Cultivation : Castor is an essential crop of the tropics and to some extent of sub-tropics. It is grown on sandy or clayey deep red loams and on good light alluvial loams. Generally seeds are sown in September-October. Affication of organic manures such as farmyard manure, groundnut or castor cake, and inorganic fertilizers is beneficial. The harvesting period varies between 4 and 9 months. The harvested spikes are stacked in heaps till the capsules blacken. They are dried in the sunlight. The seeds are beaten out of the capsules by sticks, or thrushed under the feet of bullocks.

Characters of Seeds : The seeds are oval, anatropous, compressed, 0.8-1.8 cm long, 0.4-1.2 cm broad with variable size and colour. The testa is smooth, thin and brittle. The colour is grey, brown or black with brown or black mottled. At one end there is a small yellowish caruncle from which the raphe extends on the flat or ventral side, to the chalazal at the opposite end. The testa is easily removable exposing the large white and oily endosperm bearing thin, flat foliaceous cotyledons, one on either side of a central, lenticular cavity, and connected with the short caulicle and radicle.

Castor oil Preparation : The seed coat is removed by passing the seeds through a decorticator. The rollers with sharp cutting edges break testa but do not injure the kernel. The tasta are removed by sieves and compressed air. The kernels are cold expressed with 1-2 pressure per sq. inch to get about 30% oil. The oil is filtered and steam is passed through the oil to destroy toxic proteins albumins (ricin). The oil is bleached and sold.

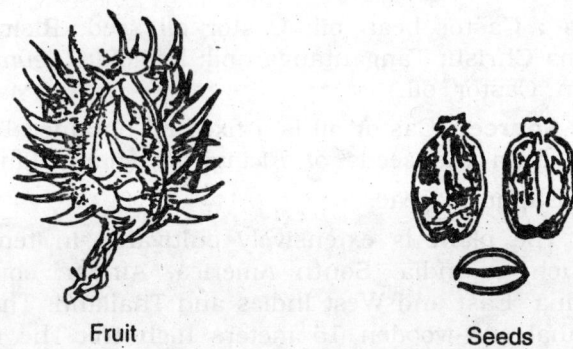

Fruit   Seeds

Fig. 9.1. Castor *(Ricinus communis)*

Characters : Castor oil is a colourless or pale yellow viscous liquid. It has slight somewhat characteristic (nauseating) odour. The crude oil tastes slightly acrid with a decidedly nauseating after-taste. It has excellent keeping qualities, and does not turn rancid unless subjected to excessive heat. When exposed to the air, it gradually thickens, darkens in colour and develops more intense odour and taste. It is dextrorotatory, $(\alpha)_D$ 0.96, viscosity 6-8 poises, acid value <4, saponification number 176-187, iodine number 81-91, acetyl value 144-150, hydroxyl value 161-169. It is miscible with alcohol, ether, chloroform and glacial acetic acid. It dissolves in its own volume of petroleum ether and in 95% alcohol due to the presence of hydroxyl group in ricinoleic acid. When heated to 300° for several hours it polymerizes and becomes miscible with mineral oil.

Chemical Constituents : Castor seeds contain fixed oil (45-55%), proteins (20%) consisting of globulin, albumin, nucleoalbumin, glycoprotein and ricin (a toxalbumin), ricinine alkaloid and some enzymes. The fixed oil consists of the glycerides of ricinoleic (87%), isoricinoleic, stearic (1%), dihydroxystearic (traces), linoleic (3%), oleic (7%), and palmitic (2%) acids. The purgative nature of the oil is due to free ricinoleic acid and its stereoisomers which are produced by hydrolysis of triricinolein by lipases in the duodenum.

Uses : Castor oil is purgative and emollient. It is used as ointment base, for the preparation of flexible collodion, to prepare undecylenic acid which is a fungistatic preparation, to manufacture lipsticks, perfumed hair oil and hair fixers. As an industrial raw material it is used for the preparation of chemical derivatives used in coating, urethane derivatives, surfactants and dispersants, cosmetics, lubricants, paints, varnishes, grease, polishes, etc. It is the chief raw material for the production of sebacic acid.

SHARK LIVER OIL

Synonym : Oleum selachoide.

Biological Source : Shark liver oil is the fixed oil obtained from the fresh and healthy livers of shark fish, *Hypoprion brevirostris.*

Order : Selachii.

Habitat : Shark is found on seacoasts of many European countries and in India in Tamil Nadu, Maharastra and Kerala.

Preparation : Livers are removed from the fishes, cleaned thoroughly, freed from fatty substances and attached tissues like gall-bladders. Then the livers are heated in water at about 80°C. The oil exudes, floats on the top, and is separated, washed and water is removed. The dehydrated oil is cooled to separate stearin. The suspended materials are removed by centrifugation. The oil is supplemented with vitamins A and D in desired amount.

Characters : Shark liver oil is pale yellow to brownish yellow viscous liquid with fishy odour and bland taste. It is insoluble in water, sparingly soluble in alcohol and freely miscible in non-polar solvents such as petroleum ether, chloroform and benzene. Its acid value is about 2, saponification value 150-200 and iodine value 160-350.

Chemical Constituents : The active principle of Shark liver oil is vitamin A which varies from 15,000-30,000 I.U. per g of the oil. It contains glycerides of saturated and unsaturated fatty acids.

Chemical Tests

1. A solution of Shark liver oil (1 drop) in chloroform (1 ml) is treated with sulphuric acid (1 drop). A violet colour changing to purple or brown is formed due to the presence of vitamin A.

2. Shark liver oil (1 ml) is dissolved in chloroform (10 ml). Few drops of saturated solution of antimony trichloride in chloroform are added to the solution. A blue colour is formed due to the presence of vitamin A.

Uses : Shark liver oil is used to treat xerophthalmia (abnormal dryness of the surface of conjunctiva) occurring due to deficiency of vitamin A. The oil is nutritive and used as tonic.

Storage : The oil is sensitive to light and air. It should be stored in air tight, completely filled, coloured containers.

ARACHIS OIL

Synonyms : Groundnut oil; Monkeynut oil; Peanut oil; Katchung oil; Earth-nut oil.

Biological Source : Arachis oil is obtained by expression of shelled and skinned seeds of *Arachis hypogaea* Linn.

Family : Leguminosae.

Habitat : South America (Brazil) is the original home of ground nut and now found in South and Central America, Peru, Argentina, Nigeria, Australia, Gambia, and other reasonably warm regions of all countries.

Groundnut plant is a small, prostrate, diffuse, erect, branched, annual herb, 30-60 cm in height, leaves alternate with adnate stipules and yellow papilionaceous flowers. After fertilization, the pedicel elongates rapidly and enters the ground, where the ovary begins to develop into a pod maturing in about two months. Pods or nuts are cylindrical, hard, reticulated, indehiscent and inflated, 2.5-5.0 cm long, 1-3 seeded, with pericarp constricted between the seeds. The seeds are covered by a light or deep reddish brown seeds coat, and consisting of two white fleshy cotyledons rich in oil and proteins.

Fruits are dug out by raking the plants from the soil, seeds are separated by machine and expressed in a hydraulic press at ordinary temperature. The remaining oil of cakes is removed by solvent extraction. The two oil fractions are combined and purified.

Cultivation : Groundnut is predominantly a crop of the tropical and subtropical countries, up to an elevation of 1,160 m. It requires plenty of sunlight, timely and evently distributed rainfall (50-125 cm) during its growth and a long season for its maturation and harvesting. It also requires a high temperature (21-26°) particularly during the nights to induce early flowering. The plant does not stand frost, long and severe drought and water stagnation. Groundnut seeds are sown from April-May to June-July. It requires light, well-drained, loose, friable soil. No regular manuring is done by the growers and the plant is benefitted from green manuring.

Groundnut is susceptible to infection by se eral fungi, bacteria and viruses. Some important diseases in India are tikka leaf spot, collar rot, dry root rot, stem rot, rust, bud necrosis and yellow mould.

Groundnut Oil : It is a non-drying oil belonging to the oleo-linoleic acid group of oils. It is pale-yellow in colour or almost colourless liquid with a nutty odour and bland taste. Clouds are formed in the oil at low room temperature. It has acid value 0.08-6, saponification value 188-195, iodine value 84-102; thiocyanogen value 67-73 and hydroxyl value 2.5-9.5. It very slowly thickens and becomes rancid on prolonged exposure to air. It is miscible with solvent ether, petroleum ether, chloroform, carbon disulphide, benzene; very slightly soluble in alcohol.

Chemical Constituents : The important constituents of the glycerides of groundnut oil are the fatty acids palmitic (8.3%) stearic (3.1%) oleic (56%), linoleic (26%), arachidic (24%)

eicosenoic, behenic (3.1%) and lignoceric (1.1) acids. Myristic, hexacosanoic, erucic, caprylic, lauric and trace amounts of odd carbon fatty acids are also present.

The principal glycerides of the oil are triolein (11%), dioleolinolein (21%), saturated oleolinoleins (22%), dilinoleoolein (12%), saturated diolein (15%) and saturated dilinoleoolein (6%).

The yellow colour of the oil is due to the presence of carotenoid pigments, chiefly β-carotene and lutein. The unsaponifiable matter consists of sterols, (campesterol, stigmasterol, β-sitosterol and cholesterol), sterol glycosides (β-sitosterol-D-glycoside and others), and triterpenoid alcohols (β-amyrin, cycloartenol and 24-methylene cycloartenol). Tocopherols occur free in groundnut oil. Squalene, an unsaturated hydrocarbon, occurs in extremely small amounts in the unsaponifiable fraction. Two other unsaturated hydrocarbons, hypogene and arachidene, have also been reported.

The kernels contain fixed oil (40-50%), proteins (26.2%), water (1.8%), carbohyorates (20.6%), ash and high concentration of thiamine. The chief proteins are arachin and conarchin, both are globulins of different solubility. The vitamin content of groundnut is moderate, the largest being in the episperm.

Uses : Groundnut oil is used as an edible oil, in control of pasture bloat, as a substitute for Olive oil, as a solvent in pharmaceutical aid, in hydrogenated state as shortening, in mayonnaise, in confections; for the manufacture of margarine, soap, paints, liniments, plasters and ointments, as vehicle for intramuscular medication and in the laboratory as heat transfer medium in melting point apparatus.

SESAME OIL

Synonyms : Benne oil; Teel oil; Gingelli oil, Sesamum Seed oil.

Biological Source : Sesame oil is obtained by refining the expressed or extracted oil from the seeds of cultivated varieties of *Sesamum indicum* Linn.

Family : Pedaliaceae.

Habitat : The plant is widely cultivated in India, China, Japan, East Indies, West Indies and in the southern United States.

Cultivation : The plant is an annual herb, 1 m in height. Sesamum is cultivated in the plains and on elevations up to 1,200 m at temperature of 21° and above. It requires a warm climate and cannot withstand frost, continued heavy rain or prolonged drought. It grows on a light well-drained soil which is capable of retaining adequate moisture. It thrives best on typical sandy loams.

The seeds are sown broadcast. In nothern India the crop is sown in June-July and harvested in October-November. The crop is not generally manured.

The seeds are small, flat, oval, smooth and shiny, whitish, yellow or reddish brown; sweet and oily taste; odour is slight. They are pointed at one end where hilum is located, raphe runs as a line from hilum, along the centre of one flat face to the broader end. The endosperm is present as a thin layer around the embryo. The seeds contain fixed oil (45-55%), proteins (aleurone, 22%) and mucilage (4%).

Preparation : The oil is expressed by hydraulic or low and medium-powered screw presses. A good yield of the oil is obtained by three successive expression. Prior to processing in the screw press, the seed is subjected to a cooking process. If live steam is used for cooking, the cuticles separate partly from the kernels and the mixture of kernels, cuticles and seed slips in the cage and lumpy material is obtained instead of a firm cake. If the seed is heated in cooker without the addition of steam or water, and water is added at the point of entry of dried seed into the screw press cage, the efficiency of oil extraction is greatly enhanced. Alkali refining, bleaching, hydrogenation and decolourization of Sesame oil can be effected with very little loss.

The sesame oil is pale yellow liquid, almost odourless, bland taste, saponification no. 188-193, iodine no. 103-122, soluble in chloroform, solvent and petroleum ether, carbon disulphide; slightly soluble in alcohol and insoluble in water.

Chemical Constituents : Sesame oil consists of a mixture of glycerides of oleic (43%), linoleic (43%), palmitic (9%), stearic (4%), arachidic, hexadecenoic, lignoceric and myristic acids. It also contains the lignan sesamin (1%) and the related sesamolin, and vitamins A and E.

Sesamol forms pink colour when the oil (2 ml) is shaken with concentrated hydrochloric acid (1 ml) containing 1% sucrose (Bandouin's test). Furfural may be used in place of sucrose and this modified test (Villavecchia test) is widely used to detect Sesame oil in other oils and fats. The presence of sesamolin or free sesamol is responsible for this colour which are not found in other vegetable oil.

Uses: Sesame oil is used as demulcent, in dysentery and urinary complaints, as a solvent for injection of steroids, antibiotics, and hormones, as mild laxative, nutritive, emollient, pediculicide, in manufacture of oleomargarine, cosmetics, iodized oil, anti acids, ointment, etc. It is injectable as a vehicle for fat soluble substances. The oil is also used an insecticidal sprays.

Sesamin   Sesamolin

LINSEED AND LINSEED OIL

Synonyms : Flax seed, Alsi (Hindi), Linum; Semina Lini.

Biological Source : Linseed is the dried, ripe seed of *Linum usitatissimum* Linn. Linseed oil is obtained by expression of linseeds.

Family : Linaceae.

Habitat: Linseed is cultivated in many sub-tropical countries such as South America, India, USA, Canada, England, Russia, Greece, Italy, Spain and Algeria.

Collection : Linseed in an erect annual herb, 60-120 cm high with sky-blue flowers and a globular capsule. The plant is cultivated for its seeds and fibre (flax). A moderate rainfall is best suited for its growth. It grows in almost all types of soils where sufficient moisture is available, but thrives best in heavy soils with high moisture retaining capacity. As a mixed crop it is sown either on the margins of fields or in rows alternating with the other crop. Nitrogenous fertilizers yield better crop. The crop is harvested in February and March before the capsules are dried. Plants are cut close to the ground, dried in the field and threshed to separate seeds.

Morphology of Seeds : The seeds are oval, flattened, 4-6 mm long, and 2-3 mm wide. Testa is glossy, smooth, reddish-brown with minutely pitted surface. Seeds are rounded at one end. The other end is obliquely pointed where the hilum and micropyle are present in a slight depression. Raphe is present along one edge. Endosperm is narrow and encircles the embryo. It consists of two thick flattened, planoconvex cotyledons and a radicle. The seeds are odourless but possess an oily and mucilaginous taste.

Chemical Constituents : Linseed contains fixed oil (30-40%), mucilage (6%), protein (25%) (linin and colinin), small amount of enzyme lipase and linamarin which is a cyanogenetic glycoside. The carbohydrates present are sucrore, raffinose, cellulose and mucilage. Linamarin is a glucose ether of acetone cyanohydrin and is identical to phaseolunatin. Unripe seeds contain starch which is converted to mucilage on ripening the seeds. Mucilage consists of calcium salts of linseed acids which on hydrolysis produces arabinose, rhamnose, galactose, galacturonic acid and xylose. Mucilage swells with water and forms red colour with ruthenium red. Linamarin on hydrolysis yields acetone, hydrocyanic acid and· glucose. The other constituents are phytin, lecithin, wax, resin, pigments, and malic acid.

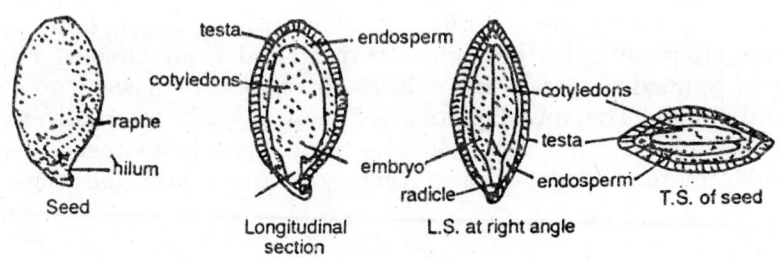

Fig. 9.2. Linseed

LINSEED OIL

Preparation : The dried seeds are crushed in rollers, moistened and heated to 80-90° C in steam to soften the seed tissues. They are then pressed through hot hydraulic press at a high pressure. The oil so obtained is treated with alkali to separate free fatty acids and bleached with fuller's earth or charcoal. On cooling the oil waxy substances are removed.

Linseed oil is a yellowish liquid, with a peculiar odour and bland taste. On exposure to air it gradually thickens, becomes darker and acquires a more pronounced odour and taste. On drying it forms a hard varnish. It has a high iodine value (~170) which indicates the presence of excess amount of glycerides of unsaturated fatty acids. The oil is slightly soluble in alcohol, miscible with chloroform, ether, petroleum ether, carbon disulphide and terpentine oil. It has density 0.925-0.935, viscocity 1.47, congealing point -20°C, saponification number 187-195, refractive index 1.47-1.48, and unsaponifiable matters not over 1.5%. A water-soluble resinous matter with antioxidant properties has been isolated from the oil.

On hydrolysis Linseed oil produces unsaturated acids like linolenic acid (30-50%), linoleic acid (23-24%), oleic acid (10-18%) together with saturated acids-myristic, stearic and palmitic (5-11%).

Uses : Linseed is used as demulcent and in form of poultices for gouty and rheumatic swellings. Internally it is used for gonorrhoea and irritation of the genito-urinary system. Linseed oil has emollient, expectorant, diuretic, demulcent and laxative properties and is utilized externally in lotions and liniments. Non-staining iodine ointment, soap, linoleum, greases, polishes, polymers, varnishes, paints, putty, oil cloths, printing inks, artificial rubber, tracing cloth, tanning and enamelling leather, etc. are prepared from Linseed oil. It is applied to paper and fabrics to render them waterproof and tough. The mucilaginous infusion is used internally as a demulcent in colds, coughs and bronchial affections, inflammation of the urinary tract, gonorrhoea and diarrhoea.

Linamarin   Vitamin A

Adulterants : When market price is high, Linseed oil is adulterated with vegetable oils, such as rape, cottonseed, soyabean, sunflower, safflower and candlenut, as well as with rosin and mineral and fish oils. Boiled linseed oil is more frequently adulterated than raw oil. Adulteration is rather difficult.

Admixture of rape and mustard oil may be detected by the presence of erucic acid; the adulterants lower the saponification value. Fish oil may be detected by the odour produced on heating and by melting points of ether - insoluble bromides. Rosin and mineral oils increase the proportion of unsaponifiable matter.

OLIVE OIL

Synonyms : Salad oil; Sweet oil, Oleum olival.

Biological Source : Olive oil is a fixed oil obtained by expression of the ripe fruits of *Olea europoea* Linn. (Fam. Oleaceae).

Geographical Source : Olive is a native of Palestine and produced extensively in the countries adjoining the Mediterranean sea, Spain being the largest producer. It is also grown in the south western United States and many other subtropical localities.

The tree is propagated by cuttings; grafting and budding of *O. europoea* or Indian olive *(O. ferruginea)*.

For proper growth the plant needs deep fertile soil and a temperature average to 13° not dropping to below -10°.

Collection and Preparation : The olive is an evergreen tree, up to 12 m in height which produces drupaceous fruits about 2-3 cm in length, purplish in colour when ripe. The fruits are collected from November to April. After grinding, the pulp is introduced into coarse, grass baskets and placed in a screw press. The oil coming out is collected into tubes containing water and the upper layer is skimmed off. The product is called as *Virgin oil* obtained by gently pressing the peeled pulp freed from the endocarp. The marc is then treated with water and again expressed to yield second grade of edible oil. Finally, the pulp is mixed with hot water and pressed again for technical oil. The pulp may be extracted with carbon disulphide to obtain "sulphur" olive oil of inferior quality. The yield is from 15 to 40 per cent. If the fruit is not fully mature, the yield of the oil is poor and its taste is bitter.

Characters : Olive oil is a pale yellow or light greenish-yellow due to presence of chlorophyll or carotenes, non-drying oily liquid with a pleasanting delicate flavour. Taste is bland becoming faintly acrid. It is miscible with ether, chloroform and carbon disulphide and is slightly soluble in alcohol. Upon cooling at +5 to 10° it becomes cloudy and at 0°C it usually forms a whitish granular mass. It becomes rancid on exposure to air. It has specific gravity of 0.914-0.919, acid value 0.2-2.8, saponification value 187-196 and iodine value 79-90.

Chemical Constituents : Olive oil contains mixed glycerides of oleic acid (83.5%), palmitic acid (9.4%), linoleic acid (7%), stearic acid (2.0%), and arachidic acid (0.9%). The minor constituents are squalene up to 0.7%, phytosterol and tocopherols about 0.2%.

Uses : Olive oil is used in the manufacture of pharmaceutical preparations, soaps, textile lubricants, sulphonated oils, liniments, cosmetics, plasters; as food in salads, with sardines for cooking and baking. It has demulcent, emollient and laxative properties.

CHAULMOOGRA OIL

Synonyms : Hydnocarpus oil; Gynocardia oil.

Biological Source : Chaulmoogra oil is the fixed oil obtained by cold expression from ripe seeds of *Taraktogenos kurzii* King, (syn. *Hydnocarpus kurzii* (king) Warb.), *Hydnocarpus wightiana* Blume, *H. anthelmintica* Pierre, *H. heterophylla* and other speices of *Hydnocarpus*.

Family : Flacourtiaceae.

Habitat : The plants are tall trees, up to 17 m high, with narrow crown of hanging branches; native to Burma, Thailand, eastern India and Indochina.

The tree bears irregular fruits which are collected once in 2-3 years when a full crop is expected. The seeds resemble brown pebbles in appearance and are of varying size and shape. Commercial oil obtained by the expression of kernels. They contains large amounts of free fatty acids which are of poor quality.

Characters : The oil is yellow or brownish yellow. Below 25°C it is a soft solid. It has peculiar odour and sharp taste. It is soluble in benzene, chloroform, ether, petrol; slightly soluble in cold alcohol; almost entirely soluble in hot alcohol and carbon disulphide.

Chemical Constituents : Chaulmoogra oil contains glycerides of cyclopentenyl fatty acids like hydrocarpic acid (48%), chaulmoogric acid (27%), gorlic acid with small amounts of glycerides of hydrocarpic acid, palmitic acid (6%) and oleic acid (12%). The cyclic acids are formed during last 3-4 months of maturation of the fruit and are strongly bactericidal towards the Micrococcus of leprosy.

CH$=$CH
| CH$-$(CH$_2$)$_{10}$$-$COOH
CH$_2$ $-$ CH$_2$

Hydnocarpic acid

CH $=$ CH
| CH$-$(CH$_2$)$_{12}$$-$COOH
CH$_2$ $-$ CH$_2$

Chaulmoogric acid

CH$=$CH
| CH $-$ (CH$_2$)$_6$$-CH=$CH $\cdot$ (CH$_2$)$_4$$-$COOH
CH$_2$ $-$ CH$_2$

Gorlic acid

Uses : The oil is useful in leprosy and many skin diseases. The cyclopentenyl fatty acids of the oil exhibit specific toxicity for *Mycobacterium leprae* and *M. tuberculosis*. The oil has now been replaced by the ethyl esters and salts of hydnocarpic and chaulmoogric acids. At present organic sulphones have replaced Chaulmoogra oil in therapeutic use.

KOKUM

Synonyms : Kokum butter; Kokum oil.

Biological Source : Kokum is the fat obtained by expression of the ripe seeds of *Garcinia purpurea* Roxb. (syn. *G. indica* Chois.).

Family : Guttiferae.

Habitat : The trees are slender evergreen with drooping branches found in tropical rain forests of Konkan, western ghats of Bombay, Malabar and Canara.

Seeds are separated from the ripe fruits. The dried pericarp is composed of fat which is known as Kokum. Its taste is sweet-sour. Seeds are expressed to get solid wax-like fat 'Kokum butter' (30%). Kokum bitter is also obtained by extracting the seeds with boiling water and skimming off the fat from the top or by churning the crushed pulp with water. It is greyish-white fat having slight odour or taste, mp. 39-42°C.

Kokum butter consists of egg-shaped lumps or cakes of light grey or yellowish colour with a greasy feel and a bland oily taste.

It contains a mixture of stearic and oleic acids; the other acids isolated are palmitic, arachidic and linoleic acids. It contains about 75% of mono-oleodisaturated glycerides. The glyceride components are as : tristearin (1.5%), oleodistearin (68%), oleopalmitostearin (8%), stearodiolein (20%), palmitodiolein and triolein. The Kokum bitter has mp. 39-42°, saponification value 299.5 and iodine value 37.4.

Uses : Kokum has emollient, nutritive, demulcent and astringent action and is used in skin diseases, dysentery, mucous diarrhoea, and phthisis pneumonia. Externally, it is employed to cure ulcers, fissures of lips and hands, chapped skin, wounds and sores. It is used as a base in ointments suppository, for the preparation of pomades, as garnish to give an acid flavour to curries and for preparing cooling syrups during hot months.

THEOBROMA

Synonyms : Cacao butter; Cocoa butter; Cacao seeds; Cacao beans; Semina Theobromatis; Cocao seeds.

Biological Source : Theobroma oil is obtained by expression of the ground kernels of Theobroma cacao Linn. (family Sterculiaceae).

Geographical Distribution : The Cocoa tree (Chocolate tree) is a native of tropical America (Mexico), and cultivated in Ecuador, Curacao, Mexico, Trinidad, Central America, Brazil, West Africa (Nigeria and Ghana), Sri Lanka, the Philippine Islands, South India and Orissa.

Good growing conditions for Cacao require high humidity, temperature range from 18-32° and clay-loams, sandy loams and loam soils. It is reproduced by seeds. Seedlings may be raised in nursery beds. The seeds germinate within a week. Transplanting is done when seedlings are 4-5 months old. Adequate shade is necessary for the establishment of young trees.

Collection and Preparation : The plant is a small evergreen with a dense rounded crown tree attaining the height of about 12 meters. The small flowers arise from the older branches or trunk. They are succeeded by large ovoid, fleshy red fruit which has ten longitudinal furrows and five rows of seeds, 10 or 12 in each row. Thus 40-50 colourless, fleshy seeds embedded in a scanty, mucilaginous pulp are present. The seeds are separated from the pod and packed in boxes, in which they undergo a process of fermentation at 42°C. They are then dried in the sun. At the end of these processes the seeds acquire a reddish–brown colour, and the taste, at first astringent and bitter, and becomes mild and oily. They are then roasted (140°C), lossing water and developing distinct odour and taste. The roasted seeds are passed through a "nibbling" machine to crack the seed coats which are separated from the kernels by air. The broken kernels (nibs) are ground between hot rollers to yield a paste containing up to 50% of fat, called *Cacao Butter*. At room temperature the paste is congealed to yield *Bitter Chocolate*. When sugar and flavouring substances, like vanilla, are added to the *Bitter Chocolate* it is known as *Sweet Chocolate*. After expressing Cacao butter, the marc, retaining some oil, is powered which is called as *Prepared Cacao* or *Breakfast Cocoa*.

Description : Cocoa seeds are flattened-ovoid, about 20-30 mm long, 15 mm wide and 7 mm thick. The seed-coat is chocolate brown in colour, brittle and thin. The kernel consists of two irregularly folded, chocolate-coloured cotyledons.

Theobroma oil is yellowish-white solid, brittle below 25°; chocolate odour and taste. m.p. 30°-35°C; insoluble in water; slightly soluble in alcohol; soluble in boiling alcohol, very soluble in chloroform, ether and benzene.

Chemical Constituents : Cocoa butter consists of the glycerides of stearic, (34%), palmitic (26%), arachidic, oleic, (37%) and other acids. These glycerides are present in the form of simple and mixed glycerides. Mono-oleo-disaturated glycerides, mainly oleo-palmitostearin, are the major constituents.

The seeds contain 35-50% of a fixed oil, 15% of starch, 15% of proteins, 1-4% of the alkaloid theobromine and 0.07-0.36% of caffeine. Cocao-red is formed by the action of a ferment on a glyceride and gives red colour to the seeds.

Theobromine is present in the kernel (1-1.7%) and the shell (0.19-2.98%).

Uses : Theobroma oil is used as lubricant in massage, base for suppositories and ointments, in manufacturing chocolate, toilet soaps, creams, etc. Cocoa, called "breakfast Cocoa" is a popular beverage.

COTTONSEED OIL

Biological Source : Cottonseed oil is obtained by expression of seeds of *Gossypium harbaceum* Linn. in hydraulic or other presses.

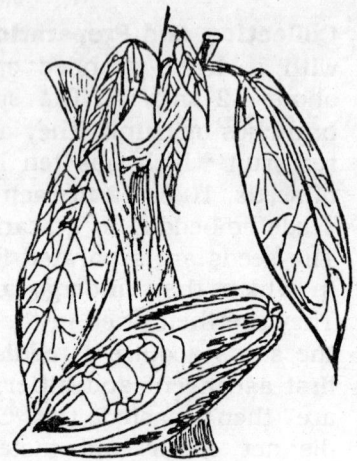

Fig. 9.3. *Theobroma cacao*

Family : Malvaceae.

Characters : The crude oil is amber to deep red or black in colour with a characteristic odour, sp. gr. 0.92, saponification value 192-200, iodine value 100-115 and unsaponifiable matter 0.6-2.0 per

Theobromine

cent. Refined Cottonseed oil is pale yellow in colour with a bland nutty taste and nearly odourless. The oil is a semi-drying substance. On cooling a sediment of olein or liquid glycerides separates out which may be collected by filtration in the cooled condition.

Cottonseed oil is graded on the basis of its acidity; refining loses flavour. Refined oil is graded according to the colour, odour and flavour.

Chemical Constituents : The important constituents of the glycerides of Cottonseed oil are linoleic (45-50%), oleic (23-29%), palmitic (20-23%), myristic (1.5-3.5%), stearic (1.1-2.7%) and arachidic acids (1.0%). The glycerides present are palmito-oleolinoleins (35-40%), palmitodioleins (20%) and trioleo- or lineo-disaturated (12-13%). The unsaponifiable fraction contains β-sitosterol, ergosterol, vitamin E and tocopherols. The phosphatides present are lecithin (29%) and cephalins (71%). The minor constituents present in the oil are free fatty acids (0.3-5.6%), gossypol (0.05%), raffinose, pentosans, resins, wax, proteoses, peptones, phospholipids, inosite phosphates, phytosteroline, xanthophyll, chlorophyll and muscilage substances.

Uses : Cottonseed oil is used for edible purposes. The oil possesses emollient properties and is used in liniments, in several pharmaceutical preparations, as a substitute of Olive oil and in large doses as lubricant cathartic. Low grade oil is used in the manufacture of soaps, lubricants, sulphonated oils and protective coatings.

Cottonseed oil is detected when present in admixture with other oils by the Halphen colour test. The oil (1 ml) is dissolved in equal volume of amyl alcohol. A 1% solution of flowers of sulphur (1 ml) in carbon tetrachloride is added and the mixture heated for two hours on water bath. A red colour indicates the presence of Cottonseed oil.

WAXES

Waxes are the esters of higher straight-chain fatty acids with long-chain or high molecular weight monohydric alcohols, some containing more than 30 carbons in the chain. Waxes may be of plant origin such as Carnauba wax or of animal origin such as Beeswax, Wool-fat, Spermaceti, etc.

In many ways, waxes are identical to fats, but they are more difficult to saponify. Fats may be saponified by aqueous or alcoholic alkalies but waxes are only saponified by alcoholic alkalies. Waxes are distinguished from fats and oils by their low saponification values and very low iodine value due to the presence of saturated acids.

Waxes usually contain esters of the free acids, hydrocarbons, free alcohols and sterols. The hydrocarbons and sterols are unsaponifiable. In plants, waxes are present on the outer cell walls of epidermal tissue. They protect the loss of water or its penetration to the inner part. Waxes are used in pharmaceuticals for hardening cosmetic creams and ointments and in preparation of cerates.

LANOLIN

Synonyms : Wool fat; Oesipos; Agnin, Alapurin; Agnolin; Lanum; Lanain; Lanalin; Lanesin; Lanichol; Anhydrous lanolin; Adeps lanae; Laniol.

Biological Source : Lanolin is the "fat like" purified secretion of the sebaceous glands of sheep, *Ovis aries* Linn. (Family

Bovidae) which is deposited into the wool fibres. It contains about 25-30% water.

Preparation : Wool is cut and washed with a soap or alkali. An emulsion of wool fat, called as wool grease, takes place in water. Raw lanolin is separated by cracking the emulsion with suphuric acid. Wool grease floats on the upper layer and fatty acids are dissolved in the lower layer. Lanolin is purified by treating with sodium peroxide and bleaching with reagents.

Characters : Lanolin is a yellowish white, tenacious, unctuous mass; odour is slight and characteristic. Practically, it is insoluble in water, but soluble in chloroform or ether with the separation of the water. It melts in between 34-40°. On heating it forms two layers in the beginning, continuous heating removes water. Lanolin is not saponified by an aqueous alkali. However, saponification takes place with alcoholic solution of alkali.

Anhydrous lanolin is a yellowish tenacious, semisolid fat, slight odour, mp 38-42°. Practically insoluble in water but mixes with about twice its weight of water without separation. It is sparingly soluble in cold, more in hot alcohol, freely soluble in benzene, chloroform, ether, carbon disulphide, acetone and petroleum ether.

Chemical Constituents : Lanolin is a complex mixture of esters and polyesters of 33 high molecular weight alcohols, and 36 fatty acids. The alcohols are of three types: aliphatic alcohols, steroid alcohols, and triterpenoid alcohols. The acids are also of three types : saturated nonhydroxylated acids, unsaturated nonhyroxylated acids and hydroxylated acids. Liquid Lanolin is rich in low molecular weight, branched aliphatic acids and alcohols while waxy Lanolin is rich in high molecular weight, straight-chain acids, and alcohols.

The chief constituents of Lanolin are cholesterol, isocholesterol, unsaturated monohydric alcohols of the formula $C_{27}H_{45}OH$, both free and combined with lanoceric($C_{30}H_{60}O_4$), lanopalmitic ($C_{16}H_{22}O_3$), carnaubic and other fatty acids. Lanonin also contains esters of oleic and myristic acids, aliphatic alcohols, such as cetyl, ceryl and carnaubyl alcohols, lanosterol, and agnosterol.

Uses : Lanolin is used as an emollient, as water absorable ointment base in many skin creams and cosmetic and for hoof dressing. Wool fat is readily absorbed through skin and helps in increasing the absorption of active ingredients incorporated in the ointment. However, it may act as an allergenic contactant in hypersensitive persons.

Cholesterol   Lanosterol

Agnosterol

BEESWAX

Synonyms : Yellow beeswax, White beeswax; Cera flava; Cara alba.

Biological Source : Beeswax is obtained by purifying the honeycomb of *Apis mellifica* or *A. mellifera* and other bees.

Family : Apidae.

Geographical Source : The beeswax is prepared in West Indies, California, Chile, Africa, Jamaica, Madagascar and India.

Preparation : Yellow Beeswax : Wax is secreted in cells on the ventral surface of the last four segments of the abdomen of worker bees. The wax comes out through pores in the chitinous plates and is used to form the comb for storing the honey. After separation of the honey, the honeycomb is melted in water and cooled. The water-soluble impurities are removed, stained and allowed to solidify in suitable moulds to get yellow beeswax.

White Beeswax : It is prepared from the yellow beeswax by bleaching with charcoal, potassium permanganate, chromic acid, chlorine, etc. or slow bleaching with sunlight, air and water. For slow bleaching the melted wax is fell on a revolving moist cylinder. Ribbon-like strips of wax are formed which are exposed to sunlight and air. The strips are frequently moistened and turned until the outer surface is bleached.

Characters : The beeswax is yellowish to brownish-yellow, or white, pieces or plates, translucent when thin, soft to brittle, honey-like odour, slight balsamic taste, density 0.95-0.96, mp 62-65°. It is practically insoluble in water, slightly soluble in cold alcohol, soluble in hot alcohol, chloroform, benzene, ether, and carbon disulphide. It is soft and brittle, but becomes plastic on warming. On cooling it hardens and breaks with a flaky granular surface.

Chemical Constituents : Beeswax consists mainly of myricyl palmitate (myricin) (~80%), myricyl stearate, free cerotic acid (15%) and its homologues, an aromatic substance cerolein, hydrocarbons, (~12%), lactones, moisture, cholesteryl ester, pollen pigments, and propolis (bee glue). The colour of the wax is due to the presence of pollen pigments and propolis. The esters consist of straight-chain monohydric alcohols with even-numbered carbon chains from C_{24} to C_{36} esterified with straight-chain acids also having even number of carbon atoms up to C_{36}. The other examples of esters are triacontanol hexadecanoate and hexacosanol hexacosanoate. These esters are mixed with about 20% of hydrocarbons having odd numbered straight carbon chains from C_{21} to C_{33}.

The other constituents are 1, 3-dihydroxyflavone, w-myristolactone, lacceryl palmitate, myricyl cerotate, myricyl hypogaeate, and ceryl hydroxypalmitate. The main components are hentriacontane and nonacosane. The unsaturated hydrocarbon, melene, is also present. The free acids present are lignoceric, cerotic, montanic and psyllic; cerotic acid being the predominant saturated free acid. Palmitic, hydroxypalmitic and hypogaeic (7-hexadecenoic) acids are also reported.

Uses : Beeswax is used to prepare plasters, ointments, cerates, face creams, wax paper, candles, modelling artificial fruits and flowers, in process engraving, shoe polish, etc.

A beeswax and vegetable oil mixture is used as a vehicle for the administration of respiratory forms of certain medicaments such as penicillin and curare. It is used in the formulation of medicinal preparations for treating skin cracks. A combination containing of tallow, olive oil, camphor, beeswax and common salt is used for ulcer and external tumour treatment.

$$C_{15}H_{31} \; COOC_{30} \; H_{61} \qquad\qquad C_{26}H_{53}COOH$$

Myricin   Cerotic acid

Adulterants : Beeswax is adulterated with chief substances such as solid paraffin, ceresin, carnauba wax, Japan wax (Fat of the fruits of *Rhus* species; family Anacardiaceae), stearic acid and colophony.

Detection of Adulteration

1. On heating the wax with aqueous sodium hydroxide, cooling and acidifying, there should be no turbidity. Beeswax is a true wax and on saponification the cerotic acid does not form soap. The adulterated substances form water soluble soap on treatment with alkali.
2. Wax is hydrolyzed with alcoholic alkali by heating, and cooled by stirring. It should be cloudy between 59-61°C and not above 61°.

QUESTIONS

1. Give official source, chemical constituents and uses of: (a) Chaulmoogra oil (b) Linseed (c) Castor oil (d) Beeswax.
2. How are fixed oils formed in the plants ? Give method of preparation and chemical tests for identification of Olive oil. What are its common adulterants and how are they detected ?
3. Give the source, preparation, chemical constituents and uses of Arachis oil.
4. How will you differentiate among fixed oils, fats and waxes. Discuss the pharmacognosy of Arachis oil.
5. Describe biological source, chemical constituents and uses of the drugs belonging to the following families : (a) Euphorbiaceae (b) Leguminosae (c) Pedaliaceae (d) Flacourtiaceae (e) Malvaceae.

10

VOLATILE OILS

Volatile or essential oils are mono- and sesquiterpenes obtained from the sap and tissues of certain plants. They are flavouring compounds and have been used in perfumery from the ancient times. On exposition to air at room temperature they evaporate. Chemically, they are composed of hydrocarbons of the general formula $(C_5H_8)_n$ and their oxygenated, hydrogenated, and dehydrogenated derivatives. All the volatile oils are of vegetable origin.

The thermal decomposition of volatile oils gives isoprene as one of the products. Therefore, essential oils are built up of isoprene units. These units are joined 'hand-to-tail' in natural terpenoids.

In most instances the volatile oil pre-exists in plant. Volatile oils may be present in particular secretory parts such as glandular hairs, parenchyma cells, vittae or oil tubes, in mesophyll (Eucalyptus leaves), sub-epidermal tissues of Lemon and Orange, in lysigenous or schizogenous passages, in all tissues (Conifers), in petals (Orange, Rose), in bark and leaves (Cinnamon), in pericarp (Umbelliferous fruits), in glandular hairs of the stems and leaves (Mint), and in rind (Orange). Plants containing essential oils usually have the greatest concentration at some particular time, e.g., jasmine at sunset. In some cases volatile oil does not pre-exist, but is formed by the decomposition of a glycoside (in Black Mustard).

as :
Four general methods of extraction of volatile oils are

1. steam distillation,
2. expression,
3. extraction by means of volatile solvents and
4. Adsorption in purified fat.

Steam distillation is one of the most widely used. In this method the plant is macerated and then steam distilled to get the oil. If some compounds are decomposed under these conditions, they may be extracted with light petrol at 50° and the solvent is removed by distillation under reduced pressure. Adsorption in fat is the alternate method used for isolation of volatile compounds. In this method, the fat is heated to 50°C and the flower petals are spread on the surface until it becomes saturated with essential oils. Then the petals are removed to dissolve the oils present in fat. Fat is removed by cooling the alcohol at 20°C. The alcoholic extract is fractionally distilled under reduced pressure to remove the solvent.

Volatile oils are colourless liquids and are lighter than water. They possess distinct odours, have high refractive indices, generally are optically active. They are immiscible with water, but the water shaken with an essential oil possesses its flavour due to slight solubility of the oil. Volatile oils are freely soluble in ether, alcohol, chloroform, acetone, etc.

Each volatile oil differs widely in chemical composition. Usually hydrocabons, alcohols, ketones, aldehydes, ethers, oxides and esters are present in volatile oils. Some of the essential oils possess high percentage of a particular compound e.g., eugenol in Clove oil (85%), allylisothiocyanate in Mustard oil (93%), menthol in Peppermint oil (~70%), and α-terpineol in Pine oil (~65%).

Volatile oils differ from fixed oils in various ways. The former oils are evaporated at room temperature, and can be distilled from their natural sources. They are not glyceryl esters of fatty acids and, therefore, cannot be saponified with alkalies. Volatile oils are not rancidified like fixed oils. On exposure to air and light, they oxidize and resins are formed.

Volatile oil containing drugs are used in perfumery, cosmetic, as insect repellants and as flavouring agents to mask the taste and smell of unpleasant medicines. They act as counterirritants in inflammation and rheumatism. They have carminative, digestive, spasmolytic, stimulant, bactericidal, antiseptic disinfectant, diuretic, expectorant and anthelmintic properties.

A volatile oil may contain hydrocarbons which are usually devoid of aroma. The other constituents of the oil are monoterpenes which are isomeric substances of the formula $C_{10}H_{16}$, but they vary considerably in structures. All terpenes are optically active. The important terpenes are pinenes, limonene, phellandrene and camphene. Sesquiterpenes of the general formula are also present in an essential oil. They are usually the highest-boiling fraction of the oil. The principal sesquiterpenes are caryophyllene and cadinene.

UMBELLIFEROUS PLANTS

Volatile oils are most frequently present in the pericarp of Umbelliferous fruits. The plants are erect and possess alternate, undivided or divided leaves, base of stalks often dilated and sheathing the stem. Flowers are small, usually less than 1.2 cm diameter, regular, polygamous, in umbels, rarely in heads. Umbels are compound or simple, with or without bracts and bracteoles at the base of the primary and secondary rays, respectively.

The Umbelliferous fruits are schizocarps (splitting), dried, consisting of two one-seeded, indehiscent carpels, which separate from a very slender, simple or forked, central axis.They have transversed longitudinal five ridges or wings, the central ridge being called the dorsal, two marginal the lateral and the remaining two the intermediate ridges.

The carpels are also often furnished with internal, longitudinal oils-canals or vittae, which are best seen in cross sections.

Schizocarps are simple dry indehiscent fruits. They split into partial fruits possessing seeds in each part. Umbelliferous fruits are cremocarps in which the fruits split into two partial fruits, called mericarps, and is derived from inferior bicarpellary biocular ovary, Each mericarp possesses a stylopod at it apex. Stylopod is a disc-like nectary with style and remains of calyx. There are two surfaces of mericarps-the outer dorsal or curved surface and the inner, ventral or commissural surface. On the surface of mericarp five longitudinal, straight or wavy, conspicuous or inconspicuous ridges are present which join apex to the base. These ridges are called primary ridges due to the presence of vascular bundles below the ridges. In Coriander, secondary ridges are present alternatively with primary ridges. Vascular bundles are not present under the secondary ridges. In between primary ridges special secretory ducts, secreting volatile oils, called vittae, are found in the mesocarp. Each vitta runs from apex to the base longitudinally through the mesocarp.

Coriander, Fennel, Caraway, Dill, and Anise, are the important drugs belonging to Umbelliferae family.

CORIANDER

Synonyms : Coriander fruit, Dhaniya (Hindi); Fructus coriandri.

Biological Source : Coriander is the dried, ripe fruits of *Coriandrum sativum* Linn.

Family : Umbelliferae.

Geographical Source : Coriander is indigenous to Italy. It is extensively cultivated in Holland, central and eastern Europe, Morocco, Malta, Egypt, China, India and Bangladesh.

Collection : Coriander is an annual herb, about 0.7 m high with small white or pinkish flowers. Fruits are collected when ripe and dried. Aromatic odour is developed on drying the fruits.

Cultivation : Coriander is generally grown as a rain-fed crop. The time of sowing varies in different localities. Before sowing the fruits are rubbed till the two mericarps are separated and sown either broadcast or in rows. The crop requires 2 or 3 weedings and the field is irrigated whenever required.

The crop matures in about 3-3.5 months after sowing. The plants are then pulled out by the roots and after drying, the fruits are threshed out. They are further dried in the sun, winnowed and stored in bags.

Morphology : The drug consists of entire cremocarps, 2.3-4.3 mm in diameter, shape sub-spherical. Cremocarps consist of two hemispherical mericarps united by their margins. Two divergent styles present on the apex. On the surface there are ten primary ridge˜ which are wavy and inconspicuous. Alternating in primary ridges there are eight more prominent, straight, secondary ridges. The colour is straw-yellow, odour is aromatic and taste is spicy. Fresh plant emits a very disagreeable odour on rubbing.

Chemical Constituents : Coriander fruits contain volatile oil (1%). The prominent constituents of the volatile oil are (+)- linalool (65-70%) and pinene. Small amounts of geraniol, borneol, p-cymene, dipentene, phellandrene, terpinolene, hydrocarbons such α-and β-terpinene, geraniol, n-decylic aldehyde, fixed oils, malic acid, esters of acetic and decylic acids, tannins, and mucilage are also present. Coriander oil is a colourless, pale yellow liquid, having characteristic odour and taste. The seeds also contain fatty oil (19-20%) which is mixture of glycerides of palmitic, oleic, linoleic and petroselinic acids.

Uses : Coriander is aromatic, stimulant, carminative, antibilious, diuretic, tonic, stomachic, refrigerant and aphrodisiac. It is used as flavouring agent to conceal the odour of other medicines and to correct the griping qualities of Rhubarb and Senna.

FENNEL

Synonyms : Large Fennel; Sweet Fennel, Fennel fruit; Saunf (Hindi); Fructus Foeniculi.

Biological Source : Fennel is the dried, ripe fruits of *Foeniculum vulgare* Mill.

Family : Umbelliferae.

Geographical Source : Fennel is indigenous to Mediterranean region of Asia and Europe. It is widely cultivated in Russia, India, Japan, Southern Europe, China and Egypt.

Cultivation : Fennel is stout, glabrous, aromatic herb and cultivated as a garden or homeyard crop at all altitudes up to 2,000 m. It grows in any good soil, but thrives best in rich, well-drained loam or

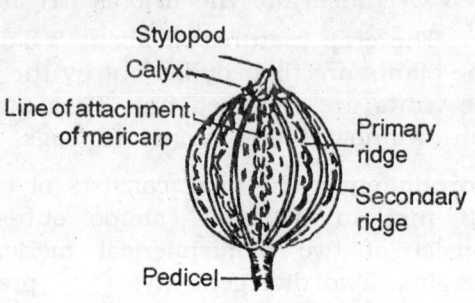

Fig. 10.1 Coriander fruit

black sandy soil containing sufficient lime. It is propagated readily by seeds, but can also be grown by root or crown division. Seeds are · sown broadcast by hand or by shallow drill in October-November in the plains and March-April on the hills. when 10 cm high.

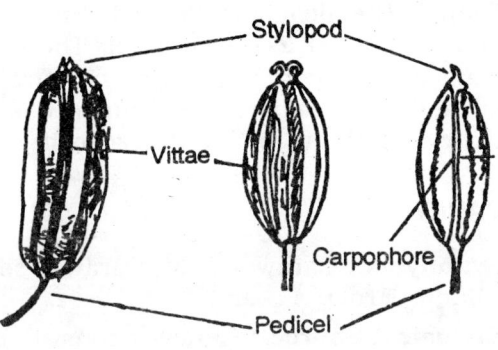

Fig. 10.2. Fennel fruit

The plants are thinned out to about 30 cm apart. Occasional weeding. and irrigation once a week are done. The crop is harvested before the fruits are fully ripe. The stems are cut with the sickle and spread out in loose sheaves to dry in the sun. The dried fruits are threshed out and cleaned by winnowing.

Fennel plant is stout, glabrous, aromatic herb, about 2 m high, leaves pinnately decompound; flowers small, yellow, in compound terminal umbels.

Morphology : The drug consists partly of whole cremocarps and partly of mericarps. The fruit is 0.5-1.0 cm long, 2-4 mm broad. Shape is slightly curved and oval. Surface is glabrous with 5 straight prominent straw-coloured primary ridges and bifid stylopod at the apex. Colour is greenish-brown, odour is aromatic and taste is distinct, sweet and aromatic.

Chemical Constituents : Fennel contains volatile oil (2-6.5%) and fixed oil (12%). The main constituent of the volatile oil are phenolic ether, anethole (50-60%) and the ketone, fenchone (18-20%) which give the fruit its distinct odour and taste; the other constituents of volatile oil are methyl chavicol, anisic aldehyde, anisic acid, α-pinene, dipentene, limonene, and phellandrene.

Uses : Fennel is used as stimulant, aromatic, stomachic, carminative, emmenagogue and expectorant. It is added to cough and stomach mixture. Anethole is used in mouth and dental preparations. Fennel is useful in diseases of the chest, spleen and kidney.

Adulterants : Fennel is generally adulterated with exhausted

Fennel. The alcohol-exhausted Fennel looks like fresh Fennel and contains 1-2% volatile oil. The steam-exhausted Fennel fruits are darker in appearance. They contain little volatile oil and are heavier than water. It is also adulterated with undeveloped or mould-attack fruits.

CARAWAY

Synonyms : Caraway fruit; Caraway seed; Carvi; Carum; Zira (Hindi); Fructus Carvi.

Biological Source : Caraway consists of the dried. ripe fruits of *Carum carvi* Linn.

Family : Umbelliferae.

Geographical Source : The plant is cultivated in European countries (Holland, Denmark, Germany, Russia, Finland, Norway, Sweden and England) and in China, Egypt, Morocco. In India the plant grows widely in northern Himalayan regions, and is cultivated in the plains as a cold season crop and in the hills of Kashmir, Kumaon, Garhwal and Chamba at altitudes of 3,000-4,000 m as a summer crop.

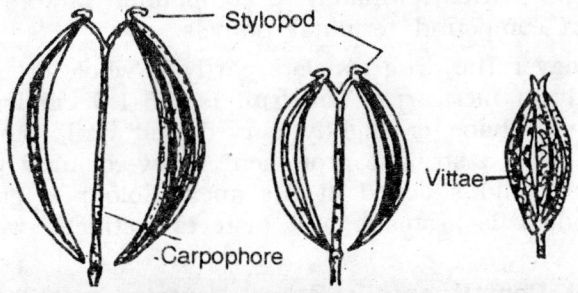

Fig. 10.3 Caraway fruit

Habitat and Morphology : Caraway is a perennial or biennial herb, about 1 m. high with thick tuberous roots and compound leaves. The fruits consist of mericarps without pedicels. They are 4-7 mm long, 1 mm broad, slightly curved, smooth and tapering at both ends. There are five primary ridges, stigma is attached and a stylopod at the apex. The colour is brown, odour and taste are characteristic and spicy.

It is cultivated in the plains as a cold season crop and in hilly areas as a summer crop. The plant requires a dry temperate climate and thrives well in soils rich in humus. The fruits may be sown either broadcast or in rows. The fruits are collected before ripening. The plants are dried and the fruits threshed out, cleaned and stored in bags.

Chemical Constituents : Caraway contains volatile oil (3-7%), fixed oil (8-20%), proteins, calcium oxalate, colouring matter, resins, sugar, tannins, and mucilage. Monoterpenes identified in the volatile oil are carvone (50-60%), dihydrocarvone, limonene, carveol, and dihydrocarveol.

Uses : Caraway is used as aromatic, carminative, stomachic, lactagogue, flavouring agent and as a spice.

DILL

Synonyms : Dil fruit; Fructus Anethi.

Biological Source : Dill is the dried, ripe fruits of *Anethum graveolens* Linn. Indian Dill consists of dried ripe fruits of *Anethum sowa* Kurz.

Family : Umbelliferae.

Source : Dilli is cultivated in England, Germany, Rumania and U.S.A. Indian dill is grown throughout India.

Cultivation : *A. graveolens* is an annual, erect, glabrous herb, 1 m in height, cultivated to a small extent in the plains. It prefers sandy loam soil of moderate fertility and avoids low lying damp areas. It is grown as a cold weather crop in Indian plains. The seeds are sown in October in rows and the seed crop is harvested by the end of April. Germination takes in 7 to 9 days. Flowering commences between 40-67 days after germination. Application of nitrogenous and phosphatic fertilizers increases yield on medium fertile lands. The crop in given 4 to 6 irrigations. The harvested umbels are dried in shade for 2 to 3 days and threshed. The dried seeds are stored in gunny bags lined with polythene to reduce storage loss of oil.

Morphology : The drug consists of separate, broadly oval mericarps, 3-4 mm long, 2-3 mm wide, 1 mm thick. The fruit is dorsally compressed and has 5 primary yellow-coloured ridges. The two lateral ridges are extended as thin wings, the remaining three are inconspicuous. Stylopod is present at the apex of each mericarp. The colour is brown; odour and taste are aromatic and spicy.

Chemical Constituents : Dill contains volatile oil (3-4%) and the principal constituent of the oil is carvone (50-60%). The other components of the oil are dihydrocarvone, d-limonene and phellandrene. The Indian variety contains essential oil from 2.5 to 6.0%, which consists of carvone (22-46%), dihydrocarvone (5-25%), dillapiol (12-15%), limonene (22-45%), isoeugenol, d-phellandrene, α-terpinene and carveol.

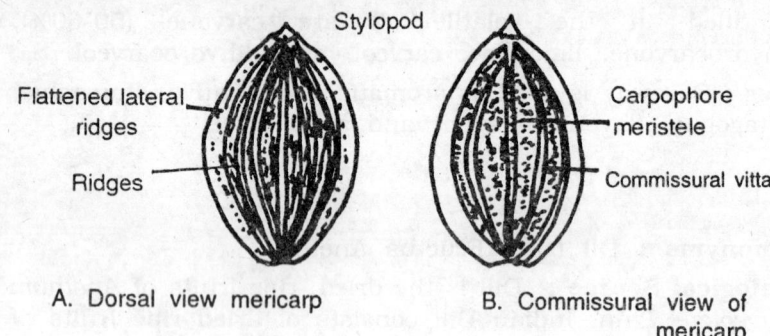

Fig. 10.4. Dill

In addition to volatile oil, the other compounds isolated from the fruits are myristicin, coumarins (bargapten, umbelliprenin scopoletin, esculetin), flavonoids (quercetin, isorhamnetin kaempferol, kaempferol-3-glucuronide, glucoflavone, dillanoside), phenolic acids (caffeic, ferulic and chlorogenic acids), sterols (γ-sitosterol, β-sitosterol glucoside) and phytofluene.

Uses : Dill is used as carminative stomachic, diuretic, anthelmintic, antiflatulant and flavour in gastric disturbances of children and for preparation of dill water and gripe water.

ANISE

Synonyms : Anise fruit, Anise seed, Star anise; Fructus Anisi.

Biological Source ; Anise is the dried ripe fruit of *Pimpinella anisum* Linn.

Family : Umbelliferae.

Geographical Source : The plant is native to Asia Minor, Egypt and Greece and widely cultivated in Spain, Germany, Italy, Russia, Bulgaria, Chile and Maxico. In India the drug is grown in north-west region, U.P., Punjab and Orissa.

Morphology : The plant is an annual herb. The fruit is pear-shaped, entired compressed cremocarps attached to pedicles, 2-12 mm in length. Cremocarps are 3-6 mm long and 2-

Linalool α-Pinene β-Pinene Borneol

Anethole Fenchone α-Terpinene β-Terpinene

3-Carene α-Terpinene Anise aldehyde (R = CHO) Anisic acid (R = COOH) Carveol

Limonene Dihydrocarveol Cineol β-Phellandrene

Carvone Dillapiole α-Phellandrene

Myrcene Cymene Carvone

.3 mm broad. There are five wavy ridges on the mesocarp. Outer surface contains short, numerous, conical epidermal trichomes (papillae). Odour is aromatic and taste is sweet.

The oil is a clear, colourless or pale yellow liquid, free from water, crushed fruit like odour and sweet and aromatic taste. It crystallizes on cooling.

Chemical Constituents : Anise fruit contains volatile oil (1.5-3.5%), starch, protein and fixed oil (30%). The principal constituent of the volatile oil is anethole (90%), rest being p-methoxyphenyl acetone, methyl chavicol, chavicol and some terpenic hydrocarbons.

Uses : Anise fruit is diuretic and carminative and used to prevent flatulence colic, as flavouring agent and in mouth and dental preparations. Anethole is employed as expectorant, aromatic, carminative and flavouring agent.

STAR-ANISE OIL

Biological Source : It is a volatile oil obtained from the fruits of the Chinese Star-anise, *Illicium verum* (Family : Illiciaceae).

Habitat : The Star-anise is an evergreen tree, about 4-5 m in height, indigenous to the south-west states of China and other tropical countries. The fruits are collected and the oil distilled locally in China and Vietnam.

The fruits consist mostly of eight one-seeded follicles. Each follicle is about 1.5 cm in length. The pericarp is reddish-brown, woody and slightly wrinkled. Each carpel has the seed which has a brittle, shining testa and oily kernel. The oil, present in both seed and pericarp, gives the drug an aromatic odour and spicy taste.

Chemical Constituents : The fruits yield a volatile oil (2.5-5%) which contains anethole (80-90%) as the main component. The other compounds present in the oil are chavicol methyl ether, p-methoxy-phenylacetone and safrole.

Uses : The oil is used as a flavouring agent and carminative.

PEPPERMINT

Synonyms : Brandy mint; Lamb mint.

Biological Source : Peppermint consists of dried leaves and flowering tops of *Mentha piperita* Linn. containing not less tha 1.2 per cent of volatile oil.

Family : Labiatae.

Geographical Source : The plant is cultivated in Asian countries, Canada, Europe and North America. It is grown in gardens.

The plant is a perennial glabrous strongly scented herb, 40-70 cm in height, and cultivated in fertile soil having capacity of holding water. If rainfall is unsufficient, water is irrigated. Much sunlight is required for better crop. The plants are propagated by rhizome cuttings. At flowering stage plants are cut, dried for sometime in sunlight and stored. Several varieties of peppermint are cultivated in various countries, e.g., *Mentha arvensis* var. *piperascens* (Japan mint), *M. piperita* var. *vulgaris* (Black mint), *M. piperita* var. *officinalis* (White mint).

Peppermint thrives well in humid and temperate climates and is sensitive to drought. It grows well on high calcareous soil or deep rich loams in open sunny situations. The cuttings of rootstocks are planted in rows 30-90 cm apart.

Farmyard manure is applied as a basal dose before planting. Planted in February or March, the plants flower in July of the second year, when the crop is harvested; a second flush may be taken in September after the rain.

Peppermint oil is colourless, pale yellow or greenish yellow liquid with a strong agreeable odour and a powerful aromatic taste, followed by a cooling sensation when air is drawn into the mouth. On ageing, the oil darkens in colour and becomes viscous. When chilled, menthol separates out.

Chemical Constituents : Peppermint contains volatile oil, resin, tannins and gum. The predominent constituent of the oil is menthol (50-90%), the other compounds identified are l-and d-menthone (10%), menthyl acetate, menthyl valerate, menthofuran, jasmone, phellandrene, α-pinene, cineole, l-limonene, terpinene, cadinene, amyl alcohol, acetic acid, isovaleric acid, acetaldehyde, isovaleric aldehyde and piperitone. American peppermint also contains acetaldehyde, isovaleraldehyde, acetic acid, valeric acid, limonene, menthyl isovalerate, cadinene, amyl alcohol and dimethyl sulphide.

Uses : The herb is considered aromatic, stimulant, stomachic and carminative, and used for allaying nausea, flatulence and vomiting. Bruised leaves are employed as an external application for relieving local pain and headache. A hot infusion in taken to allay stomach ache and diarrhoea. The drug is frequently adulterated with spearmint, which is difficult to detect.

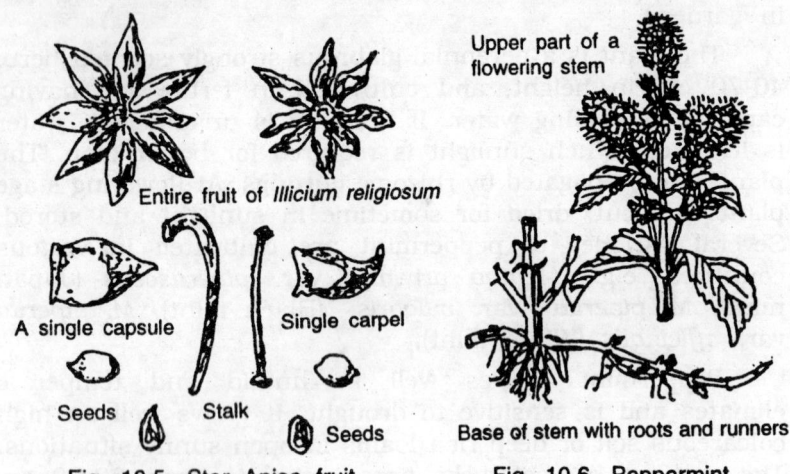

Fig. 10.5. Star Anise fruit   Fig. 10.6. Peppermint

Peppermint oil is used for flavouring in pharmaceuticals, dental preparation, mouth washes, cough, drops, soaps, chewing gums, candies, confectionery and alcoholic liquers. It is widely used in flatulence, nausea and gastralgia. The oil has mild antiseptic and local anaesthetic properties. It is used externally in rheumatism, neuralgia, congestive, headache and toothache.

Menthol is antipruritic and used on the skin or mucous membrane as a counter-irritant, antiseptic and stimulant. Internally it has a depressant effect on the heart.

Menthol   Menthone   Menthyl acetate

Menthofuran   Jasmone   1, 8-Cineole

CINNAMON BARK

Synonyms : Ceylon Cinnamon; Dalchini (Hindi), Saigon Cinnamon, Chinese Cassia; Cortex Cinnamoni.

Biological Source : Cinnamon is the dried bark of *Cinnamomum loureirii* Nees or *C. zeylanicum* Nees.

Family : Lauraceae.

Geographical Source : Cinnamon is a native of China, Japan, and Formosa and found in Sri Lanka, Java, Vietnam, Sumatra, West Indies, Jamaica, Laos, Indonesia, Brazil, and Seychelles. In India the plant occurs widely in the southern coastal regions of western India up to an altitude of 2,000 meters.

Cultivation : Cinnamon is a large handsome, evergreen, 6-10 meter high tree. It is grown in rich but light soil. It requires a rainfall of nearly 200-300 cm and temperature 32°C. The fresh seeds are sown in seed beds. The plants are transplanted at a distance of 2-3 meter apart. Two or three years old trees are coppiced few inches above the ground. From each plant 5 to 6 straight shoots are allowed to grow. Bark is separated from shoots which are about 3 cm thick. Bark is collected from April to July after heavy rainy season. The shoots and twigs are removed with a brass knife-like instrument (Catty). Leaves and twigs are separated and bark is stripped off from shoots. The bark is kept in the shade for about 24 hours and then kept in the open air wood frames. The dried bark is sorted, put into bundles and enclosed in jute cloth.

The bark as it dries, contracts and forms a quill. During the drying process, which takes about 3 days, the quills are rolled by hand and pressed to prevent swelling and splitting. The bark obtained from the central branches is superior to that from the outer shoots. The quills are graded on the basis of appearance and aroma.

Macroscopic Characters : Cinnamon occurs in single or double compound quills. Length of quill is up to 1 meter, 6-10 mm in diameter and 0.5 mm thick. The external surface is yellowish brown and shows longitudinal wavy lines (pericyclic fibres) and occasional scars and holes. The inner surface is dark brown longitudinally straited. Fracture is short and splintery. Odour is aromatic; taste in warm, sweet and aromatic.

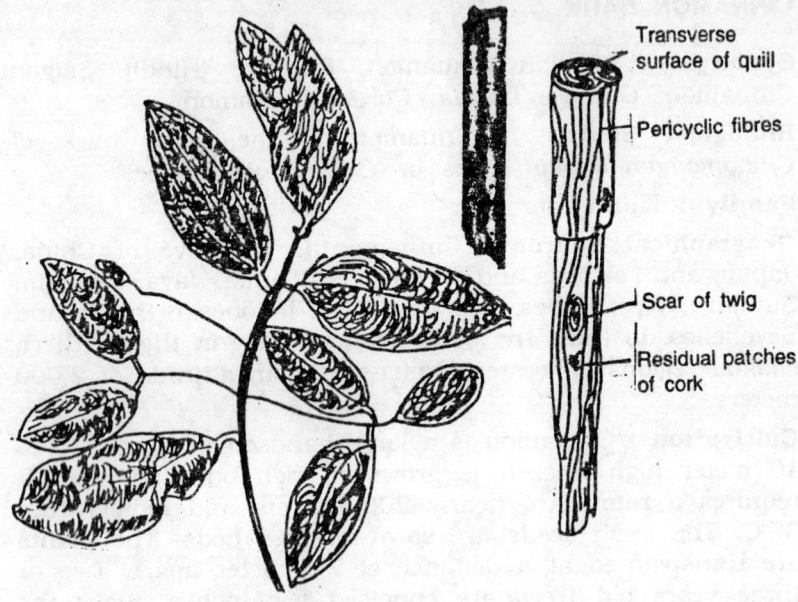

Fig. 10.7. *Cinnamomum zeylanicum* twig   Fig. 10.8. Cinnamon bark

Chemical Constituents : Cinnamon contains volatile oil (1-6%), phlobatannin, mucilage, calcium oxalate, sugar and starch. The principal constituent of the volatile oil is cinnamic aldehyde, C_6H_5 CH=CH-CHO (60-75%). The other components identified are eugenol (4%), pinene, phellandrene, caryophyllene, cinnamyl acetate and small quantities of ketones and alcohols (benzaldehyde, methyl amyl ketone, cumic aldehyde) and esters of isobutyric acid.

Chemical Tests

1. Volatile oil (1 ml) is dissolved in alcohol (5 ml) and then a drop of $FeCl_3$ is added. Ferric chloride on reaction with cinnamic aldehyde and phenolic compound, eugenol, produces pale green, colour.

2. Alcoholic extract of the bark (1 g) or volatile oil (1 ml) on treatment with phenylhydrazine hydrochloride forms red coloured phenylhydrazone of cinnamic aldehyde.

Uses : Cinnamon is pungent, aromatic, astringent, stimulant and carminative. It is useful for checking nausea and vomiting. It is employed as flavouring agent and it has antiseptic and antidiarrhoeal properties and is a powerful germicide. It is employed as a counter-irritant in the treatment of muscular strains, rheumatism and inflammations.

Allied Drug : *Saigon Cinnamon* is obtained from wild trees of *C. loureirii Nees* grown in Annam. It contains numerous starch grains and volatile oil. It is used as flavouring agent and mild astringent.

Cassia or Chinese Cinnamon : Cassia bark is obtained from *Cinnamomum cassia* Blume (Fam. Lauraceae). The plant is grown in south eastern provinces of China and Cochin. Bark is removed from 6 years old tree.

Cassia yields volatile oil (1-2%) which contains cinnamic aldehyde, caryophyllene, methyl O-cumin aldehyde and coumarin.

Java Cinnamon : It is the bark obtained from *Cassia burmanii* Blume. It is used in Holland. Its powder contains tabular crystals of calcium oxalate. The oil contains about 75% cinnamic aldehyde.

Oliver Bark or Black Sassafras : It is obtained from the Brisbane 'white sassafras' tree, *C. oliveri* Bailey, found in Queensland. The bark occurs in flat strips about 20 cm wide, 4 cm long and 1 cm thick, brown coloured outer surface. It contains 1-2.4% volatile oil.

CASSIA OIL (CINNAMON OIL)

Biological Source : Cassia oil is obtained by steam distillation of the leaves and twigs of the plant *Cinnamomum cassia* Blume. It contains not less than 1.0% of volatile oil.

Family : Lauraceae

Habitat : The plant is indigenous to China. It also occurs in Sri Lanka and Burma. In India, it is cultivated in Cochin.

Characters : The oil is a yellowish to brownish liquid that becomes darker and thicker by age or by exposure to air. It contains the typical odour and taste of Cassia Cinnamon.

Chemical Constituents : The main constituent of the oil is cinnamic aldehyde (80-95%); the other components identified are limonene, p-cymene, linalool, β-caryophyllene and eugenol.

Uses : Cassia oil is used as a flavouring agent. It has carminative, pungent, antiseptic and aromatic properties.

It should be stored in well-filled, tight, light-resistant containers and protected from excessive heat.

LEMON PEEL

Synonym : Fructus Limonis.

Biological Source : Lemon peel is obtained from the fresh ripe fruit of *Citrus limon* (L.) Burm. f. *(C. medica* var *Limon* Linn.).

Family : Rutaceae.

Geographical Habitat : It is cultivated in California. West Indies, Italy, Spain, Sicily, Portugal, Florida, California, Jamaica and Australia; grown all over India, particularly in home gardens and small-sized orchards.

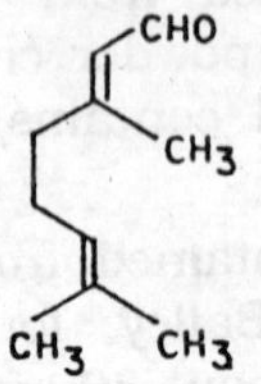

Citral

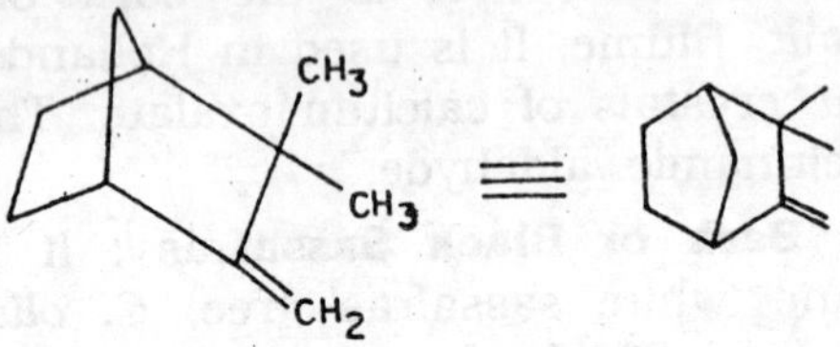

Camphene

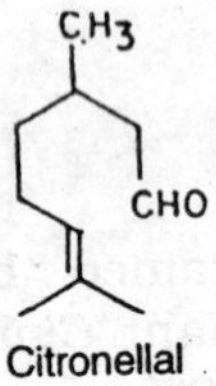

Citronellal

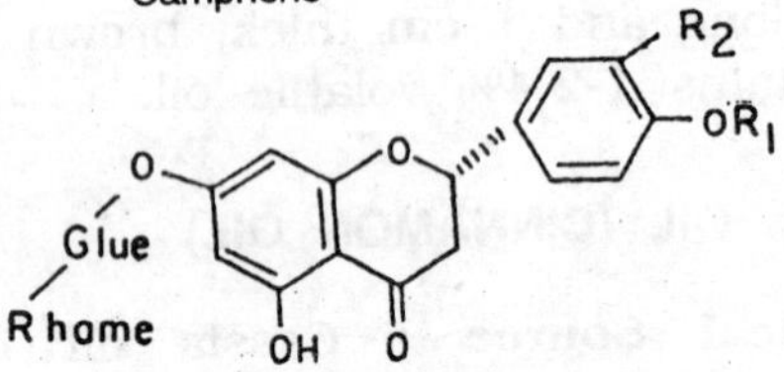

Hesperidin (R₁=OCH₃, R₂=OH)
Neringin (R₁=R₂=H)

Hesperidin (R_1=OCH$_3$, R_2=OH)
Neringin (R_1=R_2=H)

Collection : Lemon plant is a small, 3-5 m high, evergreen thorny tree with shining leaves. Fruits are collected before their green colour changes to yellow in January, August and November. The outer dark yellow peel is removed with a sharp knife. Dried lemon peel is spiral, 20 cm long, 1.5 wide, 2-3 mm thick, outer surface is rough and yellow, inner surface is pithy and white. Odour is strong and aromatic, taste is aromatic and bitter.

Chemical Constituents : Lemon peel contains volatile oil (2.5%), vitmain C, hesperidin and other flavone glycosides, mucilage, pectin, and calcium oxalate. The important constituents of the volatile oil are limonene (90%), citronellal, geranyl acetate, α-pinene, camphene, linalool, terpineol, methyl heptenone, octyl and nonyl aldehydes, etc.

Uses : Lemon peel is stomachic and carminative. It is used as a flavouring agent in medicine, also in beverages, confectionery, and cooking.

BITTER ORANGE PEEL

Synonyms : Fructus Aurantii; Seville Orange.

Biological Source : Bitter orange peel is the dried rind of nearly ripe fruit of *Citrus aurantium* var. *amara* L. and *C. aurantium* var. *sinensis* L.

Family : Rutaceae.

Geographical Source : Bitter orange is native of India. It is grown near Mediterranean Sea, Spain, West Indies, Florida, California, Sicily, Malta, etc.

Collection : Fruits are collected when they are about to ripe. The peel is removed in four 'quarters' or in a spiral band.

Characters : The bitter orange peel is spiral or irregular ribbons, 2-6 mm thick, brittle and hard, breadth is 6-12 mm. Outer surface is dark orange red, rough due to raising over oil glands, various small pits and reticulate ridges. Inner surface is yellowish white, pithy, fracture is hard and short. Odour is aromatic and taste is aromatic and bitter.

Chemical Constituents : Bitter orange peel contains volatile oil (1-2.5%), vitamin C, flavonoid glycosides hesperidine (vitamin P-factor), neohesperidine, naringin, aurantiamaric acid, aurantiamarin (1.5-2.5%); acrid resin, gum and tannin. The bitter taste of the peel is due to the presence of flavonoids aurantiamarin, aurantiamaric acid, naringin, hesperidine and isohesperidine. The dominant component of the volatile oil is limonene (90%) in addition to citral, citronellal and methyl anthranilate.

Chemical Test : Concentrated hydrochloric acid is put on a thick section of the drug. A dark green colour is obtained. This test is absent in sweet orange peel.

Uses : Bitter orange peel is used as flavouring agent, stomachic, and carminative.

SWEET ORANGE PEEL

Biological Source : Sweet orange peel is the fresh rind of fruit of *Citrus aurantium* L. var. *sinensis* (Fam. Rutaceae). The plant is about 8 m in height, and found where the bitter orange grows.

Chemical Constituents : The volatile oil of sweet orange peel contains limonene (90%), citral (5%), methyl anthranilate, decyclic aldehyde, linalool, terpineol, etc. Other constituents isolated from the peel are flavonoids aurantin, hesperidine, 5-hydroxyaurantin and 5-O-desmethyl nobiletin.

Uses : The peel is aromatic and used as carminative, tonic and flavouring agent. Fresh rind is rubbed on the face as remedy for acne.

SAFFRON

Synonyms : Crocus, Spanish Saffron, French Saffron.

Biological Source : Saffron is the dried stigma and style-tops of *Crocus sativus* Linn.

Family : Iridaceae.

Geographical Source : The drug is native of south Europe and is found in Spain, France, Macedonia, Italy, Persia, Austria, China, Germany,Switzerland and Iran. In India the plant is cultivated in Kashmir.

Cultivation and Collection :
The plant is small, perennial herb, 6-10 in high. The corms are planted in July-August in well-prepared soil. In the following year flowering takes place. Each corm is replaced by daughter corms. The flowers are collected early in the morning. The style of each flower is separated just below the stigma and dried by artificial heat for 30-45 minutes. The drug is cooled and stored in dry place. About 1 kg of drug is collected from nearly 100,000 flowers.

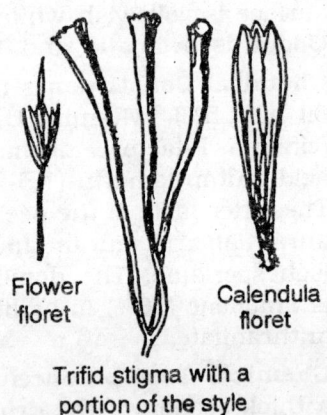

Flower floret

Calendula floret

Trifid stigma with a portion of the style

Fig. 10.9. Saffron

Saffron thrives well in cold regions with warm or sub-tropical climate. It requires a rich, well-drained, sandy or loamy soil. The plant is propagated by bulbs. No manure is applied or irrigation given once the plants are established. The bulbs continue to live for 10 or 15 years, new bulbs being produced annually and the old ones rotting away.

The plants flower in October-December. Heavy rains during this period are harmful. Styles and stigmas are separated and dried in the sun or over low heat on sieves in earthen pots.

The tripartite stigmas plucked from freshly collected flowers and dried in the sun constitute Saffron of the best quality.

Characters : Saffron is flattish-tubular, almost thread like stigmas which are about 3 cm long with slender funnel having dentate or fimbricate rim. Colour is reddish-brown with some yellowish pieces of tops of styles. Odour is strong, peculiar and aromatic; taste is aromatic and bitter.

Chemical Constituents : Saffron possesses a number of carotenoid coloured compounds such as ester of crocin (a coloured glycoside), picrocrocin (a colourless bitter glycoside), crocetin (an aromatic compound), gentiobiose, α-and γ-carotenes, crocin-2, crocin-3, lycopene, zeaxanthin and crocin-4. Picrocrocin is made of Safranal (aldehyde) and glucose. The drug contains volatile oil (1.3%), fixed oil and wax. Crocin is the chief colouring principle in Saffron. On hydrolysis it yields, digentiobiose and the carotenoid pigment crocetin. The colourless glycoside, picrocrocin, gives on hydrolysis, glucose and the aldehyde, safranal. Stearoptene (m.p. 106°) has been isolated from the essential oil.

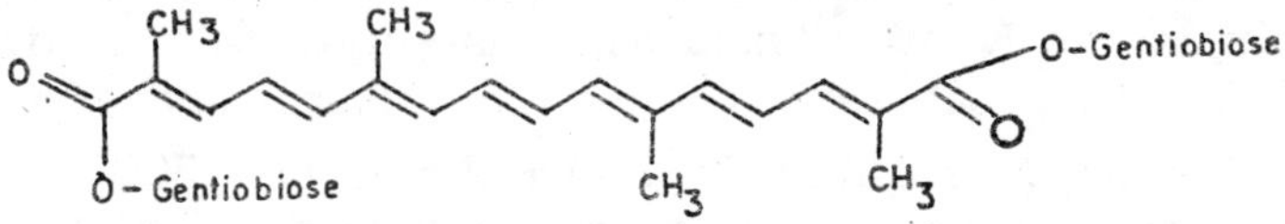

Crocin

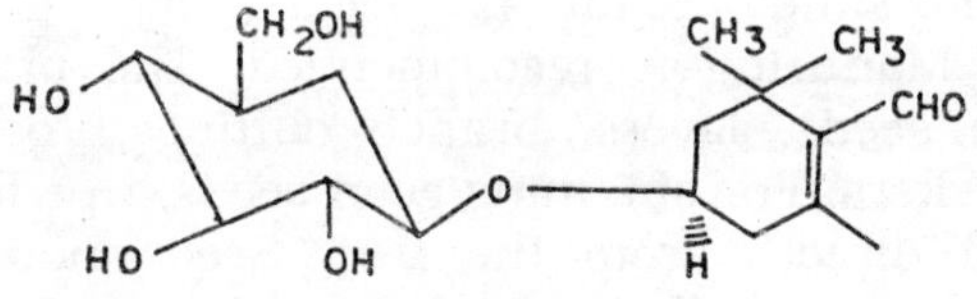

Prcrocrocin

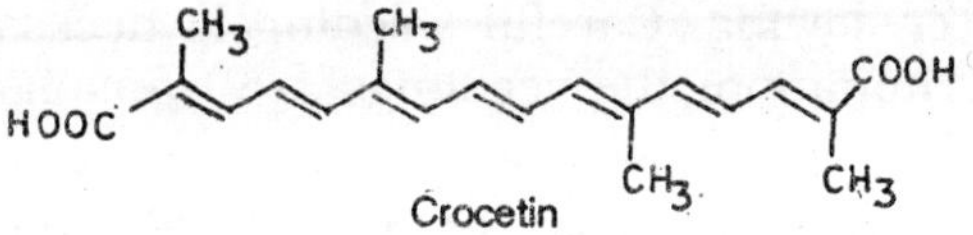

Crocetin

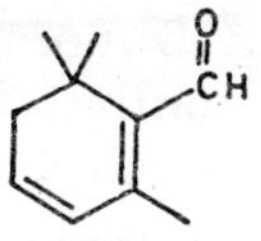

Safranal

About 34 more components, especially terpenes, terpene alcohols and esters, have been identified in the essential oil.

Uses : Saffron is used in fevers, cold, melancholia and enlargement of the liver; as colouring and favouring agent, catarrhal, snake bite, cosmetics and pharmaceutical preparation and as spice. Saffron has stimulant, stomachic, tonic, aphrodisiac, emmenagogue, sedative and spasmolytic properties. Saffron has been employed as an abortifacient.

Adulterant : Saffron is frequently adulterated with styles, anthers and parts of carolla of Saffron. Exhausted Saffron, flowers and floral parts of some *Compositae* like *Calendula* species and *Carthamus tinctorius*, corn silk, and various materials coloured with coal tar dyes, are also used as adulterants. Water, oil or glycerine is added to increase the weight. Coke Saffron of commerce often contains safflower florets with adhesive sugary substances.

CAMPHOR

Synonyms : 2-Bornanone, 2-Comphanone, Gum Camphor, Japan Camphor.

Biological Source : Camphor is a solid ketone obtained from the volatile oil of *Cinnamomum camphora* (L.) Nees et Eber.

Family : Lauraceae.

Geographical Source : The plant is a big tree native to Eastern Asia. It is found widely in Mediterranean region, Sri Lanka, Egypt, South Africa, Java, Sumatra, Brazil, Jamaica, Florida, Formosa, Japan, South China and California. In India the tree is planted in some gardens up to 1300 meters height in the N. W. Himalayas. It is successfully cultivated at Dehradun, Saharanpur, Calcutta, Nilgiris and Mysore.

The plant is cultivated at elevations of 1,500 - 2,000 m provided the temperature does not full below 15°F. A fertile, well-drained, sandy loam is needed for its successful cultivation. Manuring is recommended. The plants can be raised from seeds, layers, branch cuttings, roots cuttings, and root-suckers. For obtaining good seeds, ripe fruits should be collected directly from the tree. Seed should be sown immediately after collection. Germination takes place in about 3 months after sowing. Careful weeding is necessary. Six months after germination, the seedlings are transplanted into seeds baskets.

Preparation : Old trees possess high concentration of Camphor. The small wood chips are treated with steam. Camphor is sublimed and liquid volatile oil passed away into the receiver. Excess of Camphor is obtained from the volatile oil. Camphor is purified by treating it with lime and charcoal and resublimation into large chambers. The collected Camphor is made into blocks by hydraulic pressure.

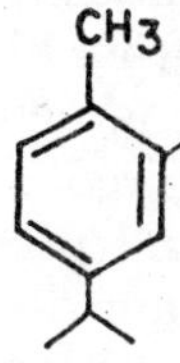

Carvacrol 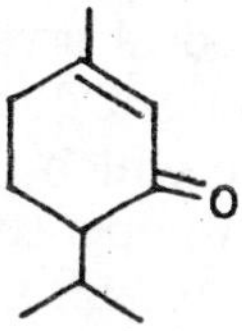   Piperitone 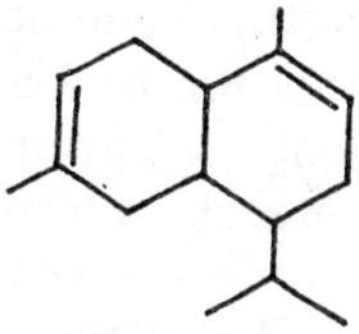   β-Cadinene 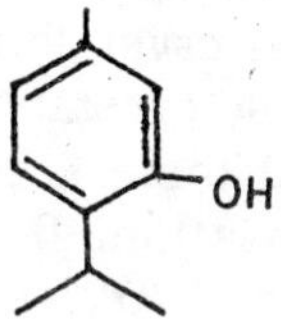   Thymol

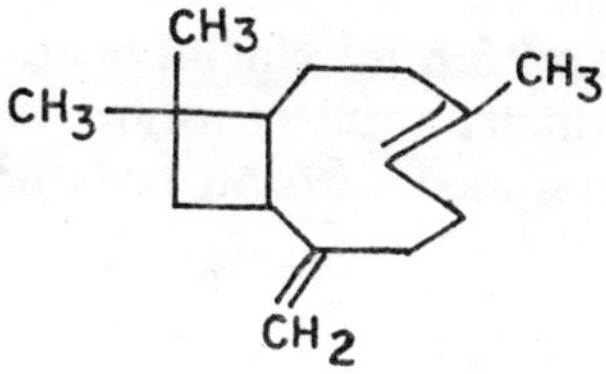

Caryophyllene 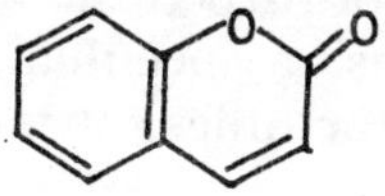   Coumarin 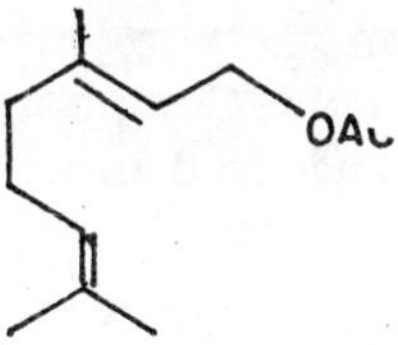   Geranyl acetate

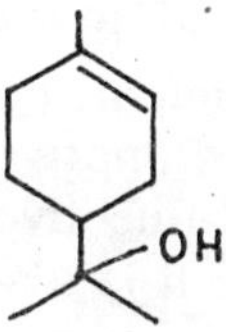

α-Terpineol 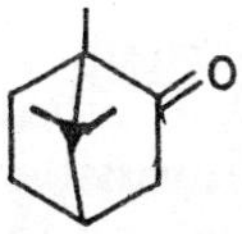   Camphor 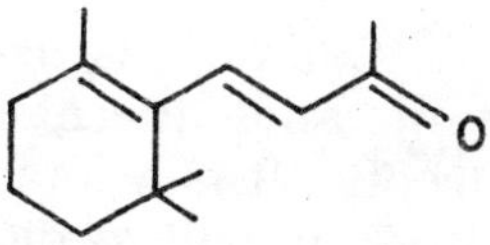   α-Ionone

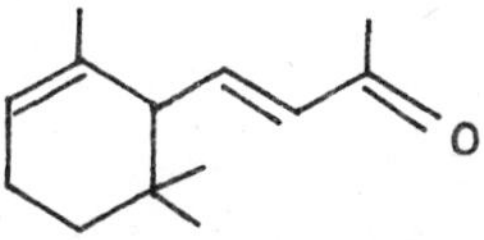

β-Ionone 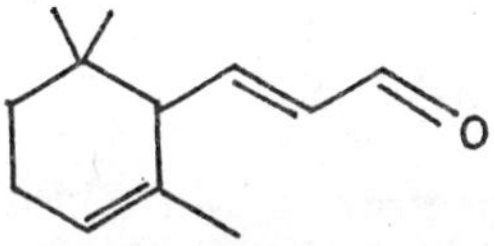   α-Irone

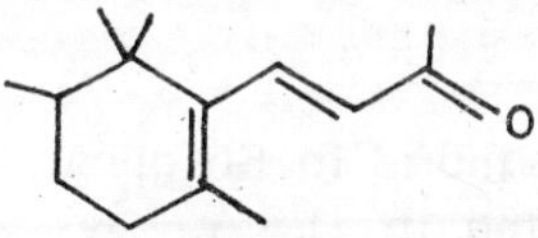

β-Irone 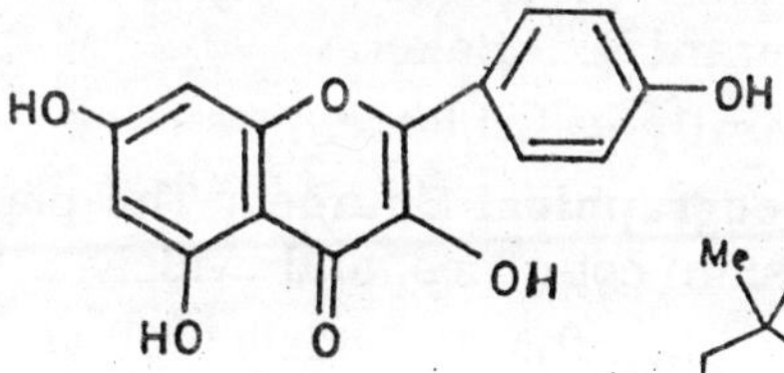   Kaempferol

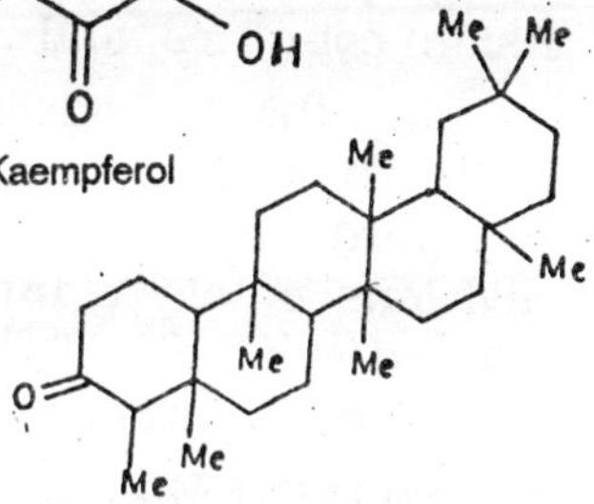

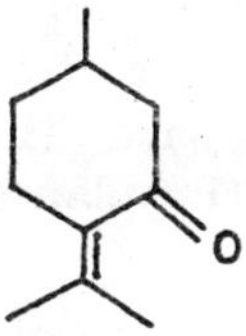

Pulegone 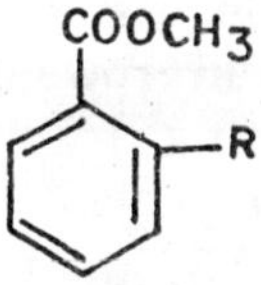   Methyl anthranilate (R=NH₂)   Friedelin
Methyl salicylate (R=OH)

Characters : Natural Camphor is colourless translucent mass with crystalline fracture, rhombohedral crystals from alcohol, cubic crystals by melting and chilling. Odour is characteristic and taste is pungent and aromatic which is followed by cold sensation. It evaporates at room temperature and pressure, m.p. 180°, very volatile in steam. At 25°, one gram dissolves in about 800 ml water (giving a colloidal solution), in 1 ml alcohol, 1 ml ether, 0.5 ml chloroform, 0.4 ml benzene, 0.4 ml acetone, 1.5 ml of turpentine oil, and 0.5 ml glacial acetic acid. Camphor has a peculiar tenacity and cannot be powdered in a mortar unless it is moistened with an organic solvent.

Chemical Constituents : Comphor oil contains camphor, cineol, aldehyde, pinene, camphene, phellandrene, limonene and diterpenes. Camphor is entirely a monoterpenic ketone, $C_{10}H_{16}O$. Its basic carbon framework is related to borneol.

Uses : Camphor is used externally as a rubefacient, counter-irritant and internally as a stimulant, carminative, and antiseptic. It is a topical antipruritic and anti-infective, used as 1-3% in skin medicaments and in cosmetic. It is also used to manufacture some plastics, in lacquers, varnishes, explosives, pyrotechnics, as moth repellent and in embalming fluids.

SPEARMINT

Synonyms : Mint, Pudina (Hindi).

Biological Source : Spearmint consists of the dried leaf and flower tops of *Mentha spicata* L. (*M. viridis* L.) or *M. cardiata.* Gerard ex. Baker.

Family : Labiatae.

Geographical Source : The plant is found in European and Asian countries and widely cultivated in U.S.A.

Mentha is widely cultivated throughout the plains of India. It thrives best in heavy loams well supplied with farmyard manure. It is usually propagated by planting divisions of old plants in rows 30 cm apart. The field is weeded and watered during dry weather. The plants produce leaves for a number of years.

Characters : Mint is a glabrous herb identical to peppermint, 30-90 cm high, with creeping rhizomes, but the stems are usually more purple, leaves are more or less crumpled, opposite, ovate-lanceolate, 3-7 cm long. The apex is acute or acuminate, and the margin unequally serrate. The leaves are almost sessile with bright green colour free from purple. Inflorescence is slender, interrupted cylindrical spikes or crowded lanceolate spikes with 7-10 mm long bracts. Odour and taste are aromatic and characteristic without any cooling sensation.

Chemical Constituents : Spearmint contains volatile oil (0.5%), resin and tannin. The principal component is carvone (50-55%) along with some other monoterpenic constituents like limonene, phellandrene, dipentene, dihydrocarveol, dihydrocarveol acetate, cineol, α-pinene, linalool, etc.

Uses : Spearmint is used as flavouring agent, spice and carminative. It has stimulant, digestive, spasmolytic and diuretic properties. It is given in fever, vomiting and bronchitis and employed as a lotion in aphthae.

Green leaves are used for making chutney and for flavouring clinary preparations, vinegar, jellies and cold drinks.

A soothing tea is brewed from the leaves. A sweetened infusion of the herb is given as a remedy for infantile troubles, vomiting in pregnancy and hysteria.

BUCHU LEAVES

Synonyms : Bucco; Bucku; Buku; Folia Buchu.

Biological Source : Buchu is the dried leaf of *Barosma betulina* Barti & Wendl (short or round Buchu) or of *B. crenulata* (L.) Hook. (oval Buchu) or of *B. serratifolia* Willd (long Buchu).

Family : Rutaceae.

Geographical Source : South Africa

Characters : Leaves of *B. betulina* are 12-20 mm long, 4-5 mm broad, rhomboid-ovate in shape, with a blunt and recurved apex. The margin is dentate towards upper side and serrate towards the base. Dried leaves are brittle and coriaceous. Odour and taste are strong and characteristic.

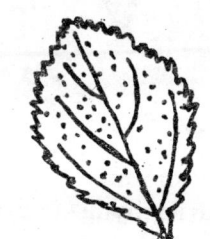

Fig. 10.10. Buchu Leaf of *Barosma betulina*

Chemical Constituents : Buchu leaves contain volatile oil

(30%), diosmin (flavonoid), mucilage, resin and calcium oxalate. The important constituent of the oil is a phenolic camphor, diosphenol (buchu camphor), d-limonene, dipentene, 1-menthone and p-menthane-8-thio-3-one. Diosmin on hydrolysis yielded diosmetin, glucose and rhamnose.

Uses : Buchu is used as a urinary antiseptic, diuretic and carminative.

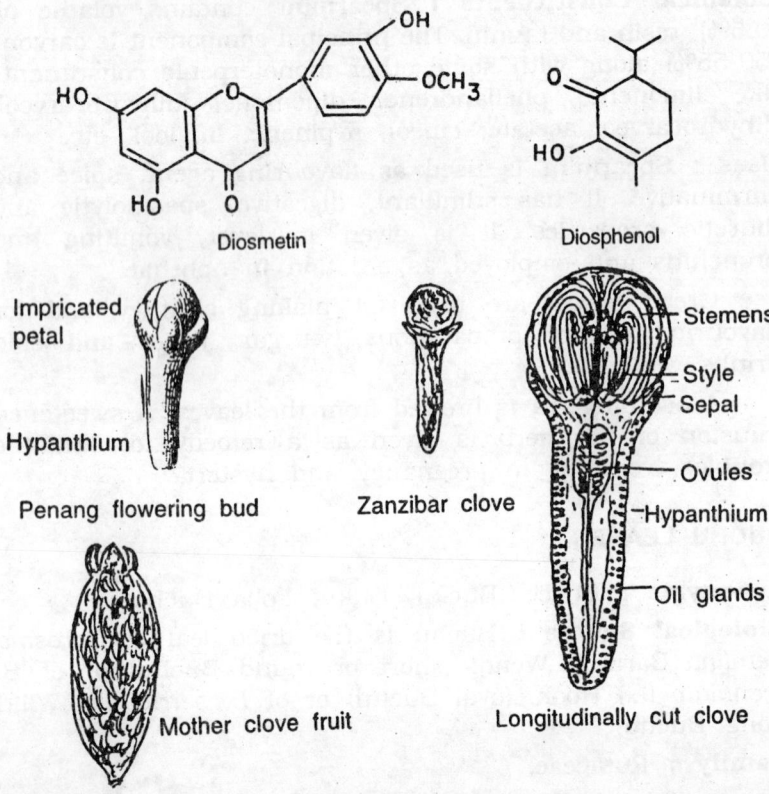

Diosmetin   Diosphenol

Impricated petal

Hypanthium

Penang flowering bud   Zanzibar clove

Stemens

Style
Sepal

Ovules

Hypanthium

Oil glands

Mother clove fruit   Longitudinally cut clove

Fig. 10.11. Clove

CLOVE

Synonyms : Caryophyllus, Clove buds, Caryophyllum; Caryophylli; Laung (Hindi).

Biological Source : Cloves are the dried flower buds of *Eugenia caryophyllus* Bull. et Harri. (Syn. *Syzygium aromaticum* (L.) Merr.

Family : Myrtaceae.

Geographical Source : The clove tree is native of Molucca Island. It is cultivated in Zanzibar, Sumatra, South America, West Indies, Zanzibar, Brazil, Pemba, Ambon, Madagascar, Mauritius and South India.

Cultivation : Clove is pyramidal or conical evergreen plant, 10-20 meters in height, grown in well-drained soil. The plant is propagated from seeds sown during August-October. Dehusked seeds are immediately sown, as their viability deteriorates rapidly. Ripe fruits may be sown without removing the skin, but the germination is poor. Germination takes place in 4-5 weeks. Seedlings are transplanted when they attain a height of about 25 cm during rainy season.

It requires moist, warm and equable climate and suitable rainfall. The plants are protected from pests, diseases and direct sunlight. When seedlings are 9 months old, they attend the height of about 1 meter and then transplanted at a distance of 6 meters in the beginning of rainy season. The plants are shaded by banana planting up to 3 years.

Collections : Flower buds are collected when their base turns into crimson-red in colour in dry weather from August to December. Natives climb on the tree or put ladder for the collection. The cloves are dried in open air and their stalks are separated. On drying about 70% water is lost. Dried cloves are graded according to size, packed into bales and exported.

Morphology : Cloves are reddish-brown, 1-1.7 cm long, consisted of lower solid stalk called hypanthium and upper crown or cap. Hypanthium is swelling, subcylindrical, slightly flattened, tapering below, 10-13 mm long, 4 m wide and 2 mm thick. A bilocular ovary containing numerous ovules attached to axile placentae is present above the stalk. Various schizolysigenous oil glands are present in the hypodermis.

The crown consists of calyx, corolla, stamens and style. Calyx contains four slightly projecting teeth. Corolla is dome-shaped, which is made of four pale yellow-coloured, imbricate, immature, membraneous petals. Many free, introse and tetradelphous stamens are enclosed in the crown.

Ovary contains numerous ovules with axile placentation. A single, erect, firm style reaching up to corolla is present. A nectar-disc (nectary) is present at the base.

Clove has a strong fragrant and spicy odour and pungent, aromatic taste.

Chemical Constituents : Clove contains volatile oil (14-21%), tannins (10-13%), triterpenic acids (e.g. oleanolic acid) and esters, glucosides of sitosterol, stigmasterol and campestrol, vanillin, chromone, eugenin, gum and resin. The important chemical constituents of the volatile oil are eugenol (85-90), acetyl eugenol (3%), α- and β-caryophyllenes, methyl amyl ketone, methyl furfural, dimethyl furfural, carbinol, vanillin and methyl-n-heptyl ketone. Eugenol is a colourless or pale yellow liquid, b.p. 255°. It becomes dark and thick on exposure to air. It has the odour of cloves and spicy, pungent taste. Other substances present in traces are methyl salicylate, methyl benzoate, methyl alcohol, benzyl alcohol, furfuryl alcohol, furfural, methyl furfuryl alcohol, β-pinene, 2-heptanol and 2-nonanol.

Uses : Clove has antiseptic, aromatic, carminative and stimulant action. It is used in flatulence, dyspepsia, throat infection, baking, confections and as flavouring agent. Clove oil is used in toothache, dental preparation and in mouth washes.

Chemical Tests

1. Treatment of hypanthium of Clove or clove oil with potassium hydroxide solution (50%) forms needle-shaped crystals of potassium eugenate.

2. To clove oil (1 ml) in alcohol (5 ml) add $FeCl_3$ solution (1 ml). The solution turns blue due the presence of phenolic hydroxyl group.

3. Add $FeCl_3$ solution to aqueous extract of Clove. Blue-black colour is formed due to the presence of tannins.

Adulterants

1. **Exhausted Clove :** Exhausted cloves are oilless, darker in colour, more shrunken, and float on water surface. The volatile oil is removed by distillation.

2. **Clove Stalks :** Clove stalks are subcylindrical, longitudinally wrinkled, jointed, sometimes branching, brown, and less aromatic than Clove. They contain 4-7% of volatile oil.

   During collection buds are collected along with stalks and some stalks remain attached to the buds after separation. Clove stalks contain calcium oxalate and stone cells which are not present in clove buds.

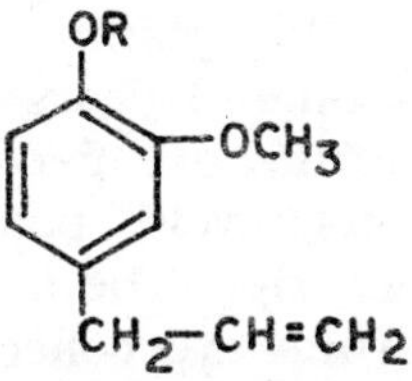

Eugenol (R=H)
Acetyl eugenol (R-COCH₃)

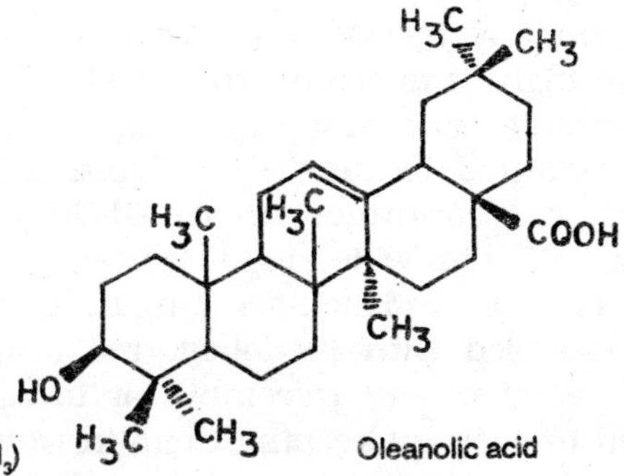

Oleanolic acid

3. **Clove Fruits** : Clove fruits are ripened fruits, about 2 cm long, ovate and tapering below, dark brown in colour with rough outer surface. Each fruit possesses a single firm seeds. It is slightly aromatic and contains starch. Small amount of volatile oil is present in the Clove fruit and adulterated with clove buds.

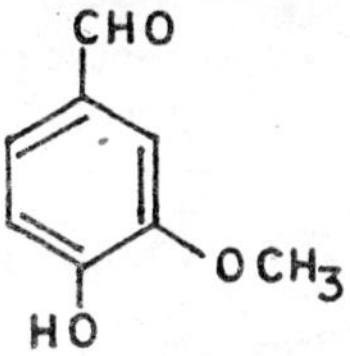

Vanillin

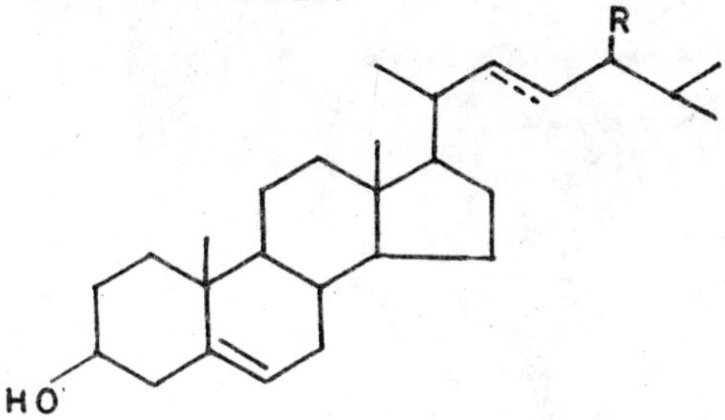

Campesterol (R=Me)
Sitosterol (R=Et)
Stigmasterol (R=Et, $\Delta^{22,23}$)

NUTMEG

Synonyms : Jaiphal; Jayepatri; Myristica; Nux moschata; Nuces (Semen) nucistae; Myristicae semina.

Biological Source : Nutmeg is the dried, ripe seed of *Myristica fragrans* Houtt deprived of its seed coat and with or without a thin coating of lime.

Family : Myristicaceae.

Natural Distribution : The plant is native of eastern Moluccas Island near Indonesia. Now it is cultivated in Malay, Sumatra, Java, Sri Lanka, West Indies and other tropical countries. In India it is found only as a specimen tree in southern region.

Cultivation and Collection : Nutmeg is a dioecious or occasionally monoecious evergreen aromatic tree, usually 9-20 m high. It is grown from fresh seeds which are germinated in about one month. The 6-months old plants are transplanted to the fields. Fruiting begins on 8-9 years old trees and continues up to 20-30 years. Fruits are 5-7 cm long, 4-5 cm wide, light yellow, drupaceous, ovoid, peach-like berries, and dehisce longitudinally when ripe. The seeds are exposed with its lobed, red arillus. Fruits are collected in November and December or in April-June. The seeds are dried in oven by keeping them in trays. The testa is separated with the help of a wooden mallet or special machine and the Nutmeg is extracted. After cracking, the Nutmeg are graded according to size and external appearance and exported in barrels.

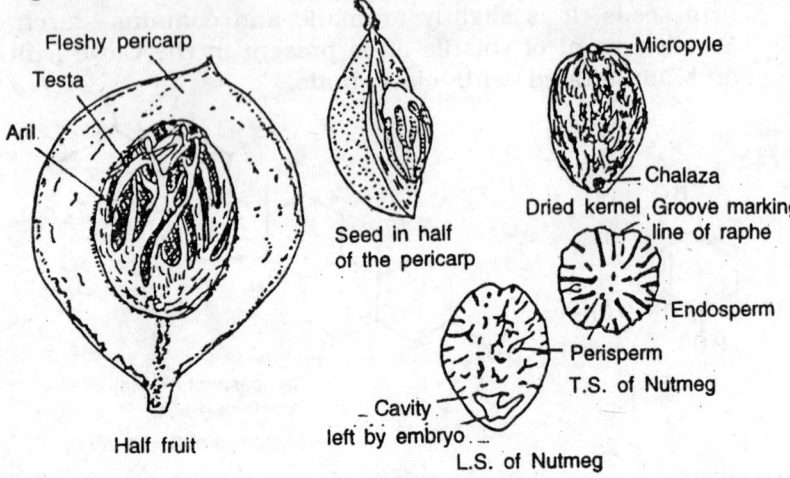

Fig. 10.12 Nutmeg

Morphology : The kernels consist of perisperm, endosperm and embryo. They are 2-3 cm long and about 2 cm in breadth. Shape is ovoid. Outer surface is rough, dark-brown with reticulate furrows. At one end there is a small projection. Micropyle and hilum are present near the projection. The hilum is surrounded by a raised ring. From hilum light furrow runs to chalaza which indicates the position of raphe. The odour is strong and aromatic, taste is pungent and slightly bitter.

Chemical Constituents : Nutmegs contain volatile oil (5-10%), fat or nutmeg butter (30-40%), proteins, phytosterin, starch, amylodextrin and colouring matter. The important constituents of volatile oil are myristicin, elemicin, eugenol, p-cymene and isoeugenol. The myristicin fraction of the volatile oil together with elemicin (>25%) is supposed to be responsible for the signified hallucinogenic properties of Nutmeg seed. Nutmegs contain 15% free myristic acid. Neolignans, polyphenols, tannins, epicatechin, cyanidin, thiamine, riboflavin and niacin have also been reported in Nutmegs.

Uses : Nutmegs are carminative, astringent, aphrodisiac, and stomachic useful in flatulency, nausea and vomiting and as a source of myristica oil. The essential oil from *M. fragrans* showed antibacterial activity. Ingestion of large quantities causes drowsiness, stupor and death.

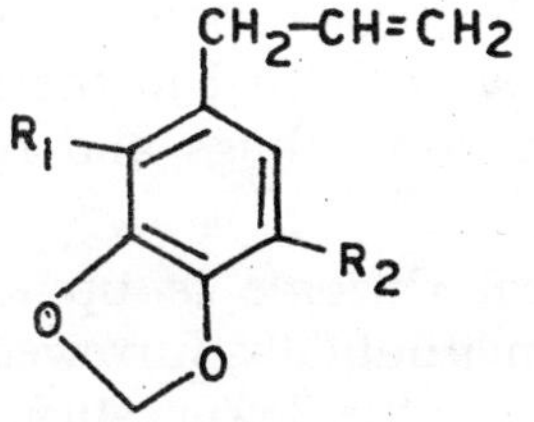

Safrol (R₁=R₂=H)
Myristicin (R₁=H, R₂=OCH₃)
Apiole (R₁=R₂=OCH₃)

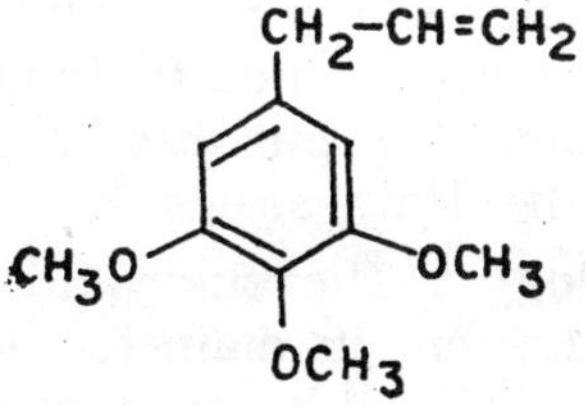

Elemicin

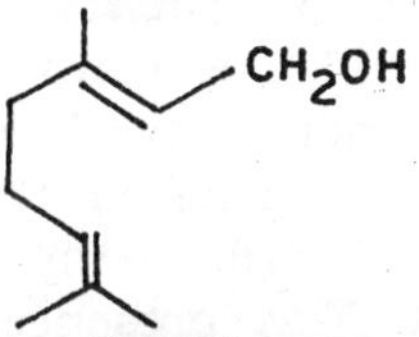

CH₃-(CH₂)₁₂-COOH
Myristric acid

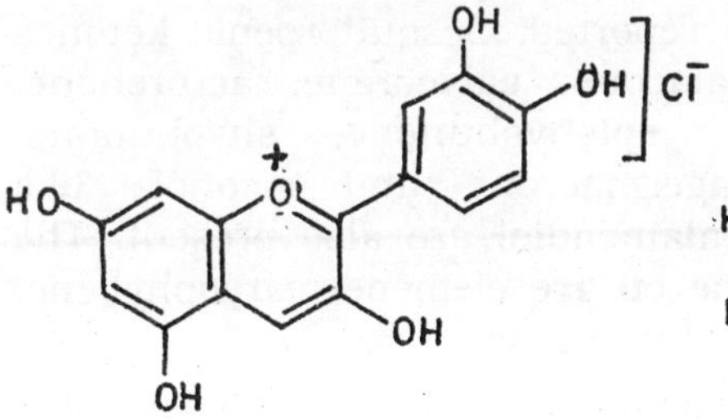

Geraniol

Cyanidine chloride

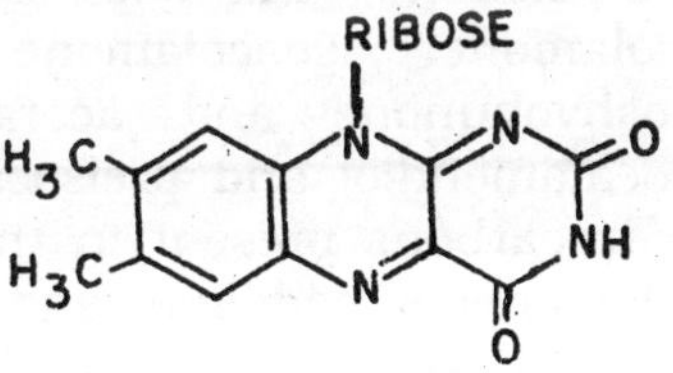

Riboflavine

CALAMUS

Synonyms : Sweetflag; Bach (Hindi); Calamus rhizome; Vaj, Godavaj; Rhizoma Acori Calami.

Biological Source : Dried peeled or unpeeled rhizomes of *Acorus calamus* Linn. are called Calamus (Family Araceae).

Giographical Source : The plant widely occurs in Asia, Europe and North America. It is found throughout India and Sri Lanka.

As a semi-aquatic, perennial, erect, aromatic herb with creeping rhizomes, it grows wild and also is cultivated. Rhizomes are horizontal, joined, somewhat vertically compressed.

The plant is grown in clayey loams and light alluvial soils of river banks. The field is irrigated and ploughed with green manure before planting. The crop is ready for harvest in about a year. The plants are dug out, rhizomes removed and the tops kept for the next planting. The rhizomes are cut into pieces of 5-8 cm and all fibrous roots are removed. The pieces are washed thoroughly and dried in the sun. The dried material is put into rough gunny bags and rubbed to remove the leafy scales.

Morphology : The subcylindrical rhizome is up to 20 cm long and 2 cm in diameter, longitudinally furrowed on the upper surface with root scars on the lower surface.

Chemical Constituents : Calamus contains volatile oil (2-4%) from which α-asarone, β-asarone, calamene, calamenol and calamenone have been identified. Glucoside acorin has also been reported in the rhizome. Other constituents of Calamus oil are methyl eugenol, eugenol, α-pinene and camphene. The presence of small amounts of palmitic, heptylic and butyric acids, asaronaldehyde, calamol, calamone and azulene has also been reported. Sesquiterpenic ketones like acorone, calarene, calacone, calacorene, acrorenone, acolamone, isoacolamone, epishyobunone, shyobunone, isoshyobunone and acoragermacrone and alcohols like isocalamendiol and preisocalamendiol are also present. The hydrocarbons present in the oil are elemene, caryophyllene, calamenene, cadalene and humulene.

Uses : Calamus is nauseant, aromatic, antispasmotic, nervine stimulant, expectorant, carminative, emetic, stomachic, sedative drug and used in dyspepsia, colic, intermittent fevers, nervine tonic, in bronchitis, dysentery of children, insectifuge, in snake-bite, mental ailments, diarrhoea, bronchial catarrh, glandular tumors, and anthelmintic.

α-Asarone

β-Asarone

They are employed for kidney and liver troubles, rheumatism, and eczema. The rhizomes are used in the form of powder, balms, enemas and pills.

Calamus oil is credited with carminative, anti-spasmodic and antibacterial properties. Asarone is a mild sedative, tranquillizer and hypotensive substance. The powdered rhizome is used as an insecticide for the destruction of fleas, bedbugs, moths, lice, etc.

Substitution : They are sometimes substituted for the rhizomes of *Alpinia galanga* (Bach) and *Aconitum* species (Bish).

EUCALYPTUS OIL

Synonyms : Gum wood oil; Australian fever tree oil; Blue-gum tree oil.

Biological Source : Eucalyptus oil is a volatile oil obtained by steam distillation of the fresh leaves of various species of *Eucalyptus* such as *E. globulus* Labill, *E. polybractea, E. smithii, E. viminalis, and E. australiana.* It contains not less than 65% of caneole.

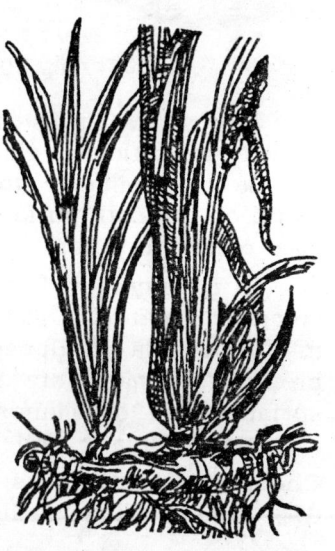

Fig. 10.13. *Acorus calamus*

Family : Myrtaceae.

Habitat : *E. globulus* is a native of Australia and Tasmania. Now it is cultivated in South France, Spain, Portugal, Brazil, Zaire and India (Nilgiri hills).

E. globulus is a large tree attaining a height of 100 m or more with a clean straight bole under forest conditions.

It grows well in Nilgiris (1,700-2,700 m), Annamalai and Palni hills in South India. A cool, moist, equitable climate and deep fertile soil, which is not calcareous or saline, are favourable for the growth of *E. globulus*. It is propagated by seeds.

Morphology : In *E. globulus* leaves are bifacial, lanceolate, scythe-shaped, glabrous, sessile, thin and wax-coated. A coating of wax is present over the thin cuticle, stomata of ranunculaceous type are present on the lower surface and few round internal oil glands are present. Prismatic and rosette type crystals of calcum oxalate are present.

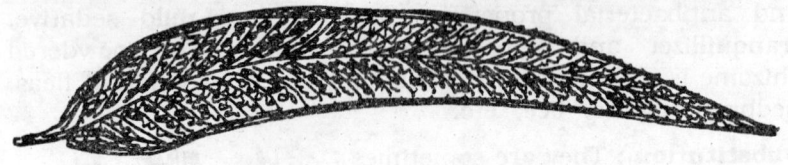

Fig. 10.14. Eucalyptus leaf

E. rostrata leaves are bifacial, lanceolar, sickle-shaped, coriaceous, petiolate, glaucous, ovate with distinct venation. Cuticle is papillate, stomata are of ranunculaceous type found on the both surfaces; many oil glands are present and also rosette crystals.

In *E. viminalis*, leaves are bifacial, elongated or falcate-lanceolate, glabrous, glaucous and sessile. Thick cuticle with minute papilla in upper and marked in lower surface is present; stomata are ranunculaceous present on both surfaces and oil glands are also present. Both types of crystals, prismatic and rosette, are present.

Chemical Constituents : Eucalyptus contains volatile oil (3-6%), resins, tannic acids, dihydroflavanol, aromadendrin-7-

$$HO-\langle\ \rangle-CH=CH\cdot COOH$$

p-Coumaric acid

Dihydroflavanol

Rutin

methyl ether, p-coumaric acid, cinnamic acid, eucalyptic acid and rutin.

Eucalyptus oil is a colourless or pale yellow liquid having a typical, aromatic, camphor-like odour and pungent, spicy cooling taste. The oil contains cineole (70-85%) as the predominent compound. Other components identified in the oil are pinene, camphene, butyric aldehyde, valerenic aldehyde, caproic aldehyde, aromadendrene, cuminaldehyde, pinocarveol, and phellandrene.

Uses : Eucalyptus oil is antiseptic, disinfectant, diuretic, diaphoretic, expectorant, and flavouring agent. It is used in infections of the upper respiratory tract, malaria, certain skin diseases, in ointment for burns and as mosquito repellant. Internally, it is used as a stimulating expectorant in chronic bronchitis and asthma. Eucalyptus increases the flow of saliva, gastric and intestinal juices and thus increases appetite and digestion. It increases the rate of heart beats, lowers the arterial tension and quickens respiration. In toxic doses it is a narcotic poison. It paralyses the respiratory centre in the medulla. Oil obtained from Indian species does not contain butyric and valerinic aldehydes; it is less likely to produce cough and other unpleasant side effects. Mixed with an equal amount of olive oil, it is useful as a rubefacient for rheumatism.

CHENOPODIUM OIL

Synonyms : American Wormseed oil, Mexican Tea oil, Spanish Tea oil, Jerusalem Tea oil, Ambrosia oil.

Biological Source : Chenopodium oil is the essential oil collected by steam distillation of fresh aerial parts of *Chenopodium ambrosioides* L. variety *anthelminticum.*

Family : Chenopodiaceae.

Habitat : Chenopodium plant is an erect, much-branched aromatic herb with glandular hairs, about 30-60 cm in height commonly found in eastern USA and cultivated in Maryland, Carroll Country and South India. It is indigenous to the West Indies. The oil is formed in glandular hairs occurring on the leaves, flowers, and fruits but it is found in excess on pericarp and ovary.

Chemical Constituents : Chenopodium contains volatile oil (1-4%) which is light yellow in colour with a characteristic unpleasant odour and a bitter burning taste. The chief active constituent of the oil is ascaridol (70%) which is an unsaturated terpene peroxide. It explodes on heating or on treating with certain acids. Other constituents of the oil are limonene, myrcene, methyl salicylate, pinene, p-cymene, l-limonene and d-camphor.

Uses : Chenopodium oil is an anthelmintic, particularly for roundworms, hookworms and intestinal amoebae. It is generally used in veterinary practice.

$$CH_3$$

Ascaridol

CARDAMOM

Synonyms : Grains of Paradise, Cardamom Fruit, Ilayachi (Hindi).

Biological Source : Cardamom consists of the dried ripe seeds of *Elettaria cardamomum* Maton var. *minuscula*.

Family : Zingiberaceae.

Geographical Source : Cardamom is cultivated in Sri Lanka, south India (Mysore and Kerala) and Guatemala.

Cultivation : Plant is reedlike 3-4 meters high herbaceous perennial herb. Seeds are planted in nurseries. After one year the young seedlings are transplanted in fields. Fruits are developed on 3-4 years old plants. The nearly ripe capsules, when their colour turns from green to yellow, are collected, washed to remove sand and dried quickly to get green Cardamom. Bleaching takes place when the fruits are dried for longer time in sunlight or by placing trays of the fruits over burning sulphur. Stalk, calyx and split fruits are removed and graded according to size and quality.

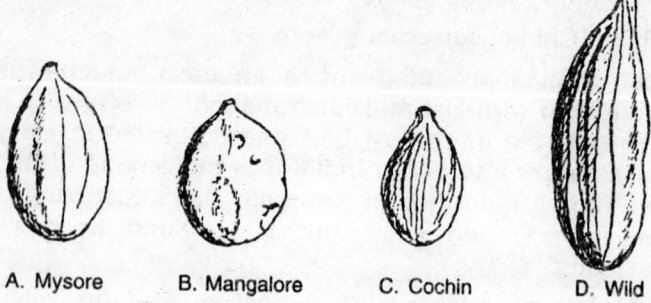

A. Mysore   B. Mangalore   C. Cochin   D. Wild

Fig. 10.15. Cardamom fruits

Morphology : The Cardamom fruit is an inferior, ovoid or oblong, trilocular capsule, 1-2 cm long, apex is beak-shaped, base is rounded with remains of stalk, surface is longitudinally striated, and colour is light green. In each cell there is a double row of seeds attached to axial placenta. The seeds are up to 4 mm in length, irregularly angular, dark reddish brown and wrinkled surface. The odour is aromatic and taste is aromatic, pleasant and somewhat pungent.

Chemical Constituents : Cardamom contains volatile oil (3-8%), resin, fixed oil (1-2%), starch and calcium oxalate. The essential oil possesses eucalyptol (cineole) (50%), borneol, sabinene, terpineol and its acetate, limonene, terpinene, 1-terpinen-4-ol and its formate and acetate and dipentene. The fixed oil consists of the glycerides of oleic, stearic, linoleic, palmitic, caprylic and caproic acids. The unsaponifiable matter from the fixed oil contains β-sitosterol. The seeds contain vitamin B_1.

Uses : Cardamom is aromatic, stimulant, stomachic, carminative, diuretic and used as flavouring agent for pharmeceutical syrups, curries and cake and for preparation of Compound Cardamom Tincture.

Allied Drug

1. *Elettaria cardamomum var.* **major :** This species is the source of the long wild native Cardamom of Sri Lanka. They are 4 cm long, pericarp is dark brown and coarsely striated. Its volatile oil is used in liquors.

2. *Amomum aromaticum* **and** *A. subulatum* **:** *A. aromaticum* is obtained from Bengal and Assam and known as Bengal Cardamom. *A. subulatum* is obtained from Nepal, Bengal, Sikkim and Assam and known as Nepal or Greater Cardamom.

   Malabar Cardamom is characterized by a short leafy shoot, 3 m in height, the fruit shape is roundish or elongated, smaller than the Mysore Cardamom.

   Mysore Cardamom is a robust with leafy steam, up to 5 m high. Mysore Cardamom fruits are elongated, 1-2 inch long, yellowish green when ripe, slightly arched and darkish brown when dry; seeds are numerous, large and less aromatic. Ceylon Cardamom is also a robust variety with shorter pinkish stems and broader leaves.

Adulteration : Cardamom fruits are often adulterated with orange seeds and unroasted coffee grains. The adulterants of seeds are small pebbles and seeds of *Amomum* spp. Powdered seeds are adulterated with the powder of hulls.

VALERIAN

Synonyms : Valeriana; Valerian rhizome; Valerian root; European Valerian; Rhizoma Valerianae.

Biological Source : Valerian is the dried roots, rhizome and stolons of *Valeriana officinalis* L.

Family : Valerianaceae.

Habitat : England, Holland, Germany, France, Belgium, Japan, eastern U.S.A. and India (Kashmir).

Collection : Valerian is about 1 meter high glabrous and perennial herb. Valerian grows well in all ordinary soils, but prefers a rich and heavy loam with moisture. It is often found to flourish in damp and shady places. The plant is propagated by portions of the old rootstocks or from the seeds. The nursery - raised seedlings are first transplanted at a spacing of 18-20 cm in rows. Early in the spring, the seedings may be re-transplanted to their permanent sites at the same spacing. Application of farmyard manure favours the growth of the plants and roots.

The rhizomes and roots of the plants are harvested in the autumn, though the yield is low. The bud-raised plants do not attain a suitable size up to second year. Their tops are cut at the ground-level before the rhizomes are dug up. The rhizomes and roots are thoroughly washed, dried in the sun and the longer rhizomes are longitudinally cut into pieces and the drug is dried below 40°. Fresh drug is odourless but dried drug becomes darker in colour and develops a typical smell of isovaleric acid produced by hydrolysis of borneol isovalerianate which is one of a constituent of the drug.

Morphology : The drug consists of rhizomes, stolons and roots. The rhizomes are 2-4 cm in length and 1-2.5 cm wide. The roots are up to 10 cm in length and 2 mm in diameter, usually matted and broken. Longitudinal slices are also present. Roots are longitudinally striated. The fracture is short and horny. The odour is characteristic valerianaceous and taste is camphoraceous and slightly bitter.

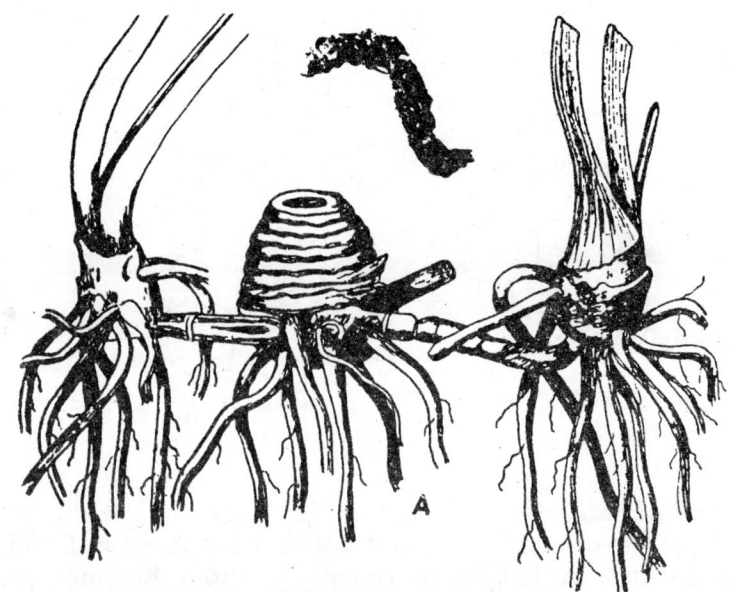

Fig. 10.16. *Valeriana officinalis* - Rootstock with two stolons.

Chemical Constituents : Valerian contains volatile oil (1%), alkaloids (0.05-0.1%) like chatinine, valerine, 2-acetylpyrrol ketone and valerianine; valeric, formic and malic acids, tannins, resin and epoxy-iridoids called as valepotriates (e.g. valtrate, didrovaltrate, acevaltrate, and isovaleroxyhydroxy didrovaltrate). On prolonged storage, hydrolysis of these valepotriates takes place to yield isovaleric acid and activity of the drug is changed. The composition of the valeopotriate mixture differs greatly according to the variety. Valerenic and acetoxyvalerenic acids are the characteristic constituents of the official drug.

Volatile oil contains esters, like bornyl isovalerianate, bornyl acetate, bornyl formate, eugenyl isovalerate, isoeugenyl isovalerate, alcohols, eugenol, terpenes and a sesquiterpene alcohol (valerianol).

Uses : Valerian is carminative, antispasmodic, tranquillizer and sedative and used to cure hysteria, epilepsy, shell shock and neurosis, insomnia, nervous excitement and palpitation of heart. Valepotriates possess mild but definite tranquillizing activity in animals. The drug is also utilized in the perfumery industry, in fevers and for asthenic inflammations.

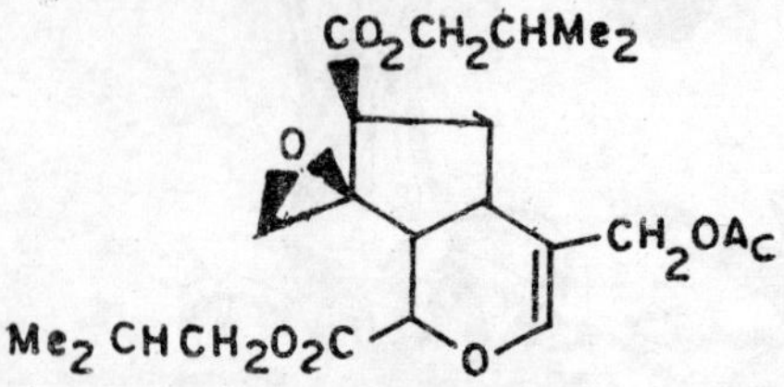

H_3C [structure] CH_2R

$CO_2CH_2CHMe_2$

O

CH_2OAc

$Me_2CHCH_2O_2C$

Valtrate

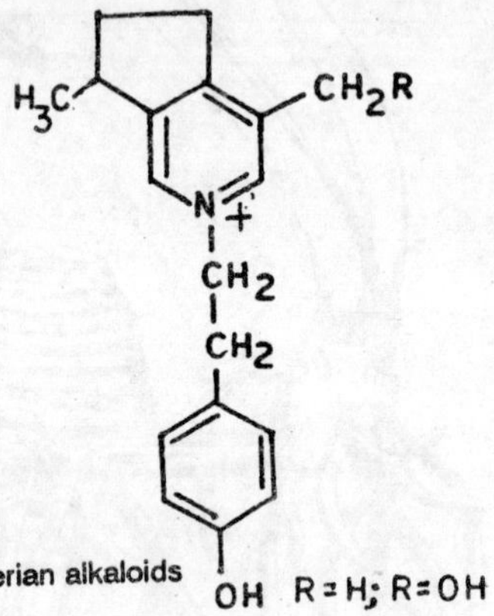

Valerian alkaloids OH $R = H; R = OH$

N^+

CH_2

CH_2

OH

Allied Drug

Indian Valerian (Syn. Mushkbala or Tagar in Hindi). It consists of the dried rhizome and roots of *Valeriana wallichii* DC. It occurs in temperate Himalayas, from Kashmir to Bhutan and Khasia Hills. It consists of yellow-brown rhizomes, size is 4-8 cm long, about 1 cm thick. The size of roots is variable which may be up to 7 cm in length and 1-2 mm thick.

There is no branching of the rhizome and it is somewhat flattened dorsiventrally. Leaf scars are present on the upper surface while roots or root scars exist on the lower surface. The fracture is short. The odour is valerianaceous and the taste is bitter and camphoraceous. The drug possesses volatile oil (0.3-1.0%) which contains esters of isovalerianic and formic acids. Medicinal properties are similar to *V. officinalis* for which it is a good substitute.

Valepotriates of Valerian have also been isolated from *Centranthus ruber* root (Fam. Valerianaceae).

Japanese valerian or Kesso *(V. angustifolia)* contains about 8% volatile oil which is different from the oil of *V. officinalis*.

GARLIC

Synonyms: Allium; Lasan (Hindi).

Biological Source : Garlic is the ripe bulb of *Allium sativum* Linn. (Family Liliaceae).

Habitat : Garlic occurs in central Asia, Southern Europe, and U.S.A. It is widely cultivated in India.

Morphology : It is a perennial herb having bulbs with several cloves, enclosed in a silky white or pink membraneous envelop.

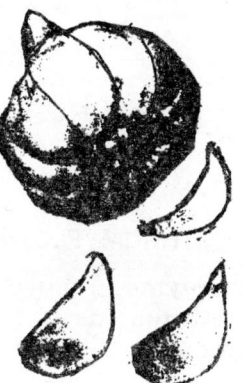

Fig. 10.17. Garlic bulb

Cultivation : The cultivation of Garlic is similar to that of onion. It is generally grown as an irrigated crop throughout the year. It can be grown under a wide range of climatic conditions but it succeeds best in mild climates without extremes of heat and cold. It is grown on a wide variety of soils. It requires a rich well-drained clay loam to grow well. The land in well ploughed to a fine tilth and beds and channels are made. Garlic is planted during October-November in plains and during February-March in the hills. The cloves are separated and pressed lightly into the soil. Garlic requires heavy manuring.

Chemical Constituents : Allicin, a yellow liquid responsible for the odour of garlic, is the active principle of the drug. It is miscible with alcohol, ether and benzene and decomposes on distilling. The other constituents reported in Garlic are alliin, volatile and fatty oils, mucilage and albumin. Alliin, another active principle, is odourless, crystallized from water-acetone and practically insoluble in absolute alcohol, chloroform, acetone, ether and benzene. Upon cleavage by the specific enzyme alliinase, an odour of garlic develops, and the fission products show antibacterial action similar to allicin. Essential oil (0.06-0.1%) contains allyl propyl disulphide, diallyl disulphide and allicin. γ-Glutamyl peptides are isolated from the Garlic. The amino acids present in the bulb are leucine, methionine, S-propyl-L-cysteine, S-propenyl-L-cysteine, S-methyl cysteine, S-allyl cysteine sulphoxide (alliin), S-ethyl cysteine sulphoxide and S-butyl-cysteine sulphoxide.

Uses : Garlic is carminative, aphrodisiac, expectorant, stimulant and used in fevers, coughs, febrifuge in intermittent fevers, respiratory diseases such as chronic bronchitis, bronchial asthma, whooping cough and tuberculosis. It is also used in atherosclerosis and hypertension

$$CH_2=CH-CH_2-\underset{\underset{O}{||}}{S}-S-CH_2 \; CH=CH_2$$

Allicin

$$CH_2=CH-CH_2 \; \underset{\underset{O}{||}}{S}-CH_2 \; \underset{\underset{NH_2}{|}}{CH}-COOH$$

Alliin

PYRETHRUM FLOWERS

Synonyms : Dalmatian insect powder; Persian insect powder, Pyrethrum Insect flowers; Pyrethrum; Flower Heads; Flores pyrethri.

Biological Source : Pyrethrum flowers are the dried flower heads of *Chrysanthemum cinerariaefolium* Visiani or *C. coccineum* Willd. (*C. roseum* Weber et Mohr.) or *C. marschallii* Asch.

Family : Compositae.

Habitat : The plant is indigenous to the Dalmatia (Yugoslavia-Balkans). It is widely grown in Kenya, Japan, Ecuador, Yugoslavia, east central Africa, Brazil, Tanzania, and Zaira. In India the plant is cultivated in Kashmir, Nilgiris and north-west Himalayas.

Cultivation and Collection : Pyrethrum is a 1 meter long glaucous perennial herb with finely cut leaves and numerous flower head. It is cultivated by planting seeds and transplating in calcareous soil. The plant grows better at an altitude of 1900-2700 m (as in Kenya) and annual rainfall of 76-180° cm. Pyrethrum thrives best in a dry climate on well-drained sandy soil. It can grow on mountain slopes and waste lands. Sowing is usually done in spring or in autumn in shade. Before sowing, the seeds are soaked in water, wrapped in cloth, and buried in damp sand. The seeds germinate in 10-15 days and the shading is removed after the shoots appear. The land must be well-drained. Application of excessive nitrogen manures suppresses flowering. The plants flower within one year of transplanting but the yield in poor. The flower heads are gathered when the last florets are about to open. The active principles in over-mature flowers decompose more rapidly than in immature or nearly mature flowers. A low night temperature (5-15°C) stimulates high bud production. Pyrethrum flowers are collected from 2-6 years old plants by hand. The flowers are immediately dried in sunlight or in ovens below temperature 55°C. Fresh flowers are not toxic to insects. Dried flowers are packed tightly in bales and sent to the market.

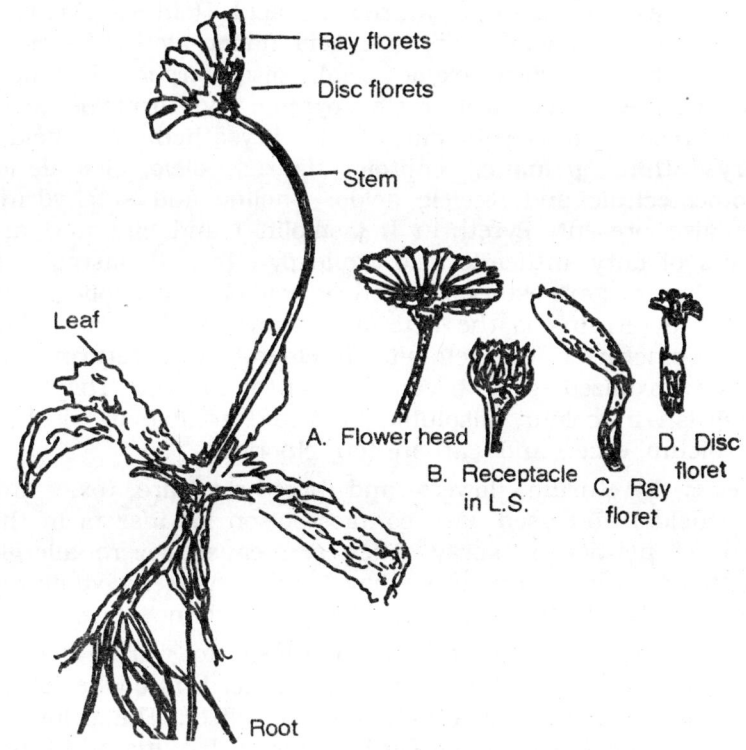

- Ray florets
- Disc florets
- Stem
Leaf
A. Flower head
B. Receptacle in L.S.
C. Ray floret
D. Disc floret
Root

Fig. 10.18 Pyrethrum plant

Morphology : The closed heads of Pyrethrum flowers are nearly 6-9 mm in diameter and open-heads are 9-12 mm in diameter. Peduncle is short, striated longitudinally, receptacle is 4-8 mm in diameter, flat and without paleae, surrounded by an involucre of two or three rows of yellowish or greenish yellow lanceolate, hairy bracts with a membraneous margin. The receptacle contains various tubular florets and a single row of 15 to 23 white, cream or straw-coloured ligulate florets which are 10-20 mm in length and have about 17 veins and three rounded teeth. The central teeth is very small and suppressed. Calyx is tubular and membraneous. Ovary is inferior, achenes are 5-ribbed, style is filiform and stigma is bifid. Calyx and gynaecium in tubular florets are identical to ligulate florets.

The colour is rose-like of ray florets and ten-ribbed fruits. The odour is slightly aromatic and taste is bitter and acrid. **Chemical Constituents :** Pyrethrum contains volatile oil (1-1.5%), esters of chrysanthemic acid (chrysanthemum monocarboxylic acid), pyrethric acid (mono-methyl ester of chrysanthemum dicarboxylic acid), sesquiterpene lactones, the triterpene pyrethrol, resin, pyretol, pyrethrotoxic acid, pyrethrosin, chrysanthemine and chrysathemumic acids, chrysanthin, palmitic, caproic, lauric, oleic, isovaleric, protocatechuic and linoleic acids. Choline and stachydrine are also present. Pyrethrin I, jasmolin I and cinerin I are esters of chrysanthemic acid while pyrethrin II, jasmolin II and cinerin II are esters of pyrethric acid. The alcoholic group of the pyrethrins is the keto-alcohol pyrethrolone and that of the cinerins is the keto-alcohol cinerolone. Pyrethrins are readily oxidized and become inactive in air. They are yellowish in colour, insoluble in water, soluble in alcohol, petroleum ether and carbon tetrachloride.

Uses : Pyrethrum flowers and pyrethrins are toxic and insecticidal and used as a contact poison for insects in the form of powder or spray. They can cause severe allergic reactions. Large amounts may cause nausea, vomiting, tinnitus, headache and other CNS disturbances.

Pyrethrins are practically non-toxic to warm blooded animals when ingested, but if introduced into the blood circulation, they have a marked toxic effect. The principal site of action is the spinal cord. Cases of dermitis and other skin affections are reported.

Pyrethrum is a contact poison, highly toxic to insects. 'It is used as a livestock spray orgainst parasitic insects.

The efficacy of Pyrethrum compositions against specific organisms is greatly enhanced by certain additives. Sesome oil, sesamin, isosesamin and asarinin are effective activators against house flies. Derivatives of alkanamides, piperic and phthalic acids, and a number of other compounds function as synergists. Pyrethrum is effective as an external application in pediculosis and scabies.

Pyrethrum powder is adulterated with the stem and leaf ot the pyrethrum plant, and powdered flowers of other members of *Compositae*, perticularly *C. laucanthemum* Linn. Lead chromate, Turmeric and fustic are used for imparting a yellowish tinge to the powder.

Pyrethrum concentrates should be stored after the addition of antioxidants in sealed containers.

	R_1	R_2
Pyrethrin I	Me	$CH=CH_2$
Jasmolin I	Me	CH_2-CH_3
Cinerin I	Me	CH_3
Pyrethrin II	CO_2Me	$CH=CH_2$
Jasmolin II	CO_2Me	CH_2-CH_3
Cinerin II	CO_2Me	CH_3

SANTONICA

Synonyms : Levant wormweed; Artemisia; Flores cinate; Santonica flowers; Semen cinae; Semen contra.

Biological Source : Santonica consists of the dried unexpanded flower heads of *Artemisia maritima* (Berg) Willkomm.

Family : Compositae.

Habitat : Santonica is found in Turkestan, Pakistan, Iran, Tibet, Nepal and India (from Kashmir to Kumaon) at altitudes of 2,100-2,700 m.

Collection : Santonica is a small decidous perennial shrub with much branched woody rootstalk, up to 100 cm in height. It is distinguished by its short, white-tomentose, 2-pinnatisect leaves with linear segments. Dried close flower heads are 2.4 cm long and nearly 1 mm broad, green. The unexpanded flower heads are collected in July-August and dried quickly.

Artemisias flower at different times in different areas. The age of the individual plant and stage of growth affects the santonin content. The plants should be harvested during spring and summer both for the luxuriant growth. Stripping the leaves and flower buds directly off the plant by hand is suggested. This enables the plants to put on fresh growth. It is bitter in taste.

Chemical Constituents : Santonica possesses α-santonin (2-4%), volatile oil (2-3%), artemisin,and resin. Santonin is the principal anthelmintic constituent which is a sesquiterpene lactone. Its concentration is maximum in closed flower heads and decreased quickly in mature and developed flower heads. It becomes yellow on exposure to light and is insoluble in water, but slightly soluble in alcohol, ether and chloroform. Indian plant besides santonin contains two more constituents, β-santonin with very weak anthelmintic properties and pseudo-santonin devoid of anthelmintic properties. Artemisin (8-hydroxysantonin) is responsible for the bitter taste of the drug and resin.

Uses : Santonica is anthelmintic and santonin is more effective on roundworms than threadworms. It is used as deobstruent, stomachic, laxative and tonic. A decoction of the fresh plant is used to treat intermittent and remittent fevers.

Santonin (R=H)
Artemisin (R=OH)

Sesquiterpene lactone

SAUSSUREA

Synonyms : Kuth, Kut, Costus.

Biological Source : Saussurea is the dried roots of *Saussurea lappa* C.B. Clarke.

Family : Compositae.

Habitat : The plant is found in Kashmir at altitudes from

2700 m to 4300. It is cultivated in the Himalayan region of Kullu, Manali, Lahul and Garhwal.

Cultivation : Saussurea is a robust, erect, perennial herb, 1-2 meters in height, with large cordate, radical and alternate leaves. It requires a cool and humid climate. A deep rich porous soil is preferred and plants growing on such soils develop long and thick roots. It can be propagated either by root cuttings or by seeds. Seeds for propagation purposes are collected in September from the crop. The seeds retain their viability for a year or more. In nature kuth seed is shed in autumn, lies under the snow in winter and begins to sprout during April-June as the snow melts. For propagation by seed under cultivation the same time table is adopted or seed can be sown in spring also. Seeds can be sown in a nursery and the seedlings transplanted at a spacing of 8.9 m x 0.9 m when they are one year old. Direct sowing also gives successful results. The shoots die back each winter and recommence growing when the winter snow melts in the following spring. Roots are harvested during October. They are dried and cut into pieces 10 cm long and dried in the sun.

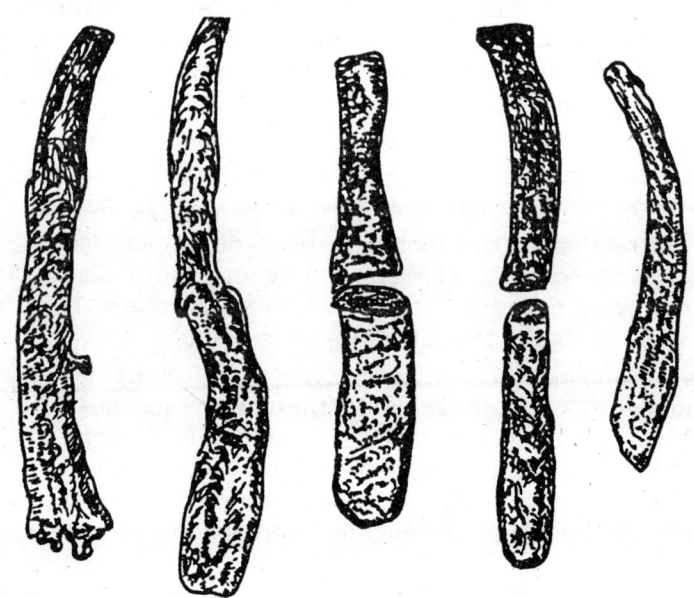

Fig. 10.19. *Saussurea lappa* root

Morphology : Saussurea roots are 7-15 cm long, 1-5.5 cm wide. The roots are fusiform or conical and tapering, collapse in the centre; thin roots are cylindrical, broad, light and stout, usually contain longitudinal wrinkles with anastomose or ridges running straight or spiral; fresh roots are dirty grey to light yellow, dried ones are brown or dull-red; fracture is short and horny; odour is strong, sweet and aromatic and taste is bitter.

Chemical Constituents : Saussurea contains volatile oil (1.5-2.5%), nitrogenous base saussarine (0.05%), inulin (15%), potassium nitrate, sugars, kushtin, and bitter resin. The essential oil is the mixture of sesquiterpene lactones like costuslactone and its dihydro derivatives, costusic acid, 12-methoxy dihydrocostunolide, costol, aplotoxin, α-and β-costenes, phellandrene, camphene, and terpene alcohol. Saussurea also contains β-sitosterol, stigmasterol, betulin, aplotaxene, β-selinene, β-elemene, α- and β-ionones, etc.

The oil is a pale yellow to brownish, very viscous liquid. It has a peculiar soft but tenacious odour. The oil blends well with α-decanolide and its isomers, cinnamic alcohol, isoeugenol, methylionones, etc.

The essential oil is valued in high class perfurmery and cosmetics where it is used for blending purposes. The oil is expensive, and is therefore. extensively adulterated with elecampane oil.

The essential oil of Kuth has strong antiseptic and disinfectant properties especially against *Streptococcus* and *Staphylococcus*. It has marked carminative properties.

Extraction of the root with benzene or petroleum ether produces a concrete of rich and true natural odour. It is commercially called the costus resinoid. Alcoholic extract of the root contains the alkaloid saussurine.

Uses : Saussurea roots have tonic, disinfectant, stomachic, spasmolytic, carminative and stimulant properties and are used as spasmodic in asthma, cough and cholera and as alterative in chronic skin diseases and rheumatism. It is also used for preserving silk and expensive wool fabrics, as an incense in religious ceremonies and as insect repellent.

LEMONGRASS OIL

Synonyms : East India lemongrass, Malabar or Cochin Lemongrass.

Biological Source : Lemongrass oil is obtained from *Cymbopogon flexuosus* Stapf. (syn. *Andropogon nardus* var. *flexuosus* Hack.). It contains not less than 75% of aldehydes calculated as citral.

Family : Gramineae.

Habitat : Lemongrass is indigenous to India and is found in Tinnevelli, Travancore, and Cochin. Two principal varieties of Lemongrass are recognized as the red-stemmed variety, the true *C. flexuosus*, which is a source of East Indian Lemongrass oil and the white-stemmed variety which is designated as *C. flexuosus* var. *albescens*. The oil from the latter is low in aldehyde content and is slightly soluble in 70% alcohol.

Cultivation : Lemongrass grows best in well-drained sandy loam or in light sandy soil. Dark, heavy, rich soil, gives a higher yield of grass, but the oil obtained from it has a lower citral content. Warmth and sunshine favour oil development. The grass grown on lower slopes, less exposed to heavy rains, is rich in oil content.

The grass is cultivated in forest clearings or on hill slopes at an altitude of about 2,000 ft. The ground is ploughed in March-April and seeds are sown at random. The grass come up with the first shower of the monsoon. Weeding is carried out systematically in the plantation. Protection against grazing is necessary. The grass is ready for cutting at the end of May or early in June and may be harvested every 35-40 days till November or December. The citral content of the oil is high (83%) when it is obtained from grass harvested during September-December. After cutting, the stubbles are burnt before the sporadic April monsoon shower. Fresh shoots come up from the roots with the start of regular monsoon, and the grass is ready for harvesting by the end of May. Plantations are renewed every 6-8 years.

Characters of Oil : A light coloured oil, rich in citral content, is obtained by steam distillation. The yield varies form 0.25 to 0.5% per acre.

Chemical Constituents : Lemongrass oil is the principal source of citral (68-85%) from which ionone is derived. The oil also contains methyl heptanone, decyl aldehyde, geraniol, linalool, limonene and dipentene.

Uses : The oil is used in perfumery, soaps, and cosmetics and as a mosquito repellent. Ionones obtained from citral are required for synthetic violet perfumes.

SANDALWOOD OIL

Synonyms : Chandan oil, Sandal oil; Yellow Sandalwood oil; Liginum.

Biological Source : Sandalwood oil is obtained by distillation of sandalwood, *Santalum album* Linn.

Family : Santalaceae.

Habitat : Sandal is a small to medium sized, evergreen semi-parasitic tree found in the dry regions of peninsular India from Vindhya Mountains southwards, especially in Mysore and Tamil Nadu. It has also been introduced in Rajasthan, parts of U.P., M.P. and Orissa.

Cultivation : Sandal tree grows mostly on red, ferruginous loam overlying metamorphic rocks, chiefly gneiss, and tolerates shallow, rocky ground and stony or gravelly soils, avoiding saline and calcareous situations. It is not found on the black-cotton soil. The growth is luxuriant on rich and fairly moist soils, such as garden loam and on well-drained deep alluvium along the river banks, but the heartwood from these trees is deficient in oil. The trees grown on poor soils, particularly on stony or gravelly soil, produce more highly scented wood, giving a better yield of the oil.

It reproduces from seeds dispersed by birds. Germination is profuse in the forests immediately after the monsoons. For artificial regeneration, it is necessary to provide suitable climatic, and ecological conditions. For procuring seeds, the fruits are collected during January-March. Germination is up to 80%. Just after the first monsoon showers, the sandal seeds are dibbed and protected by thorny bushes. The seeds germinate in about 8-14 days. The seedlings grow rapidly, i.e. up to 20-30 cm high, at the end of the first year.

Properties : Sandalwood oil is viscous, yellowish liquid having a peculiar, heavy, sweet and very lasting odour. It has sp. gr. 0.97-0.98, viscosity 1.5, and acid value 0.5-0.8.

Chemical Constituents : The main odorous and medicinal constituent of Sandalwood is santalol ($C_{15}H_{24}O$). This primary sesquiterpene alcohol forms more than 90% of the oil and is present as a mixture of two isomers, α-santalol and β-santalol, the former predominating. The other constituents reported are hydrocarbons santene, nor-tricycloekasantalene, α- and β- santalenes, the alcohols santenol and teresantalol, the aldehyde nor-tricyclo-ekasantalal, and isovaleraldehyde, the ketones l-santalone and the acids teresantalic acid and α and β-santalic acids.

Uses : Sandalwood oil is highly used in perfumery creations and finds an important place in soaps, face creams, toilet powders etc.

Substitutes and Adulterants : Oil from several plant sources are either used as substitutes for or as adulterants of natural sandalwood oil. Oil obtained from the Australian plant *Fusanus spicatus* is used as a substitute for genuine Sandalwood oil. Wood and oil of *Santalum yasi* have a feeble odour which is not delicate like that of Indian Sandalwood oil. East Africa markets the wood and oil derived from *Osyris tenuifolia*, the wood is similar to sandal and is used as an adulterant. An oil from Mauritius is reported to possess most of the characteristics of the Indian oil. In West Indies an oil derived from *Amyris balsamifera* Linn. is marketed as a cheap substitute for Indian Sandalwood oil. In India, the wood of *Erythroxylum monogynum* Roxb is used as an adulterant. The wood of *Mansonia gagei* Drum. resembles Sandalwood closely in its physical and other characteristics. Another species, which is common in southern India and used as an adultrant, is *Ximenia americana* Linn.

α-Santalol   β-Santalol

BLACK PEPPER

Synonyms : Kalimirch; Golmirch.

Biological Source : Black pepper consists of the dried, fully developed unripe fruits of *Piper nigrum*   L.

Family : Piperaceae.

Habitat : Pepper is cultivated in the hills of south-western India from North Kanara to Kanyakumari.

Cultivation : Black pepper is cultivated mostly as a mixed crop in homestead gardens. The pepper plant is a climbing vine found growing up to an altitude of 1,500 m. Supports or standards have to be provided for the plant to grow on. The standards usually preferred are quick growing trees, which not only provide support but also shade. Planting is done in April-May during the early rains so that their standards grow sufficiently to allow pepper vines to be planted in July-September. When planted as a mixed crop in coconut, arecanut, tea or coffee plantation, the main crop or the shade trees serve as standards besides providing the shade.

The Pepper vine can be propagated either vegetatively or by seeds. The planting of the pepper vine is done either in July or August. The pits for planting are made perferably on the north and north-eastern sides of the standard so that the severe western sun is avoided. Pepper is an exhausting crop and the soil needs high level of nitrogenous substances.

The wilt and *pollu* are the two important diseases of Pepper. The Pepper vine starts bearing from the third year of its growth. Usually there are two crops in a year, one in August-September and the other in March-April. The harvest season of Pepper extends from the middle of December to the middle of March in coastal areas.

Morphology : It is nearly globular in shape, about 4-5 mm in diameter with a characteristic coat with deep set wrinkles. The pericarp is thin and encloses a single seed with a hollow centre. The perisperm is horny in the outer part and floury around the central cavity.

For preparing Black Pepper, the freshly harvested spikes are spread on mats or concrete floors and dried in sun for about a week with frequent turning over to prevent infection by mildew. During drying, the green or red fruits gradually change in colour to dark brown or almost black and their skin becomes tough and wrinkled. The fruits are detached from the stalks by beating the heaped up material with sticks or treading upon it barefood. Impurities are picked by hand.

Composition : Black Pepper contains the alkaloids piperine, chavicine, piperidine and piperetine. The characteristic aromatic odour of Pepper is due to the presence of a colourless volatile oil (1-2.6%) in the cells of pericarp which contains phellandrene, caryophyllene, piperonal, dihydrocarveol, caryophyllene oxide, cryptone, α-and β-pinenes, epoxydihydro-caryophyllene, phenylacetic acid, and citronellol. Starch (45-63%) is the predominant constituent of pepper. It also contains thiamine, riboflavin, nicotinic acid, ascorbic acid and carotene.

Uses : Black Pepper is mostly used for its characteristic delicate penetrating aroma and pungent, biting taste. It is employed as an aromatic stimulant in cholera, weakness following fevers, vertigo, coma, etc., as a stomachic in dyspepsia and flatulence, as an antiperiodic in malarial fever and as an alterative in paraplegia and arthritic diseases. Externally it is valued for its rubefacient properties and as a local application for relaxed sore throat, piles and some skin diseases.

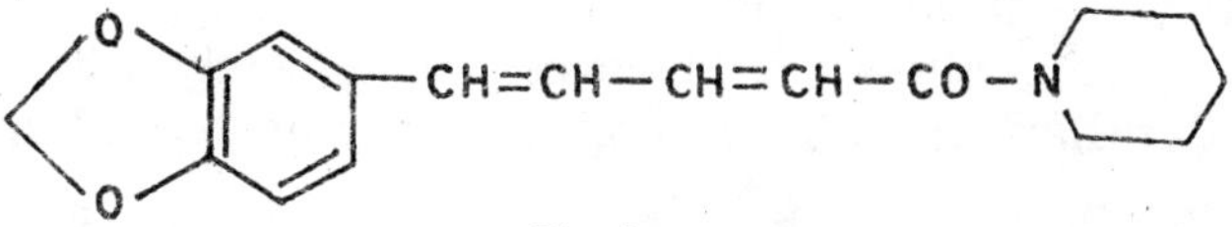

Piperine

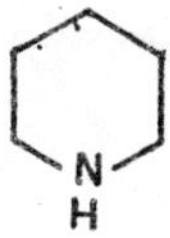

Piperidine

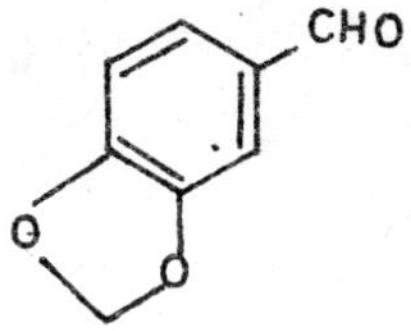

Piperonal

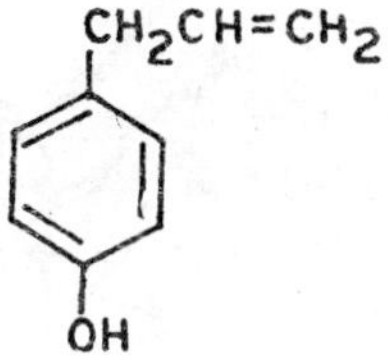

Chavicol

CANTHARIDES

Synonyms: Spanish fly; Blistering fly; Blistering beetle, Russian flies; Cantharizo.

Biological Source : Cantharides are the dried insects, *Cantharis vesicatoria* (Linn.) De Geer.

Family : Meloidae.

Habitat : Spain, Italy, Poland, Sicily, South Russia, and Romania.

Collection : Cantharides are found on some shrubs of the families Caprifoliaceae and Oleaceae. The mature insects have brilliant green colour with metallic luster. They appear in June-July and their presence can be detected from a distance due to strong unpleasant odour. Due to cold night, the insects become sluggish in the early morning. A large piece of cloth is spread under plants and the shrubs are shaken or beaten with a stick. The insects fall on the cloth and are collected. As the insects cause irritation on touching, the collector protects his body parts from them. The insects are killed by putting them in dilute vinegar, chloroform or ether or by exposing to the fumes of ammonia or sulphur dioxide. Then the insects are dried carefully below 40°C, stored in air tight containers and preserved from attack of other insects by adding few drops of chloroform or carbon tetrachloride.

Characters : Cantharides are 1.5-2.5 cm long, 5-8 mm broad, wings are brown, transparent and membraneous and protected by wing covers known as elytra which are copper green in colour; their body consists of three parts, viz, head, thorax and abdomen. A pair of antennae and two small black eyes are present on the head. Three pairs of legs are attached to the thorax. Abdomen is covered completely with wings. Dried Cantharides have strong unpleasant typical odour.

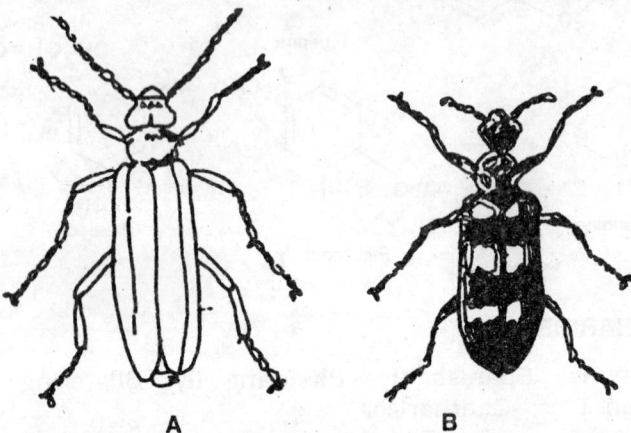

A   B

Fig. 10.20. (A) *Cantharis vesicatoria* (B) *Mylabris sidoe.*

Chemical Constituents : Cantharides contain the vesicating principle cantharidin (0.6-1%), fat (10-15%), resinous mass, acetic and uric acids. Cantharidin, mp 218°C, is a crystalline lactone or anhydride of cantharidic acid, sublimes at about 110°, insoluble in cold water, soluble in acetone, chloroform, ether and ethyl acetate.

Uses : Cantharides are vesicant, counter-irritant and rubefacient. Cantharidin is used externally in a solution form as a counter-irritant and to remove certain types of warts,

Cantharidin

in some hair tonic formulations and as an aphrodisiac.

Allied Drug

Mylabris (syn. Chinese Cantharides, Chinese blistering flies) is the dried blistering bettle of *Mylabris sidoe* Fabr (Fam. Meloidae). The beetles are found in China and some parts of eastern India and used as substitute for cantharides. These beetles are blackish brown in colour, cylindrical body, rounded above, flattish below; two black antennae with eleven segments at the globular head and abdomen containing black wings covered with black elytra with three tawny bright yellow bands and wing cases marked with a spot at point of insertion. Mylabris contains cantharidin (1-2%) and fixed oil. It is used as a substitute of cantharides.

AJOWAN

Biological Source : Ajowan is the ripe dried seeds of *Trachyspermum ammi* (L.) Spr. (syn. *Carcum copticum).*

Family : Umbelliferae

Habitat : It is a native of Egypt and grown through out India, Mediterranean region and in south-west Asian countries such as Iraq, Iran, Afghanistan and Pakistan.

Ajowan is an erect, glabrous or minutely pubescent, branched annual herb, up to 90 cm tall. The crop is grown in cold weather, both as a dry crop and under irrigation. It grows on all kinds of soil, but does well on loams or clayey loams. Seeds are sown broadcast in the moist soil from September to November. Germination takes in 5-15 days, depending upon climatic conditions. First irrigation should be light. The flowering takes place in about two months. The harvesting period is February or March. The fruits become ready for harvesting when the flower heads turn brown. The plants then pulled out by the roots and dried. The dried fruits are separated by carefully rubbing with hands or feet.

The drug occurs as entire cremocarps or separated mericarps. Cremocarps are ovoid-cordate to ovate, laterally compressed; 1.7 - 3.0 mm long; 1.5 - 2.4 mm broad, dirty yellow to yellowish brown in colour and half to two-thirds apical portion has slight purplish tinge. At the top of the cremocarp is a bifid stylopod surrounded by five minute sepals. Each mericarp shows five light-coloured ridges and is covered with light yellow protuberances. The drug has an aggreeable odour and aromatic and warming taste.

Chemical Constituents : Ajowan contains an essential oil (2-3.5%), protein (17.1%), and fat (21.8%). Ajowan oil is a colourless or brownish yellow liquid possessing a characteristic odour of thymol and a sharp taste. The principal constituents of the oil are phenol, mainly thymol (35-60%), carvacrol, p-cymene, γ-terpinene, α- and β-pinenes and dipentene. The fatty oil is composed of palmitic, petroselinic, oleic, linoleic and 5, 6-octadecenoic acids.

Uses : Ajowan is widely used as a spice in curries; in pickles, certain types of biscuits, confectionery, beverages and in *pan*-mixtures. It is valued for its antispasmodic, stimulant, tonic and carminative properties. It is given in flatulence, atonic dyspepsia, diarrhoea and cholera. It is used most frequently in conjunction with asafoetida, myrobalans and rocksalt. Ajowan is also effective in relaxed sore throat and in bronchitis, and often constitutes an ingredient of cough-mixture. It is taken with buttermilk for relieving difficult expectoration due to dried up phlegm. Externally, a paste of the crushed fruit is applied for relieving colic pains, and as a hot and dry fometation of the fruits on the chest in asthma. It is also used to prepare lotions and ointments and applied for checking chronic discharge. It has antibiotic activity.

Ajowan oil is used as an antiseptic and aromatic carminative, for perfuming disinfectant soaps and as an insecticide. The action of the oil and its uses are similar to those of thymol. The oil is useful as an expectorant in emphysema, bronchial pneumonia and some other respiratory ailments.

The fatty oil is recommended as an external application in cases of rheumatism.

TURPENTINE OIL

Synonyms : Oleum Terbinathae; Rectified oil of Turpentine.

Biological Source : Turpentine oil is obtained by distillation of oleoresin of *Pinus palustris* (long leaf pine) and other species of *Pinus* such as *P. longifolia* Roxb., *P. elliottii, P.*

radiata, etc.

Family : Pinaceae

Geographical Source : The oil is prepared on commercial scale in India, France, Russia and U.S.A.

Cultivation and Collection : In India *Pinus longifolia* and *P. insularis* are found naturally in Himalayas from Kashmir to Bhutan. *P. longifolia* is cultivated in Himachal Pradesh, Jammu, Punjab and Uttar Pradesh. The plant grows well at altitude 600 to 2400 m, in rainfall between 100 to 175 cm, temperature 30 to 38°C and on variety of soils like limestone, quartz and clay, stand stone and on bare rocks. It is grown by seed germination in March and April. The 20-25 year old plants are used for the collection of the Colophony (resin) and the volatile oil.

Preparation : Suitable number of blazes are made and then heavy tapping is done. The resin flows which is collected in earthenware or other suitable containers. It continues for 8 to 10 years. This type of tapping produces schizogenous ducts. The crude oleo-resin is purified by heating in a steam jacketed vessel with spiral tube. Vegetable debris, sand particles and other impurities are removed by setting or floating. The clear resin is re-distilled in a distillation plant after treatment with sodium hydroxide or lime water to remove resins, acids, phenols, etc. It is then dried over sodium sulphate and packed in suitable containers. The oleoresin produces Turpentine oil (25%) and Colophony (70%). The Terpentine oil after treatment with alkalies is known is *rectified turpentine oil.* U.S.A. is main producer of the total world production which is about 70%.

Description : The oil is colourless or slightly yellow in colour, clear, transparent liquid. Odour is strong, characteristic and becomes much stronger on storage with less pleasantness; taste is bitter and pungent. It is insoluble in water, soluble in alcohol, chloroform, carbon disulphide, glacial acetic acid, benzene, petroleum ether and fixed oils.

Chemical Constituents : About 40 monoterpenes are reported in the oil. The major components are α-pinene (20-30%), β-pinene (5-10%), camphene, β-phellandrene, δ-3-carene, p-cymene, longifoline, estragol, limonene, etc. Americal oil contains α-pinene (65%) and β-pinene (30%) as the principal constituents.

Uses : Externally it is used as a counter-irritant and rubefacient. For inhalation, terebene is used which is prepared from the oil by the action of cold sulphuric acid. It is used in the treatment of chronic bronchitis. Commercially, it is used to prepare synthetic pine oil, disinfectants, denaturants, insecticides, paints, varnishes fragrances, vitamins, etc.

Adulterants : The common adulterants are resin oil, wood turpentine and petroleum jelly. The last adulterant is detected low weight per ml of the oil and resin oil leaves the stain of fatty matters on staining on a paper.

CITRONELLA OIL

Biological Source : It is a volatile oil obtained by steam distillation from the fresh leaves of *Cymbopogon nardus* (Linn.) Rendle.

Family : Gramineae.

Habitat : The plant is native of Sri Lanka and now cultivated in Burma, Malaysia, Indonesia, Fiji and India.

Cultivation and Collection : It is tall, 1.75 m high, perennial plant with throwing dense leaves growing from a short rhizome. The leaves are linear and tapering, up to 60-70 cm long, glabrous green and lower ribs are red in colour. It is cultivated by vegetative propagation. Regular irrigation is required during winter and summer. The crop is ready for harvesting after 8 months and it can be harvested several times with regular intervals. About 20 tonnes of grass can be harvested per hectare. It contains about 0.5% of volatile oil.

Description : The oil is pale-greenish yellow in colour. It has pungent taste. It is insoluble in fixed oils.

Chemical Constituents : Citronella grass contains 0.3 to 0.9% of volatile oil. The main constituents of the oil are geraniol (40-60%) and citronellal (15-20%). Other constituents are d-camphene, limonene, dipentene, borneol, linalool, cadinene, elemicin, and methyl eugenol. Java variety possesses citronellal (25-50%), geraniol (25-40%), camphene, limenene and dipentene.

Uses : The oil is used as perfume for soap, brilliantines, in mosquito-repellent ointments and sprays and as a flavouring agent for liniments, lotions and cosmetics.

QUESTIONS

1. How are volatile oils prepared ? Give a general scheme for the biosynthesis of volatile oil components.

2. What are umbelliferous fruits ? Describe the morphological and anatomical features of Cardamom. Mention its chemical constituents and uses (Jamia Hamdard, 1994).

3. Give the structural formula of the following constituents. Mention the source and uses of drugs in which these constituents are found (a) Menthol (b) Citral (c) Dilapiole (d) Carvone (e) Podophyllotoxin (f) Piperine (g) Abietic acid (h) Curcumin (Jamia Hamdard, 1994).

4. Mention plant sources of the following terpenes : (a) α-Pinene (b) α-Ionone (c) Citronellal (d) Cineol (e) Car-3-one (f) Carvone (g) Fenchone (h) β-Ionone.

5. Give the comparative account of umbelliferous fruits you have studied (Delhi university, 1987).

6. Write structural differentiation of the following phytoconstituents and give the major plant source of each constituent : (a) α-Pinene and α-terpineol (b) Linalool and linalyl acetate (c) Citronellol and citral (d) Eugenol and thymol (C.C.S.U., Meerut, 1995).

7. (a) Name the volatile oil drugs which contain phenolic esters. Give the constituents of Fennel and Nutmeg.

   (b) Give official source, chemical constituents and uses of Clove and Cardamom. (Delhi University, 1988)

8. What are essential oils ? How are they isolated ? Give source, constituents and uses of Lemongrass oil.

9. Describe Cardamom under suitable pharmacognostical scheme.

11

RESINS

Resins are solid or semisolid plant exudates formed in schizogenous or schizolysigenous ducts or cavities. They are complex mixtures of compounds like resin alcohols (resinols), resin acids, resinotannols, (resinphenols), esters and resenes. Some resins(e.g. Benzoin and Balsam of Tolu) are formed when the plant is injured. These resins are called as pathological resins.

The resins commonly used in pharmacy are derived from natural sources, and almost are plant products -Shellac, an insect secretion, being an important exception.

Resins are classified on the basis of their occurrence in combination with another compounds as :

Balsams : Balsams are resinous substances which contain large proportions of benzoic or cinnamic acids either free or in combination or their esters. Tolu Balsam contains 35 to 50% of balsamic acids (chiefly benzoic and cinnamic acids) which are present partly in the free state and partly in combination with complex 'resin alcohols'. Benzoin, Peru Balsam and Storax, are another examples of balsams.

Oleoresins : When resins occur with volatile oils, the mixture is called as oleoresins. Turpentine, Capsicum, Ginger, Male Fern, Canada Balsam and Copaiba are oleoresins.

Gum Resins : When resins are found in combination with gums, then such resins are known as *gum resins*. These resins are purified by dissolving the associated gum in water. Asafoetida, Gambage and Myrrh are gum-resins.

Oleo-gum Resins : Oleo-gum-resins are associated with gum and volatile oil both. The volatile oil is removed by steam distillation while gum is separated by dissolving in water, e.g., Myrrh, Ipomoea.

Glycoresins (Glucoresins) : Some resins are found in combination with glycosides. These resins occur in Ipomoea, Scammony, Jalap and Podophyllum. On hydrolysis they produce sugars and complex resin acids as aglycones.

Formation of Resins

In many instances a resin in plants is formed in special passages or tubes called resin ducts, which are usually anastomose . Thus a single incision may drain the resin from a considerable area of the plant. The cells lining the ducts possess a layer (called the resinogenous layer) of slimy matter bounded by a fine cuticle and resin is secreted in this layer. It is excreted through the cuticle layer into the resin duct.

In some cases, e.g. Copaiba, numerous resin ducts are present. Tapping is necessary to drain the ducts. Such resin is called as normal or physiologically-produced resin. In other instances, e.g. turpentine, only a few resin ducts are normally present, but following injury to the cambium the new or secondary wood subsequently formed which contains very large number of ducts. The resin from these ducts is called wound, traumatic or pathologically-produced resin.

Resin may continue to flow for a considerable period from wounding, or in some cases it may be necessary to inflict wounds at frequent intervals. Further, invasion of the wound by fungi and bacteria sometimes plays an important part in the composition of the resin exuded. For example, the simple wound resin of Styrax and Benzoin differs materially from the resin exuded after fungal invasion of the wound.

Characters : Purified resins are amorphous, brittle, transluscent, hard solids. On heating they are softened and then melted. They are practically insoluble in water but dissolve in organic solvents like alcohol, ether and chloroform. Varnish-like film is formed on evaporation of the solvent. They produce smoky flame on burning.

Chemical Constituents : Chemically, the resins are complex mixtures of the following compounds :

1. **Resin Acids :** Resin acids are the mixture of oxyacids, carboxylic acids and phenolic acids. They are present in the free state or as esters. They are soluble in aqueous alkaline solutions which form soap-like froth on shaking. Abietic acid in Rosin or Colophony, copaivic acid and oxycopaivic acid in Copaiba, guaiaconic acid in Guaiac, pimaric (pimarinic) acid in Frankincense, sandaracolic acid in Sandarac, aleuritic acid in Shellac and commiphoric acid in Myrrh are the examples of resin acids.

2. **Resin Alcohols :** Resin alcohols are complex molecules with high molecular weight. They are present in the free state or as esters of simple aromatic acids, e.g. benzoic acid, salicylic acid and cinnamic acid. They are further sub-divided as :

   (i) *Resinotannols :* They are tannins and form blue colour with ferric chloride, e.g., aloeresinotannol from Aloe, amoresinotannol and galbaresinotannol from Ammoniac, peruresinotannol from Balsam of Peru, siaresinotannol and sumaresinotannol from Benzoin.

   (ii) *Resinols :* Resinols do not contain tannins. Benzoresinol from Benzoin, storesinol from Storax and guaiacresinol from Guaiac resin are the examples of resinols.

3. **Resenes :** Resenes are complex neutral compounds which do not respond to any chemical reaction. They are insoluble in acids and alkalies and do not form any salts or esters, e.g., alban and fluavil from Gutta percha, copalresene from Copal, dammaresene from Dammar, dracoresene from Dragon's blood and olibanoresene from Olibanum.

Resin containing drugs possess purgative (Podophyllum), cathartic (Colocynth, Gamboge, Ipomoea), hydragogue (Jalap), sedative (Cannabis), counter-irritant (Capsicum, Turpentine), anthelmintic (Asphidium), expectorant (White Pine, Copaiba, Storax, Tolu Balsam, Benzoin) and laxative (Asafoetida) properties. Externally resins are used as mild antiseptic in the form of cerates, ointments and plasters. They are employed in the preparation of emulsions.

COLOPHONY

Synonyms : Rosin, Yellow resin; Abietic anhydride; Colophony resin; Amber resin; Resin; Coloponium.

Biological Source : Colophony is a solid residue left after distilling off the volatile oil from the oleoresin obtained from *Pinus palustris* (long leaf pine) and other species of *Pinus* such as *P. elliottii* (slash pine), *P. pinaster* (syn. *P. maritima*), *P. halepensis*, *P. massoniana*, *P. tabuliformis*, *P. carribacea* var. *hondurensis*, *P. oocarpa*, *P. radiata.* and *P. roxburghii* (syn. *P. longifolia*).

Family : Pinaceae.

Habitat : The genus *Pinus* is widely found in many countries including U.S.A., France, Italy, Portugal, Spain, Greece, New Zealand, China, India (Himalayan region), and Pakistan.

Colophony is chiefly produced in U.S.A. contributing about 80% world supply. Other countries producing resin are China, France, Spain, India, Greece, Morocco, Honduras, Poland and Russia.

Collection : The collection of the oleoresin is very laborous procedure. Although Colophony is a normal (physiological) resin of *Pinus* species, its amount is increased by injuring the plant. For its collection a few-feet long groove or blaze is made in the bark with the help of knife or some other instrument. A metal or earthenware cup is attached below the groove by nails. The cup is adjusted accordingly when the size of groove increases. The resin is taken out at different intervals and sent for further processing.

The flow of oleoresin is increased by applying sulphuric acid (50%), plant hormones or cultures of *Fusarium* species to the grooves. By such treatment the living xylem cells produce excess amount of oleoresin which is leaked to the adjacent cells.

Preparation : The crude oleoresin is mixed with turpentine, heated in a stainless steel vessel and filtered. The filtrate is allowed to stand to separate water and other impurities. The diluted oleoresin is steam distilled in copper or stainless steel stills to remove turpentine. After distillation the molted resin is transferred into barrels, cooled and exported.

Characters : Colophony occurs as translucent, hard, shiny, sharp, pale yellow to amber fragments, brittle fracture at ordinary temperature, burns with smoky flame, slight turpentine-like odour and taste, melts readily on heating, density 1.07-1.09. Acid number is not less than 150. It is insoluble in water but freely soluble in alcohol, benzene, ether, glacial acetic acid, oils, carbon disulphide and alkali solutions.

Chemical Tests

1. To a solution of powdered resin (0.1 g) in acetic acid (10 ml) one drop of conc. sulphuric acid is added in a dry test tube. A purple colour, readily changing to violet, is formed.

2. To a petroleum ether solution of powdered Colophony twice its volume of dilute solution of copper acetate is shaken. The colour of the petroleum ether layer changes to emerald-green due to formation of copper salt of abietic acid.

3. To alcoholic solution of Colophony water is added. It becomes milky white due to precipitation of chemical compounds.

4. Alcoholic solution of Colophony turns blue litmus to red due to the presence of diterpenic acids.

Abietic acid   Pimaric acid

Chemical Constituents : Colophony contains resin acids (about 90%), resenes and fatty acid esters. Of the resin acids about 90% are isomeric α-, β-and γ-abietic acids (sylvic acid, $C_{20}H_{30}O_2$);the other 10% is a mixture of dihydroabietic acid and dehydroabietic acid. Before distillation the resin contains excess amounts of (+) and (-) pimaric acids. During distillation the (-) pimaric acid is converted into abietic acid while (+) pimaric acid is stable. On heating at 300°C abietic acid is transformed into *neo*-abietc acid. The other constituents of Colophony are sipinic acid and a hydorcarbon.

Uses : Colophony is used as stiffening agent in ointments, plasters and cerates and as a diuretic in veterinary medicine. Commercially it is used to manufacture varnishes, printing inks, cements, soap, sealing wax, wood polishes, floor coverings, paper, plastics, fireworks, tree wax, rosin oil; for water proofing cardboard, walls, etc.

BALSAM TOLU

Synonyms : Tolu Balsam; Thomas Balsam; Opobalsam; Resin Tolu; Balsam of Tolu; Balsamum tolutanum.

Biological Source : Balsam Tolu is obtained by incision of stem of *Myroxylon balsamum.* (L.) Harms.

Family : Leguminosae.

Habitat : Colombia (near lower Magdalena river), West Indies, Cuba, Venezuela and Peru.

Collection : Balsam Tolu is a pathological resin and is formed in trunk tissues as a result of injuries. It is collected all the year except the period of heavy rains by making V-shaped incisions in the bark and sap wood. Calabash cups are placed to receive the flow of balsam. Many other incisions are made on higher portion on the trees. Collected balsam is transferred into larger tin containers and exported.

Characters : Tolu Balsam occurs as soft, yellowish-brown or brown, semi-solid or plastic solid, transparent in thin layers, brittle when old, dried or kept in cold, aromatic odour, and taste is aromatic, vanilla-like and slightly pungent. It is insoluble in water and petroleum ether; soluble in alcohol, benzene, chloroform, ether, glacial acetic acid and partially soluble in carbon disulphide and NaOH solution.

Chemical Tests

1. Alcoholic solution of Balsam Tolu (1g) gives green colour with ferric chloride due to toluresinotannols.
2. Alcoholic solution of Balsam Tolu is acidic to litmus paper.
3. To filtered solution of Balsam Tolu (1 g) in water (5 ml) aqueous potassium permanganate solution is added and heated for 5-10 minutes. Odour of benzaldehyde is produced due to oxidation of cinnamic acid.

Chemical Constituents : Tolu Balsam contains resin (~80%) which is a mixture of resin alcohols combined with cinnamic and benzoic acids. The aromatic acids are also present in free state in   proportions 8-15 per cent. The other constituents reported in the drug are benzyl benzoate, benzyl cinnamate, vanillin, styrene, eugenol, ferulic acid, 1,2-diphenylethane (bibenzyl), mono-and sesquiterpene hydrocarbons and alcohols.

Uses : Balsam of Tolu is used as an expectorant, stimulant and antiseptic. It is an ingredient of cough mixtures and Compound Benzoin tincture. It is also used as a pleasant flavouring agent in medicinal syrups, confectionery, chewing gums and perfumery.

Adulteration : Commercial preparations are usually adulterated with rosin but the general sophistication is the natural balsam from which the aromatic substances have been isolated.

PERU BALSAM

Synonyms : Peruvian Balsam; Indian Balsam; China oil; Black Balsam; Honduras Balsam; Surnam Balsam; Balsam of Peru; Balsamum peruvianum.

Biological Source : Peru Balsam is obtained by incision of the stem of *Myroxylon balsamum* var. *pereirae* (Royle) Klotsch.

Family : Leguminosae.

$C_6H_5COOCH_2C_6H_5$
Benzyl benzoate

C_6H_5 CH=CH COOCH$_2$C$_6$H$_5$
Benzyl cinnamate

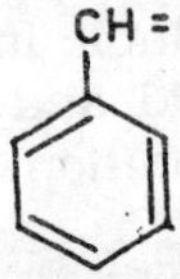

CH = CH$_2$

Styrene

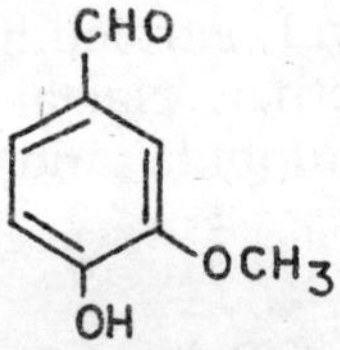

CHO

OCH$_3$

OH

Vanillin

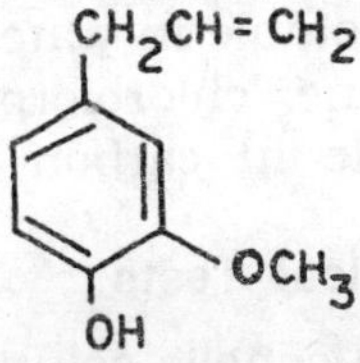

CH$_2$CH = CH$_2$

OCH$_3$

OH

Eugenol

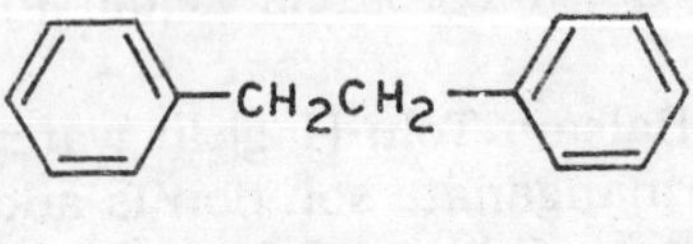

$-CH_2CH_2-$

1,2-Diphenyl ethane (Bibenzyl)

CH$_2$OH

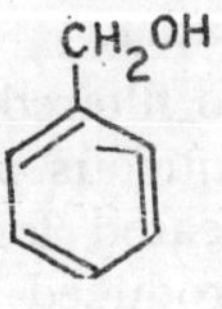

Benzyl alcohol

$C_6H_5CH=CH$ COO CH$_2$ CH=CH-C$_6$H$_5$
Cinnamyl Cinnamate
(Styracin)

$$(CH_3)_2 \ C=CH(CH_2)_2 \ \overset{\overset{\displaystyle CH_3}{|}}{C}=CH(CH_2)_2 \ \overset{\overset{\displaystyle CH_3}{|}}{C}=CH \ CH_2OH$$

Farnesol

$$(CH_3)_2 \ C=CH(CH_2)_2 \ \overset{\overset{\displaystyle CH_3}{|}}{C}=CH(CH_2)_2 \ \underset{\underset{\displaystyle OH}{|}}{C}-CH=CH_2$$

Neroiidol (Peruviol)

Habitat : The plant is most widely found in Colombia, Venezuela, Central America (San Salvador), in forests near Pacific coast and cultivated in West Indies, Cuba, Florida and Sri Lanka.

Collection : *M. pereirae* is a large tree, about 25 meters in height. Peru balsam is a pathological resin and is formed when the plant is injured. The 10 years old tree is beaten on four sides in November or December. The cracked bark is scorched with torch to separate it from the trunk. Within a week the bark is dropped from trunk and the balsam begins to flow from the exposed wood. The injured part is covered with cloths or rags in which the resin is absorbed. When the cloths are saturated with exudate, they are removed from time to time and boiled with water. On cooling the water extracted balsam is settled out which is removed, strained, packed in tin cans and exported.

Characters. : Fresh Peru. Balsam is a soft, yellow, viscous liquid or semi-solid. On keeping it becomes dark brown, or nearly black, brittle solid. It softens on heating in which crystals of cinnamic acid may be visible under microscope. It does not stick, has an empyreumatic, aromatic, vanilla-like odour and a bitter, acrid, persistent taste. It is insoluble in water and olive oil but soluble in alcohol, chloroform, and glacial acetic acid, usually with a slight opalescense.

Chemical Constituents : The drug contains balsamic esters (56-66%) like benzyl cinnamate (cinnamein), C_6H_5 CH=CH COOCH$_2$ C_6H_5 (50-60%), benzyl benzoate and cinnamyl cinnamate (styracin), resin (28%) consisting of peruresinotannol combined with cinnamic and benzoic acids, alcohols [nerolidol (peruviol) farnesol and benzyl alcohol] and small amounts of vanillin, and free cinnamic acid.

Uses : Peru Balsam is used as miticide, to aid in healing of indolent wounds, as scabicide and parasiticide, in skin ulcer therapy, as local protectant and rubefacient. It is an antiseptic and vulnerary and as a stimulating expectorant. It is also employed in perfumery and some chocolate flavourings, also in making of odours.

SUMATRA BENZOIN

Synonyms : Gum Benjamin; Benzoinum; Benzoin; Luban (Hindi).

Biological Source : Sumatra Benzoin is obtained from the incised stem of *Styrax benzoin* Dryander and *Styrax paralleloneurus* Perkins. It contains about 25% of total balsamic acids, calculated as cinnamic acid.

Family : Styraceae.

Habitat : Sumatra, Malacca, Malaya, Java and Borneo.

Collection : The plants are medium size trees. Sumatra Benzoin is a pathological resin which is formed by making incision and by attack of fungi. In Sumatra the seeds are sown in rice fields. The rice plants provide protection to benzoin plants during first year. After harvesting of the rice crop the trees are allowed to grow. When they are 7 years old, three triangular wounds are made in a vertical row about 40 cm apart from each other at the base exposing the xylem. A yellow, soft, sticky resin exudes after a week which is known as Almond Tears. The first secretion is sticky and rejected. Further new wounds are made above the earlier wounds at a distance of 4 cm at 3-monthly intervals. Second exudation is milky white and is used for medicinal purpose. The stem is incised four times during one year. All types of exudations are sent to industry for further processing. A single tree yields about 10 kg of resin per year and is completely exhausted by the 19th year of its life.

Characters : Sumatra Benzoin consists of hard opaque, whitish or reddish blocks or tears, brittle, softening on warming and gritty on chewing. The matrix is translucent, reddish-brown or greyish-brown. Odour is balsamic and taste is slightly acrid, aromatic and resinous.

Chemical Constituents : Sumatra Benzoin consists of free balsamic acid (cinnamic and benzoic acids) (25%) and their esters. The amount of cinnamic acid is usually double that of benzoic acid. It also contains triterpenic acids like siaresinolic acid (19-hydroxyoleanolic acid) and sumaresinolic acid (6-hydroxyoleanolic acid); traces of vanillin, phenylpropyl cinnamate, cinnamyl cinnamate and phenylethylene.

Uses : Sumatra Benzoin possesses expectorant, antiseptic, carminative, stimulant and diuretic properties. It is used in cosmetic lotions, perfumery and to prepare Compound Benzoin. It forms an ingredient of inhalations in the treatment of catarrh of upper respiratory tract in the form of Compound Benzoin Tincture. Benzoin is used as an external antiseptic and protective, and is one of the main ingredients of Friar's Balsam. It is also used to fix the odour of incenses, skin-soaps, perfumes and other cosmetics and for fixing the taste of certain pharmaceutical preparations. Benzoin retards rancification of fats and is used for this purpose in the official benzoinated lard.

Benzoic acid   Cinnamic acid

SIAM BENZOIN

Biological Source : Siam Benzoin is a balsamic resin derived from stem of *Styrax tonkinensis* Craib.

Family : Styraceae.

Habitat : North Laos, North Vietnam, Annam, and Thailand.

Collection : Siam Benzoin is also a pathological resin produced by incising the bark and by fungus attack. The stem of 6-8 years old plant is incised when balsam exudates. The resin is obtained in the form of liquid which is solidified.

Sumaresinolic acid

Characters: Siam Benzoin occurs as tears or in blocks of variable sizes and reddish brown externally, but milky-white or opaque internally. Matrix is glassy, reddish-brown, resinous, brittle but softening on chewing and become plastic-like on chewing. It has vanilla-like odour and a balsamic taste.

Chemical Constituents : The principal constituent of Siam

Benzoin is coniferyl benzoate (60-70%) (3-methoxy-4-hydroxycinnamyl alcohol). Other constituents are free benzoic acid (10%), triterpene siaresinolic acid (6%) and vanillin.

Chemical Tests

1. Heat Sumatra Benzoin (5 g) with 10% aqueous potassium permanganate solution. A bitter almond-like odour is produced due to oxidation of cinnamic acid present in Sumatra Benzoin. This test is negative in case of Siam Benzoin.
2. To a petroleum ether solution of Benzoin (0.2 g), 2-3 drops of sulphuric acid are added in a China dish. Sumatra Benzoin produces reddish-brown colour while Siam Benzoin shows purple-red colour on rotating the dish.
3. To alcoholic solution of Benzoin ferric chloride solution is added. A green colour is produced in Siam Benzoin due to the presence of phenolic compound coniferyl benzoate. This test is negative in case of Sumatra Benzoin which does not contain sufficient amount of phenolic constituents.

Uses : Siam Benzoin acts as antiseptic and expectorant; it is used to prepare benzoinated lard, cosmetics, fixatives and in perfumery. It is superior to the Sumatra Benzoin with respect to antioxidative effect in Lard and other fats.

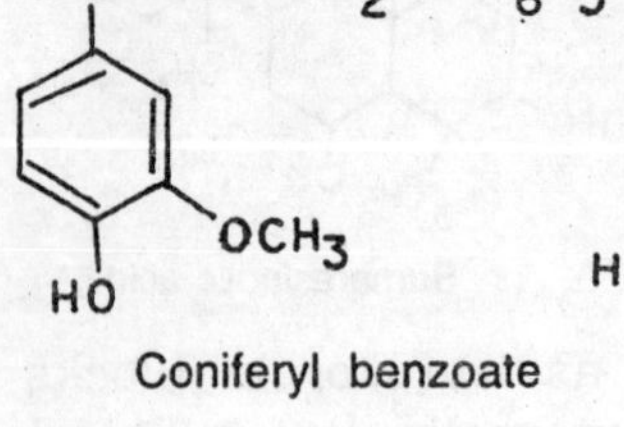

CH=CH·CH$_2$OCOC$_6$H$_5$

Coniferyl benzoate

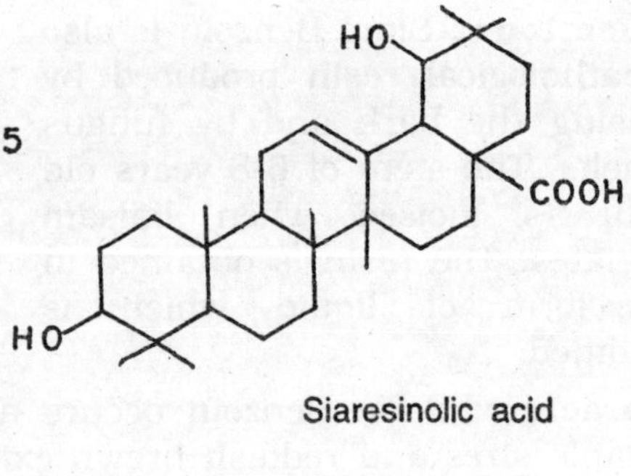

Siaresinolic acid

STORAX

Synonyms : Styrax; Sweet oriental gum; Prepared Storax; Liquid Storax; Styrax preparatus.

Biological Source : Storax is a balsam obtained from the trunk of *Liquidambar orientalis* Miller, commercially known as Levant Storax, or of *Liquidambar styraciflua* Linn, known as American Storax. The balsam is subsequently purified.

Family : Hamamelidaceae.

Habitat : Levant Storax is a native to Asia Minor. American Storax is produced chiefly in Honduras; found along the Atlantic coast from Connecticut to Central America.

Collection : Levant Storax and American Storax are medium-sized trees attaining the height of 15 m and 40 m, respectively. Levant Storax is a pathological resin. In the early summer the bark of 3-4 years old tree is injured by bruishing. Cambium is activated to produce new wood with balsam secreting ducts. The bark is gradually saturated with balsam which is peeled off. The pieces of bark are pressed to get the product. The bark is boiled in hot water and re-pressed. The crude balsam is poured into casks or cans and exported.

American Storax exudes into natural spaces present in between the bark and the wood. The presence of balsam in spaces may be detected by excresences on the outside of the bark. From these pockets the balsam is tapped with gutters into containers which is exported in tin cans.

Storax is purified by dissolving the crude balsam in alcohol, filtering and evaporating the solvent under low temperature not to lose volatile compounds. The alcohol-insoluble part consists of vegetable debris and a resin.

Chatacters : Levent Storax is a viscous, semiliquid greyish, sticky, opaque mass which deposits as a dark-brown, heavier, oleoresinous product on standing. American Storax is a semisolid, sometimes solid mass softened by warming, becoming hard, opaque, and darker coloured. Storax is transparent in thin layers, has characteristic taste and odour, and is denser than water. It is insoluble in water; almost completely soluble in warm alcohol, ether, acetone, and carbon disulphide. Odour is agreeable and taste is balsamic.

Chemical Constituents : Storax is rich in two resin alcohol (50%), α-storesin and β-storesin and balsamic acids (30-47%). The alcohols occur partly free and partly as esters of cinnamic acid (10-20%). Storax also contains cinnamyl cinnamate or styracin (5-10%), phenylpropyl cinnamate (10%); ethyl cinnamate, benzyl cinnamate, free cinnamic acid (5-15%), styrene, traces of vanillin and volatile oil (0.5-1%).

Steam-distillation of Storax yields a pale yellow or dark brown oil (0.5-1.0%), known as oil of Storax. It has a pleasant but peculiar odour.

Uses : Storax is used as a stimulant, expectorant, parasiticide, topical protectant and an antiseptic. Pharmaceutical preparations like Compound Benzoin Tincture, Friars' Balsam and Benzoin Inhalation are also prepared from the Storax.

COPAIBA

Synonyms : Balsam Copoiba; Balsam of Copaiba; Balsam Capivi; Jesuit's Balsam, Copaiva.

Biological Source : Copaiba is an oleoresin obtained from trunks of South American species of *Copaifera (Copaiba)* like *Copaifera lansdorfii* Dest.

Family : Leguminosae.

Habitat : Brazil, Venezuela, Colombia, especially the Amazon valley and banks of Orinoco.

Collection : Copaiba is a physiological resin. The tree is 18 meters in height which is tapped and the oleoresin conducted directly to containers. About 20-24 litres of the product is collected from one tree.

Characters : Copaiba is a transparent, viscid, pale yellow to brown-yellow liquid, peculiar odour; bitter acrid, nauseating taste. It is insoluble in water but soluble in benzene, chloroform, ether, oils, carbon disulphide, absolute alcohol, and petroleum ether.

Chemical Constituents : Copaiba contains volatile oil, resin, illuric acid ($C_{20}H_{28}O_3$), metacopaivic acid (in Maracaibo Copaiba), copaivic acid and oxycopaivic acid (in Para Copaiba). These acids are the diterpenes relating to abietic or pimaric acid.

Uses : Copaiba has diuretic, antiseptic, expectorant and disinfectant properties and is used in leucorrhoea, gonarrhoea, in varnishes and for manufacturing photographic paper.

ASAFOETIDA

Synonyms : Devil's dung; Food of the gods; Asafoda; Asant; Hing (Hindi).

Biological Source : Asafoetida is an oleo-gum-resin obtained as an exudation by incision the decapitated rhizome and roots of *Ferula asafoetida* L., *F. foetida*, Royel, *F. rubricaulis* Boiss. and some other species of *Ferula*.

Family : Umbelliferae.

Habitat : Iran, Turkestan, Afghanistan. (Karam and Chagai districts).

Collection : The plant is a perennial branching, 3 m high herb possessing large schizogeneous ducts and lysigenous cavities containing milky liquid. Upon exudation and drying of the liquid, Asafoetida is obtained. For the collection of the drug the upper part of the root is laid bare and the stem cut off close to the crown in March-April. The exposed surface is covered by a dome-shaped structure made of twigs and earth. After separating each slice, exudation of oleo-gum-resin, present as whitish gummy resinous emulsion in the schizogenous ducts of the cortex of the stem, takes place. It hardens on the cut surface which is collected, packed in tin-line cases and exported. Removal of the exudation and exposure of fresh surface proceeds until the root is exhausted. The yield is usually soft enough to agglomerate into masses when packed.

Characters : Asafoetida occurs as a soft solid mass or irregular lumps or "tears", sometimes almost semiliquid. Tears are rounded or flattened and about 5-30 mm in diameter, greyish-white or dull yellow or reddish brown in colour.

Asafoetida mass is mixed with fruits, fragments of root, sand and other impurities. Asafoetida has a strong garlic-like (alliaceous) odour and a bitter, acrid and alliaceous taste. When triturated with water, it makes a milky emulsion. It should not have more than 50% of matter insoluble in alcohol (90%) and not more than 15% of ash.

Chemical Constituents : Asafoetida contains volatile oil (4-20%), resin (40-65%) and gum (~25%). The garlic-like odour of the oil is due to the presence of sulphur compounds of the formulae $C_7H_{14}S_2$, $C_{16}H_{20}S_2$, $C_8H_{16}S_2$, $C_{10}H_{18}S_2$, $C_7H_{14}S_3$ and $C_8H_{16}S_3$. The main constituent of the oil is isobutyl propanyl disulphide ($C_8H_{16}S_2$). The three sulphur compounds, viz. 1-methylpropyl 1-propenyl disulphide, 1-(methylthio)-propyl 1-propenyl disulphide and 1-methylpropyl 3-(methylthio)-2-propenyl disulphide have also been isolated from the resin; the latter two have pesticidal properties. Resin consists of ester of asaresinotannol and ferulic acid, pinene, vanillin and free ferulic acid. On treatment of ferulic acid with hydrochloric acid, it is converted into umbelliferone (a coumarin) which gives blue fluorescence with ammonia.

Ferulic acid   Umbelliferone

Chemical Tests

1. On trituration with water it produces a milky emulsion.
2. The drug (0.5 g) is boiled with hydrochloric acid (5 ml) for sometime. It is filtered and ammonia is added to the filtrate. A blue fluorescence is obtained.
3. To the fractured surface add 50% nitric acid. Green colour is produced.
4. To the fractured surface of the drug, add sulphuric acid (1 drop). A red colour is obtained which changes to violet on washing with water.

Uses : Asafoetida is used as carminative, expectorant, antispasmodic and laxative as well as externally to prevent bandage chewing by dogs; for flavouring curries, sauces and pickles; as an enema for intestinal flatulence, in hysterical and epileptic affections, in cholera, asthma, whooping cough and chronic bronchitis.

Adulteration : Asafoetida is adulterated with gum Arabic, other gum-resins, rosin, gypsum, red clay, chalk, barley or wheat flour, slices of potatoes, etc.

MYRRH

Synonyms : Gum-resin Myrrh; Gum Myrrh; Arabian or Somali Myrrh; Myrrha.

Biological Source : Myrrh is an oleo gum-resin obtained from the stem of *Commiphora molmol* Eng. or *C. abyssinica* or other species of *Commiphora*.

Family : Burseraceae.

Habitat : Arabian pennisula, Ethiopia, Nubia and Somaliland.

Collection : Myrrh plants are small trees up to 10 meters in height. They have the phloem paranchyma and closely associated ducts containing a yellowish granular liquid. The tissues between these ducts often collapse, thereby producing large cavities similarly filled, i.e., schizogenous ducts become lysigenous cavities. The gum-resin exudes spontaneously or by incising the bark. The yellowish-white, visc nus fluid is solidified readily to produce reddish-brown masses which are collected by the natives.

Characters : Myrrh occurs as irregular masses or tears weighing up to 250 g. The outer surface is powdery and reddish-brown in colour. The drug breaks and is powdered readily. Fractured surface is rich brown and oily. Odour is aromatic and taste is aromatic, bitter and acrid.

Chemical Constituents : Myrrh contains resin (25-40%), gum (57-61%), and volatile oil (7-17%). Large portion of the resin is ether-soluble which contains α-, β-and γ-commiphoric acids, resenes, the esters of another resin acid and two phenolic compounds. The ether insoluble portion is a mixture of α-and β-heerabomyrrholic acids. The volatile oil is a mixture of cuminic aldehyde, eugenol, meta-cresol, pinene, limonene, dipentene and two sesquiterpenes The disagreeable odour of the oil is due to mainly the disulphide, $C_{11}H_2OS_2$. The gum contains proteins (18%) and carbohydrate (64%) which is a mixture of galactose, arabinose, glucuronic acid and an oxidase enzyme. From the essential oil of *Commiphora abyssinica* the sesquiterpenes like elemol, furanodiene, furanodienone, isofuranogermacrene, curzerenone and linderstrene have been isolated.

Chemical Tests

1. A yellow brown emulsion is produced on trituration with water.
2. Ethereal solution of Myrrh turns red on treatment with bromine vapours. The solution becomes purple with nitric acid.

Uses : Myrrh is used as carminative and in incense and perfumes. It has local stimulant and antiseptic properties and is utilized in tooth powder and as mouth wash. Topically it is astringent to mucous membranes.

OH

Elemol

It is used as a tincture, paint, gargle and rinse due to its disinfecting, deodourizing, and granulation-promoting actions in inflammatory conditions of the mouth and throat. Alcoholic extracts are used as fixatives in the perfumery industry.

MALE FERN

Synonyms : Aspidium, Male shield-fern, Filix mas (B.P.); Male fern rhizome; Rhizoma filicis maris.

Biological Source : Male Fern consists of the rhizome, frond bases and apical bud of *Dryopteris filix-mas* (L.) Schot, known as European Aspidium or Male Fern, or of *Dryopteris marginalis*, known as American Aspidium or Marginal Fern collected late in autumn, divested of the roots and dead portions, and carefully dried, retaining its internal green colour.

Family : Polypodiaceae.

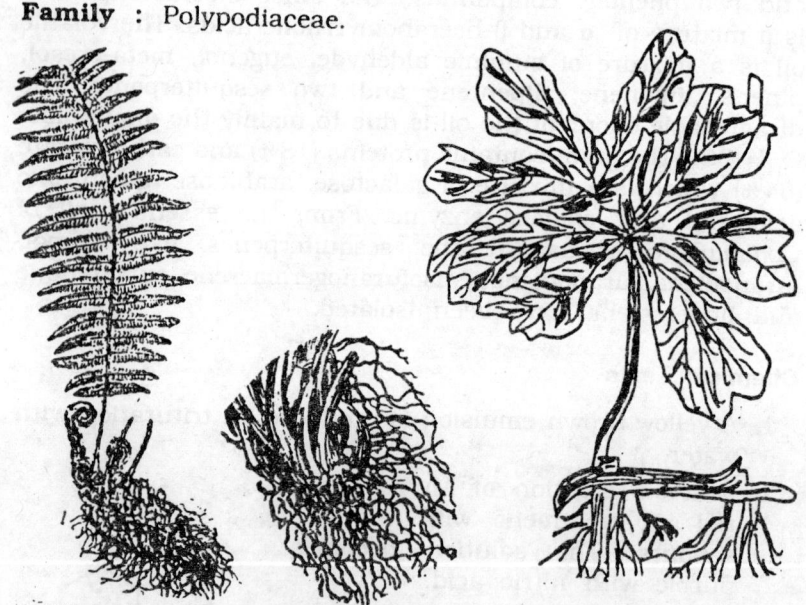

A. Whole drug   B. Entire ramentum   Fig. 11.2. *Podophyllum peltatum*
Fig. 11.1 Male Fern   entire plant

Habitat : *Dryopteris filix-mas* is native of Europe, Northern Africa, Northern Asia, North America, Rocky Mountains and Andes of South America. *Dryopteris marginalis* occurs in eastern and central U.S.A. and India.

Collection : Male Fern is a perennial wood fern. The underground parts of the plant are collected in late autumn; roots, and dead portions are removed, dried and preserved carefully.

Characters : The drug occurs in pieces, 7-25 cm in length, 2 cm in diameter. It is surrounded by frond bases which are brown externally and densely covered with ramenta. Internally the frond bases are green. Larger pieces are generally cut into small slices. The rhizome is brown externally and yellow-green internally. On long storage the internal part of rhizome turns brown and the activity decreases. Odour is slight and taste is sweet in the beginning and bitter and nauseous later on.

Chemical Constituents : The drug contains oleoresin (6.5-15%) which is a mixute of active constituents derived from phloroglucinol. The compounds possess mono-, bi-, tri-, and tetracyclic ring structures. The monocyclic derivatives are aspidinol, filicinic acid and filicinyl butanone which condense to yield bicyclic components like albaspidin and flavaspidic acid or tricyclic derivative like filixic acid. In addition to these aromatic compounds, volatile oil asbaspidin, filicin, filmaron, and filix red have been isolated from the Male Fern.

The chief active principle of the Male Fern is the complex dibasic acid, filmarone, an amorphous brownish yellow acid.

The crude drug deteriorates rapidly in storage. The oleoresin, which is comparatively more stable, is extracted from the drug. The oleo-resin is obtained by exhausting the fresh coarsely powdered drug with ether in a perculator and evaporating the extract into a thick syrup. The official oleo-resin should contain 24-26% filicin by weight.

Uses : Male Fern is used as taenicide due to its anthelmintic properties. The side effects of the drug are stomach pains, colic, diarrhoea, blood in stool, albuminuria, nervous excitement, mental disturbances and defects in vision and blindness.

Filicin is an active vermifuge, especially effective for the expulsion of tapeworm. It is administered in capsules or in pills. Taenia are expelled in a few hour after administration. In combination with calomel, both vermifugal and purgative actions are ensured.

PODOPHYLLUM

Synonyms : May apple; Mandrake root; Indian apple; Vegetable calomel; Podophyllum rhizome, American Mandrake; Rhizoma podophylli.

Biological Source : Podophyllum consists of the dried rhizome and roots of *Podophyllum peltatum* Linn.

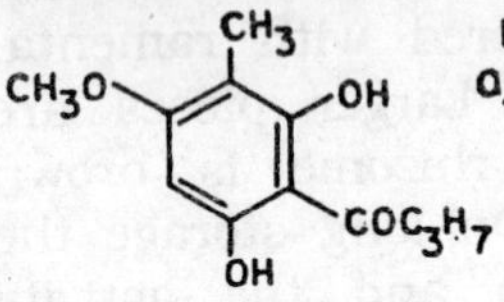

Aspidinol

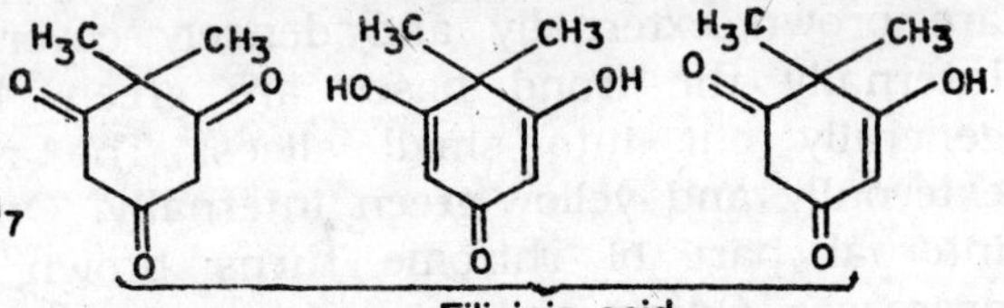

Filicinic acid

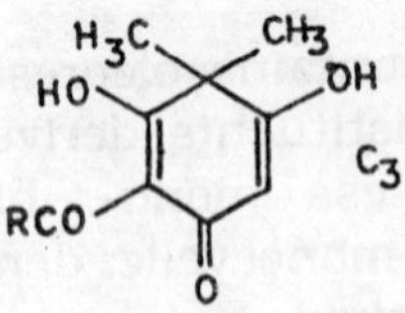

Acylfilicinic acid (R=CH₃; C₂H₅; C₃H₇)

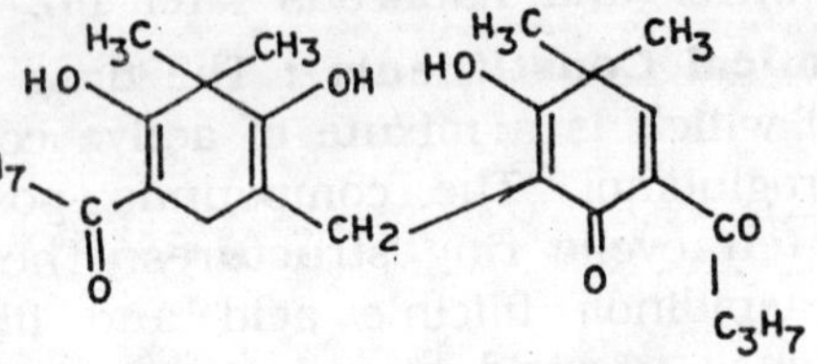

Albaspidin

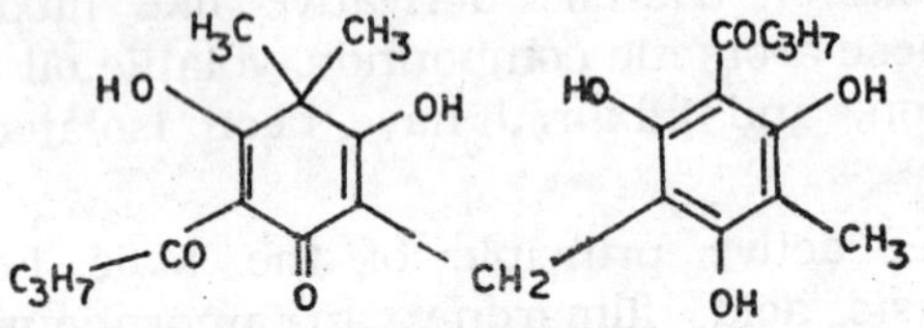

Flavaspidic acid

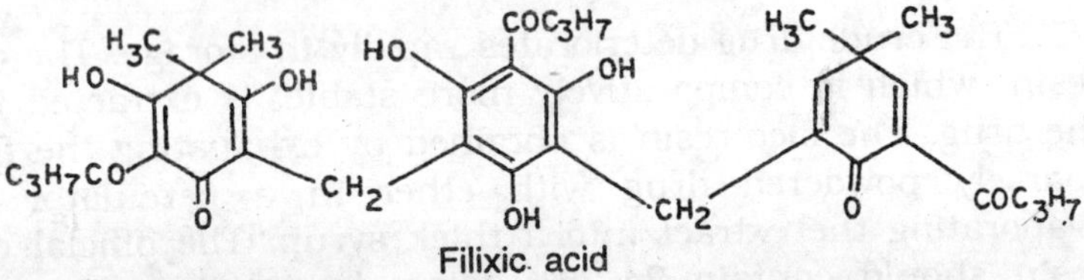

Filixic acid

Family : Berberidaceae.

Habitat : Podophyllum is found in eastern parts of Canada and the U.S.A.

Collection : The plant is a perennial herb growing in marshy, shady situations. It bears a single rhizome which is a meter in length. This is dug up, cut into 10 cm long pieces and dried. The bulk of the crop is gathered in late summer and autumn, cut into pieces 10-20 cm long, dried, and the rootlets usually removed. The rhizomes are reported to contain a higher percentage of active constituents in late spring and early summer, but drug collected at these times contains very little starch and abundance of water, and consequently there is considerable shrinkage upon drying.

Characters : Podophyllum occurs in subcylindrical reddish-brown pieces, length 5-20 cm, breadth 5-6 mm. The nodes are elongated. Outer surface is wrinkled in case of summer rhizome or smooth in autumn rhizome. Stem scars are present on the upper surface while on the lower side of each node 5-12 root scars or root portions exist. The fracture is short and starchy.

Chemical Constituents : Podophyllum contains resin (3.5-6%) whose active principles are lignans (C_{18} compounds). The important lignans are podophyllotoxin (~20%), β-peltatin (~10%) and α-peltatin (~5%) occurring in free state and as glucoside. In addition to these lignans, the other closely related compounds like dimethyl podophyllotoxin and the glucoside, desoxypodo-phyllotoxin and podophyllotoxone are present in the drug. All these compounds possess cytotoxic or antitumour activity. Treatment of lignans with alkali produces epimerization with formation of the stable cis-isomers which are physiologically inactive.

Fig. 11.3. Podophyllum roots and rhizome

Picropodophyllin and quercetin are also present in Podophyllum.

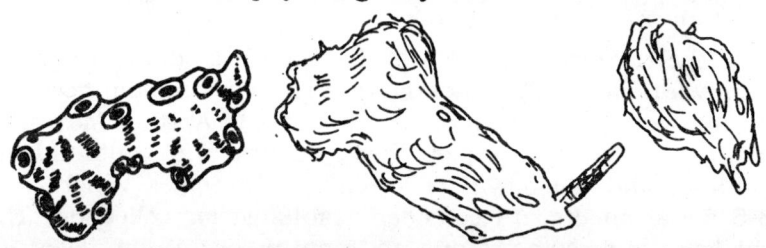

Podophyllotoxin, $R_1=CH_3$, $R_2=OH$, $R_3=H$

α-Peltatin, $R_1=R_2=H$, $R_3=OH$

β-Peltatin, $R_1=CH_3$, $R_2=H$, $R_3=OH$

Demethylpodophyllotoxin, $R_1=R_3=H$, $R_2=OH$

Podophyllotoxone $R_1=CH_3$, $R_2=OH$, $R_3=H$

Desoxypodophyllotoxin, $R_1=CH_3$, $R_2=R_3=H$

Uses : Podophyllum possesses purgative and anti-cancer properties. It has a cytotoxic action and is used as a paint in the treatment of soft venereal and other warts.

INDIAN PODOPHULLUM

Synonyms : Papra (Hindi); Rhizoma Podophylli indici; Indian Podophyllum rhizome.

Biological Source : Indian Podophyllum consists of the dried rhizome and roots of *Podophyllum hexandrum* Royle (syn. *P. emodi* Wall. ex Hook). It contains 40-50% of podophyllotoxin.

Family : Berberidaceae.

Habitat : Podophyllum is found in the interior ranges of Himalayas at   3000-4600   m from Sikkim to Hazara descending to 2,000 m in Kashmir. It is cultivated in Punjab, Uttar Pradesh and N.W. Frontier Provinces.

The plant fluorishes well as an undergrowth in the fir forests, rich in humus and decayed organic matter. It is generally associated with species of *Rhododendron, Salix, Juniperus* and *Viburnum*, but it also met with in open alpine meadows. The plant loves moist and shady localities situated between 2,500 and 4,000 m.

The rhizome and roots of the plant are obtained entirely from wild plants. The underground rhizomes remain dormant during winter and produce aerial shoots in April or May after melting of ice. The shoots bear flowers and fruits during summer and die down in November. Rhizomes which bear 3-5 aerial shoots are considered suitable for collection. The rhizomes and roots are dug up in spring or autumn, cleaned, dried in the sun, packed and stored in gunny bags; sometimes they are cut into cylindrical pieces and carefully dried. Rhizomes collected in spring contain a higher resin content than those obtained in autumn. Freshly collected rhizomes possess more amount of active compounds which are lost on prolonged storing.

Characters : The plant is an erect, glabrous, succulent, perennial herb bearing 2-8 cm and 1-2 cm thick, subcylindrical, tortuous and irregular rhizomes. Internodes of the rhizomes are very short appearing knotty. Upper surface bears 3-4 cup-shaped or oval or circular depressed stem scars with an occasional bud or bud-scar on the lateral surface, lower surface contains numerous roots which are about 10 cm in length and 3 mm thick. The roots may be longitudinally wrinkled, nearly straight, curved or tortuous. Colour is earthy brown. Roots are broken off easily. Fracture is short and starchy. Odour is slight but distinct; taste bitter and acrid.

Chemical Constituents : Indian podophyllum contains excess amount of resin (6-12%) and the concentration of podophyllotoxin is up to 40 per cent. No peltatins are reported but the other constituents are almost the same as reported in the American Podophyllum. The drug also possesses quercetin, berberine, starch and calcium oxalate.

It also contains kaempferol, astragalin (kaempferol-3-glucoside), an essential oil (3.7%) responsible for the odour, wax (8.6%) and mineral salts.

The lignan compounds of podophyllin from *P. hexandrum* are podophyllotoxin, podophyllotoxin glucoside, picropodophyllin, 1-O-glucopyranosyl-picropodophyllin, 4'-dimethyl podophyllotoxin, 4'-demethylpodophyllotoxin glucoside, dehydropodophyllotoxin, podophyllol, podophyllic acid and 4'-demethyl deoxypodopohyllotoxin glucoside.

Uses : Podophyllum resin (podophyllin) is used to treat soft venereal and other warts. The drug has been reported to possess anticancer, cholagogue, purgative, alterative, emetic and bitter tonic properties.

CANNABIS

Synonyms : Indian hemp; Indian Cannabis; Marihuana; Marijuana; Bhang; Ganja; Charas; Kif; Hasach; Pot; Cannabis indica.

Biological Source : Cannabis is the dried flowering tops of pistillate plants of *Cannabis sativa* Linn. (Syn. *C. indica* Linn.). It contains not more than 10% of its fruits, large foliage leaves, and stems over 3 mm in diameter.

Family : Moraceae. Some authors have mentioned family as Cannabinaceae and Urticaceae.

Habitat : Cannabis occurs in India. Bangladesh, Pakistan, Iran, Central America, U.S.A., East Africa, South Africa and Asia Minor.

Cannabis Products : The following products are prepared from Cannabis.

1. **Ganja :** It contains up to 10% of its fruits, large foliage leaves and stems over 3 cm. It is known as *Flat-* or *Bombay ganja* when 30 cm long pieces of the herb are made into bundles and pressed. *Round* -or *Bengal ganja* is prepared by rolling the wilted tops between the hands.

2. **Bhang-or Hashish :** It consists of the larger leaves and twigs of both male and female plants. It is smoked with or without tobacco. It is unfit for medicinal use owing to deficiency of resin.

3. **Charas :** It is the crude resin obtained by rubbing the tops between the hands and beating them on a piece of cloth. This is an inferior product. It may be collected by beating the flowering tops in coarse cotton cloths spread on the ground. A greenish-brown soft mass adheres, and may be purified by pressing it through the cloths. The resin is scraped off. It is mixed with many smoking mixtures.

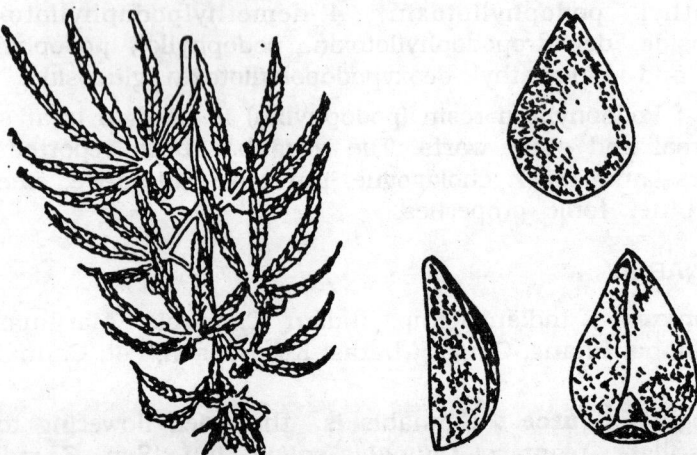

Fig. 11.4. *Cannabis sativa* branch   Fig. 11.5 Kaladana seeds

Morphology : Cannabis occurs in flattened, rough, dull dusky green masses. The dried resin is hard, brittle and does not stick. The flat-ganja is flattened mass of a dull green colour. The odour is very marked in the fresh drug and becomes faint alterwards; taste is slightly bitter.

Chemical Constituents : Cannabis yields resin (15-20%) which is brown, amorphous, semi-solid, soluble in alcohol, ether and carbon disulphide. It contains more than 60 compounds (cannabinoids). Some principal active compounds

are cannabinol, tetrahydrocannabinol, cannabidiol, cannabidiol
-carboxylic acid, cannabigerol and cannabichromene. The
tetrahydrocannabinols (Δ^8-and Δ^9-THC) possess euphoric
activity. In addition to cannabinoids the plant also contains
volatile oil which is a mixture of 30 compounds; the bases
choline, trigonelline, spermidine and cannabisativine (alkaloid);
flavonoid O-glucosides of both vitexin and orientin, and
calcium carbonate.

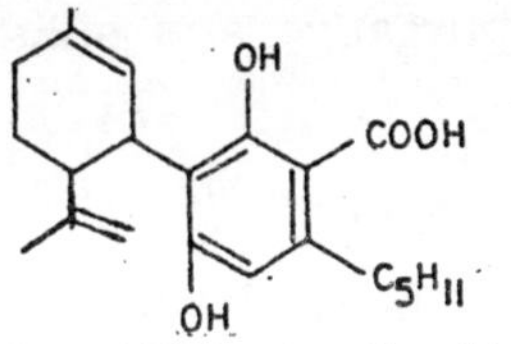

Cannabidiol-carboxylic acid

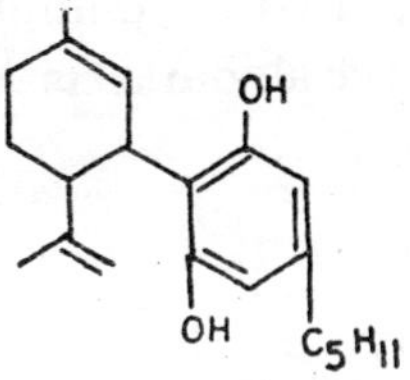

Cannabidiol

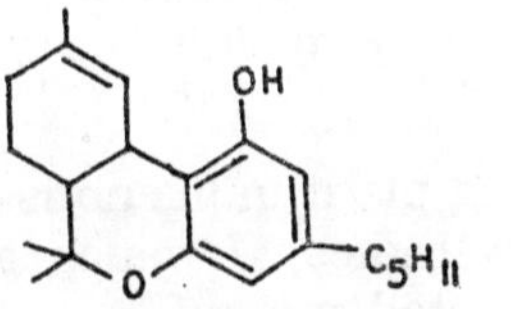

Δ^1-Tetrahydro-cannabinol

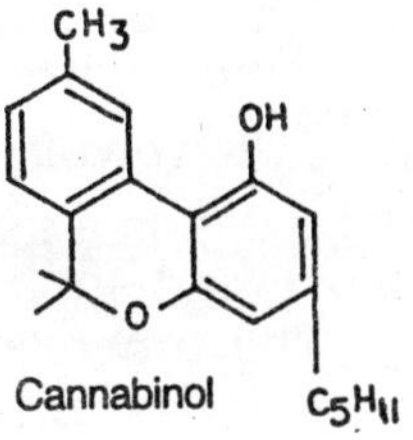

Cannabinol C_5H_{11}

$(CH_3)_2 \overset{+}{N}+CH_2 \, CH_2 \, OH]$ OH⁻
Choline

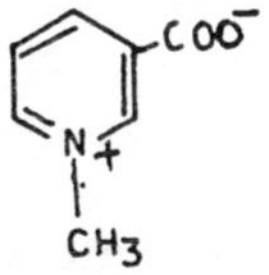

Trigonelline

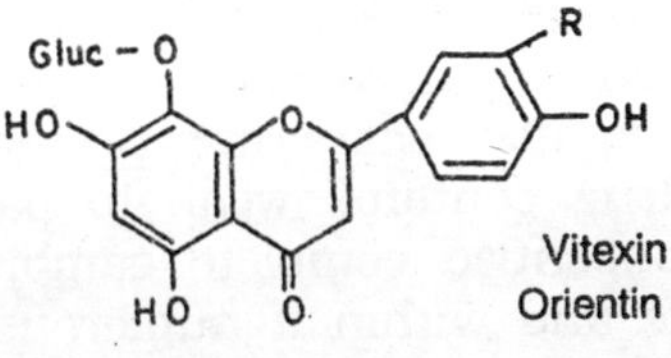

Vitexin (R=H)
Orientin (R=OH)

Uses : Cannabis is used as tonic, intoxicant, stomachic,
antispasmodic, analgesic,narcotic, anticonvulsant, anti-anxiety
and antitussive agent. When ingested or inhaled as smoke,
it may cause euphoria, delirium, hallucinations, weakness,
hyporeflexia, and drowsiness. It is a drug of abuse.

KALADANA

Synonyms : Mirchi (Hindi), Krishnabija (Sanskrit).

Biological Source : Kaladana consists of the dried ripe seeds
of *Ipomoea hederacea* (L.) (syn *I. nil* Roth.).

Family : Convolvulaceae.

Habitat : Throughout India both cultivated and apparently
wild, up to 2,000 m in the Himalayas.

Morphology : The seeds are 5-6 mm long, 3.7 mm wide, triangular, brownish black in colour. Each seed has two flat faces joining at an angle of 60 to 80°. At the base of joint there is a cordate hilum. Testa is dull black, hard, smooth and glabrous. Taste is first sweetish then acrid.

Chemical Constituents : Drug contains resin (about 15%), mucilage, fixed oil and saponin. Hydrolysis of the resin affords hydroxypalmitic acid and sugar.

Uses : Kaladana is used as purgative and substituted for Jalap.

JALAP

Synonyms : Jalap root; Radix jalapae; Mexican or Vera cruz Jalap.

Biological Source : Jalap is the dried tubercles or tuberous roots of *Ipomoea purga* Hayne (syn. *Exogonium purga* Benth).

Family : Convolvulaceae.

Habitat : Jalap is a large, twining plant indigenous to Mexico. It is also found in India, West Indies, Jamaica and South America. The tubercles are collected mainly in autumn. The larger specimens are cut into pieces to facilitate drying.

Characters : Jalap is fusiform, napiform or irregularly ovoid or pyriform in shape and length is 3-15 cm. The drug is very hard, compact, resinous, and heavy. The surface is covered with a dark brown, wrinkled cork. Lighter-coloured transverse lenticels and rootlet scars are present on the surface. Internally the drug contains weak to pale brown, with dark secondary, concentric complete cambium zones fairly close to the outside and within it numerous irregular dark lines. The drug has slight smoke-like odour, taste is starchy and sweet in the beginning and acrid afterwards.

Chemcial Constituents : Jalap contains resins (8-12%), volatile oil, starch, gum and sugar. The main constituent of Jalap resin is convolvulin which contains 8 hydroxy groups esterified with valeric, tiglic and exogonic acids. It also contains ipurganol, jalapin, β-methyl esculetin, palmitic and stearic acids, and mannitol. Convolvulin on hydrolysis gives glucose, rhamnose and convolvulinic acid.

Uses : It is a hydragogue cathartic and drastic purgative.

$$C_{45}H_{72}O_{20} (OH)_8$$

Convolvulinic acid

$$CH_3\ CH_2\ CH_2\ CH_2\ COOH$$

Valeric acid

CH₃CH=C(CH₃) COOH   C₁₀H₁₄O₃   CH₃(CH₂)₄CH-(CH₂)₉-COOH
                                                        OH

Methylcrotonic acid   Exogonic acid   Jalapinolic acid
                                            (11-Hydroxyhexadecanoic
                                            acid)

INDIAN JALAP

Synonyms : Turpeth root; Nishodh (Hindi); Black Nishodh.

Biological Source : Indian jalap consists of dried roots of *Ipomoea turpethum* R. Br.; syn. *Operculina turpethum (L.)* Silva Mansó.

Family : Convolvulaceae.

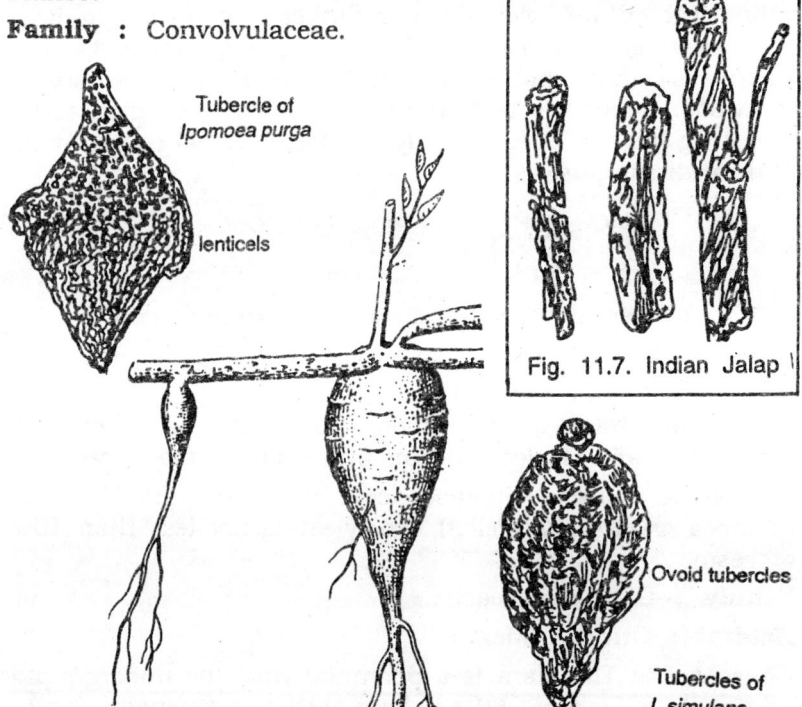

Tubercle of
Ipomoea purga

lenticels

Fig. 11.7. Indian Jalap

Ovoid tubercles

Tubercles of
I. simulans.

Fig. 11.6. Jalap

Habitat : Throughout India up to 1000 m.

Characters : Indian jalap occurs in cylindrical or spirally twisted form, length 2-15 cm, diameter 3-5 mm. Outer surface is greyish-brown containing longitudinal wrinkles. Fracture is irregular. Roots are darker and longitudinally furrows are present. Odour is slight and distinct; taste is unpleasant.

Chemical Constituents : Indian jalap contains resin (7-8%) and volatile oil. Alcoholic soluble portion of the resin is a mixture of gluco-gluco-rhamnosides of turpethinic acids like 11-hydroxypalmitic acid (jalapinolic acid), 3,12-dihydroxypentadecanoic acid (operculonic acid); 4, 12-dihydroxypentadecanoic acid; and 4, 12-dihydroxypalmitic acid.

Uses : Indian jalap is used as purgative.

Allied Drug : In Indian system of medicine white Nishoth is also used as purgative. It consists of roots of *Marsdenia tenacissima.* (Family : Asclepiadaceae). The plant is a large twinning shrub occurring throughout India. Roots are cylindrical, cut into pieces. Outer surface contains longitudinal furrows, ridges, and irregular cracks. Colour is yellow to buff, fracture is short and starchy in the bark and splintery in the wood. Odour is musty and taste is bland first, then acrid. The drug has not been investigated for chemical constituents and medicinal uses.

$$CH_3 \ (CH_2)_3 \ \underset{\underset{OH}{|}}{CH} \ (CH_2)_8 \underset{\underset{OH}{|}}{CH}\text{-}CH_2 \ COOH$$

Operculinolic acid (3:12-Dihydroxyhexadecanoic acid)

IPOMOEA

Synonyms : Mexican Scammony (root); Orizaba Jalap root; Orizaba Jalap; Mexican Scammony root; Ipomoea radix.

Biological Source : Ipomoea consists of the dried root of *Ipomoea orizabensis* (Pellet) Led. yielding not less than 15% of resin.

Family : Convolvulaceae.

Habitat : Orizaba, Mexico.

Characters : The plant is a perennial vine, the underground portion is a fusiform 60 cm long root. Drug usually occurs as transversely cut slices of 3-12 cm in diameter and 1-5 cm thick. Outer surface is brown to grey, longitudinally wrinkled, fracture is short, irregular and resinous; texture is hard and tough, breaking with difficulty. Odour is slight; taste is acrid and resinous.

Chemical Constituents : Ipomoea contains resin (10-20%), scopoletin (coumarin), volatile fatty acids, sugars, sitosterol, and calcium oxalate. The 65 per cent of the resinous mass is ether soluble. The prominent constituents of Ipomoea resin

(Jalapin) are the methyl pentosides and other glycosides of jalapinolic acid and its methyl ester, phytosterol glycosides, (ipuranol), ipurolic acid and convolvullinic acid. Other compounds reported in ipomoea are 3, 4-dihydroxycinnamic acid, cetyl alcohol and gum.

Uses : Ipomoea is used as cathartic with hydragogue activity and for preparation of resin.

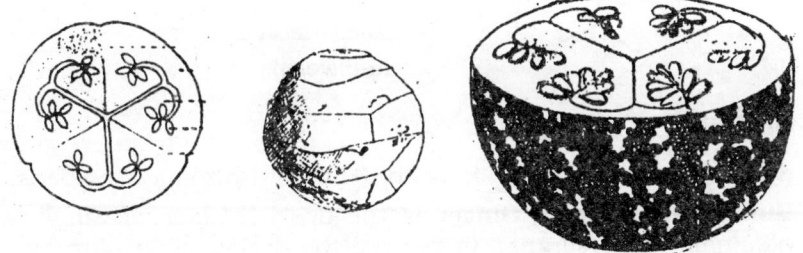

Scopoletin   Ipurolic acid

COLOCYNTH

Synonyms : Bitter apple; Bitter cucumber; Bitter gourd; Colocynth pulp; Indrayan (Hindi); Colocynthis; Fructus Colocynthidis.

Biological Source : Colocynth is the dried pulp of the unripe but fully grown fruit of *Citrus colocynthis* Schrad.

Family : Cucurbitaceae.

Habitat : The plant occurs in Syria, Cyprus, Sudan, North Africa, Turkey, Spain and widely throughout India.

Collection : The plant is a perennial herbaceous vine. The collected fruits are peeled to separate the epicarp and immediately dried in the sun.

A. Whole fruit   B. T.S. of fruit showing placenta and seeds

Fig. 11.8. Colocynth   Peeled fruit

Morphology : The fruit is almost a globular berry, 4-10 cm in diameter. The peeled fruits are 4-8 cm in diameter, subspherical, nearly white, light in density and show sometimes small patches and impressions due to cuts occurred by knife. Transverse section of the fruit shows three segments, divided by the radiating placentas, with seeds attached to the internal margins. Pulp is light, pithy and spongy, easily broken white or light yellow in colour.

Flat, ovoid seeds, 200-300 in each fruit, are present which are compressed, brown or orange in colour, one end somewhat pointed with rounded margin, 7 mm long and 4.5 mm wide. Fruit is odourless and taste is very bitter.

Chemical Constituents : Colocynth contains ether-chloroform soluble resin, a phytosterol glycoside, citrullol, pectin, colocynthin, colocynthetin, albuminoids and other glycosides. The glycosides on hydrolysis form cucurbitacin E (α-elaterin), and cucurbitacin L (dihydroelatericin B). Choline and two alkaloids have also been isolated from the drug.

Uses : Colocynth is very powerful cathartic. Cucurbitacin E is reported to possess anticancer activity.

Cucurbitacin E
(α-Elaterin)

GINGER

Synonyms : Zingiber, Saunth (Hindi); Rhizoma zingiberis.

Biological Source : Ginger is the dried rhizome of *Zingiber officinale* Rosc, scraped to remove the darker outer skin and dried in the sun.

Family : Zingiberaceae.

Habitat : Southern Asia, West Indies. China, Africa, India, cultivated in all tropical countries.

A number of commercial varieties of Ginger are available. *Nigerian Ginger* is darker in colour, small size and more pungent taste. *Cochin Ginger* is usually larger, well scraped, contains more starch and breaks with a shorter fracture.

African Ginger is darker in colour, more pungent in taste and less flavour than *Jamaica Ginger*.

African Ginger is mostly unpeeled, much of the ventral and dorsal surfaces bear patches of wrinkled cork of an earthy-brown colour. It is darker than Cochin Ginger in bulk, and appears discoloured due to lack of care during preparation. The fracture is short, odour strongly aromatic and taste pungent.

The rhizomes of *Jamaican Ginger*, the best quality ginger, are unbleached and devoid of outer suberized layers. The rhizome is pale yellowish brown to yellowish orange. The fracture is short and uneven, fibrous and resinous. It is pleasantly pungent and aromatic. An inferior grade of Jamaican Ginger, known as *Rotoon Ginger*, is also marketed.

Indian Ginger is considered only second to *Jamaican* in quality. There are two main types of Indian Ginger : (i) *Cochin Ginger*, which comes from central Kerala, is the peeled type, light brown to yellowish grey externally; and (ii) *Calicut Ginger*, from Malabar, is orange or reddish brown, resembling *African Ginger*, but the periderm is usually removed. It is inferior to *Cochin Ginger* in quality. Another type, *Calcutta Ginger*, is greyish brown to greyish blue externally. Indian Ginger is more strachy and is almost as pungent as *Jamaican Ginger*, but is less agreeable in odour. *Indian Ginger* has a faint lemon-like odour due to the presence of citral.

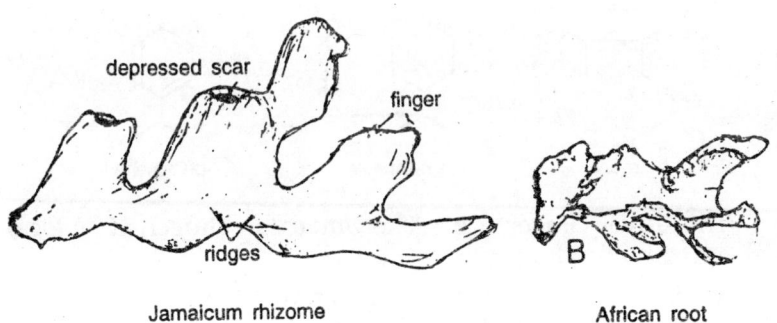

Jamaicum rhizome   African root

Fig. 11.9. Ginger rhizome

Chinese Ginger is white and is free from fibre. It is inferior in aroma to the *Jamaican Ginger* and consists of rhizomes which are not fully ripe. The fibres are absent.

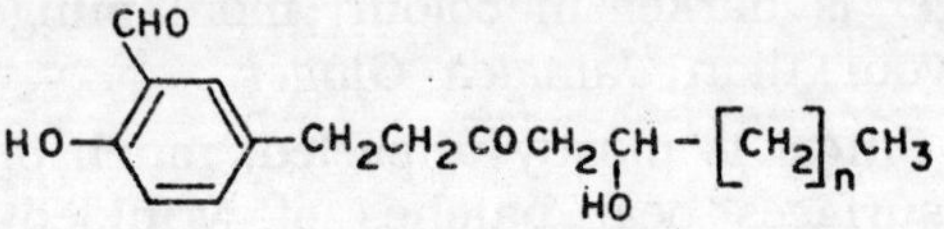

Gingerol (n=3, 4 or 5)

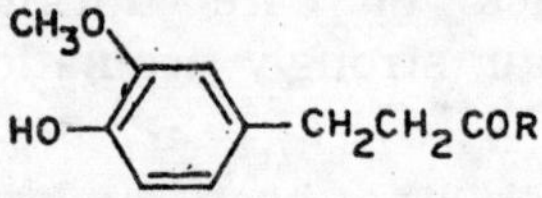

Zingerone, R=CH₃
Shogaol, R=CH=CH-[CH₂]₄-CH₃

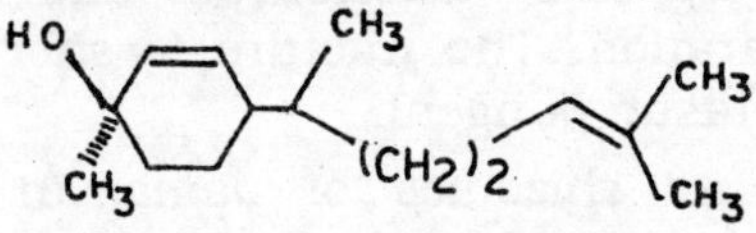

Zingiberenol

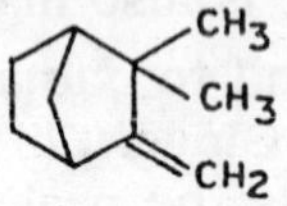

Camphene

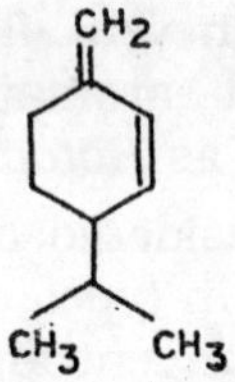

β-Phellandrene

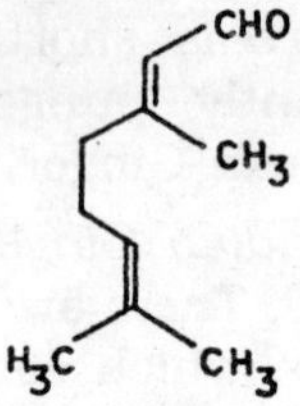

Citral

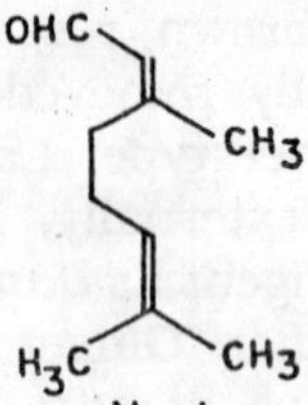

Neral

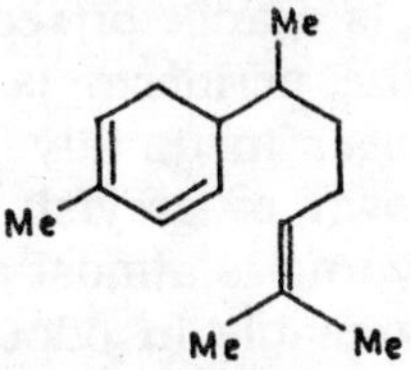

Zingiberene

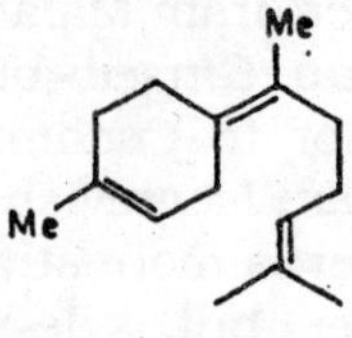

Bisabolene

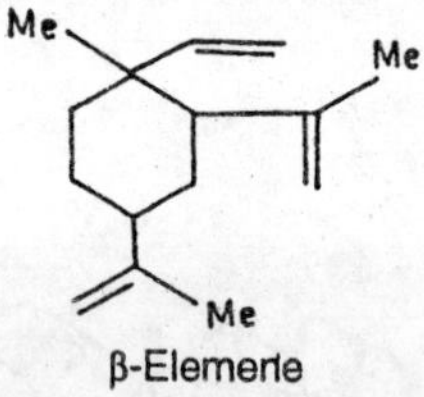

β-Elemene

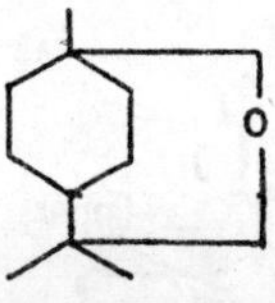

1,8-Cineole

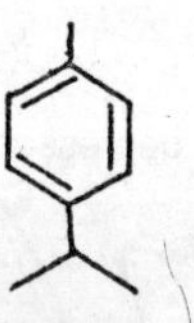

p-Cymene

The other Ginger are : The *Japanese Ginger (Z. mioga)* and *Martinique Ginger (Z. zerumbet).*

Cultivation : Ginger plant is a perennial herb about 1 m high with branching rhizome. The plant is propagated by rhizome cuttings each bearing a bud. The pieces of rhizome are planted in holes during March or April in a well-drained clayey loam. In December or January rhizomes are collected. For getting scrapped drug rhizomes are boiled with water, peeled, washed and dried in sun by turning them up and down from time to time.

Ginger requires a warm and humid atmosphere. A well distributed rainfall is required for its cultivation. If areas receiving less rainfall, the crop needs regular irrigation.

Morphology : Rhizomes are thick, horizontal, laterally compressed, often palmately branched, each having at its apex a depressed scar, showing longitudinal striations and occasional loose fibres, size 5-15 cm long, 3-4 cm wide and 1-15 cm thick: fracture-short, and starchy with projecting fibres. Fractured surface shows a narrow cortex, a well marked endodermis and a wide stele; the whole showing numerous scattered greyish points. Colour is buff; odour is agreeable and aromatic; taste is pungent.

Chemical Constituents : Ginger contains acrid resinous substances (5-8%), volatile oil (1-3%), starch (50%), protein (2-3%) and sugars such as sucrose, raffinose and glucose. The pungency of Ginger is due to gingerol [n=4]. The pungency is lost by boiling with 2% KOH. The other minor constituents of resin are gingediols, methylgingediol, gingediacetates and methylgingediacetates. Gingerols and shogaols are non-volatile phenolic compounds with different side-chains.

Volatile oil is a mixture of more than 25 components of monoterpenes (β-phellandrene, camphene α-and β-pinenes, cumene, myrcene, limonene, cineole, citral, borneol, p-cymene, 1,8-cineol, linalool, neral, etc.) and sesquiterpenes (zingiberene, farnesene, γ-selinene, ar-curcumene, β-sesquiphellandrene, β-eudesmol, β-elemene and bisaboline). Zingerone is also found in rhizome which is also pungent and has sweet odour. Dehydration of gingerol produces shogaol which is not present in fresh rhizomes. The oxygenated monoterpenes are 2-heptanol, 2-nonanol, n-nonanal, n-decanal, methyl heptenone, borneol, bornyl acetate, etc.

Uses : Ginger is used as an aromatic stimulant, carminative, condiment and flavouring agent. It is prescribed in dyspepsia, flatulent colic, vomiting spasms, as an adjunct to many tonic and stimulating remedies; for painful affections of the stomach, cold, cough and asthma. Sore-throat, hoarseness and loss of voice are sometimes benefited by chewing a piece of ginger.

Ginger stimulates the flow of saliva, raises the tonus of the intestinal musculature, and activates peristalsis.

Adulteration : Ginger may be adulterated by addition of 'wormy' drug or 'spent ginger' which has been exhausted in the extraction of volatile oil. This adulteration may be detected by the official standards, for alcohol-soluble portion, water-soluble portion, total ash and water-soluble ash. Sometimes pungency of exhausted Ginger is increased by the addition of Capsicum or seeds or *Aframomum melequeta* (grains of paradise, fam. Zingiberaceae). Such type of pungency is not destroyed by boiling with an alkali.

TURMERIC

Synonyms : Saffron Indian; Haldi (Hindi); Curcuma; Rhizoma curcumae.

Biological Source : Turmeric is the dried rhizome of *Curcuma longa* Linn. (syn. *C. domestica* Valeton).

Family : Zingiberaceae.

Habitat : The plant is native of southern Asia (Probably India) and is cultivated extensively in temperate regions. It is grown on a larger scale in India, China, East Indies, Pakistan, and Malaya.

Cultivation : Turmeric plant is a perennial herb, 2-3 ft high with a short stem and tufted leaves; the rhizomes, which are short and thick, constitute the Turmeric of commerce. The crop requires a hot and moist climate, a liberal water supply and a well-drained soil. It thrives on any soil-loamy or alluvial, but the soil should be loose and friable. The field should be well prepared by ploughing and turning over to a depth of about one ft. and liberally manured with farmyard and green manures. Sets or fingers of the previous crop with one or two buds are planted 3-inches deep at distance of 12-15 inches from April to August. The crop is ready for harvesting in about 9-10 months when the lower leaves turn yellow. The rhizomes are carefully dug up with hard picks, washed and dried.

Characters : The primary rhizomes are ovate or pear-shaped, oblong or pyriform or cylindrical and often short branched. The rhizomes are known as 'bulb' or 'round' turmeric. The secondary, more cylindrical, lateral branched, tapering on both ends, rhizomes are 4-7 cm long and 1-1.5 cm wide and called as 'fingers'. The bulbous and finger-shaped parts are separated and the long fingers are broken into convenient bits. They are freed from adhering dirt and fibrous roots and subjected to curing and polishing process. The curing consists of cooking the rhizomes along with few leaves in water until they become soft. The cooked rhizomes are cooled, dried in open air with intermittent turning over and rubbed on a rough surface. Colour is deep yellow to orange, with root scar and encircling ridge-like rings or annulations, the latter from the scar of leaf base. Fracture is horny and the cut surface is

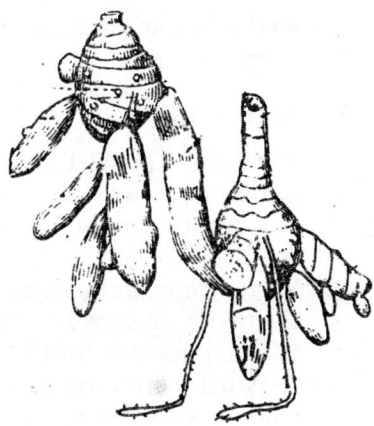

Fig. 11.10. Turmeric roots and rhizome

waxy and resinous in appearance. Outer surface is deep yellow to brown and longitudinally wrinkled. Taste is aromatic, pungent and bitter; odour is distinct.

Chemical Constituents : Turmeric contains yellow colouring matter called as curcuminoids (5%) and essential oil (6%). The chief constituent of the colouring matter is curcumin I (diferuloylmethane) (60%) in addition with small quantities of dicaffeoylmethane (curcumin III), caffeoylferuloylmethane (curcumin II) and dihydrocurcumin. The volatile oil contains mono- and sesquiterpenes like zingiberene (25%), α-phellandrene, sabinene, turmerone, ar-turmerone, borneol and cineole. Choleretic action of the essential oil is attributed to p-tolylmethyl carbinol. Turmeric also contains arabinose (1%), fructose (12%), glucose (28%), starch grains, p-α-dimethylbenzyl alcohol, 1-methyl-4-acetyl-1-cyclohexene, and caprylic acid.

Uses : Turmeric is used as aromatic, stomachic, uretic, anodyne for billiary calculus, stimulant, tonic, carminative, blood purifier, antiperiodic, alterative, spice, colouring agent for ointment and a common house-hold remedy for cold and cough. Externally, it is used in the form of a cream to improve complexion. Dye-stuff acts as a cholagogue causing the contraction of the gall bladder. It is also used in menstrual pains. Curcumin has choleretic and cholagogue action and is used in liver diseases.

Curcuminoids have antiphlogistic activity which is due to inhibition of leukotriene biosynthesis. ar-Turmerone has anti-snake venom activity and blocks the haemorrhagic effect of venom.

Chemical Tests

1. Turmeric powder on treatment with concentrated sulphuric acid forms red colour.
2. On addition of alkali solution to Turmeric powder red to violet colour is produced.
3. With acetic anhydride and concentrated sulphuric acid Turmeric gives voilet colour. Under U.V. light this colour is seen as an intense red fluorescence.
4. A paper containing Turmeric extract produces a green colour with borax solution.
5. On addition of boric acid a reddish-brown colour is formed which, on the addition of alkalies, changes to greenish-blue.
6. A piece of filter paper is impregnated with an alcohol extract, dried, and then moistened with boric acid solution slightly acidified with hydrochloric acid, and re-dried. Pink or brownish-red colour is developed on the filter paper which becomes deep blue on addition of alkali.

All these tests are due to the presence of curcuminoids in the drug.

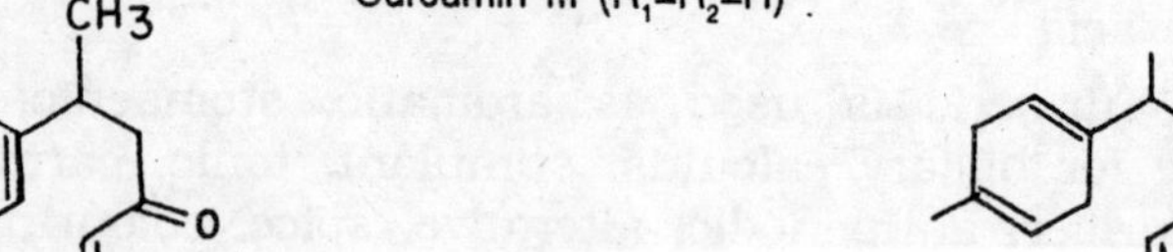

HO—⟨R₁⟩—CH=CH–CO–CH₂–CO–CH=CH—⟨R₂⟩—OH

Curcumin I (R₁=R₂=OCH₃)
Curcumin II (R₁=OCH₃, R₂=H)
Curcumin III (R₁=R₂=H)

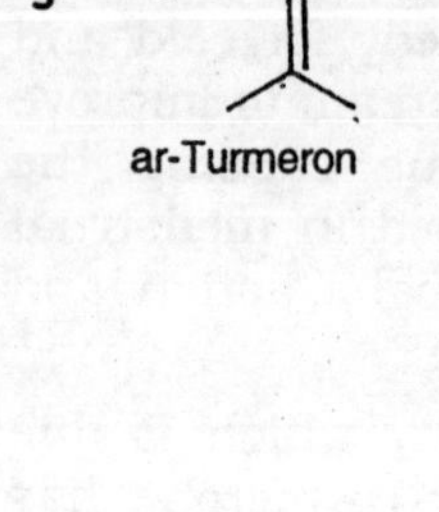

ar-Turmeron

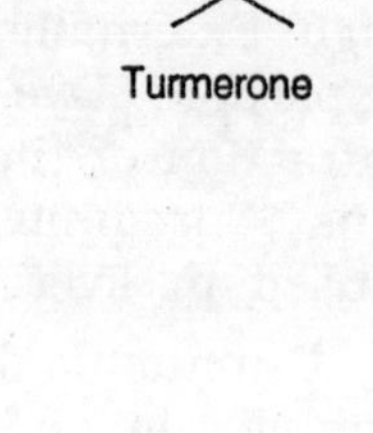

Turmerone

Borneol

Sabinene

GALANGA

Synonyms : Galangal; Colic root; East India root; Chinese ginger; Ganlang rhizome; Rasna; Barakulanjan (Hindi); Lesser galangal; Galangal rhizome; Rhizoma galangae.

Biological Source : Galanga consists of dried rhizome of *Alpinia officinarum* Hance.

Family : Zingiberaceae.

Habitat : Galanga is grown in China, Thailand, eastern Himalayas, Bengal and south-west India.

Morphology : The plant is 1-2 m long perennial herb bearing rhizomes. The drug consists of irregularly branched cylindrical rhizomes, about 2-8 cm long and 1-2 cm thick. They are marked with fine, wavy annulations of lighter colour than the general surface which is reddish or rusty brown in colour. Taste is aromatic, and pungent; odour is aromatic, distinct, spicy and agreeable. Fracture is very tough and fibrous, the exposed surface is lighter orange or brown in colour.

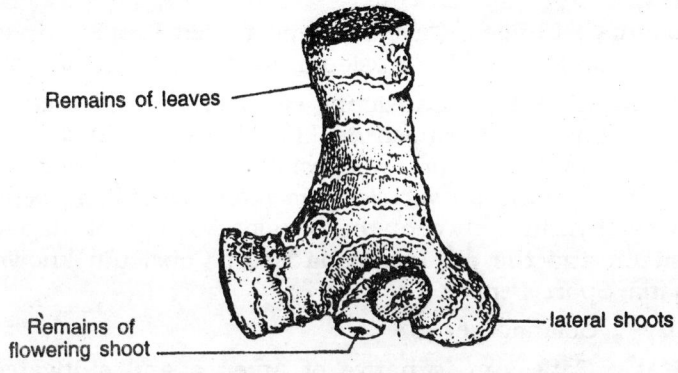

Remains of leaves

Remains of flowering shoot

lateral shoots

Fig. 11.11. Rhizoma of *Alpina officinalis* (Galanga)

Chemical Constituents : Galanga contains volatile oil (0.5-1%), resin (20%), kaempferol, galangin, dihyoxyflavanol, galangol, phlobaphene tannins and starch in abundance. The volatile oil is a mixture of 1, 8-cineole, α-pinene, β-pinene, methyl isovalerate, camphene, limonene, p-cymene, camphor, β-elemene, α-bergamotene, terpinen-4-ol, δ-cadinene, γ-cadinene, methyl cinnamate and eugenol. Kaempferol, galangin and alpinin are the flavonoids.

Uses : Galanga is used in rheumatism, fever, catarrahal affections specially in bronchial catarrah, stomachic, stimulant, aphrodisiac, carminative and as flavouring agent. It has antifungal and antibacterial properties.

Allied Drugs : *Alpinia galanga* (Greater galanga) rhizome, a native of Java and Sumatra and cultivated in India, is substituted to the *A. officinarum*. Greater galanga is larger is size, colour deep orange brown externally and pale buff internally. The drug does not contain any flavonoid. Alcoholic extract of the drug on filter paper does not show any fluorescence under U.V. light due to absence of flavonoids.

Adulteration : The genuine drug is not available in sufficient quantities and most of it is adulterated with the rhizomes of *Acorus calamus*.

Kaempferol (R=OH)
Galangin (R=H)

CAPSICUM

Synonyms : Chillies; Cayenne Pepper; Red Pepper; Spanish Pepper; Mirch (Hindi); Capsicum fruits; Fructus Capsici.

Biological Source : Capsicum consists of the dried, ripe fruits of *Capsicum frutescens* Linn (African Chillies) or of *Capsicum annuum* Linn. var. *conoides* (Tabasco pepper) or of *Capsicum annuum* var. *longum* (Lonusiana Long pepper), or of a hybrid between the Honka variety of Japanese Capsicum and the old Louisiana Sport Capsicum known as *Loisiana Sport Pepper*.

Family : Solanaceae.

Habitat : Capsicum is native of America and cultivated in tropical regions of India, Japan, Southern Europe, Mexico, Africa (Kenya, Tanzania, and Sierra Leone) and Sri Lanka.

Cultivation : Capsicum is cultivated mostly as a rain-fed crop. In the gangetic area, it is a cold weather crop. The crop is raised on a variety of soils, e.g. ordinary red loams, black soils and clayey loams. Good drainage is essential and water-logging is detrimental. Seedlings are first rainsed in a nursery. Seeds obtained from selected pods and mixed with ashes are sown by broadcasting. Germination occurs in about a week. The field is ploughed and manured with compost. The field is irrigated once a day until the plants are established. Flowering starts when the plants are 2.5 3.5 months old. Dew and heavy rain at flowering time are injurious. Ripe and nearly ripe fruits are picked at intervals of 5, 10 and 20 days.

Characters : Capsicum is 5-12 cm long, 2-4 cm wide, globular, ovoid or oblong in shape, surface is shrievelled, orange or red in colour, pedicel is prominent and bent. Internally the fruits are divided into two halve parts by a membranous dissepiment to which the seeds are attached. Capsicum has characrteristic odour and an intense pungent taste.

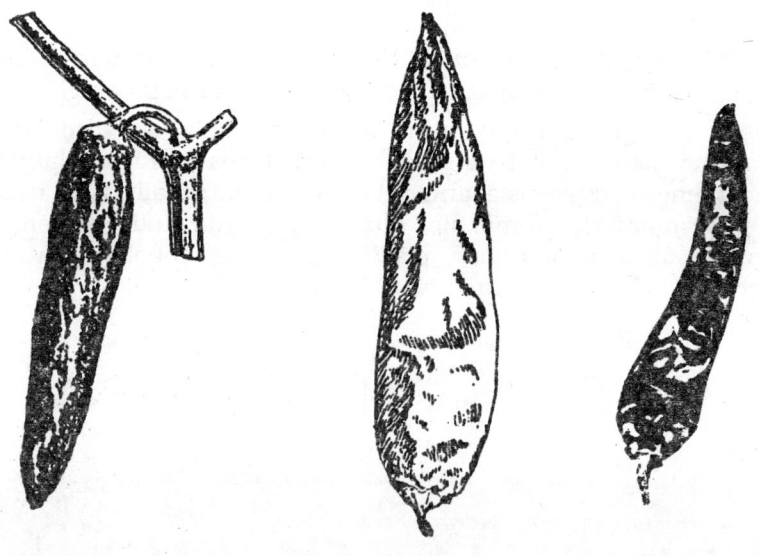

Fig. 11.12. Capsicum

Collection : The fruits are picked as they become fully ripe. The quality of the drug is in part determined by its colour. The unripe fruits fade to pale buff upon drying. The fruits are dried in sun, graded by colour; occasionally oil is rubbed on the fruits to give a glossiness to the pericarps. Most of the calices and pedicels are removed.

Chemical Constituents : Capsicum contains fixed oils (0.1-1%), oleo-resin, carotenoids, capsacutin, capsico (a volatile alkaloid), volatile oil (1.5%) and ascorbic acid (0.2%). The resin contains an extremely pungent principle, capsaicin, (decylenic vinillyl amide) (about 0.5%). Capsaicin retains its characteristic pungency in a dilution of 1 part in 10 million parts with water. The maximum concentration of capsaicin is in the inner walls. Its pungency is uneffected by alkalies but is destroyed by oxidising agents. Capsanthin is the main carotenoid of red fruits. It also occurs as monoester and diester along with cryptocapsin. Other carotenoids include zeaxanthin, lutein, cryptoxanthin, α- and β-carotenes and few xanthophylls. The carbohydrates reported in chillies are fructose, galactose, sucrose, fructosyl-sucrose, planteose, planteobiose, etc. Tocopherol (vitamin E) is present in trace amounts (~2.4 mg/100 g).

The pungent compounds of *C. annuum* are capsaicin (69%), dihydrocapsaicin (22%), nordihydrocapsiacin (7%), homo-capsaicin (1%) and homodihydrocapsaicin (1%).

Uses : Capsicum has been used externally as stimulant, counter irritant, rubefacient, in sore throat and scarlatina, hoarseness, dyspepsia and yellow fever. Internally it is used as carminative, stomachic, atonic dyspepsia and flatulence. In the form of ointment, plaster, medicated wool it is used for the relief of rheumatism, lumbago, etc.

Capsaicin (Vanillyl amide of isodecenoic acid)

Capsanthin

QUESTIONS

1. What are Resin and Resin combinations ? Write official source, chemical constituents and uses of Podophyllum, Cannabis and Male Fern.
2. What are balsams ? How is Balsam of Peru obtained ? Give chemical tests and constituents of it.

3. Give the sources, chemical constituents and uses of the following drugs : (a) Benzoin (b) Asafoetida (c) Ipomoea (d) Cannabis.

4. Give natural occurrence, chemistry, isolation and pharmaceutical uses of podophyllotoxin and curcumin.

5. Write short but informative notes on : (a) Ginger, (b) Podophyllum, (c) Turmeric.

6. Discuss chemistry and isolation of Curcumin from Turmeric and give its biological activities.

7. Write short notes on : (a) Balsam of Tolu (b) Sumatra Benzoin (c) Turmeric (d) Podophyllum.

8. How are the following drugs identified : (a) Myrrh (b) Asafoetida (c) Colophony (d) Benzoins.

9. Describe the biological source, chemical constituents and uses of the resin drugs belonging to the following family : (a) Berberidaceae (b) Styraceae (d) Zingiberaceae (d) Bureseraceae.

10. Describe different commercial varieties of Ginger, its chemical constituents and uses.

11. Discuss turmeric under a pharmacognostic scheme. Write its chemical constituents and tests of identification.

12. Give the physical characters, chemical constituents and chemical tests for : (a) Colophony (b) Myrrh (c) Asafoetida.

12

PROTEINS

Proteins are highly complex molecules which contain the elements of carbon, hydrogen, nitrogen, and usually sulphur. They are synthesized by living cells and are an essential part of the structure of the cell and its nucleus. The plant proteins are more easily isolated in crystalline form. Proteins are stored in plants in the form of aleurone grains. They are required for animals as the source of nitrogen in food.

The molecular weight of most proteins can be estimated only approximately by centrifugal sedimentation methods for soluble proteins, which vary from few thousand to many millions. Other methods are osmotic pressure measurements, X-ray diffraction, light scattering effects, gel filtration and chemical analysis.

Soluble proteins form colloidal solutions which are generally viscous and may form gel. Many of them (e.g. egg albumin) are coagulated by heat or action of acids, alkalies or certain chemicals or by U.V. light. This process is known as 'denaturation' in which solubility of the protein in decreased.

Proteins are hydrolyzed to form simpler substances and ultimately amino acids. The hydrolytic process takes place during digestion by proteolytic enzymes or in laboratory by hot acids or alkalies :

Protein → Polypeptide → Peptide → Amino acids

Proteins are built up from amino acids linked together in chains or rings. The carboxylic group of one molecule is condensed with an amino group of the adjacent molecule with the formation of the amide linkage commonly known as peptide linkage.

$$RCH - COOH + R' - CH - COOH \xrightarrow{-H_2O}$$
$$\quad | \qquad\qquad\qquad\quad | $$
$$\quad NH_2 \qquad\qquad\qquad NH_2$$
$$\text{Amino acid} \qquad\qquad \text{Amino acid}$$

$$R - CH - CO - NH - CH - R'$$
$$\quad | \qquad\qquad\qquad\quad |$$
$$\quad NH_2 \qquad\qquad\qquad COOH$$
$$\text{Dipeptide}$$

Natural compounds formed in this way are called as 'polypeptide' if they have molecular weight below 10,000. Molecules with molecular weight above ~ 10,000 are known as proteins. In general, proteins and polypeptides differ in chemical and physical properties. Both type of compounds often exhibit physiological activity as in case of enzymes and hormones.

Proteins may be classified as :

(i) Fibrous proteins which serve as structural materials for animals, e.g., collagen, horn, feathers, nails, fibroin (silk), and

(ii) Globular proteins which are soluble in water and dilute acids and alkalies.

In another classification proteins are divided as

(i) Simple proteins, which yield only amino acid on hydrolysis, e.g., protamines, albumin, globulins, etc.,

(ii) Conjugated proteins, which contain a non-protein group, known as prosthetic group, e.g., nucleoproteins, chromoproteins, glycoproteins, phosphoproteins, lipoproteins, and metalloproteins, and

(iii) Derived proteins, which are the degradation products obtained by the action of acids, alkalies or enzymes on proteins. For example, denatured proteins, metaproteins, secondary proteoses, peptones, polypeptides, simple peptides and amino acids are the derived proteins.

Since proteins are present in all living organisms, they are of great importance in biochemistry. They form an important class of food, e.g. meat, fish and egg are important source of animal proteins. Cereal grains, e.g., wheat, pulses, etc., are plant protein foods. Whole glandular products, oil-bearing plant seeds, antitoxins, serums, and globulins contain proteins in combination with other biochemical substances. These products possess therapeutic activity. Allergens are usually proteinaceous materials producing allergic reactions.

Certain proteins are highly poisonous. Among them are plant toxalbumins, ricin from castor beans, robin from locust bark, abrin from jequirty seeds, hemolysins from salamanders and various toxins, e.g., neurotoxoids from snake venum.

Properties of Proteins : Proteins are amphoteric in nature. At some definite pH, characteristic for each protein, the positive and negative charges are exactly balanced and the molecules do not migrate in an electrical field. This condition is known as 'isoelectric point' and at this pH the protein has its least solubility. All proteins are optically active and may be coagulated and precipitated from aqueous solution.

Colour Reactions : Proteins exhibit a variety of colour reactions, e.g.,

1. **Biuret Reaction** : To alkaline solution of protein (2 ml), a dilute solution of copper sulphate is added. A red or violet colour is formed with peptides containing at least two peptide linkages. A dipeptide does not give this test.

2. **Xanthoproteic Reaction** : Proteins usually form a yellow colour when warmed with concentrated nitric acid. This colour becomes orange when the solution is made alkaline. The colour is due to nitration of aromatic ring present in phenylalanine, tyrosine and tryptophan.

3. **Millon's Reaction** : Millon's reagent (mercuric nitrate in nitric acid containing a trace of nitrous acid) usually yields a white precipitate on addition to a protein solution which turns red on heating. This reaction is characteristic of phenols (e.g. the phenolic amino acid tyrosine).

4. **Ninhydrin Test** : To an aqueous solution of a protein an alcoholic solution of ninhydrin is added and then heated. Red to violet colour is formed.

5. **Nitroprusside Test** : Proteins containing sulphur group form red colour with nitroprusside solution.

6. **Lead sulphide Test** : Alkaline solution of sulphur containing proteins, on addition to lead acetate, produces a black precipitate.

GELATIN

Synonyms : Gelfoam; Puragel; Gelatinum.

Biological Source : Gelatin is a heterogenous mixture of water-soluble proteins of high average molecular weight obtained by treating specific animal tissues like skin, tendons, ligaments and bones with hot water. Gelatin is not found in nature but derived from collagen by hydrolytic action.

Preparation : For preparation of Gelatin, the insoluble collagens are converted into soluble gelatin which is then purified and concentrated to a solid form. Commercially, gelatin is obtained from by-products of slaughtered cattle, sheep, and hogs. The starting materials, e.g. bones, are defatted with an organic solvent. Sometimes these are decalcified with hydrochloric acid. The material is then heated with water at 85°C to convert collagens to Gelatin. The solution is decolourized, filtered by electro-osmosis, concentrated under reduced pressure, allowed to set into gel in shallow trays and dried rapidly in drying-rooms at 30, 40, 50 and 60° for some weeks.

Characters : Gelatin is colourless or slightly yellow, transparent, brittle, practically odourless, tasteless sheets, flakes or course powder. In water it swells and absorbs 5-10 times its weight of water to form a gel in solutions below 35-40°. It is soluble in hot water, glycerol, acetic acid; insoluble in organic solvent and is amphoteric. In dry condition it is stable in air, but when moist or in solution, it is attacked by bacteria. The gelatinizing property of Gelatin is reduced by boiling for long time.

Commercially two types of gelatin , A and B, are available. Type A has an iso-electric point between pH 7 and 9. It is incompatible with anionic compounds such as acacia, agar and tragacanth. Type B has an isoelectric point between 4.7 and 5 and it is used with anionic mxtures. Gelatin is coloured with a certified colour for manufacturing capsules or for coating of tablets. It may contain various additives.

Chemical Constituents : Gelatin consists of the protein glutin which on hydrolysis gives a mixture of amino acids. The approximate amino acid contents are : glycine (25.5%), alanine (8.7%), valine (2.5%), leucine (3.2%), isoleucine (1.4%), cystine and cysteine (0.1%), methionine (1.0%), tyrosine (0.5%), aspartic acid (6.6%), glutamic acid (11.4%), arginine (8.1%), lysine (4.1%) and histidine (0.8%). Nutritionally, gelatin is an incomplete protein lacking tryptophan. The gelatinizing compound is known as chondrin and the adhesive nature of Gelatin is due to the presence of glutin.

Uses : Gelatin is used to prepare pastilles, pastes, suppositories, capsules, pill-coatings, gelatin sponge; as suspending agent, tablet binder, coating agent, as stabilizer, thickener and texturizer in food; for manufacturing rubber substitutes, adhesives, cements, lithographic and printing inks, plastic compounds, artificial silk, photographic plates and films, matches, light filters for mercury lamps; clarifying agent; in hectographic matters; sizing paper and textiles; for inhibiting crystallization in bacteriology, for preparing cultures and as a nutrient.

It forms glycerinated gelatin with glycerin which is used as vehicle and for manufacture of suppositories. Combined with zinc, it forms zinc gelatin which is employed as a topical protectant. As a nutrient, Gelatin is used as commercial food products and bacteriologic culture media.

Absorable Gelatin Sponge : It is a water-insoluble gelatin based sterile sponge. It is prepared from purified, specially treated gelatin to form a light, white porous, pliable, non-antigenic matrix. It is sterlized by heat. It absorbs about 50 times its weight of water and about 45 times its weight of blood. It is local haemostatic and used to control capillary oozing, bleeding of veins and operative wounds. The sponge is applied to the bleeding area, held for about 15 seconds and left.

Absorbable Gelatin Film : It is a specially prepared cellophane-type gelatin product in neurosurgery and in thoracic and ocular surgery. It consists of a thin, nonantigenic, pliable absorbable film of purified gelatin. It occurs in pieces of about 2.5 x 5 cm or 10 x 12.5 cm in size and about 0.075 mm in thickness. It is moistened by immersion in salt solution for cutting into the shape required to fit into the contours of the incision.

Chemical Test

1. Biuret test is positive.
2. Xanthoproteic test is positive.
3. Millon's test is positive.
4. Ninhydrin test is positive.
5. On heating Gelatin (1 g) with soda lime, smell of ammonia is produced.
6. A solution of Gelatin (0.5g) in water (10 ml) is precipitated to white buff coloured precipitate on addition of few drops of tannic acid (10%).
7. With picric acid Gelatin forms yellow precipitate.

$CH_2 - COOH$
$|$
NH_2
Glycine

$CH_3 CH - COOH$
$|$
NH_2
Alanine

$(CH_3)_2 CH CH - COOH$
$|$
NH_2
Valine

$(CH_3)_2 CH CH_2 CH - COOH$
$|$
NH_2
Leucine

$CH_3 CH_2 CH (CH_3) CH - COOH$
$|$
NH_2
Isoleucine

$HS CH_2 CHCOOH$
$|$
NH_2
Cysteine

$[-SCH_2 CH - COOH]_2$
$|$
NH_2
Cystine

$CH_3 S - CH_2 CH_2 CH - COOH$
$|$
NH_2
Methionine

$CH_2 CH-COOH$
$| \quad |$
$HO \quad NH_2$
Serine

$CH_3 CH - CH - COOH$
$| \quad |$
$HO \quad NH_2$
Threonine

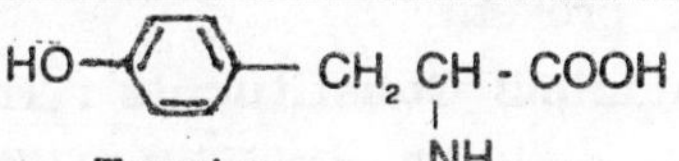

$HO-\langle \rangle- CH_2 CH - COOH$
$|$
NH_2
Tyrosine

$HOOC - CH_2 CH - COOH$
$|$
NH_2
Aspartic acid

$HOOC - (CH_2)_2 CH - COOH$
$|$
NH_2
Glutamic acid

$NH_2 - C - NH(CH_2)_3 CH COOH$
$\quad ||$
$\quad NH \qquad NH_2$
Arginine

$NH_2 - (CH_2)_4 CH - COOH$
$|$
NH_2
Lysine

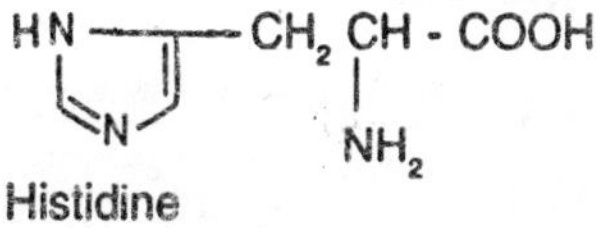

$HN-\langle \rangle- CH_2 CH - COOH$
$\quad \searrow_N \qquad |$
$\qquad NH_2$
Histidine

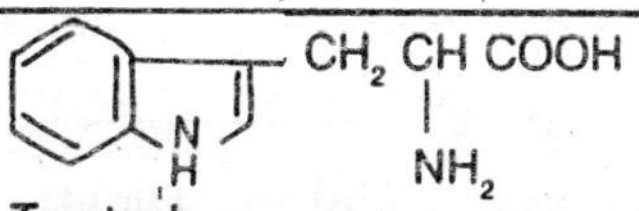

$CH_2 CH COOH$
$|$
NH_2
Tryptophan

YEAST

Synonyms : Dried yeast; Cerevisiae fermentum; Faex medicinalis.

Biological Source : Yeast are unicellular organisms, consists of the cells of a suitable strain of *Saccharomyces cerevisiae* Hansen (Fam. Saccharomycetaceae) dried to preserve the vitamins present.

Collection and Preparation : Yeast are commercially available as 'Brewer's yeast' which is viscid, semifluid frothy mass and consists of living cells of *S. cerevisiae* and related species. 'Compressed yeast' is the purer strain of yeast, partially dried by expression of water and admixed with a starch. 'Dried yeast' is the dried cells of *S. cerevisiae*. Dried yeast is usually obtained as a by-product from the brewing beer made from an extract of cereal grains and hops. The yeast cells are washed to free beer and dried, and may be debittered. Dried yeast may also be obtained by growing suitable strains of yeast, using media other than those required for the production of beer, and under appropriate environmental conditions. Dried yeast is obtained by heating the compressed yeast at 30°C until the moisture content is reduced to below 9 per cent.

Characters : Dried yeast occurs as a pale buff to weak yellowish orange flakes, granules or powder with characteristic indicative odour. Due to the presence of dead cells, dried yeast is inactive in fermentation process. Under microscope spherical, elliptical or ovate cells up to 8 μm long are present.

Chemical Constituents : The principal compounds of yeast are vitamins 'B-group' such as aneurine, nicotinic acid, riboflavine, folic acid and B_{12}. In addition to these yeast contains proteins (46%), carbohydrates (36%) particularly glycogen, fats, sterols and enzymes like zymase complex, glucogenase, invertase, maltase, emulsin and diastase, nucleoproteins, etc.

Uses : Yeast is used as dietary source of B vitamins and proteins, and in the treatment of furunculosis. Mostly yeast is used in baking bread, brewing; producing alcohol by fermentation of sugar, molasses, and cereals.

DIASTASE (MALT EXTRACT)

Synonyms : Maltin, Diastase of malt.

Biological Source : Diastase is a mixture of amylolytic enzymes obtained from malt.

Malt is obtained by artificially germinated barley grains, *Hordeum vulgare* Linn. (Fam. Gramineae). Barley is grown throughout the world in favourable climate. For preparing malt, wet barley grains in heaps are kept in warm room for germination until the caulicle protrudes. The grain is dried quickly to kill the embryo. The enzyme diastase in the moist warm grains converts starch to maltose which stimulates the embryo for germination. Dry malt contains maltose sugar (50-70%), dextrins (2-15%), proteins (8%), diastase and peptase enzyme. It resembles barley but is more crisp with an agreeable odour and sweet taste. It is used mainly in the brewing and alcohol industries.

Malt extract is prepared by extracting the partially germinating grains of *H. vulgare*. It contains dextrin, maltose, glucose and amylolytic enzymes. Diastase converts at least 50 times of its weight of potato starch into sugars (dextrin and maltose) in 30 minutes.

Diastase is a yellowish white amorphous powder or translucent scales obtained from an infusion of malt. It loses amylolytic power on keeping, on heating its solution at 85°, or on adding excess of acid. It is soluble in water with some turbidity; almost insoluble in alcohol.

Diastase in used to manufacture starch, converting starch into sugar and to remove starch from fabrics.

PAPAIN

Synonyms : Papayotin; Vegetable pepsin; Arbuz; Nematolyt; Caroid; Summetrin; Tromasin; Velardon; Vermizym.

Biological Source : Papain is the dried and purified latex of the green fruits and leaves of *Carica papaya* L. (Fam. Caricaceae). The plant is cultivated in Sri Lanka, Tanzania, Hawai and Florida. The plant is 5-6 m in height bearing fruits of about 30 cm length and a weight up to 5 kg.

Preparation : It is distributed throughout the plant, but mostly concentrated in the latex of the fruit.

The latex is obtained by making 2-4 longitudinal incisions, about 1/8 inch deep, on the surface of nearly mature but green fruits while still on the tree. The incisions are made early in the morning, at intervals of 3-7 days. The exudate is collected in non-metallic containers or on cloth of *americani* type stretched wooden frames clamped to the tree. The latex is dried as soon as possible after collection. Rapid drying or exposure to sun or higher temperature above 38°C produce dark colour product with weak in proteolytic activity. The final product should be creamy white and friable. It is sealed in air-tight containers to prevent loss of activity. If 10% common salt or 1% solution of formaldehyde is added before drying, the product retains its activity for many months.

Fully grown fruits give more latex of high enzyme potency than smaller or immature fruits. The yield of Papain varies from 20 to 250 g per tree. The yield of commercial Papain from latex is about 20%.

Papain can also be obtained from the juice of stems, leaves and petioles. The enzyme has nearly the same activity as that obtained from the fruit latex.

A highly active product is obtained by dissolving the commercial product in water, saturating with hydrogen sulphide, precipitating with alcohol and drying the precipitate at low temperature.

Commercial Papain is often adulterated with arrowroot starch, dried milk of cactus, gutta percha, rice flour and pepsin. Bleaching is done for improving the colour, but this lowers the enzyme activity of the product.

Papain possesses both milk clotting and protein digesting properties. The milk clotting property is lost through oxidation with hydrogen peroxide and is regained on reduction with hydrogen cyanide or hydrogen sulphide. The pepton hydrolyzing activity is lost on oxidation with hydrogen peroxide and is regained on reduction. Oxidation, however, does not affect the Gelatin hydrolyzing activity.

Characters : Papain occurs as white or greyish - white, slightly hygroscopic powder. It is incompletely soluble in water and glycerol. It may digest about 35 times its weight of lean meat. Best-grades render digestion of 200 - 300 times their weight of coagulated egg albumin in alkaline media. A temperature range of 60-90° is favourable for the digestive process with 65° the optimum point. Best pH is 5.0, but it functions also in neutral or alkaline media. It is activated by reduction (HCN, H_2S, etc.) and inactivated by oxidation

(H$_2$O$_2$, iodoacetate).

Chemical Constituents : Papain contains several enzymes such as proteolytic enzymes peptidase I capable of converting proteins into dipeptides and polypeptides, renninlike enzyme, clotting enzyme similar to pectase and an enzyme having a feeble activity on fats.

Two enzymes, papain and chymopapain, have been isolated in crystalline form from the latex. Papain is a typical protein digesting enzyme with isoelectric point. It contains 15.5% nitrogen and 1.2% sulphur. Crystalline Papain is most stable in the pH range 5 - 7 and is rapidly destroyed at 30° below pH 2.5 and above pH 12.

Uses : Papain is used to prevent adhesions; in sloughing and infected wounds; internally as protein digestant, as anthelmintic (nemotode), to relieve the symptoms of episiotomy (incision of vulva) and in meat industry for tenderizing beef, used for treatment of dyspepsia, intestinal and gastric disorders; for the treatment of diphtheria, for dissolving diphtheria membrane; in surgery to reduce incidence of blood clots where thromboplasma is undesirable; for local treatment of buccal, pharyngeal and laryngeal disorders.

It is used in digestive mixtures, liver tonics, for reducing enlarged tonsils, in prevention of post-operative adhesions, carbuncles and eschar burns. It is an allergic agent causing severe paroxysmal cough, vasomotor rhinitis and dyspnea. It is a powerful poison when injected intravenously. In industry it is used in the manufacture of proteolytic preparations of meat, lever and casein, with dilute alcohol and lactic acid as meat tenderizer, as a substitute for rennet in cheese manufacture, in brewing industry for making chill-proof bear, for degumming natural milk, in preparation of tooth pastes and cosmetics and in tanning industry for bating skin and hides.

BROMELAIN

Synonyms : Bromelin; Ananase; Extranse; Inflamen; Traumanase.

Biological Source : Bromelain is a protein-digesting and milk clotting enzyme found in pineapple fruit juice and stem tissues of *Ananas comosus* (L.) Merr.

Family : Bromeliaceae.

Enzymes from fruit juice and stem tissue are distinguished as fruit Bromelain and stem Bromelain. From pineapple juice the enzyme is obtained by precipitation with acetone and also with ammonium sulphate. Stem Bromelain has molecular weight of about 33,000 and is probably the first proteolytic enzyme of plant origin to be established as a glycoprotein.

Unlike Papain, fruit Bromelain does not disappear as the fruit ripens. Fruit and stem Bromelains are acidic and basic proteins, respectively.

Bromelain is used as adjunctive therapy to reduce inflammation and edema and to accelerate tissue repair. Bromelain is also used to produce protein hydrolysates, in tenderizing meats, in leather industry and chill proofing agent in beer.

It is also used as food additive and bating reagent of hides. It is useful in determining antibody substances, dissolving necrogenic tissues, treating digestive troubles; when applied as an antiphlogistic it shows less after-effects.

FICIN

Synonyms : Ficus proteinase; Ficus protease; Debricin; Higueroxyl delabarre.

Biological Source : Ficin is a concentrate prepared by filtering and drying the latex of *Ficus glabrata* (Fam. Moraceae). It is a proteolytic enzyme of molecular weight about 23,800-25,500 which requires a free sulphydryl group for activity and as such as a member of a group which includes Papain and Bromelain.

Ficin occurs as a buff to cream-coloured hygroscopic powder. It has acrid odour, which grows stronger with age. It is bulky, nearly 3 ml/g, not free-flowing. It appears dry, even when 15% water is present. It is not completely soluble in water; insoluble in usual solvents. It loses about 10-20% activity when stored 1-3 years at ordinary temperature and atmospheric conditions. Aqueous solutions are inactivated at 100°, solid partially inactivated within a few hours. Solutions are relatively stable between pH 4-8.5; incompatible with iron, copper and aluminium. Gelatin coagulates egg white;

casein, meat and most proteins are hydrolyzed with aqueous Ficin solution. Ficin has tissue - dissolving property. Therefore, it must be handled with care. Ficin is 10-20 times more active as Papain in regard to milk clotting; 4-10 times as active in general.

Ficin is used as protein digestant in the brewing industry, as a chill-proofing agent in beer; in cheese industry as a substitute for rennet in the coagulation of milk; in meat industry as a meat tenderizer and as an agent for removing castings from formed sausage. In leather industry it is used for the bating of leather; in the textile industry for shrink proofing wool, for removing gelatin from sized thread, and mixed with amylases and maltases as a spot remover. It is also used in the preparation of peptones, for determining protein material in spent grains and in determination of the Rh factor. It speeds 10 times the agglutination of human blood cells by the Rh factor when in contact with the anti-Rh serum. It has been used as a trichuricide.

Ficin causes irritation to skin, eyes and mucous membranes. Large doses by mouth cause purging.

QUESTIONS

1. Give sources, methods of preparation and uses of Gelatin and Papain.
2. Write notes on the following :
   (a) Papain (b) Malt extract (c) Ficin (d) Yeast.
3. Give the methods of preparation of Gelatin and Malt extract. What chemical tests will you perform to characterize them ?
4. What do you know about proteins ? How are they classified and identified ? Discuss Papain in detail.

13

ALKALOIDS

The term alkaloid is applied to naturally occurring basic compounds and is difficult to define. The term is derived from 'vegetable alkali' (alk = alkali; oid = like). They may be defined as organic nitrogenous substances of plant origin exhibiting well-defined physiological actions. A true alkaloid has a nitrogen atom as a part of heterocyclic system; it has a complex molecular structure; it manifests significant pharmacological activity and it is restricted to the plant kingdom.

Alkaloids have been reported in various plant parts such as in whole aerial plant (Lobelia, Tylophora, Ephedra), in leaves (Datura, Belladonna, Coca), in bark (Kurchi, Cinchona), in stem (Withania), in rhizomes and roots (Ipecac, Rauwolfia, Aconite); in flowering buds (Hyoscyamus) and in seeds (Nux vomica, Physostigma, Colchicum). Several alkaloids have been found in cultures of microorganisms, e.g., in bacteria, fungi (Ergot) and algae. Amphibian alkaloids such as toad venous (bufotoxin) and salamander alkaloids (salamandarine) are of animal origin. Alkaloids with complicated chemical structures (strychnine) are less widespread in nature than simple compounds (nicotine). About 100 families out of 283 possess alkaloids.

The names of alkaloids have been derived from the plants yielding them (atropine, tylophorine, cocaine, nicotine); from physiologic activity (emetine, morphine) and from the discoverer (pelletierine, alihirsutine). As per chemical rules the names of all alkaloids should end in "ine".

Alkaloids exhibit a variety of physical and chemical properties. All of them possess carbon, hydrogen and nitrogen and in most cases oxygen as elements. Like basic compounds they form their crystalline salts with acids like hydrochloric acid, sulphuric acid, citric acid, and tartaric acid. The free alkaloids are insoluble or slightly soluble in water but their salts are freely soluble. However, they are soluble in non-polar solvents such as ether or chloroform. Therefore, alkaloids are separated from non-polar compounds by salt formation, extracting the lipid soluble portion and basifying the solution with an alkali carbonate or ammonia. Most of the alkaloids are crystalline solids with definite melting points, some of them are amorphous and few (coniine, nicotine) are liquids. They are generally colourless compounds but few are coloured substances, e.g., berberine (yellow), betaine (red), tylophorine (dull yellow), and conessine (pale yellow). They are generally bitter in taste and optically active. On treatment with phosphotungstic acid, phosphomolybdic acid, picric acid, potassium mercuri-iodide and tannic acid, they yield insoluble precipitates (double salts). The following colour tests are used to detect the presence of an alkaloid :

1. **Mayer's Reagent** (Potassium mercuri-iodide solution) : It gives a white or pale yellow precipitate except with alkaloids of the purine group and few others.

2. **Dragendorff's Reagent** (Potassium iodide + bismuth nitrate): Alkaloids form orange coloured precipitate with the reagent.

3. **Wagner's Reagent** (iodine solution) : It gives a brown or reddish brown precipitate with alkaloids.

4. **Hager's Reagent** (A saturated solution of picric acid in cold water) : It gives characteristic crystalline precipitate with many alkaloids.

5. **Tannic Acid Test :** A freshly prepared aqueous solution of tannic acid (5%, w/v) gives a precipitate with most of the alkaloids which is soluble in dilute acid or ammonia solution.

6. **Ammonia Reineckate Test :** A saturated aqueous solution of ammonia reineckate slightly acidified with hydrochloric acid gives a pink flocculent precipitate with most of the alkaloids.

In plants alkaloids act as poisonous and stimulating agents. Sparteine acts as stimulant to an aphid when feeding on *Sarothamus scoparius*. The insect changes its feeding site according to where the highest concentration of alkaloid occurs within the host plant. Tomatin, the major alkaloid of tomato, acts as repellent. Nicotine and anabasine act as powerful repellents for many insect groups and thus protects plants from insects and herbivorous. They also act as regulatory growth factors, and reserve substances for nitrogen and other elemental supply and as end products of detoxification reactions. They occur as pigments, such as pteridine and betalains, and attract animals for pollination.

Alkaloids are capable to exhibit extensive and well-marked pharmacological activities like analgesic (cocaine, morphine, codeine), antiamoebic and emetic (emetin), anticholinergic (atropine, hyoscyamine, scopolamine), antihypertensive (reserpine, deserpine), antimalarial (quinine, cinchonine), antitumor (vinblastine, vincristine), antitussive (codeine, noscapine), cardiac depressant (quinidine), central nervous stimulant (caffeine, strychnine, brucine), diuretic (theobromine, theophylline), oxytocic (ergometrine, ergotamine) ophthalmic and cholinergic (physostigmine, pilocarpine), skeletal muscle relaxant (tubocurarine) and smooth muscle relaxant (papaverine, theophylline).

Classification

No systematic structural classification exists for alkaloids. The most widely accepted classification system is as :

1. **True Alkaloids :** True alkaloids are toxic, show a wide range of physiological activity; contain nitrogen in a heterocyclic ring, derived from amino acids and normally occur in plants, e.g., colchicine, quinine, morphine, emetine, etc.

2. **Protoalkaloids :** Protoalkaloids are relatively simple amines in which the amino acid nitrogen is not in a heterocyclic ring, e.g., mescaline and ephedrine.

3. **Pseudoalkaloids :** These alkaloids are not derived from amino acid precursors and are usually basic in nature, e.g., steroidal alkaloids (conessine) and purines (caffeine).

Alkaloids are generally arranged in order of increasing rings, e.g., pyrrolidine group (hygrine, tropinone), pyridine-piperidine group (coniine, pseudopelletierine, lobelia alkaloids, lupine alkaloids, nicotine), isoquinoline group (papaverine, dauricine), tetrahydroisoquinoline group (aporphine alkaloids, berberine, crytopine, emetine), phenanthrene or morphine

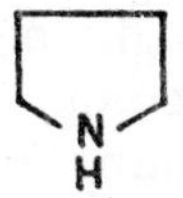

Pyrrolidine

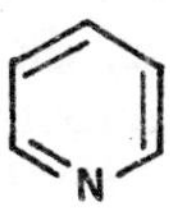

Pyridine

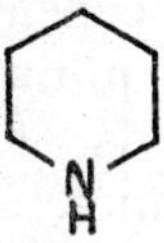

Piperidine

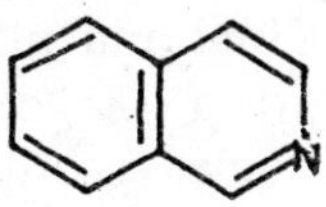

Isoquinoline

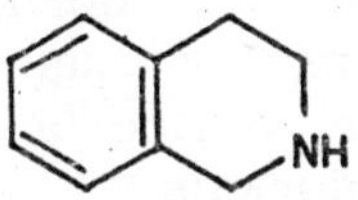

Tetrahydroisoquinoline

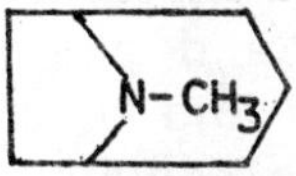

Tropane

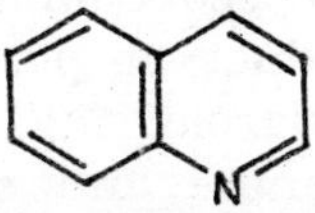

Quinoline

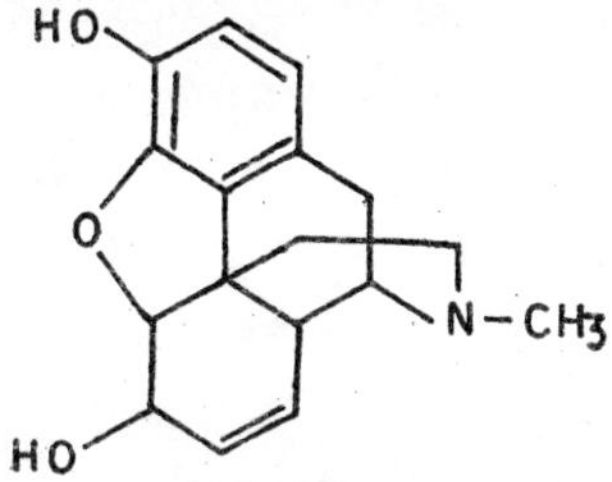

Morphine

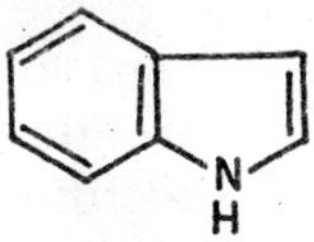

Indole

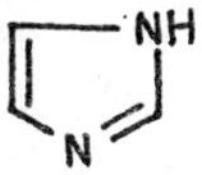

Imidazole

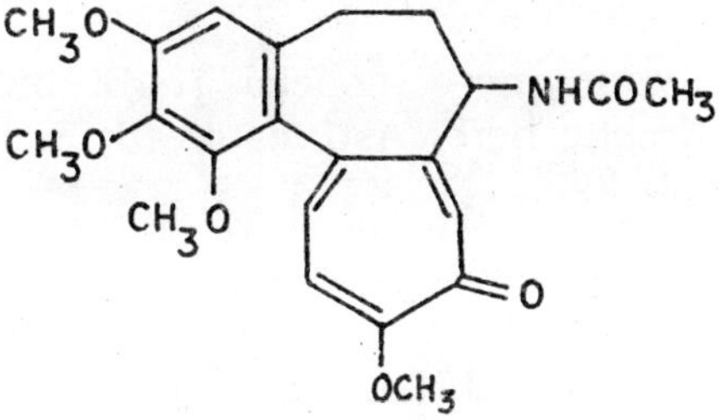

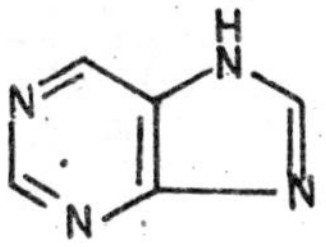

Purine

Colchiceine

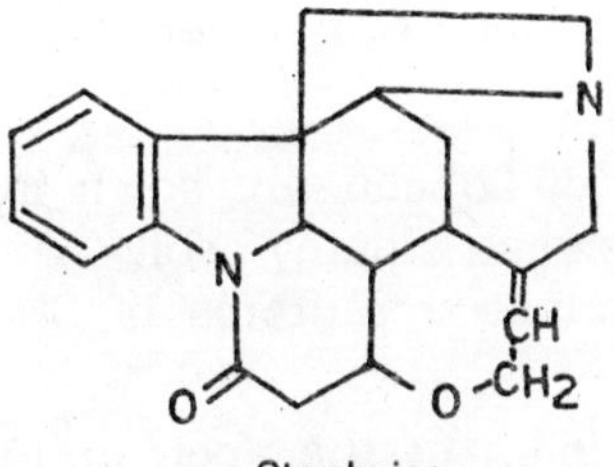

Strychnine

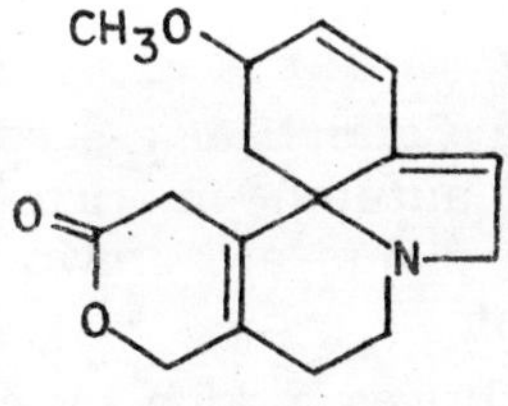

Erythroidine

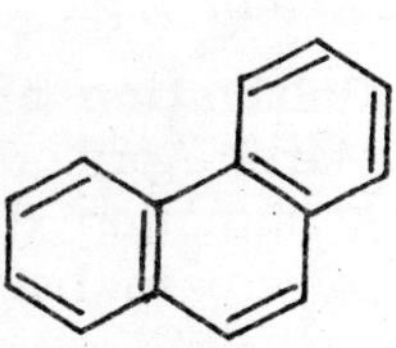

Phenanthrene

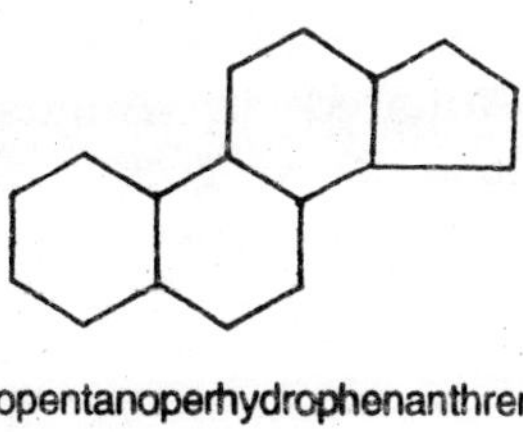

Cyclopentanoperhydrophenanthrene

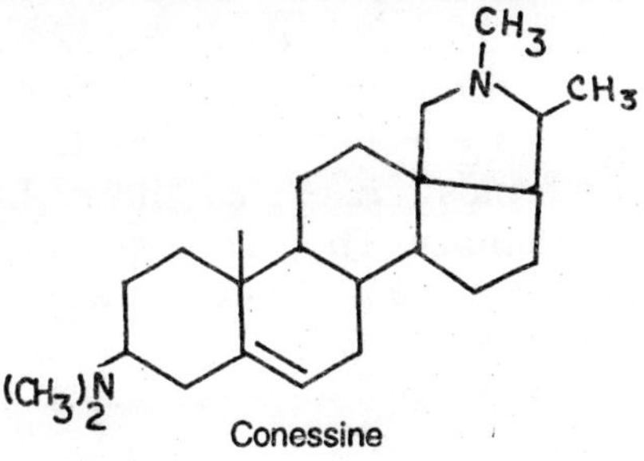

Conessine

group (morphine, codeine, thebaine), quinoline group (Cinchona alkaloids, quinine, cusparine, dictaminine), indole group (Ergot alkaloids, harmine, physostigmine), complex indole group (brucine, strychnine), erythrina group (β-erythroidine, erysopine) and colchicine. Atropine, hyoscyamine and scopolamine are derived from tropane, a condensed product of pyrrolidine and piperidine. Pilocarpine has the imidazole ring, caffeine and theobromine are purine bases, solanine and conessine contain steroidal nucleus.

PYRIDINE-PIPERIDINE ALKALOIDS

Reduction of pyridine coverts it into piperidine. This group includes alkaloids containing piperidine, α-propylpiperidine and   of nicotinic acid.

LOBELIA

Synonyms : Lobelia Herb; Indian tobacco; Wild tobacco; Emetic herb; Asthma weed; Bladder pod; Vomit wort; Herba lobeliae.

Official Source : Lobelia consists of the dried aerial parts of *Lobelia inflata* Linn. of which 60 per cent is the stem.

Family : Lobeliaceae.

Geographical Source : The plant is indigenous to the eastern USA, Canada and Holland. It is an erect annual herb, 30-90 cm high.

Cultivation and Collection : Seeds of Lobelia are sown in March-April or autumn in rich, moist, loamy soil. On germination the plants are grown to produce stems of 30-50 cm in height.

The plant thrives in rich moist loam in the open or in partial shade. Seeds are sown in well prepared ground in rows 20 cm apart. Sometimes seeds are sown in beds and seedlings transplanted in the field. Leaves and flowering tops are collected when the plants are in flower and the lowermost capsules have become inflated in August - September. They are dried in shade to preserve green colour and compressed into rectangular cakes and wrapped in paper for export.

Macroscopical Characters

General Appearance : Entire aerial part including stems, leaves, flowers, fruits and seeds.

Stem : Stems are greenish purple, winged and very hairy in the upper part. The lower part is more rounded, channelled, and less hairy.

Leaf : Leaves are 2 cm long, broken or entire with bristly hairs, sessile, ovate to ovate-lanceolate in shape. The margin is irregularly serrate, dentate and the teeth contain water-pores; acute and yellowish green in colour, slightly pubescent with characteristic odour and taste. Hairs are present on

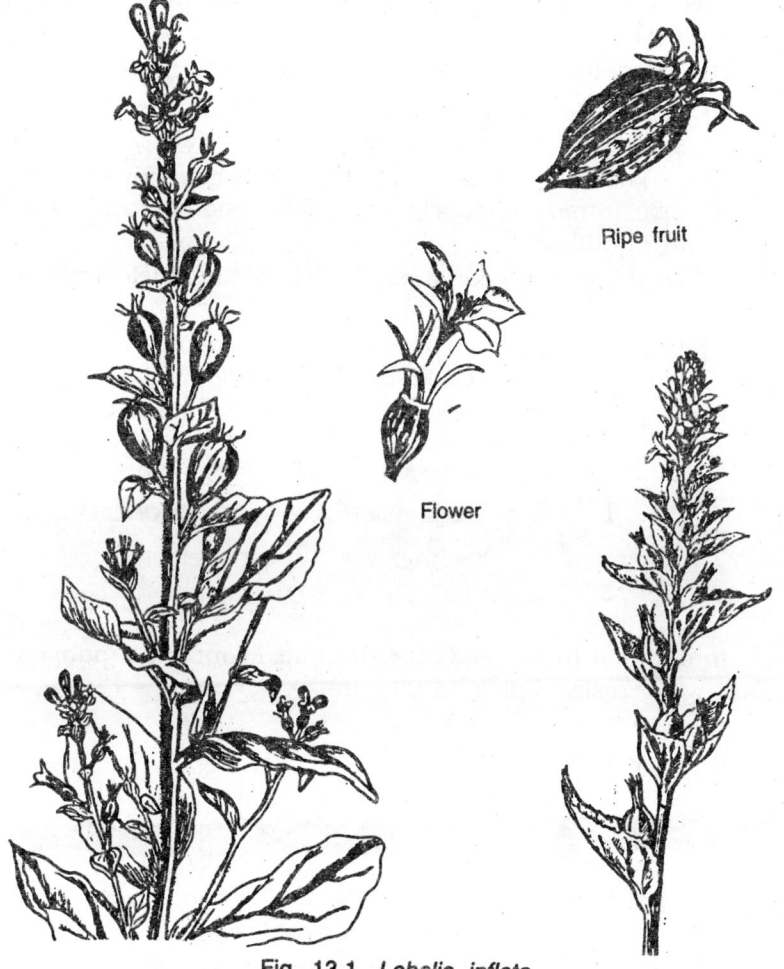

Ripe fruit

Flower

Fig. 13.1. *Lobelia inflata*

lamina. Base is wedge- shaped, entire. The upper epidermis lack stomata with very few or no trichomes whereas the lower one shows numerous ranunculaceous stomata with few-hairs. Trichomes are unicellular with rounded base and pointed tips.

Fruits are yellowish green capsule and inflated, 7-8 mm long, ovate and bilocular. Seeds are 0.5 - 0.7 mm in length, about 0.3 mm broad and brown in colour. Outer surface is covered with elongated, polygonal lignified reticulation. Odour is irritating and taste is acrid.

Chemical Constituents : Lobelia contains about 0.4 per cent alkaloidal constituents of which lobeline is the important active base.

The alkaloids of Lobelia are classified into there groups:

(i) Lobeline, the most active alkaloid of the drugs is similar to nicotine in action but weaker.

Lobeline group includes l-lobeline, dl-lobeline, lobelanine, norlobelanine, lobelanidine and nor-lobelanidine.

(ii) Lelobine group contains dl-lelobanidine, l-lelobanidine I and II and norlelobanidine.

(iii) Lobinine group contains the alkaloids lobinine, isolobinine, lobinanidine and isolobinanidine.

These alkaloids possess a piperidine nucleus.

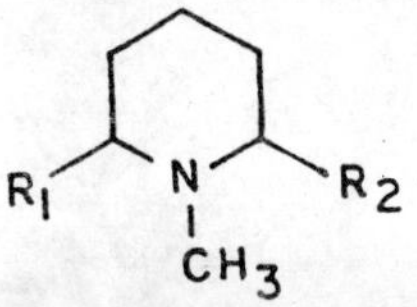

Lobelanine, $R_1 = R_2 = C_6H_5 \ COCH_2$-

Lobelanidine, $R_1 = R_2 = C_6H_5 \ CH(OH)CH_2$-

Lobeline, $R_1 = C_5H_6 \ CH \ (OH)CH_2$-

$R_2 = C_5H_6 \ COCH_2$-

In addition to alkaloids the drug also contains a pungent volatile oil, resin, lipids, and gum.

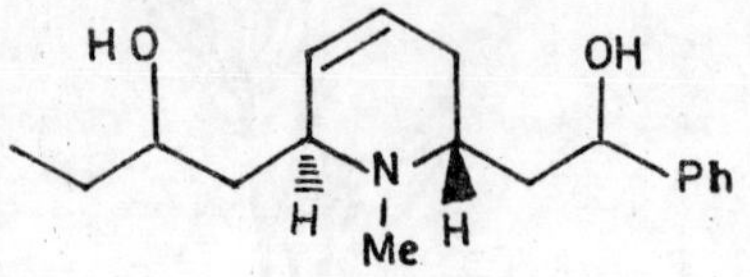

Lobinanidine

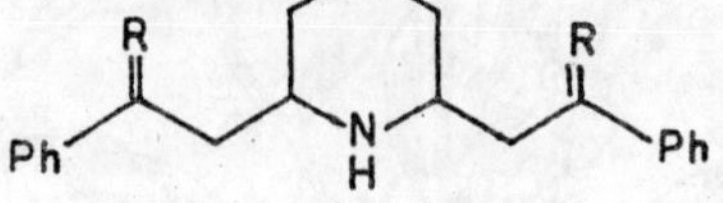

Norlobelanidine (R = H, OH)
Norlobelanine (R = O)

Uses : Lobelia is an expectorant used to treat spasmodic asthma and chronic bronchitis. Lobeline is a respiratory stimulant, relaxant and is given in the resuscitation of newborn infants; in gas, alcohol and narcotic poisoning; in drowning in water, electric shock and collapse. Lobelia in also used to discontinue smoking habit.

INDIAN LOBELIA

Synonyms : Nala; Narasala (Hindi); Nali (Gujrati); Badanala (Bengali).

Biological Source : Indian Lobelia consists of dried aerial parts of *Lobelia nicotianaefolia.* (Fam. Lobeliaceae). The drug is collected in October-November and dried in shade.

It is a large biennial or perennial herb, 1.2-3.6 m high, found in western ghats from Bombay to Travancore at altitudes of 700-2200 m. The leaves and stems are larger in size than those of American Lobelia. The lower leaves are up to 30 cm long and 7 cm broad while the upper leaves are smaller up to 10 cm long and 2 cm wide. They are green in colour, have apex acute to acuminate, margin serrulate, venation reticulate, upper surface glabrous, lower surface glabrous to pubescent, upper epidermis has ranunculaceous stomata and few or no hairs mainly on prominent veins . Hairs and trichomes are absent in older leaves. The stomata are many on the lower epidermis. The stem is cylindrical, greenish-yellow, straight and hollow in the centre. Longitudinal striations and scars of leaf bases are present on the upper surface. Flower pedicels are up to 3 cm long, smaller in thin stems. The odour in similar to tobacco and the taste is acrid and nauseous.

The leaves of the species can be distinguished from American Lobelia on the basis of trichomes, stomata and quantitative values.

Chemical Constituents : Up to 0.4% total alkaloids are present in Indian lobelia. Lobelanidine, non-lobelanidine, lobeline and d-lobelanidines II and III have been isolated from the drug. The alkaloid content in *L. nicotianaefolia* plant showed seasonal variation, being in highest concentration in October and November.

Uses : Indian lobelia is used as respiratory stimulant and antispasmodic agent. An infusion of leaves is used as an antiseptic.

ARECA NUTS

Synonyms : Betel nuts; Pinang; Semina Areacae; Supari (Hindi).

Biological Source : Areca nuts are the seeds of *Areca catechu* Linn.

Family : Palmae (Palmaceae).

Habitat : The tree is cultivated in tropical India, Sri Lanka, Malay states, South China, East Indies, Philippine Islands and parts of East Africa (including Zanzibar and Tanzania). In India it is cultivated in the coastal regions of southern Bombay and Madras, Mysore, Bengal and Assam.

Cultivation : Areca palm is mostly propagated by seeds. The palm requires a moist tropical climate for luxuriant growth; it is very sensitive to drought. It grows in areas with heavy rainfall in between temperature of 15° to 38°. It is cultivated in plains, hill-slopes and low lying valleys. The seeds are collected from 25-50 years old trees.

Collection : Areca nut is a handsome palm with a tall, slender stem crowned by large elegant leaves. Each tree contains about 100 fruits per year which are detached by means of bamboo poles, and the seeds extracted. The pericarp is fibrous and surrounds a single seed which is easily separated. The seeds are usually boiled in water with the addition of a little lime and dried.

Characters : Areca nuts are about 2.5 cm in length, bluntly rounded, conical in shape and 2-3 cm wide at the base. The testa is brown and marked with a network of small depressed lines. The ruminate endosperm is opal-white. Patches of a silvery coat, the inner layer of the pericarp, occasionally adhere to the testa. The deep - brown testa is marked with a network of depressed fissures; the colour of the testa is due to the presence of tannin. In the centre basal part of the endosperm, the small embryo is situated and an external pale area indicated its position. The seed is very hard, has a faint cheese - like odour when broken and an astringent, acrid taste.

Chemical Constituents : Areca nut contains a number of alkaloids of a piperidine series such as arecoline (methyl ester of arecanine), arecaine (N - methyl guvacine), guvacine (tetrahydronicitinic acid), arecaidine, guvacoline, arecolidine and choline. Arecoline is present in about 0.1 - 0.5 per cent yield and is medicinally important. In addition to alkaloids, Areca nuts contain fat (14%), amorphous red tannin (15%) known as areca red of phlobaphene nature, and α-catechin. The fat consists mainly of the glycerides of lauric, myristic and oleic acids.

Uses : Powdered Areca is used as anthelmintic, and vermifuge for dogs. It has aphrodisiac action and useful in urinary disorders, as nervine tonic and emmenagogue. The chewing of Areca nut may cause mouth cancer.

Substituents and Adulterants : Nuts from other plants, *vis. Areca caliso, A. concinna, A. ipot, A. laxa, A. nagensis, A. triandra, Caryota cumingii, Heterospathe elata,* etc. are used as substituents for Areca nuts. Sago palm nuts *(Metroxylon* species). dried tapioca *(Manihot esculenta)* and slices of sweet potato *(Ipomoea batatas)* form cheap adulterants that are mixed with slices of Areca nuts, and prove a serious menace affecting the industry. Nuts of *Caryota urens,* cut to various shapes and sizes resembling genuine Areca nuts, and coated with concentrated Areca nut extract *kali,* form the principal adulterant. Adulteration above 10% significantly increases the fibre content of the sample, which can be used as a measure of detecting adulteration.

Arecoline   Arecaidine   Guvacine

TROPANE ALKALOIDS

Condensation of tropane ring with piperidine constitutes the basic carbon framework of tropane nucleus. Plants of Solanaceae family are the major source of tropane alkaloids. The principal alkaloids of therapeutical interest are hyoscyamine, its more stable racemate atropine, and hyoscine. The compounds occur as esters of tropic acid with tropine (tropan-3α-ol).

Tropine   Tropic acid

HYOSCYAMUS LEAF

Synonyms : Insane root; Hog's bean; Poison tobacco; Black Henbane; Henbane; Hyoscyamus herb; Khurasani-ajvayan (Hindi); Folia Hyoscyamus; Kurasani-Yomam (Tamil); Kurashanivaman (Telgu).

Official Source : Hyoscyamus leaf consists of the dried leaves and flowering tops of *Hyoscyamus niger* Linn. containing not less than 0.05% alkaloids calculated as hyoscyamine. Egyptian henbane *(H. muticus* L.) contains about 0.5% alkaloids.

Family : Solanaceae.

Geographical Source : Hyoscyamus is cultivated in England, U.S.A, Germany, Poland, Russia and in India from Kashmir to Garhwal.

Characters : Hyoscyamus is an erect, hairy, viscid, biennial or annual herb found widely. The biennial plant has the following characteristics; stem up to 1-5 m high, leaves sessile, ovate-oblong to triangular-ovate, stalked, up to 20 cm long, margin dentate or pinnatifid, very hairy, flowers (May-June), corolla yellowish with deep purple veins. The stem of annual species is robust up to 0.5 m in height, leaves-sessile, smaller with fewer hairs than the biennial variety with less incised margin. Flowers (July-August), corolla funnel-shaped, pale in colour with less deeply veined. Drug is collected from biennial herb.

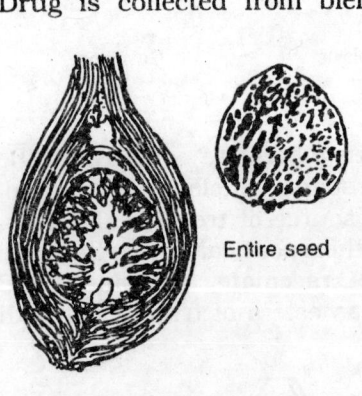

Entire seed

Vertical section of fruit and seed

Fig. 13.2. Areca nut

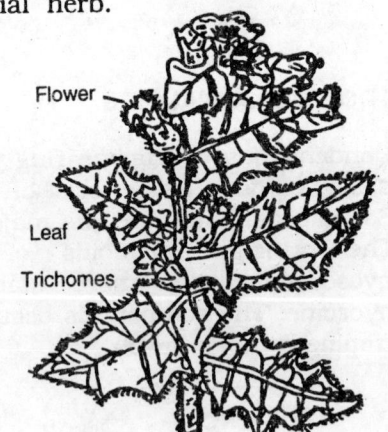

Flower

Leaf

Trichomes

Fig. 13.3. *Hyoscyamus niger*

Cultivation : The Henbane is grown by sowing seeds in June or July. The germination of seeds is slow and often erratic.

In the first year the stem is very short, leaves are in a rosette and hairy. The plant is sprayed with an insecticide if attacked by the potato beetle. The leaves and flowering tops are collected and dried rapidly at 40-50°C.

Morphology : The leaves are usually broken, crumpled, sessile, oblong to ovate, colour greyish-green, very flat broad midrib with lateral veins forming acute angles, hairy. Crowded flowers, about 2 cm long, with 4 mm long pedicel. Fruits are small, 1.5 cm long, ovoid, oblong, contain numerous dark grey-coloured flat and reniform seeds. Taste of the herb is bitter.

Chemical Constituents : Hyoscyamus contains tropane alkaloids (0.045-0.14%). l-Hyoscyamine (atropine) and hyoscine (scopolamine) are the predominent alkaloids. The petioles contain more alkaloid than the lamina and stem. During isolation optical activity of hyoscyamine is lost and racemic mixture of atropine is obtained which contains a mixture of d-and l-hyoscyamine. Hyoscipicrin and choline are also present. The alkaloid content of seeds is less than that of the leaves.

| Hyoscyamine or atropine | Hyoscine or scopolamine |

Uses : Hyoscyamus is smooth muscle relaxant, sedative, narcotic, anodyne, antiseptic, mydriatic and purgative agent and used in asthma and whooping cough. Atropine has stimulant action on the central nervous system. Atropine and hyoscine are used as ophthalmintic to dilate the pupil of the eye. The parasympatholytic action of Hyoscyamus is weaker than Stramonium and Belladonna.

Allied Drugs : *H. muticus* Linn (Egyptian Henbane) is a perennial herb allied to *H. niger*, distributed in the sandy parts of Egypt. It differs from Hyoscyamus obtained from *H. niger* by its striated cuticle and usually branched trichomes with unicellular heads. It contains a higher percentage of total alkaloids than *H. niger*. The leaves of *H. muticus* are smoked in Africa and India for inducing intoxication.

H. albus is a herb with white flowers, found in the Mediterranean region. Its properties are similar to those of official Henbane, for which it is often substituted.

H. pusillus, a herb occurring in Ladakh, has been reported to be poisonous.

BELLADONNA

Synonyms : Belladonna herb; Belladonna leaf; Deadly night shade leaves; Banewort; Death's herb, Dwale; Poison black cherry; Folia belladonnae.

Official Source : Belladonna consists of the dried leaves and flowering tops of *Atropa belladonna* Linn. (European Belladonna) containing about 0.3% of total alkaloids calculated as hyoscyamine.

Family : Solanaceae.

Location : *Atropa belladonna* is cultivated in U.S.A., Canada, U.K., Germany and India.

Plant : The plant is an erect, glandular-pubescent or near glabrous, perennial herb, about 1.5 meter high. Leaves on the upper part are in pairs of two, among which one leaf is larger and the other smaller.

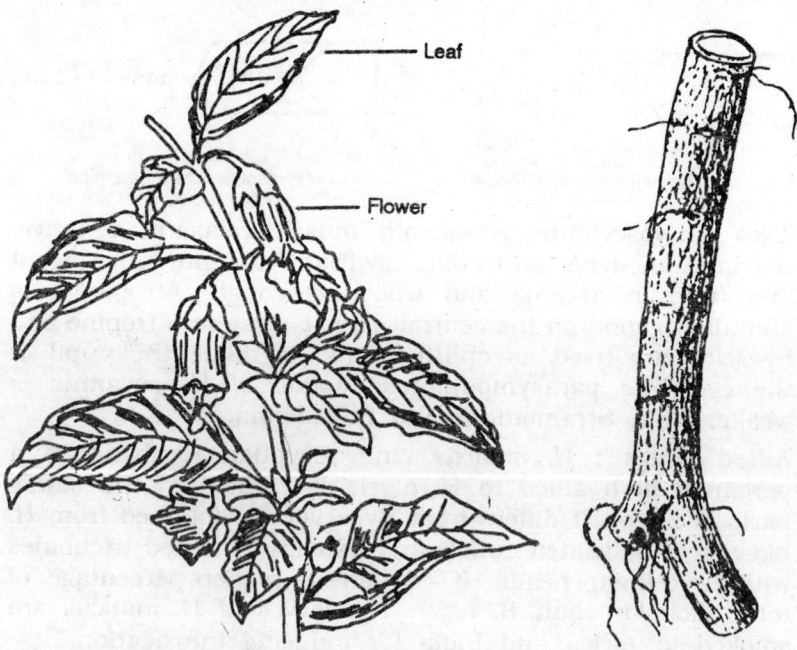

Fig. 13.4. Belladonna flowering and fruiting shoot

Fig. 13.5 Belladona root

Cultivation and Collection : Plants are cultivated by sowing seeds in nurseries and seedlings are transplanted in April to moist, calcareous and loamy soil. Weeds are removed and manure is applied for proper growth of the crop. During flowering session leaves and flowering tops are cut at least three times in a year at an interval of two months from one to three years old plants. When the plant is four years old, roots are dug out. The collected drug is dried at 40-50°C. Undried leaves deteriorate and give off ammonia. Belladonna plant infected with the fungus *Phytopthora belladonnae* should be destroyed to prevent further infection. Sometimes the leaves are damaged by flea-bettle insect and the roots by a fungus.

Morphology : The drug contains leaves, smaller stems of about 5 mm diameter, flowers and fruits. Leaves are stalked, brittle, thin, entire, long-pointed, 5-25 long, 2.5-12 cm wide, ovate lanceolate, slightly decurrent lamina, margine entire, apex acuminate, colour dull-green or yellowish-green, surface glabrous, lateral veins join the mid-rib at an angle of 60°, curving upwards and are anastomose. Flowers are pale purple, tinged with yellow or green, 1.5 cm diameter, single on drooping.

Chemical Constituents : Belladonna contains 0.3-0.6 % total alkaloids, the prominent base is l-hyoscyamine. The other components are atropine, apoatropine, asparagine, choline, chrysatropic acid, volatile bases such as pyridine; atroscine, leucatropic acid; phytosterol, N-methylpyrroline, scopoletin (β-methylaesculetin), calcium oxalate, 14% acid soluble ash and 4% acid-insoluble ash. Addition of ammonia to the alcoholic solution of scopoletin shows blue florescence. This test is useful to detect Belladonna poisoning.

Uses : Belladonna is anticholinergic, narcotic, sedative, diuretic mydriatic and used as anodyne and to check secretion. Other uses are similar to Hyoscyamus. It relieves spasm of gut or respiratory tract. Consumption of Belladonna checks excessive perspiration of patients suffering from tuberculosis.

INDIAN BELLADONNA

Synonyms : Sag-angur (Hindi); Yebruti (Bengali); Girbuti (Bombay), Bantanaku (Panjabi); Mait-brand (Kashmiri).

It consists of dried leaves and other aeiral parts of *Atropa acuminata* Royle ex Lindley (Solanaecae). The plant in found in Kashmir, Shimla, Chamba, Kangra and Kulu.

The plant is a perennial herb, 2-5 ft high, erect with dichotomous branching, leaves oblong elliptical, brownish green, 7.5-13 cm long, 4-6.5 cm wide, tapering towards apex and base, flowers are yellowish brown, drooping, funnel-shaped, solitary, fruits globular berries.

As a winter annual, it is cultivated in plains in the sub-tropical climate and in hilly areas. The plant can be propagated from seeds or from cuttings of the young shoots or from fresh rootstocks. The seeds are very small, brownish black and are obtained from berries. Seeds pre-treated with sulphuric acid, ethyl alcohol or petroleum ether give better germination than the untreated ones. The seeds are sown in well prepared nursery beds during May and July. It requires a porous, slightly acidic soil rich in mineral nutrients. The seedlings are transplanted in spring. Shading the transplants with twigs is necessary. Irrigation is required during the dry summer.

Total alkaloidal contents in Himalayan plant are 0.5% in leaves. The constituents of Indian Belladonna leaves resemble those of the European species.

Uses : Indian Belladonna is used as sedative, tranquillizers, in labour, delirium tremens, toxic psychoses and maniacal states. Atropine and other Belladonna alkaloids are common constituent of proprietary medicines for the common cold and acute rhinitis. They induce bronchial dilation and give relief in bronchial asthma. They are employed in diseases of the gastro-intestinal tract, in heavy metal poisoning, Parkinsonism and in checking enurenis in children.

Belladonna preparations are reputed as local anodynes and counter irritants for external application for treating intercostal pains, rheumatism, lumbago, neuralgia and pleurisy. They are made into plasters and liniments for local application and into suppositories employed to relieve the spasm of anal fistula.

Belladonna leaves extract is used as proprietary pharmaceutical preparations to treat gastro-intestinal hypermotility, hyper-secretion, peptic ulcer, spastic constipation, spastic dysmenorrhoea, nocturnal enuresis, bronchial asthma and whooping cough.

Adulteration : The roots of *Althea officinalis* are sometimes mixed with Belladonna roots but they can be distinguished on the basis of their fracture and absence of starch in the exposed surface. *Phytolacca acinosa* grows side by side with Belladonna in nature and resembles the latter when not in flower. Its leaves are often substituted for Belladonna leaves. Its can be detected in commercial samples by its ovate leaves and hollow stem. The leaves of *Solanum nigrum* and other species of *Solanum* and *Datura* are often used as adulterants.

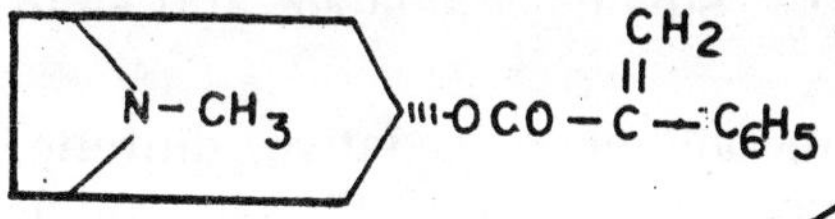

Apoatropine

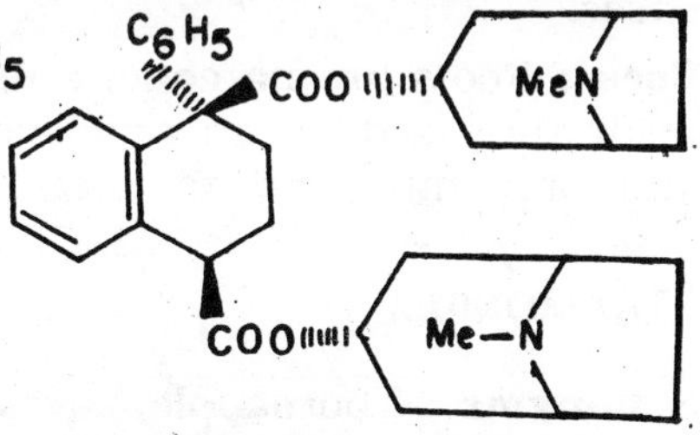

Belladonnine

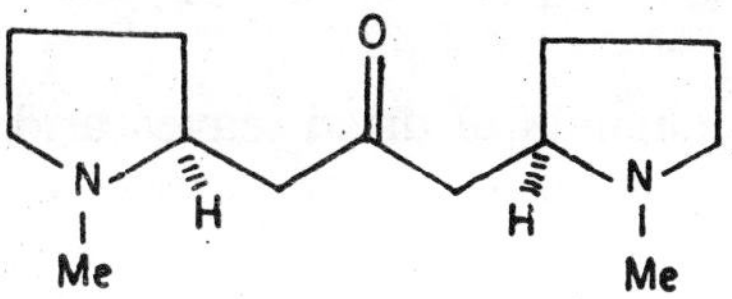

Cuscohygrine

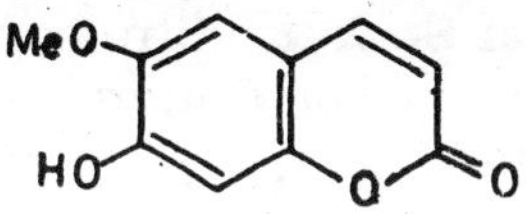

Scopoletin

BELLADONNA ROOT

Synonym : Radix belladonnae.

Biological Source : Belladonna root consists of the dried roots or rootstock of *Atropa belladonna* L. (Fam : Solanaceae).

Collection : The plant description and geographical sources are given under the heads Belladonna and Indian Belladonna. Roots of the first and second years are small in size and not collected although the percentage of alkaloid is high. The roots of three or four years old plant are collected in autumn. The roots are dug up, washed, cut into small pieces and dried at 40-50°.

Morphology : The drug occurs in small pieces or longitudinal slices, length 10-20 cm, diameter 3-4 cm; shape cylindrical and tapering; surface longitudinally wrinkled with scars of roots; fracture short; whitish or brownish interior after drying; cambium is distinct with porous xylem; colour-greenish brown; odour-distinct, taste bitter.

Chemical Constituents : Belladonna root contains 0.4 - 0.8 per cent total alkaloids. The important alkaloids isolated are hyoscyamine, atropine and scopolamine. The other chemical components obtained are apoatropine, belladonnine, cuscohygrine, and tropine along with β-methyl aesculetin, calcium oxalate and starch.

Allied Drugs : Indian Belladonna roots from *Atropa acuminata* : brownish grey roots, stolons, rootstock and stem bases.

Uses : Roots are narcotic, anticholinergic, sedative, diuretic, mydriatic used as an anodyne, local anaesthetic, in cough and bronchitis and to check perspiration of tuberculosis.

STRAMONIUM

Synonyms : Thornapple leaves; Jimson or Jamestown weed; Dhatura; Stinkweed; Devil's apple; Apple of Peru; Folia stramonii.

Biological Source : Stramonium consists of dried leaves and flowering tops of *Datura stramonium* Linn. or its variety *D. tatula* Linn.

Family : Solanaceae.

Geographical Source : Stramonium is found widely in European, Asian, and American countries and in South Africa. The plant grows commmonly in waste places throughout India from Kashmir to Malabar. It is cultivated in Germany, France, Hungary and South America.

Cultivation : Datura prefers a rich calcareous soil. It can be grown from seeds in spring in drills; the plants are later thinned to stand 3 m apart in raws. The plant is sensitive to frost and sheltered situations are preferred for cultivation. Entire plants are cut down when the fruits are mature. Nitrogen manuring, which favours the growth of plants, also favours alkaloid formation. At the end of August leaves and flowering tops are collected and dried at 45-50°C.

Plant Habitat and Morphology : *D. stramonium* is a bushy annual herb, 1.5 m high, having whitish roots and numerous rootlets. The stem is herbaceous, round, smooth, green branched, glabrous and shows dichasial branching with leaf adnation. Leaves stalked, ovate, 8-25 cm long, 7-15 wide, coarsely and irregularly lobed and toothed. Flowers are solitary, axillary, short stalk, single, white, have sweet scent, calyx tubular, 5-toothed, 5-ribbed, corolla funnel-shaped. The ripe fruits are thorny capsule about 3-4 cm long. Seeds are numerous dark brown or blackish in colour, reniform in outline, 3 mm long. The testa is reticulated and finely pitted; smell is slightly unpleasant and taste is bitter.

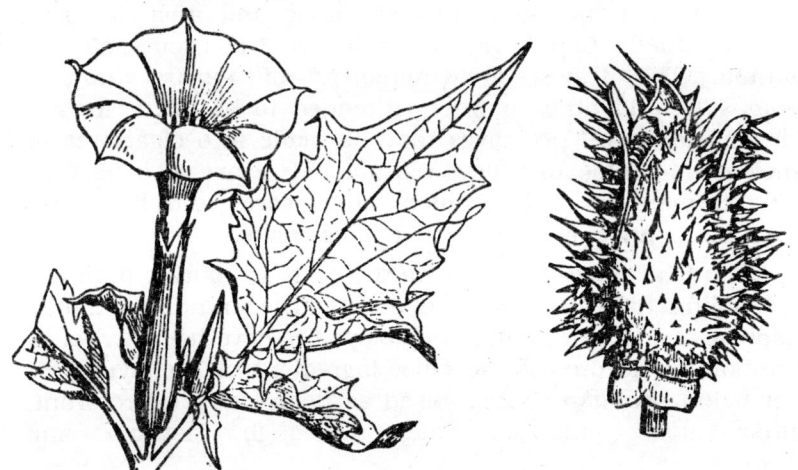

Fig. 13.6. *Datura stramonium* flowering shoot

Chemical Constituents : Stramonium contains 0.2-0.6% alkaloids. The main alkaloids are hyoscyamine and hyoscine (scopolamine). It also contains protein albumin. The Indian variety (*D. metel*) also possesses meteloidine in addition to these alkaloids. The aerial parts of *D. metel* var. *fastulosa* contains a higher percentage of total alkaloids than *D. metel*. Small amount of atropine has been reported in Stramonium. The seeds contain about 0.2% of mydriatic alkaloids and 15-30% of fixed oil.

Ditigloyl esters of 3,6-dihydroxytropane and 3, 6, 7 trihydroxytropane have also been isolated from the roots in addition to hyoscine, hyoscyamine, tropine and pseudotropine.

$$HO \underset{HO}{\overset{}{\boxed{}}} N\text{-}CH_3 \quad\rangle\!- OCO - \overset{\overset{CH_3}{|}}{C} = CH - CH_3$$

Meteloidine

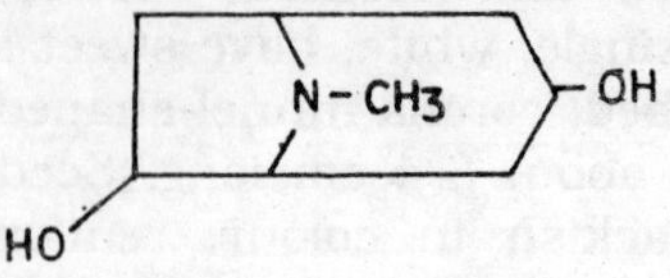

3,6- Dihydroxytropane 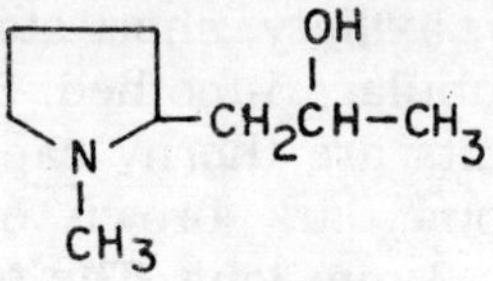   Hygroline

Uses : It is a narcotic, anti-spasmodic and anodyne, and is used chiefly to relieve the spasm of the bronchioles in asthma. The leaves are ingredient of *Pulvis stramonii compositus* and other powders intended to be burnt for the relief of asthma. The leaves may be made into cigarettes or smoked in a pipe to relieve asthma. They are also used in the treatment of parkinsonism, boils, sores and fish-bites. The flower juice is used to treat ear-ache.

The fruit juice is applied to the scalp for curing dandruff and falling hair. Stramonium ointment, containing lanolin, yellow wax and petroleum, is employed to cure haemorrhoids. Stramonium is one of the chief ingredient of the Ayurvedic prepartion, *Kanaka asaves*, used as demulcent, expectorant, antispasmodic and anodyne in cough, asthma and phthisis.

Atropine and hyoscine are used to dilate the pupil of the eye. The leaves are antispasmodic, anodyne, narcotic and applied to boils, sores and fish bites.

Adulterants : The leaves of *Datura innoxia* and *D. metel* are used as substitutes for Stramonium. The leaves of *Xanthium strumarium*, *Carthamus helenioides* and *Chenopodium hybridum* are used as adulterants.

WITHANIA (ASHWAGANDHA)

Synonyms : Ashwagandha; Withania root.

Biological Source : Withania consists of the dried roots of *Withania somnifera* Dunal.

Family : Solanaceae.

Geographical Source : Withania is widely distributed from southern Europe to Africa. In India it in found widely in the drier parts ascending to 1800

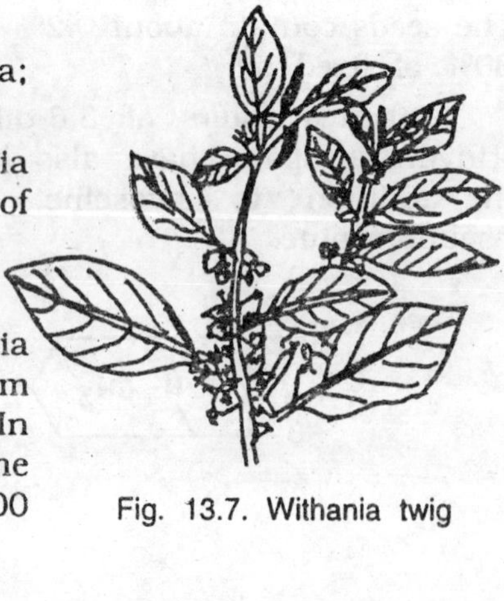

Fig. 13.7. Withania twig

meters in the Himalayas and cultivated in Neemuch near Ajmer and in Manasa (M.P.).

Plant Habitat and Macroscopy

The plant is tomentose, evergreen, perennial, branched, erect shrub. The tuberous roots are cut into small pieces and used. The roots are straight, unbianched, conical and 5-12 mm thick. The outer surface is longitudinally wrinkled and buff to greyish yellow. On the crown 2-6 stem bases are present. Taste is mucilaginous and bitter.

The plant is cultivated in soils that are unsuited for other crops. Seeds are sown broadcast in the nursery just before the onset of rainy season. Nitrogenous fertilizers promote heavy leaf growth. The plants flower and fruit in December. The entire plant is uprooted for roots, which are separated from the aerial parts cutting. They are transversely cut into smaller pieces for drying. The pieces are dark brown with a creamy interior. They are straight, unbranched and conical. The main root bears fibre-like secondary roots. Their outer surface is buff to grey-yellow with longitudinal wrinkles. The stem bases are variously thickened, cylindrical and green and have longitudinal wrinkles. The roots have a short and uneven fracture, a strong odour and mucilaginous bitter and acrid taste.

Chemical Constituents : Withania contains alkaloids and withanolides. The important alkaloids isolated are tropine, pseudotropine, hygrine (pyrolidine derivatives), isopelletierine (piperidine derivative), cuscohygrine (two pyrrolidine moieties), anaferine (two piperidine moieties), anahygrine (one pyrrolidine moiety and one piperidine moiety), and withasomnine (phenyl 1 : 5 trimethylene pyrrazole). The plant is a source of steroidal lactones known as withanolides such as withaferin A.

Uses : Withania is considered as alterative, aphrodisiac, tonic, deobstruent, diuretic, narcotic and abortifacient. It is used in rheumatism, consumption, debility from old age, emaciation of children, asthma, bronchitis, tuberculosis, leucorrhoea, and as anti-inflammatory drug.

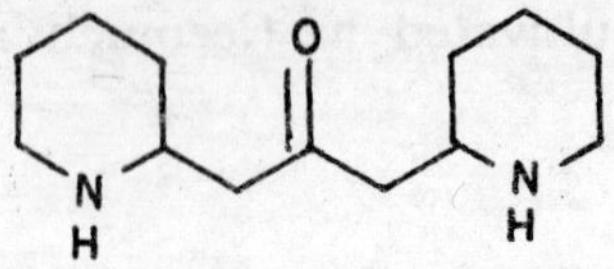

Anaferine

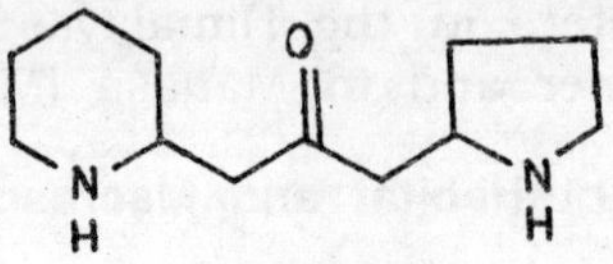

Anahygrine

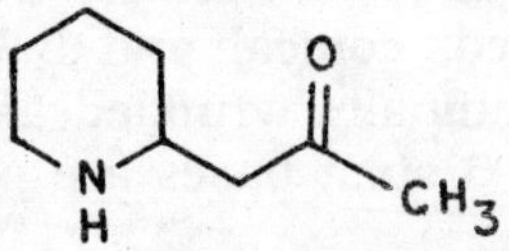

Isopelletierine

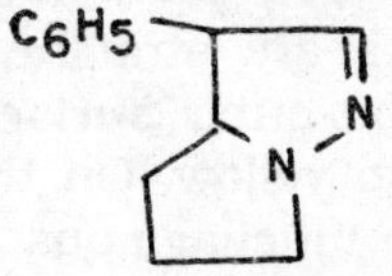

Withasomnine

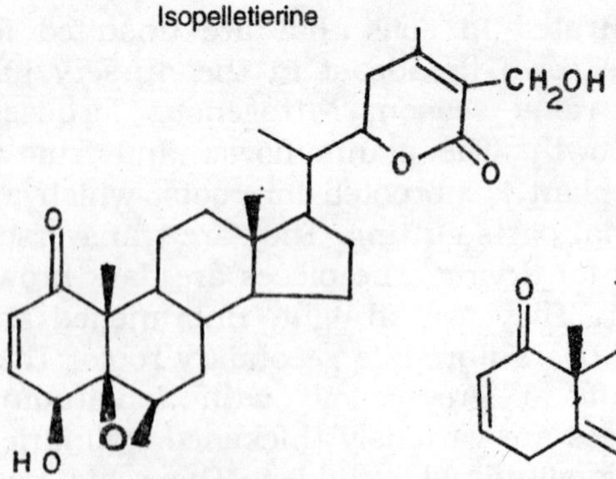

Withaferine A

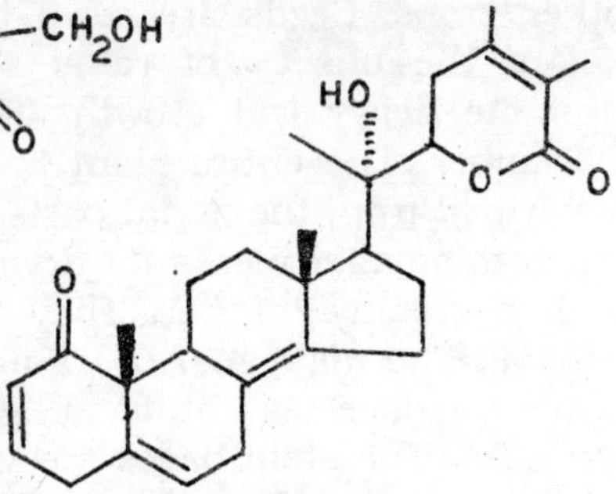

A Withanolide

COCA LEAVES

Synonyms : Coca; Huanaco coca, Truxillo coca; Java coca; Folia cocae.

Biological Source : Coca or coca leaves have been described as the dried leaves of *Erythroxylum coca* Lam (Huanaco Coca) or of *Erythroxylum truxillense* Rusby (Truxillo Coca).

Family : Erythroxylaceae.

Geographical Source : Java, Sri Lanka, Bolivia, Peru, Indonesia, and India. It is a shrub or small tree, pyramidal in shape, up to 6 m high, with dark green, ovate leaves.

Cultivation : Coca plant is grown similarly to tea-plantation. Seeds are sown in rich, light and well drained soil at an altitude of 500-2000 meters.

It requires a humid atmosphere, rainfall not below 75-80 inch and temperature between 59-68°F. It thrives best in well drained moist loams rich in humus. The plant can be propagated by cuttings, but for raising plantations, seedlings are raised in nurseries and transplanted. The first crop of leaves is gathered in 1-3 years after planting. Only the stiff ripe leaves, easily detached, are collected. The young leaves are reported to be rich in cinnamylcocaine and this is replaced in the old leaves by cocaine or truxilline.

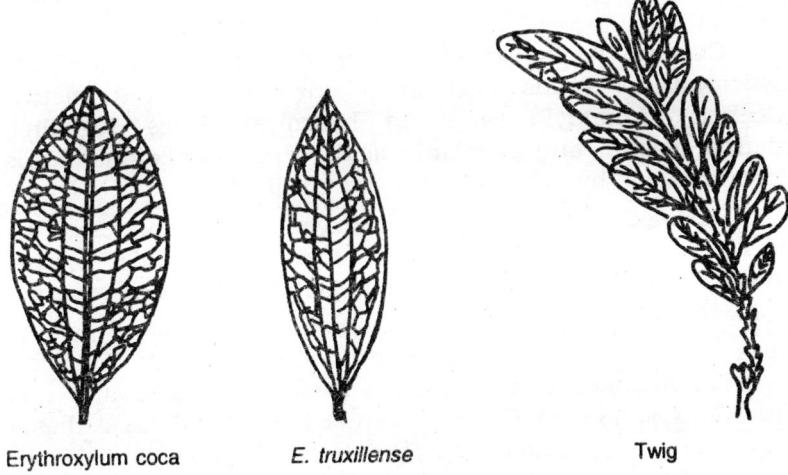

Erythroxylum coca   *E. truxillense*   Twig

Fig. 13.8. Coca leaves

Morphology

1. Huanaco or Bolivian Coca leaves are entire, 3-8 cm long, 1.5-4 cm wide, shortly petiolated, apex-acute, base tapering, lamina-brown and glabrous, margin entire, midrib prominent on the lower surface with a ridge on its upper surface, apex acute, surface-glabrous, slightly glossy, texture thin, odour-distinct, taste-bitter.

2. Truxillo or Peruvian coca are more or less broken, pale green in colour, lamina is 1.6-6 cm long, shape elliptical, margin entire, venation is identical but ridges on lower surface are conspicuous, apex acute, base tapering, surface-glabrous, not glossy, texture-thin, fragile; odour is distinct and taste is bitter.

Chemical Constituents : Coca leaves contain 0.7-1.5% of alkaloids which are of three type derivatives of :

    (i) ecgonine (cocaine, cinnamylcocaine, α-and β-truxilline)

    (ii) tropine (tropococaine, valerine) and

    (iii) hygrine (hygroline, cuscohygrine)

The alkaloidal composition varies according to the variety of the plant and stage of development of leaves.

Cocaine, cinnamylcocaine and α-truxilline are the most important alkaloids.

The constituents isolated from the leaves are simple alkaloids (hygrine, dihydrocuscohygrine), tropococaine, four yellow crystalline glycosides, cocatannic acid and essential oil.

Cocaine is the methyl ester of benzoylecgonine. On hydrolysis it yields ecgonine, benzoic acid and methyl alcohol. Cinnamyl-cocaine on hydrolysis gives ecgonine, methyl alcohol and cinnamic acid, while α-truxilline forms ecgonine, methyl alcohol and α-truxillic acid.

Besides the alkaloids, coca leaves contain an essential oil (0.06 - 0.13%), the chief constituent of which is methyl salicylate. A colouring matter, coca citrin, has been reported from the leaves.

Uses : Coca leaves are stimulant and astringent. They are used in masticatory. Cocaine is local anaesthetic and has stimulant action on C.N.S. and used in dental anaesthesia and minor local surgery of ophthalmic, ear, nose and throat.

$$CH_2 \text{——} CH \text{——} CH \text{——} COOCH_3$$
$$\quad\quad\quad\quad\quad N\text{-}CH_3 \quad\quad CH \text{—} O \text{—} CO \text{—} C_6H_5$$
$$CH_2 \text{——} CH \text{——} CH_2$$

Cocaine

Adulterants : Novocaine, boric acid, sodium carbonate and bicarbonate, lime, chalk and starch are among the adulterants of cocaine. Lactose and even quinine, have been used.

QUINOLINE ALKALOIDS

Alkaloids containing quinoline as their basic nucleus have been isolated from Cinchona, Acronychia and viridicatin. Cinchona alkaloids are the compounds of therapeutic importance.

CINCHONA BARK

Synonyms : Peruvian bark; Cinchona; Calisaya bark; Jesuit's bark; Cortex cinchonae.

Biological Source : Cinchona bark consists of dried bark of stem or of the root of *Cinchona succirubra, Cinchona calisaya, Cinchona ledgeriana* or *Cinchona officinalis* or their hybrids containing about 6.5 per cent of total alkaloids, 30-60 per cent of which are quinine-type alkaloids.

Family : Rubiaceae.

Geographical Source : Cinchona is the native of Peruvian Andes, South America. Now the plant in cultivated in Indonesia, Java, Zaire, India, Guatemala and Bolivia. In India *C. calisaya* is cultivated at elevations from 500 m - 1000 m in Sikkim and the Moyar valley in the Nilgiris. *C. officinalis* in cultivated in Ootacamund (Ooty) in the Nilgiris. *C. succirubra* is grown in the Nilgiris and Naduvattam plantation in South India, Sikkim, and in parts of Satpura range in M.P. *C. ledgeriana* is found in Bengal, on the Anamalai hills in Tinnevelly district of south India and on the Khasia and Jaintia hills.

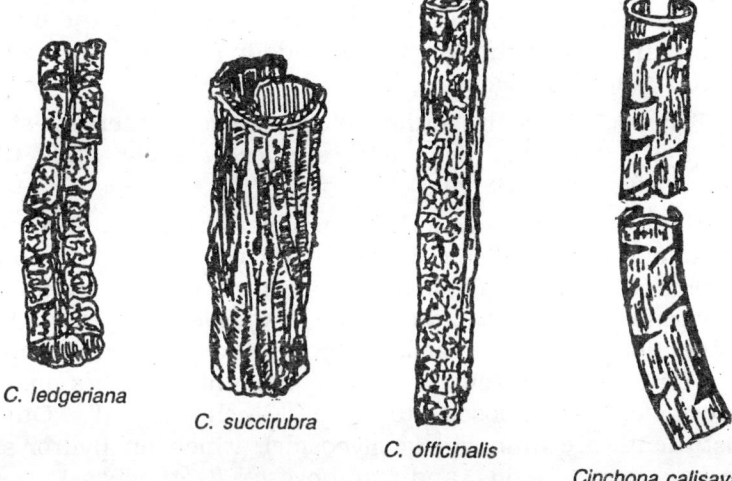

C. ledgeriana

C. succirubra

C. officinalis

Cinchona calisaya

Fig. 13.9. Cinchona bark

Cultivation : For cultivation of Cinchona the seeds are sown in tropical countries. Seedings need careful treatment and propagation to avoid diseases. The temperature should be 10-30°. A rainfall from 75" to 180" per year is required and there should be no frost. Selected stains of seedlings are transplanted at a distance of 1 meter in rich, porous and well drained soils in slopes when the plant is two years old. The plants are protected from wind by growing banana trees in between them. The hybrids of *C. ledgeriana* - *C. calisaya* produce a higher amount of alkaloids. The stems grow tall, the lower branches die and drop off and the tree crown are very close. Shade favours the higher production of quinine.

The maximum amount of alkaloid in bark is obtained when the trees are 6-9 years old. The bark of trunk and roots can be removed by hand from the uprooted plants. The young bark contains three times more alkaloids than the old trees.

General Characters : The barks of different species differ in the presence of ridges, cracks, quills and protuberances. The stem bark is curved, single or double quill. Outer rough surface contains longitudinal and transverse cracks, fissures, ridges and protuberances. Cracks and fissures are distinct for each bark. Outer surface may contain greyish patches of moss or lichen. The stem bark of *C. succirubra* is reddish-brown in colour; the other barks are yellowish to brown. Barks are usually up to 30 cm long, 1.5-2 cm in diameter and 2-8 mm thick. Inner surface is striated and reddish-brown to yellow in colour. The fracture is short in the outer part but fibrous in the inner side. Odour is slight, and taste is bitter and astringent.

The root bark is found in channelled, often twisted pieces, 2-7 cm long. The outer surface is scaly while the inner surface is striated.

Chemical Constitutents : The Cinchona bark contains about 35 alkaloids (6.5%). The cultivated bark contains 7-10% total alkaloids. The main alkaloids are quinine (70%), quinidine, cinchonine and cinchonidine. The alkaloids are present in combination with quinic acid, quinovic acid and cinchotannic acid. Cinchotannic acid is a pholobatannin and its major amount is decomposed to give 'Cinchona red'. Other constituents are quinovin (a glycoside), which on hydrolysis gives quinovic acid and quinovose (isorhodeose), red colouring oxidase, calcium oxalate and starch. *C. succirubra* and some other varieties contain more cinchonidine and cinchonine and sometimes quinidine than the cultivated variety. A white crystalline substance, cinchocerotin, is present in the bark of *C. calisaya*. A green colouring matter, tschirchin, different from chlorophyll, is present in the bark of *C. succirubra*.

Chemical Tests

1. Cinchona, slightly moistened with glacial acetic acid, on heating in a test tube gives blood-red drops on the side of the tube.

2. Cinchona bark moistened with sulphuric acid shows a blue fluorescence in U.V. light.

Uses : Cinchona bark has antimalarial, antipyretic, and analgesic properties. Quinidine is used to treat prophylaxis of cardiac arrhythmias and atrial fibrillation. The barks and all preparations of Cinchona are specially valuable in intermittent fever. They have been prescribed as tonic in dyspepsia, gastric catarrh, adynamia and convalescence from fever, as a tonic and antiperiodic; it has been used in the prophylaxis and treatment of malaria. Ten grain dose-has been given in whooping cough, hay-fever, enlargement of spleen, hemicrania and other neuralgic affections. It has also been used in small pox, septic fevers, pneumonia, acute rheumatism, tonsillitis, nasal catarrh, pyaemia, etc. As an antiseptic it has been recommended in abscesses, cavities, ulcers, as a wash and gargle in sore-throat. The indiscriminate use of quinine in continuous and large doses produces weakness of heart, restlessness and cachexia. It is a good ingredient in dentifrice. The Cinchona alkaloids cause disturbances of C.N.S. system, deliriant conditions, spasm, convulsion, and collapse. The most usual menifestations of cinchonism are abdominal pains, cholera, nostras, paralysis of limbs, regors, cold sweats, somnolence, icterus, albuminuria, fever, cyanosis, in chronic cinchonism, emaciation and cachexia. Quinine may cause blindness and deafness preceded by violent noises in the ears. It destroys the erythrocytes and causes quinine haemolysis.

Quinine (R$_1$ = OCH$_3$, R$_1$ = α-H)
Quinidine (R$_1$ = OCH$_3$, R$_2$ = β-H)
Cinchonidine (R$_1$ = H, R$_2$ = α-H)
Cinchonine (R$_1$ = H, R$_2$ = β-H)

Quinic acid

Substitutes : Barks of *Cinchona lancifolia*, (Colombian bark), *C. ovata* (Naranjada bak), *Remija pedunculata* (Cuprea bark) and *Remija purdieana* are often used as substitutes for Cinchona.

Quinovic acid (R = H)
Quinovin (R = quinovose)

Quinovose

ISOQUINOLINE ALKALOIDS

Alkaloids containing the isoquinoline structure have been isolated from Ipecac, Hydrastis, Berberis, Sanguinaria, Curare, and Opium.

IPECAC

Synonyms ; Ipecacuanha; Brazilian or Johore Ipecac; Hippo; Ipecacuanha root; Radix ipecacuanhae.

Biological Source : Ipecac consists of the dried root or rhizome of *Cephaelis ipecacuanha* (B.) A. Rich. (Rio or Brazilian Ipecac) or of *Cephaelis acuminata* Karst. (Cartagena, Nicaragua or Panama Ipecac). It should contain about 2% of ether soluble alkaloids calculated as emetine.

Family : Rubiaceae.

Geographical Source : The plant is indigenous to Brazil and also found in Colombia, Cartagena, Nicaragua, Savanilla, Malaya, Burma, Panama and west Bengal. In India it is cultivated at Mungpoo (Darjeeling), on Nilgiris near Kollar and in Sikkim.

Collection : The plant is a low, straggling shrub containing slender rhizome with annulated wiry roots.

The roots are smooth, slender and whitish when young, develop on maturation, a thick brownish bark with numerous closely placed transverse furrows.

The plant is unusually slow-growing. It thrives best in forest areas on sandy loams in humus, potash, magnesia and lime. A maximum rainfall of 90 inch is required throughout the year, a temperature between 15-40°C shaded situations are essential for successful cultivation. Temperature fluctuations should be narrow and the soil should be well drained. Propagation is by stem or root cuttings planted about a foot apart each way. Roots are harvested when the plants are about 2.5 years old and the alkaloid content exceeds 20 per cent. The plant may be dug up at any time of the year and the roots washed and dried in shade.

Morphology : The rhizome is thin, or sometimes thick and annulated. Rhio Ipecac is 5-15 cm long, 6 mm in diameter, shape is cylindrical, slightly tortuous, external surface is broadly annulated, brick red to brown in colour, the ridges are rounded and encircle the root, fracture of root is short and shows a thick, greyish bark and small dense wood. Odour is slight and taste is bitter and acrid.

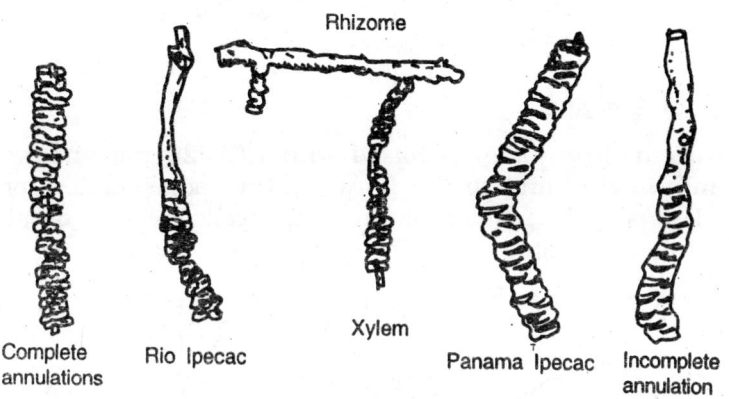

Fig. 13.10. Ipecacuanha

Cartagena Ipecac is 4-6.5 mm in diameter greyish-brown in colour, less crowded and less projecting annulations, has transverse ridges. Half of the portion contains bark.

Chemical Constituents : Ipecac contains 2-2.5% alkaloids of which 30-75% is emetine. The predominant alkaloids are emetine (40-70%), cephaeline, psychotrine, psychotrine methyl ether, protoemetine and emetamine. A crystalline glucosidal tannin, known as ipecacuanhin or ipecacuanhic acid, a neutral monoterpenoid isoquinoline glycoside (ipecoside), traces of ipecamine and hydroipecamine, malic acid, citric acid, saponins, starch, calcium oxalate and resin have also been reported from the root. Indian root contains 1.98% of total alkaloids and 1.39% emetine. The Cartagena or Nicaragua Ipecac generally contains 2.6 - 3% total alkaloids, cephaeline present to a larger extent than in Rio Ipecac. The Rio variety contain total 2% alkaloids of which about 60-75% is emetine. The Cartagena variety contains 40-50% emetine.

Emetin (R = CH₃)
Cephaeline (R = H)

Test of Emetine

Powdered drug (0.5g) is mixed with HCl (20 ml) and water (5 ml), filtered and to the filtrate (2 ml) potassium chloride (0.01) is added. If emetin is present, a yellow colour develops which on standing for 1 hour gradually changes to red.

Psychotrine (R = H)
Psychotrine methyl ether (R = CH₃)

Emetamine

Uses : Ipecac is emetic and used as an expectorant and diaphoretic and in the treatment of amoebic dysentery. The alkaloids have local irritant action.

Adulterants : The chief adulterant of the drug is the aerial stem of the plant. It can be distinguished from the root by the longitudinal striation, presence of distinct pith composed of cells with lignified walls and by the surface scars. The drug is often substituted by stem and roots of *Richardsonia scabra,* *Cryptocoryne spiralis, Psychotria emetica, Manettia ignita, Hybanthus ipecacuanha, Asclepias curassavica, Anodendron paniculatum, Calotropis gigantea* and others. The powdered drug is often adulterated with almond meal.

Ipecoside

HYDRASTIS

Synonyms : Golden seal; Yellow Root; Orange root; Yellow puccoon; Indian Turmeric; Hydrastis rhizome; Rhizoma hydrastis.

Hydrastine

Biological Source : Hydrastis consists of the dried rhizome and roots of *Hydrastis canadensis* Linn. containing not less than 2.5% ether soluble alkaloids.

Family : Berberidaceae or Ranunculaceae.

Canadine

Geographical Source : Canada, eastern USA and Europe.

Characters : The plant propagates from rhizome buds. In autumn the terminal buds are replanted. The

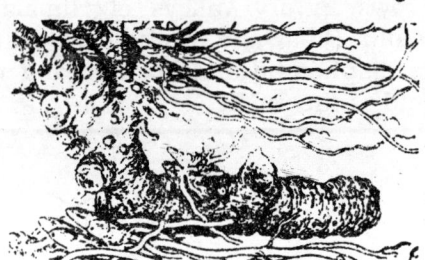

Fig. 13.11 : Hydrastis

rhizomes are cylindrical, 1-5 cm long and 2-10 mm in diameter. They possess numerous, short branches, which terminate in cup-shaped scars and bear encircling

cataphyllary leaves. Scale leaves are present on the rhizome.
The outer surface of rhizome is yellowish-brown or greyish
brown. The roots originate on the ventral and lateral surface,
are long and wiry. The fracture of the drug is short and waxy.
The odour is slight and distinct and taste in bitter.

Chemical Constituents : Hydrastis possesses the alkaloids
hydrastine, (1.5-4%), berberine (0.5-6.0%) and canadine;
some volatile oil and resin.

Uses : Hydrastis is used as astringent in inflammation of
the mucous membrane to check uterine haemorrhage and
in the treatment of caterrhal conditions of the genito-urinary
tract.

BERBERIS

Synonyms : Oregon Grape Root; Berberis aquifolium; Indian
or Nepal or Ophthalmic burberry; Tree-Turmeric; Holly-leaved
burberry; Mountain grape.

Biological Source : Berberis consists of dried rhizome and
roots of *Mahonia* species chiefly from *Mahonia aquifolium*
Nuttall (Family : Berberidaceae).

Geographical Source : Rocky mountains of British Columbia,
U.S.A.

The plants are law trailing shrubs. The chief chemical
constituents of Berberis are berberine, oxycanthine, and
berbamine which is an isomer of oxycanthine.

The root bark of *Berberis vulgaris* Linn. found in U.S.A.,
B. asiatica Roxb ex. DC of Himalayan region and *B. aristata*
DC of India are similarly used as *Mahonia* species. *B. asiatica*
grows in dry valleys of Himalayas in Bhutan, Gharhwal,
Kullu, Bihar and on the Parasnath Hill, Afghanistan. Its stem
is diaphoretic and laxative and the roots are used as tonic
and antiperiodic.

Palmatine (R = CH₃)
Jatrorrhizine (R = H)

Berberine

B. *lycium* Royle grows in dry hot places of western Himalayas. From the roots of B. *asiatica* berberine, palmatine, jatrorrhizine, columbamine, tetrahydropalmatine, berbamine, oxyberberine, and oxycanthine have been isolated. Berberine and palmitine occur as chlorides. B. *lycium*, a good source of berberine, contains all these compounds in addition to berberine acetone complex.

Uses : Roots of *Berberis lycium* has antipyretic, febrifuge, carminative, aperient, anticancer and antiprotozoal properties. They are used in eye diseases, piles, diarrhoea and menorrhagia. Berberine has anti-inflammatory activity and is effective in intestinal and hepatic amoebiasis, in cholera and for controlling gastroentritis.

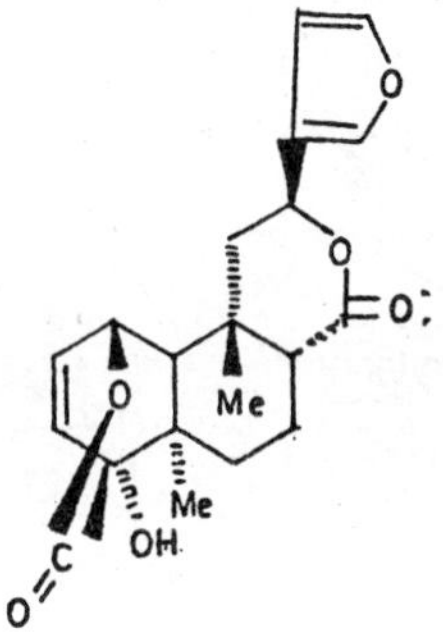

Columbin

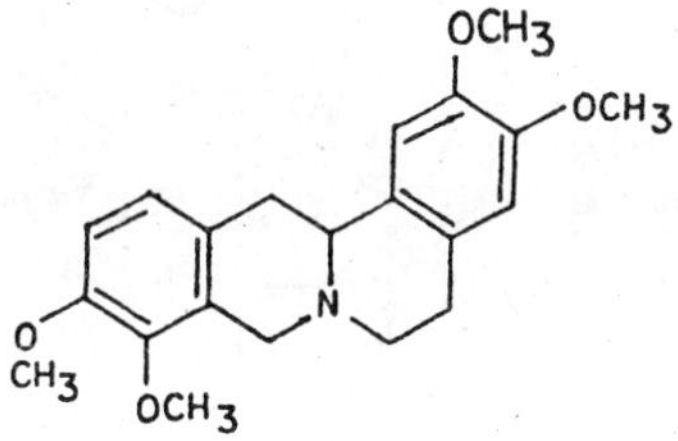

Tetrahydropalmatine

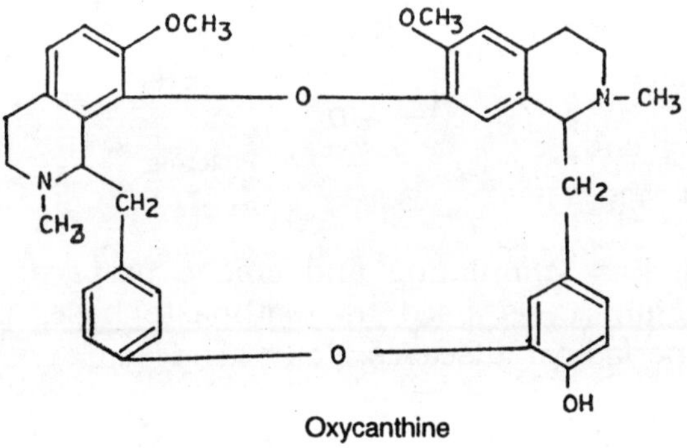

Oxycanthine

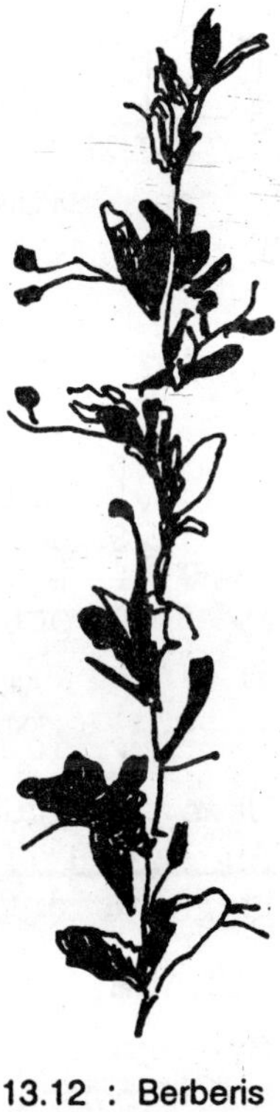

Fig. 13.12 : Berberis

SANGUINARIA

Synonyms : Blood root; Red puccoon; Ped root; Puccoon root; Tetterwort; Rhizoma sanguinariae.

Biological Source : Sanguinaria consists of dried rhizome of *Sanguinaria canadensis* Linn. (Fam. Papaveraceae).

The plant is found in Canada. It is a low perennial herb with horizontal branching rhizome.

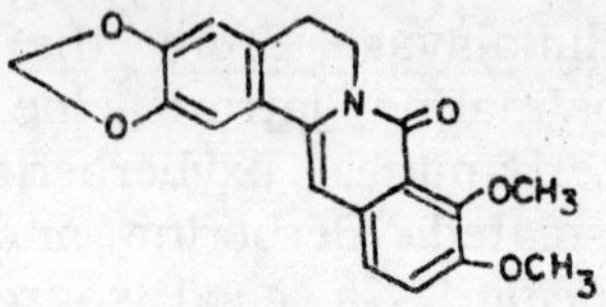

Chemical Constituents : Alkaloids of protopine series have been isolated from Sanguinaria in addition to sanguinarine (1%), chelerythrine, protopine, allocryptopine, homochelidonine and resin.

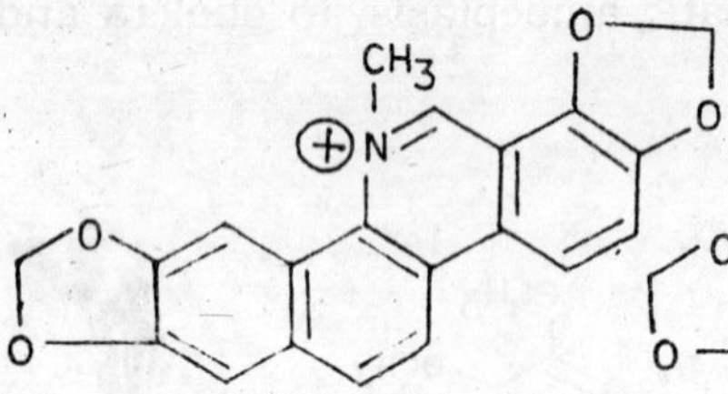

Oxyberberine

Sanguinarine

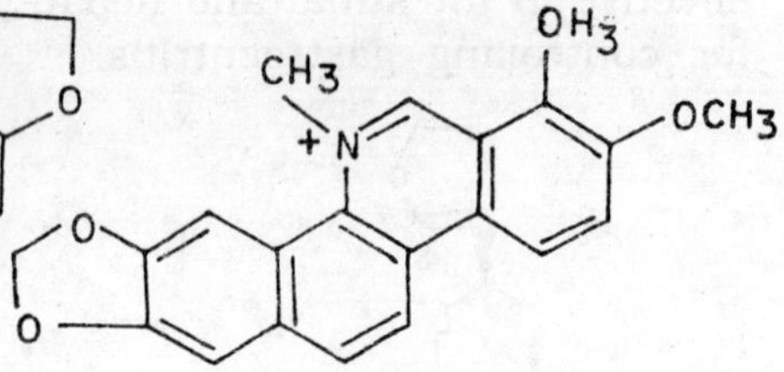

Chelerythrine

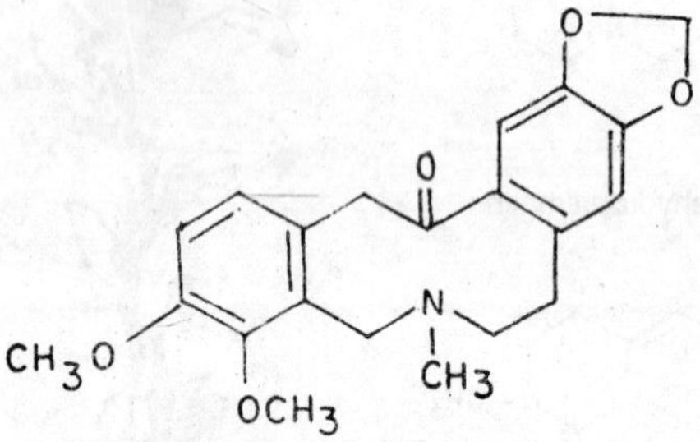

Allocryptopine
(β-Homochelidonnine)

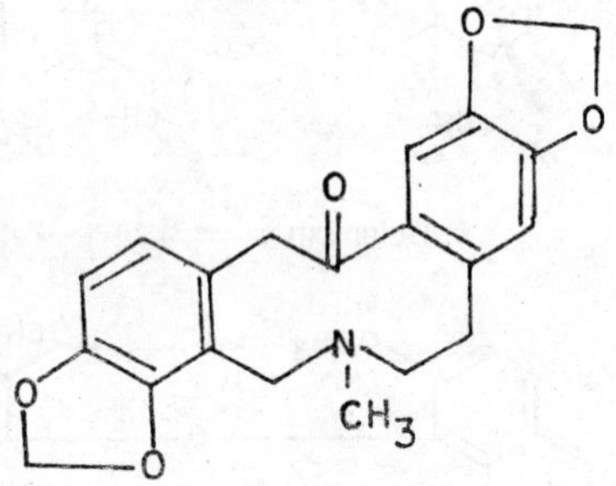

Protopine

Uses : Sanguinaria has stimulating and emetic properties. An extract of Sanguinaria is used as toothpaste base, in gingivatis and in periodical diseases.

CURARE

Synonyms : Ourari; Urari; Woorari; Woorali, South American arrow poison; Wourara.

Biological Source : Curare is a crude dried extract from the bark and stems of *Strychnos castelnaei*, Wedd., *S. toxifera*, Benth., *S. crevauxii* G. Planchon, *S. jobertiana* (Family. Loganiaceae) and from *Chondodendron tomentosum* Ruiz et Pavon and *C. microphylla.* (Fam. Menispermaceae).

The plants generally occur in Southern America.

Chemical Constituents : The drug contains several alkaloids and quaternary compounds. The most important constituent is d-tubocurarine which is a quaternary compound of *bis* benzylisoquinoline structure. *C. microphylla* possesses non quaternary base (+) - bebeerine while (-) - bebeerine has been isolated from *C. tomentosum*. Menispermaceous curare has (+) - tubocurarine, (+) - isochondrodendrine, isochondrodendrine dimethyl ether, curine (bebeerine), and (+) - chondrocurine.

Loganiaceous curare contains 12 crystalline quaternary alkaloids, the toxiferines I-XII.

Bebeerine   Tubocurarine chloride

Uses : Curare is used as a source of alkaloids. Tubocurarine chloride has muscular relaxation in surgery and is used to control convulsions of strychnine poisoning and of tetanus.

OPIUM

Synonyms : Crude Opium; Raw Opium; Gum Opium; Afim; Post.

Biological Source : Opium is the air dried milky latex obtained by incision from the unripe capsules of *Papaver somniferum* Linn. or its variety *P. album* Decand. It contains not less than 2.5 per cent of morphine in its moist conditions as anhydrous morphine.

Family : Papaveraceae.

Geographical Source : Turkey, Russia, Yugoslavia, Tasmania, India, Pakistan, Iran, Afghanistan, China, Burma, Thailand, Laos, etc. In India Opium is cultivated in M.P. (Neemuch) and U.P.

Plant Habit : The opium is an annual herb. The flowers are large, regular, terminal, solitary, white to pink in colour. It contains about eight capsules. Laticiferous vessels are found in all aerial parts which are maximum in capsule.

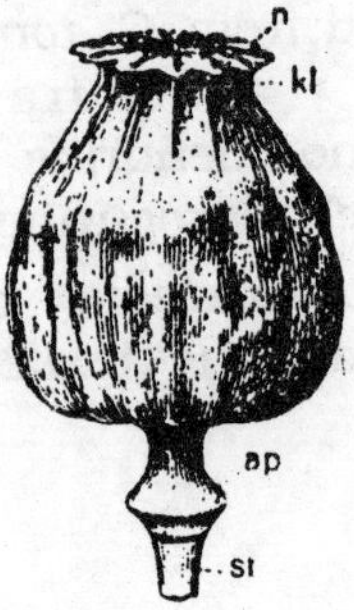

Cultivation and Collection : Opium is cultivated under licence from the government. Its seeds are sown in October or March in alluvial soil. After germination of seeds snow falls. In spring the

Fig. 13.13. *Papaver somniferum* capsule

thin plant attains the height of 15 cm. Fertilizers are used for better crop. The poppy of first crop blossoms in April or May and the capsule mature in June or July. When the capsules are about 4 cm in diameter, the colour changes from green to yellow; they are incised with a knife about 1 mm deep around the circumference between midday and evening. The incision must not penetrate into the interior of the capsule otherwise latex will be lost. The latex tubes open into one another. The latex, which is white in the beginning, immediately coagulates and turns brown. Next morning it is removed by scrapping with a knife and transferred to a poppy leaf. The dried latex is kneaded into balls, wrapped in poppy leaves and dried in shade. The principal commercial varieties of Opium are Turkish Opium, Indian Opium, Chinese Opium, Yugoslavian Opium and Persian Opium.

Characters : Opium occurs in rounded or flattened mass which is 8-15 cm in diameter and weighing from 300 g to 2 kg each. The external surface is pale or chololate-brown, texture is uniform and slightly grannular. It is plastic like when fresh and turns hard and brittle after sometime. Fragment of poppy leaves are present on the upper surface. Internal surface is coarsely granular, reddish brown, lustrous; odour is characteristic; taste is bitter and distinct.

Chemical Constituents : Opium contains about 25 alkaloids among which morphine (10-16%) is the most important base, The alkaloids are combined with meconic acid. The other alkaloids isolated from the drug are codeine (0.8-2.5%), narcotine, thebaine (0.5-2%). noscapine (4-8%), narceine, and papaverine (0.5-2.5%). Morphine contains a phenanthrene nucleus. The different type of alkaloids isolated are :

    (i) **Morphine Type** : Morphine, codeine, neopine, pseudo-or oxymorphine, thebaine and porphyroxine.

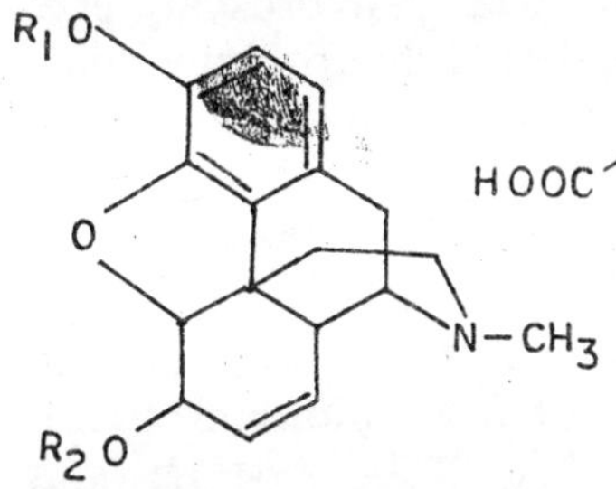

Meconic acid

Morphine ($R_1 = R_2 = H$)
Codeine ($R_1 = CH_3$, $R_2 = H$)

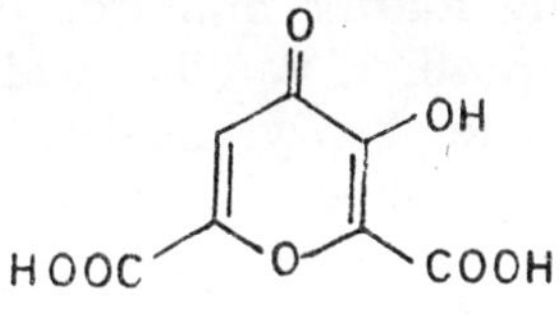

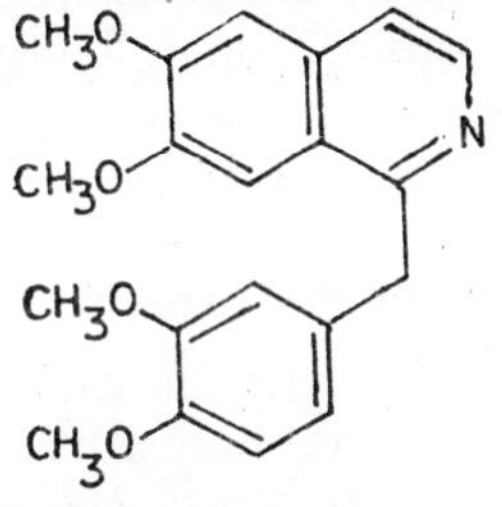

Papaverine

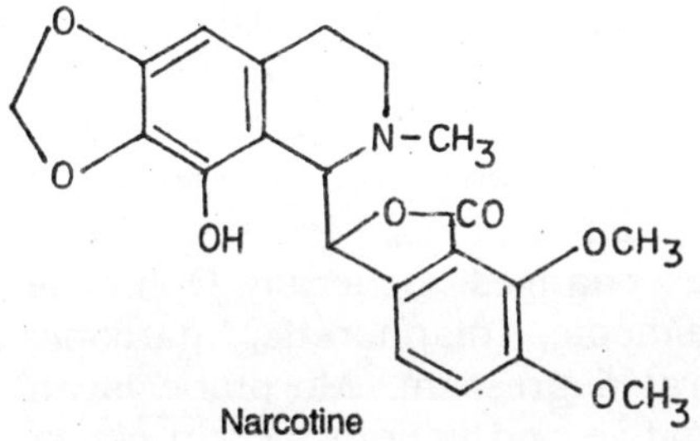

Narcotine

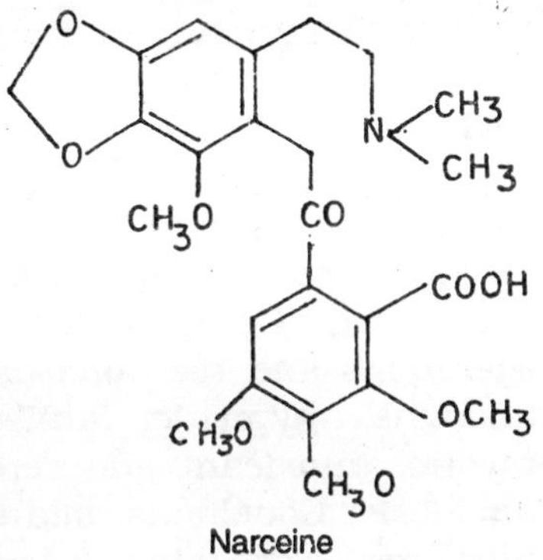

Narceine

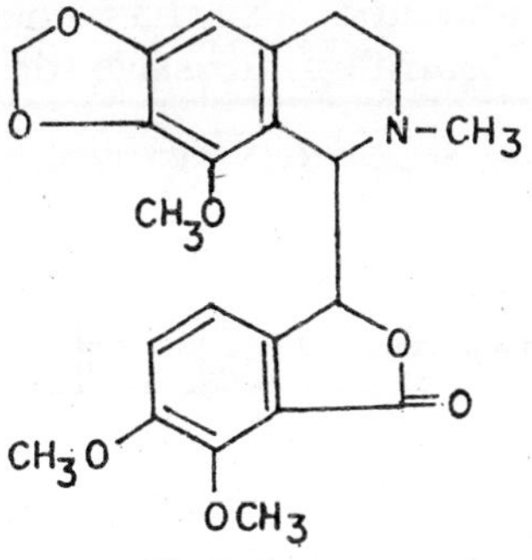

Noscapine

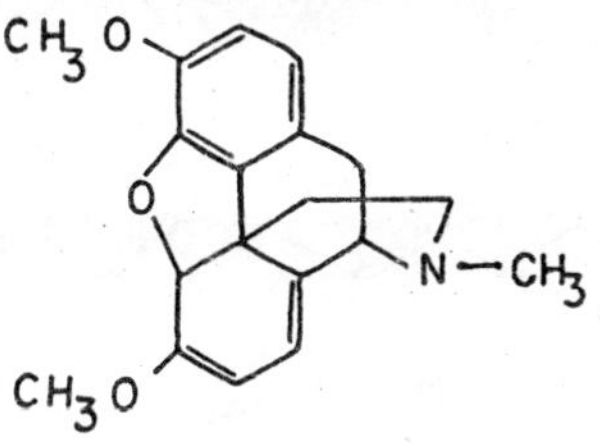

Thebaine

(ii) **Phthalide Isoquinoline Type** : Hydrocotarnine, narcotoline, l-narcotine, noscapine, oxynarcotine, and narceine.

(iii) **Benzyl Isoquinoline Type** : Papaverine, xanthaline, dl-laudanine, laudanidine, codamine and laudanosine.

(iv) **Cryptopine Type** : Protopine, cryptopine

(v) **Unknown Constituents** : Aporeine, rhodeadine, meconidine, papaveramine and lanthopine.

The drug also contains sugars, sulphates, albuminous compounds, colouring matter and moisture. In addition to these anisaldehyde, vanillin, vanillic acid, p-hydroxystyrene, fumaric acid, lactic acid, benzyl alcohol, 2-hydroxycinchonic acid, phthalic acid, hemipinic acid, meconin and an odorous compound have also been reported.

Chemical Tests

1. Aqueous extract of Opium with $FeCl_3$ solution gives deep reddish purple colour which persists on addition of HCl.

2. Morphine gives dark violet colour with conc. H_2SO_4 and HCHO.

Uses : Opium and morphine have narcotic, analgesic and sedative action and used to relieve pain, diarrhoea, dysentery and cough. Poppy capsules are astringent, somniferous, soporific, sedative and narcotic and used as anodyne and emollient. Opium is first stimulant, then narcotic, anodyne, antispasmodic, aphrodisiac, astringent and myotic. As astringent, Opium checks haemorrhages, lessens bodily secretions and restrains tissue changes. Generally Opium is anodyne, hypnotic, antispasmodic, diaphoretic, narcotic, myotic, intoxicant and cerebral depressant. Morphine is an analgesic. Codeine is mild sedative and is employed in cough mixtures. Noscapine is not narcotic and also has cough suppressant action acting as a central antitussive drug.

2-Hydroxycinchonic acid

Hemipinic acid

Meconine

Papaverine has smooth muscle relaxant action and is used to cure muscular spasms. Opium, morphine and the diacetyl derivative heroin, cause drug addiction. Abouse leads to habituation of addiction.

INDOLE ALKALOIDS

The important alkaloids possessing indole as a part of their structures are strychnine and brucine (Nux vomica), lysergic acid and its derivatives (Ergot), physostigmine (Physostigma), reserpine (Rauwolfia) and vinblastine and vincristine (Catharanthus). The compounds usually contain two nitrogens, one is present in the indole nucleus and the second is usually two carbons apart from the β-position of the indole ring.

NUX VOMICA

Synonyms : Nux vomica seeds; Kuchla (Hindi); Quaker buttons; Bachelor's buttons; Poison nut; Dog buttons; Vomit nut; Crow fig; Semina strychni.

Biological Source : Nux vomica is the ripe, dried seed of *Strychnos nux-vomica* Linn. which should contain 1.2% of strychnine.

Family : Loganiaceae.

Geographical Source : The plant is native of the East Indies and found in the forests of Sri Lanka, Malabar coast, and northern Australia. In India it also grows in forests of Gorakhpur, Bihar, Orissa, Konkan, North Kanara, North Circars, and west of Tamil Nadu up to 1300 m.

Plant Habitat and Morphology : The plant is a small tree, 12 meters in height. The fruit, collected from November to

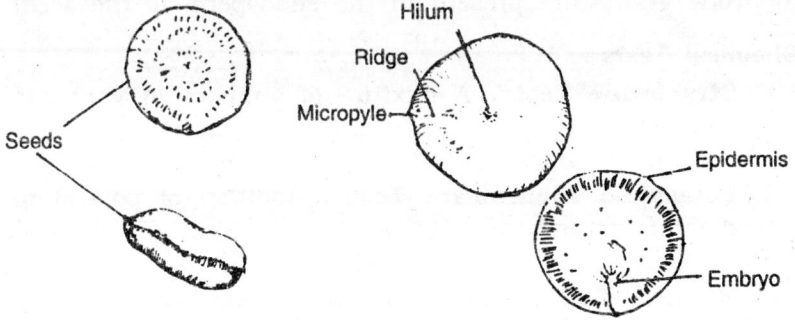

Fig. 13.14. *Strychnos nux-vomica* seeds

February by the natives, is a berry and contains 3-5 seeds which are adhered with the white and mucilaginous bitter pulp. The epicarp is separated and seeds are obtained and washed to remove adherent pulp. The dried seeds are very hard, greenish-grey in colour, disc-shaped, 10-30 mm in diameter, 4-6 mm thick, flat and some concavo-convex type. The edge is acute or rounded. Numerous silky, closely appressed, radiating hairs are present on the testa. Hilum is distinct which is present on the flattened side. From the hilum a radial ridge connects the micropyle at the circumference. A small embryo with two cordate cotyledons and a cylindrical radicle, directing towards the micropyle, is embedded in a grey, horny endosperm. A slit-like cavity is located in the centre of the seeds. The dried seeds are odourless and have a very bitter taste.

Chemical Constituents : About 1.8-5.3% of total alkaloidal base is present in Nux vomica. The main alkaloids of therapeutic importance are strychnine (1.25%) and brucine (1.5%) which are present in large thick-walled cells of endosperm. The high concentration of strychnine is present in cells near the centre of the seeds while brucine is concentrated in the outer cells near the epidermis. The other minute alkaloids present in the drug are α-colubrine, β-colubrine, icajine, 3-methoxyicajine, protostrychnine, vomicine, novacine, N-oxystrychnine, pseudostrychnine and isostrychnine. The seeds also contain chlorogenic or igasuric or caffeotannic acid (a condensation product of caffeic acid and quinic acid), loganin (a glycoside), fixed oils (3%) and proteins. Loganin is also present in the fruit pulp up to 5% along with secologanin. Hemicellulose consisting of mannan and galactan is present in the thick cell wall of endosperm. Aleurone grains are present in the endosperm of the seed.

Chemical Tests

1. **Strychnine Test :** A mixture of ammonium vanadate and sulphuric acid on addition to strychnine or a thick section of endosperm gives purple colour.

2. **Potassium Dichromate Test :** Addition of potassium dichromate and conc. H_2SO_4 with strychnine forms violet colour.

3. **Brucine Test :** Addition of conc. HNO_3 to brucine or thick section of endosperm produces yellow to orange colour.   •

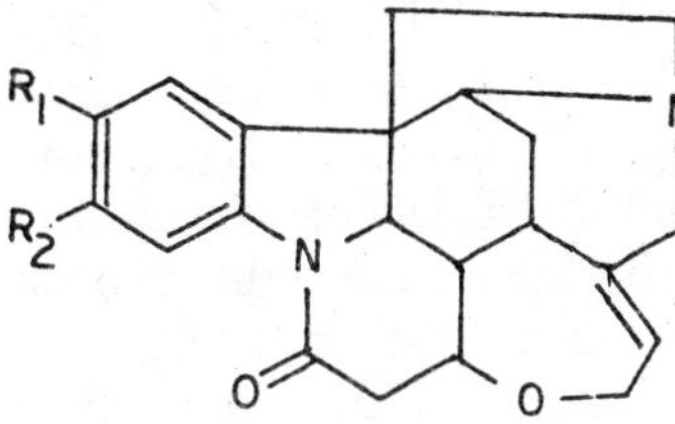

Strychnine, $R_1 = R_2 = H$
Brucine $R_1 = R_2 = OCH_3$
α-Colubrine, $R_1 = H, R_2 = OCH_3$
β-Colubrine, $R_1 = OCH_3, R_2 = H$

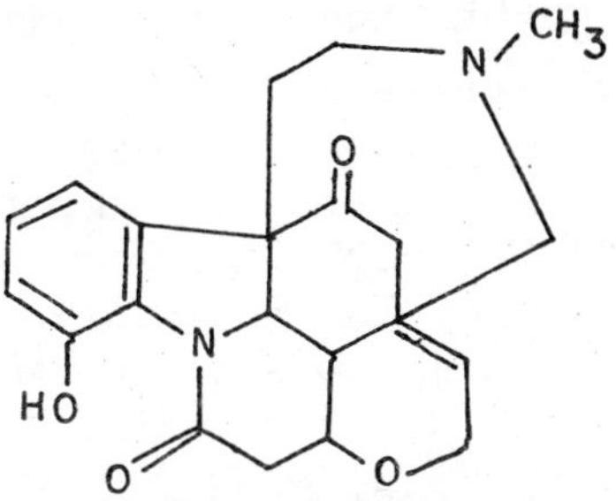

Vomicine

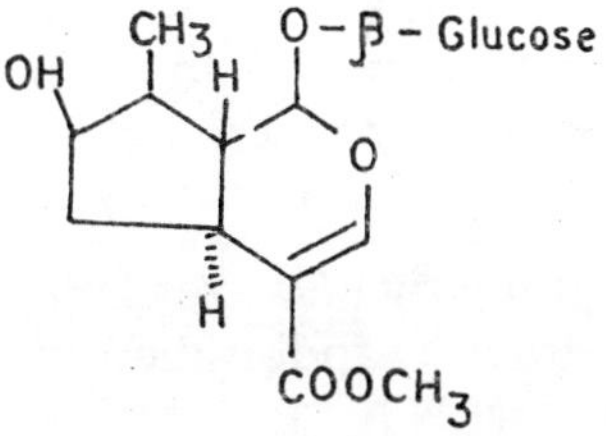

Loganin

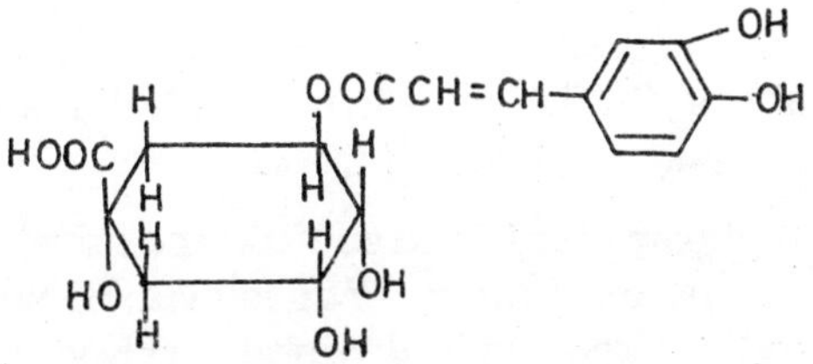

Chlorogenic acid
(Caffetannic acid)

4. **Hemicellulose Test** : When iodine and H_2SO_4 are added to a thick section, the cell walls are stained blue.

5. **Biological Test** : Strychnine (2/1000 mg) when injected to a tail of a mouse (2 weeks old), then palpitation of the tail takes place.

Uses : Strychnine is used as circulatory stimulant and bitter tonic. Nux vomica increases the tone of intestine. It is given in atonic dyspepsia, as nervine and sex tonic, circulatory stimulant in surgical shock, alcohol poisoning and as vermine killer. Strychnine improves the appetite and digestion. It is a powerful poison in large doses, producing tetanic convulsions and death.

Allied Drugs : *Ignatius beans* are dried ripe seeds of *Strychnos ignatii* Bergius (Family-Loganiaceae). The plant is found in Philippines and Vietnam. The fruits are larger than those of Nux vomica and contain about 30 seeds. The seeds are 1.5 cm long, ovoid and dark grey. They possess irregularly arranged greyish hairs. The seeds contain 2.5-3% of total basic compounds among which strychnine is 46-62 per cent.

Ignatius beans are similarly used as Nux vomica.

Strychnos tieute : It is found in Java and contains 1.4% of strychnine and small amount to brucine. *S. ligustrina*, *S. rheedii* and *S. aculeata* contain only brucine. The seeds of *S. triplinervia* from Mexico contain 1.8% of strychnine and brucine. *S. potatorum* Linn. (India) and *S. nux-blanda* (Burma), substituted for Nux vomica, do not contain strychnine and brucine.

ERGOT

Synonyms : Ergot; Rye Ergot; Secale cornutum; Spurred rye; Ergot of rye; Ergota.

Biological Source : Ergot is the dried sclerotium of a fungus, *Claviceps purpurea* Tulasne, developing in the ovary of rye plant, *Secale cereale* (Family Gramineae). Ergot should yield about 0.15% of the total alkaloids calculated as ergotoxine.

Family : Clavicipitaceae.

Geographical Source : Czechoslovakia, Hungary , Switzerland, Germany, France, Yugoslavia, Spain, Russia and India. In India Ergot is cultivated at Kodaikanal (T.N.).

Cultivation : The life cycle of the fungus, *Claviceps purpurea*, which is a parasite, passes through the following characteristic stages :

1. Sphacelia or honeydew or asexual stage
2. Sclerotium or ascigerous or sexual stage, and
3. Ascospore stage.

1. Sphacelia or Honeydew or Asexual Stage

The rye plant becomes infected by the spores of the fungus in the spring session when flowers bloom for about one week. The spores are carried by the wind or by insects to the flowers and collected at the base of the young ovary where moisture is present. There germination of the spores takes place. A filamentous hyphae is formed which enters into the wall of the ovary by enzymatic action. A soft, white mass over the surface of ovary is formed, which is known as sphacelia. A sweet viscous yellowish liquid, known as honeydew, is secreted during the sphacelia stage which contains reducing sugars (reduce Fehling solution). From the ends of some hyphae small oval condiospores (asexual spores) are abstricted which remain suspended on honeydew. The sweet taste of honeydew attracts some insects like ants and weevils.

Insects suck the sweet liquid and carry the conidiospores to the plants and spread the fungal infection in the rye plants.

2. Sclerotium or Ascigerous or Sexual Stage

During the sphacelia stage the hyphae enter only the outer wall of the ovary. On further development they penetrate into deeper parts, feed on the ovarian tissues and replace it by a compact, dark purple hard tissue known as pseudoparenchyma. It forms the sclerotium or resting state of the fungus. During summer the sclerotium or ergot increases in size and projects on the rye, showing sphacelial remains at its apex. It is collected at this stage by hands or machine and used as a drug. Ergot is then dried to remove moisture.

3. Ascospore Stage

If Ergot is not collected, it falls on the ground. In the next spring session they produce stalked projections known as stromata which have globular heads. In the inner surface of the heads there are a large number of flask-shaped pockets known as perithecia. Each of these perithecia contains many sacs (asci) which possesses eight of the thread-like ascospores. These ascospores are carried out by insects or wind to the flowers of the rye as described in the first stage. In this way life cycle of Ergot is completed.

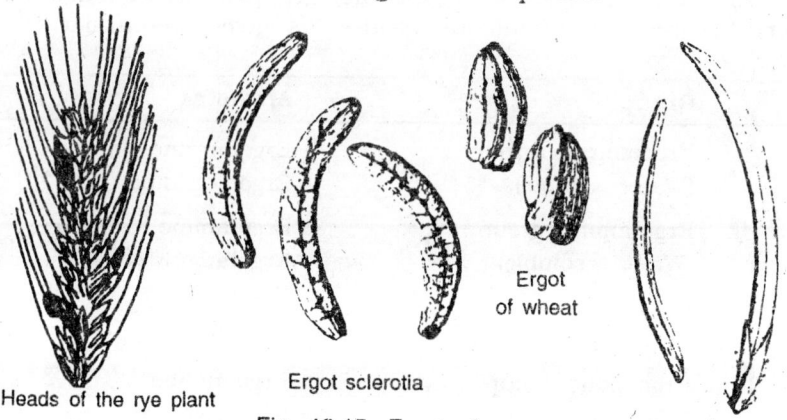

Heads of the rye plant

Ergot sclerotia

Ergot of wheat

Fig. 13.15. Ergot of rye

The ascospores may be germinated on a nutritive medium to get conidiospore-bearing cultures. The suspension of these conidiospores is usually used as a spray to infect rye plants for commercial productio.. of Ergot.

Ergot is collected from fields of rye when the sclerotia are fully developed and projecting from the spike, or they are removed from the grain by shifting. The size of the crop varies according to weather conditions.

Morphology : The size of sclerotium (Ergot) is about 1-4 cm long, 2-7 mm broad. Shape is fusiform, slightly curved, subcylindrical, tapering at both ends. The outer surface is dark or violet-black in colour, has longitudinal furrows and sometimes small transverse cracks. The fractured surface shows thin, dark outer layer a whitish or pinkish-white central zone of pseudoparenchyma in which darker lines radiate from the centre. Odour is characteristic and taste is unpleasant.

Storage : Ergot should be thoroughly dried, and the sclerotia kept entire and stored in a cool place. If the moisture content is maintained below 8 per cent, alkaloidal loss is negligible. If this figure is exceeded, deterioration is proportional to the excess moisture. The drug is liable to attack by mites and various insects, but this can be avoided by sprinkling with carbon tetrachloride.

Chemical Constituents : A large number of alkaloids have been isolated from the Ergot. The most important alkaloids are ergonovine and Ergotamine. On the basis of solubility in water the alkaloids are divided into two groups - water soluble ergometrine (or ergonovine) group or water-insoluble ergotamine and ergotoxine groups as given hereunder :

	Group	Alkaloids
I.	Ergometrine group (Water soluble)	Ergometrine Ergometrinine
II.	Ergotamine group (Water-insoluble)	Ergotamine Ergotaminine Ergosine Ergosinine
III.	Ergotoxine group (Water-insoluble)	Ergocristine Ergocristinine Ergocryptine Ergocryptinine Ergocornine Ergocorninine

Only the first group, ergometrine group, belongs to water-soluble compounds. Alkaloids of Group II and III are polypeptides in which lysergic acid or isolysergic acid is linked to amino acids. Alkaloids obtained from lysergic acid are physiologically active compounds. In the first group, e.g. ergometrine alkaloids, lysergic acid or its isomer is linked to an amino alcohol.

The other chemical components isolated from Ergot are histamine, tyramine and other amines, putrescine, cadaverine, agmatine, amino acids, acetylcholine, colouring matters, sterols like ergosterol and fungisterol, elymoclavine, sclereythrin, ergonovine, ergothioneine, clavicepsin, ergochrysin, ergoflavin, ergotic acid, histamine, choline, betaine, clavine, fat (15-30%), mannitol, lactic acid and succinic acid. The cell walls of Ergot are made up of chitinous layer in place of plant cellulose.

Chemical Tests

1. Ergot under UV light shows a red-coloured fluorescence.
2. Ergot powder is extracted with a mixture of $CHCl_3$ and sodium carbonate. The $CHCl_3$ layer is separated and a mixture of p-dimethylaminobenzaldehyde (0.1g), H_2SO_4 (35%, v/v, 100 ml) and 5% ferric chloride (1.5 ml) is added. A deep blue colour is produced.

Uses : Ergot is oxytocic, vasoconstrictor, and abortifacient and used to assist delivery and to reduce post-partum haemorrhage. Ergotamine is used to treat migraine. Lysergic acid diethylamide (LSD - 25), obtained by partial synthesis from lysergic acid is a potent specific psychotomimetic. Ergometrine is oxytocic and used in delivery. It stimulates the tone of uterine muscels and prevent postpartum haemorrhage.

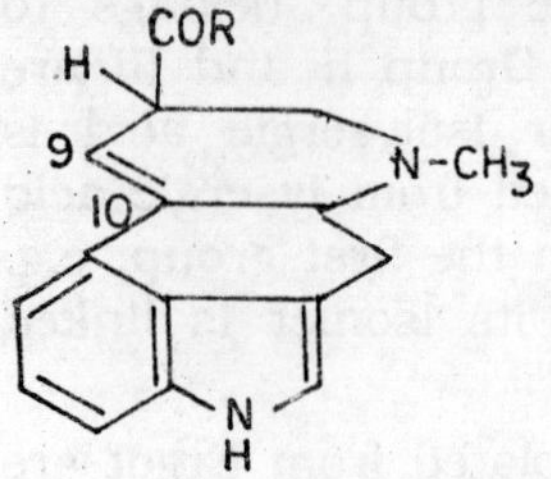

Lysergic acid, R = OH
Ergine (Lysergic acid amide), R = NH₂
Ergometrine, R = NHCH (CH₃) - CH₂OH
Methylergometrine, R = NHCH (CH₂CH₃) CH₂ OH
Ergotamine,

R=

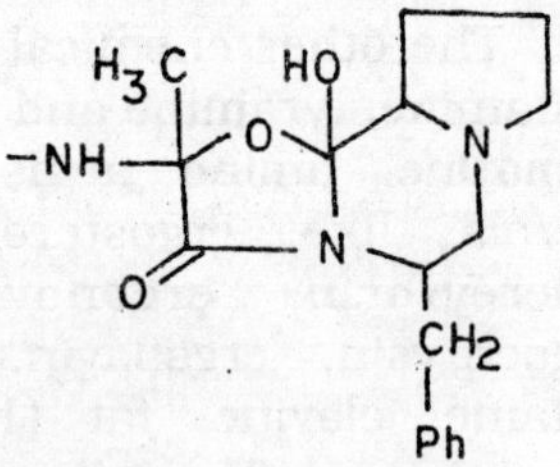

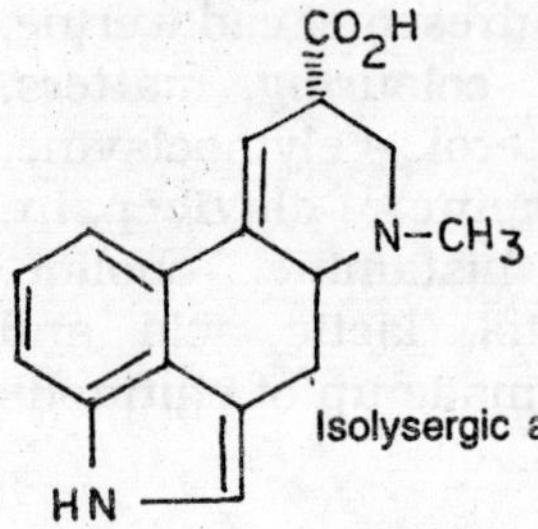

$H_2N-CH_2-CH_2CH_2-CH_2-NH_2$
Putrescine

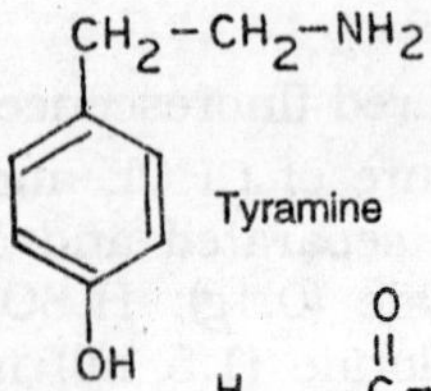

Isolysergic acid

$CH_2-CH_2-NH_2$

Tyramine

OH
$(CH_3)_3 \overset{+}{N} - CH_2 CH_2O - COCH_3$
Acetylcholine

$H_2N - (CH_2)_5 - NH_2$
Cadaverine

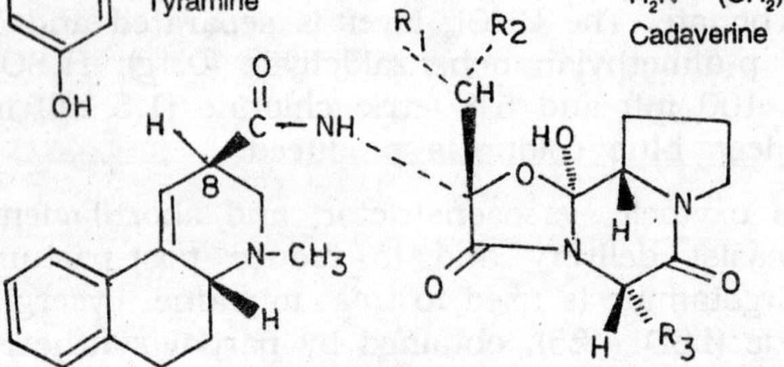

Ergosine, R₁ = R₂ = H; R₃ = CH₂ CH (CH₃)₂
Ergocornine, R = R₂ = CH₃, R₃ = CH₂ CH (CH₃)₂
Ergocristine, R₁ = R₂ = CH₃, R₃ = CH₂C₆H₅
Ergocryptine, R₁ = R₂ = CH₃, R₃ = CH₂CH (CH₃)₂

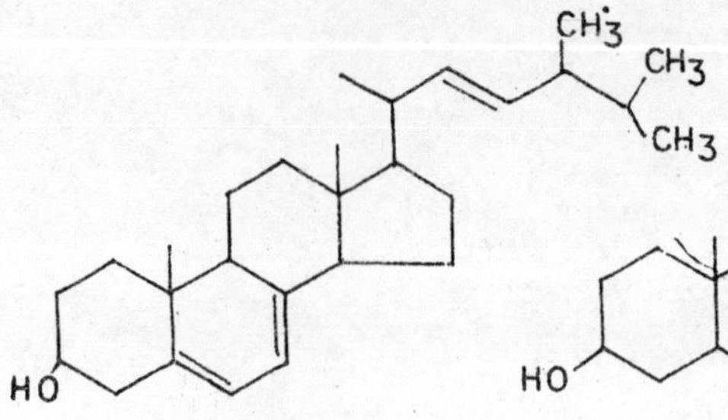

Ergosterol

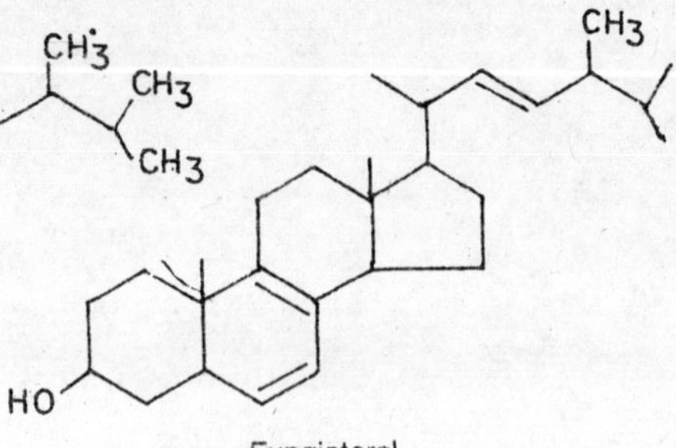

Fungisterol

$$CH_2OH$$

Elymoclavine

$$CH_2CH-COO^-$$
$$N(CH_3)_3$$

Ergothioneine

PHYSOSTIGMA

Synonyms : Calabar bean; Ordeal bean; Chop nut; Split nut; Esere nut; Semina physostigmatis.

Biological Source : Physostigma is the dried ripe seeds of *Physostigma venenosum* Balfour.

Family : Leguminosae.

It is a perennial woody climber found on the banks of streams of West Africa (near mouths of Niger and Old Calabar rivers), introduced into India and Brazil.

Characters : The plant is a perennial woody climber, bears typical papilonaceous flowers, with legumes of 15 cm length, each containing two or three seeds. The beans are flattened, reniform shape, 1.5 - 3.0 cm long, 1-1.5 cm wide and 1.5 cm thick. The seeds are very hard, dark brown testa is smooth with a grooved hilum running whole length of the convex side. Physostigma is odourless with starchy taste at first and acrid afterwards.

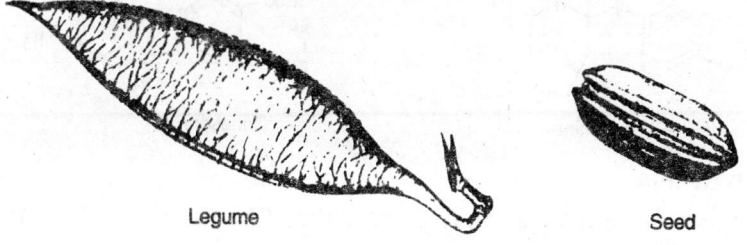

Legume   Seed

Fig. 13.16. *Physostigma venenosum*

Chemical Constituents : The seeds contain 0.15-0.3% alkoloids. Physostigmine (eserine) (0.15%), eseridine, eseramine, isophysostigmine, physovenine, geneserine, N-8-

norphysostigmine, calabatine and calabacine are the alkaloids isolated from the seeds. Exposure of the chief alkaloid, physostigmine, to heat, light or air leads to oxidation and a red compound, rubreserine, is formed. Therefore, physostigmine should be protected from air and light. Physostigmine occurs as a white, odourless, finely crystalline powder.

Uses : Physostigmine is cholinergic and miotic and used in atony of gastrointestinal tract. Its salicylate compound is used for contracting the pupil of the eye especially in mydriatics and glaucoma.

Calabar beans are odourless with starchy taste at first and acrid afterwards. The beans are extremely poisonous causing paralysis of lower limbs and death by asphyxia, and in large doses, paralysis of the heart. The poisonous principle in the seed is destroyed by boiling and scorching the seed.

Physostigmine salicylate is used in ophthalmology to reduce intraocular tension in glaucoma and to correct the dilation of the pupil. It is also used in post-operative distension and atony of the intestine or urinary bladder, and in tetanus, strychnine and atropine poisoning. It is also useful as an antispasmodic in rheumatoid arthritis, fibrositis, bruitis and in veterinary medicine for colic in horses.

Physostigmine

Physovenine

Geneserine

RAUWOLFIA

Synonyms : Sarpagandha, Chandrika; Chootachand; Indian snake-root.

Biological Source : Rauwolfia consists of dried roots of *Rauwolfia serpentina* Benth.; sometimes pieces of rhizome and aerial stem bases are attached.

Family : Apocynaceae.

Geographical Source : It is an erect, evergreen, small shrub native to the Orient and occurs from India to Sumatra. It is also found in Burma, Thailand, Philippines, Vietnam, Indonesia, Malaysia, Pakistan, and Java. In India it occurs in the sub-Himalayan tracts from Sirhind eastwards to Assam, especially in Dehradun, Siwalik range, Rohelkhand, Gorakhpur ascending to 1300 meters, east and west ghats of Tamil Nadu, in Bihar (Patna and Bhagalpur), Konkan, Kanara and Bengal.

Cultivation : Rauwolfia grows in tropical forests at an altitude of 1200-1300 meters at temperature 10-40°. There should be enough rain or irrigation for its cultivation. The soil should be acidic (pH 4-6), clayey, and manure is applied for better crop. Propagation is done by planting seeds, root-cuttings or stem-cuttings. Better drug is obtained when the propagation is carried out with fresh seeds. The plants should be protected from nematodes, fungus and *Mosaic* virus.

Collection : The drug is collected mainly from wild plants. Roots and rhizomes are dug out in October-November when the plant roots are 2-4 years old. The aerial parts and roots are separated. The roots are washed and dried in air. The roots containing moisture up to 12% should be protected from light.

Morphology : The roots and rhizomes are almost identical in external characters. The drug occurs in cylindrical or slightly tapering, tortuous pieces, 2-10 cm long, 5-22 mm in diameter. The roots are rarely branched. Rootlets, 0.5-1 mm in diameter, are rare. The outer surface is greyish-yellow, light-brown or brown. Young pieces contain slight wrinkles while old pieces have longitudinal ridges. Circular scars of rootlets are present. Bark exfoliation is present in old samples leaving

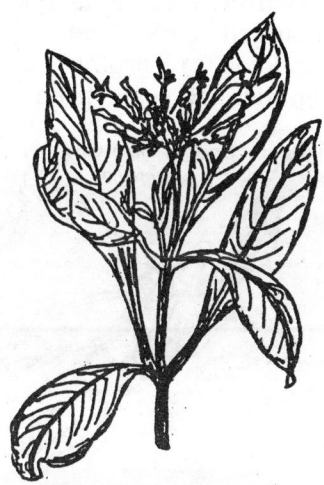

Fig. 13.17. *Rauwolfia serpentina*

behind patches of exposed wood. The fracture is short. A narrow, yellowish-brown bark and a dense pale yellow wood are present on the smooth transverse surface at both the ends. Slight odour is felt in recently dried drug which decreases with age; taste is bitter.

Chemical Constituents : Rauwolfia contains about 0.7-2.4% total alkaloidal bases from which more than 80 alkaloids have been isolated. The prominent alkaloids isolated from the drug are reserpine, rescinnamine, ψ-reserpine, rescidine, raunescine and deserpidine. The other alkaloidal components are ajmalinine, ajmaline (rauwolfine), ajmalicine (δ-yohimbine), serpentine, serpentinine, tetrahydroreserpine, raubasine, reserpinine, isoajamaline, rauwolfinine and alstonine. The other substances present are phytosterols, fatty acids, unsaturated alcohols and sugars. Raugustine and isoraunescine are the inactive alkaloids.

Uses : Rauwolfia in used as hypnotic, sedative and antihypertensive. It is specific for insanity, reduces blood pressure and cures pain due to affections of the bowels. It is employed in labours to increase uterine contractions and in certain neuropsychiatric disorders.

Allied Species : There are about 86 Rauwolfia species and most of them have been examined for reserpine and related alkaloids. *R. tetraphylla (R. canescens* Linn., *R. hirsuta)* is widely distributed in tropical areas of south America, Caribbean, India, and Australia. Its roots had been substituted for *R. serpentina.* It is recognized by its non-stratified cork, and sclereid groups in the phloem. The alkaloids reserpine and deserpidine are isolated on commercial scale from *R. tetraphylla.*

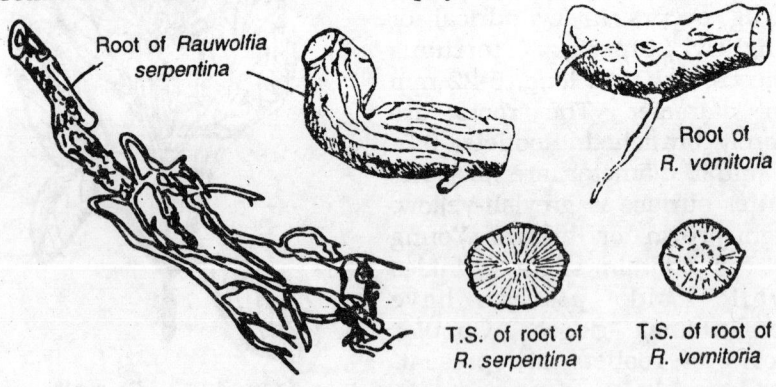

Root of *Rauwolfia serpentina*

Root of *R. vomitoria*

T.S. of root of *R. serpentina*

T.S. of root of *R. vomitoria*

Fig. 13.18. Rauwolfia

R. nitida is found in West India. From its root-bark 33 indole alkaloids have been isolated.

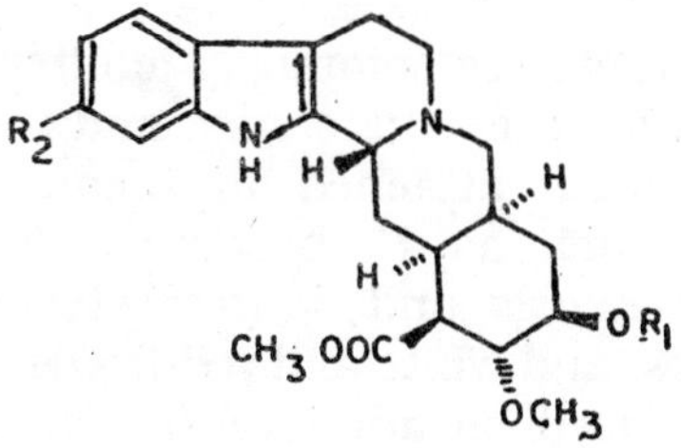

Rescimetol, $R_1 = -COCH=CH-$ (3-methoxy-4-hydroxyphenyl) $R_2 = OCH_3$

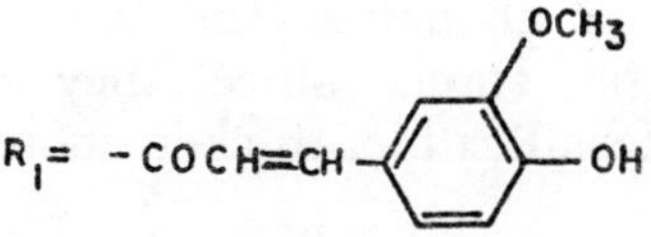

Rescinnamine, 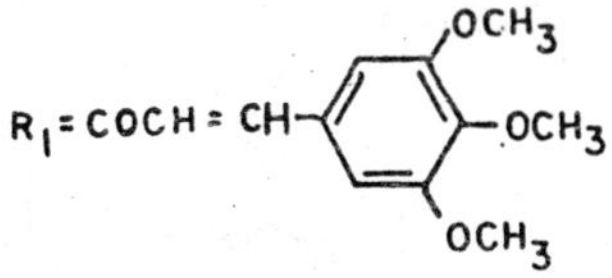 $R_1 = COCH=CH-$ (3,4,5-trimethoxyphenyl) $R_2 = OCH_3$

Reserpine, 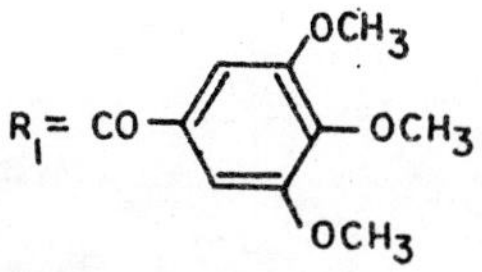 $R_1 = CO-$ (3,4,5-trimethoxyphenyl) $R_2 = OCH_3$

Deserpidine, $R_1 = CO-$ (3,4,5-trimethoxyphenyl) $R_2 = H$

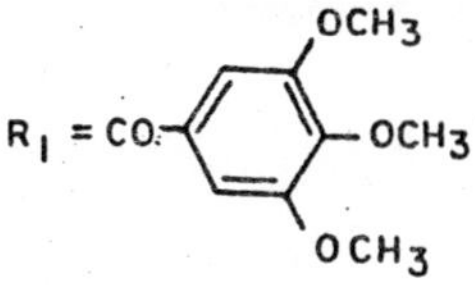

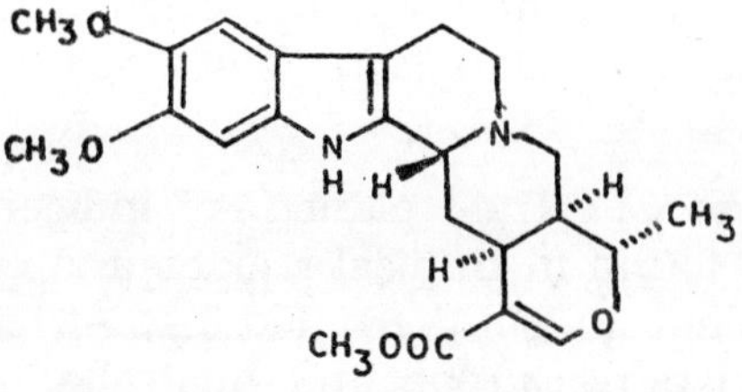

Reserpiline

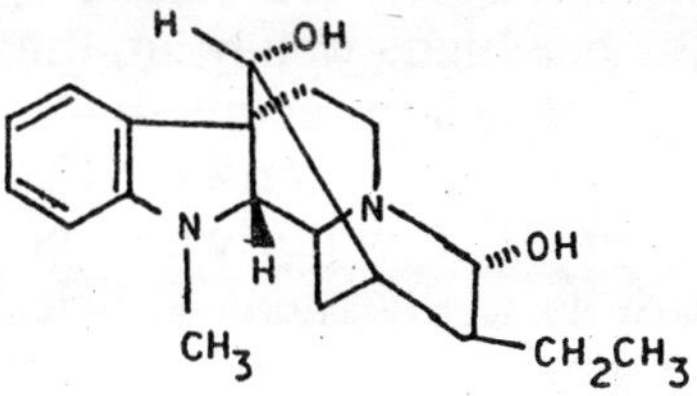

Ajmaline

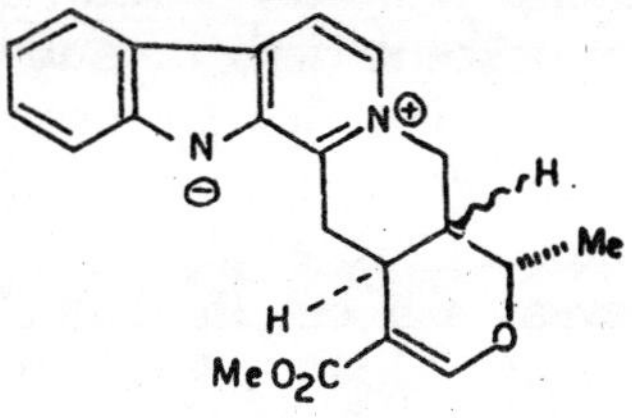

Serpentine (β-H)
Alstonine (α-H)

Adulterants : The roots are commonly adulterated with other parts of the plants such as the stems, and root stumps with some portions of stem attached to them. Roots of other *Rauwolfia* species such as *R. beddomei, R. densiflora, R. micrantha, R. perakensis* and *R. tetraphylla* and those of *Ophiorrhiza mungos*, and white and red-flowered *Clerodendrus* species have been used as adulterants. Stems of the plant contain less quantity of alkaloids. The roots can be eaisly distinguished from the stems since they have a more wrinkled surface, are less flexible, thicker, more tortuous and less branched.

Ajmalicine   Reserpinine

CATHARANTHUS

Synonyms : Vinca; Madagascar perivinkle; Shadaphul (Mar); Rattanjot (Punj.).

Biological Source : Catharanthus is the dried whole plant of *Catharanthus roseus* G. Don (syn. *Vinca rosea* Linn.).

Family : Apocynaceae.

Geographical Source : The plant is indigenous to Madagascar but now found in tropical regions and cultivated as an ornamental plant in southern Florida, Africa, India, Thailand, Taiwan, eastern Europe and Australia.

Plant Habitat : Catharanthus is an erect, everblooming pubescent herb or subshrub, 40-80 cm high, woody at the base. The leaves are oblong, with petiolate acute base, rounded apex, entire margin and oppositely arranged. The flowers are axillary, violet, rose or white or white with red eyes, 4-5 cm in diameter. The fruit is a divergent follicle. It has slight odour and taste is bitter.

Chemical Constituents : About 90 alkaloids have been reported from *C. roseus*. Vindoline, and catharanthine are indole monomeric alkaloids. The alkaloids such as ajmalicine, lochnerine, reserpine, serpentine and tetrahydroalstonine are also present in other genera of Apocynaceae. About 20 dimeric alkaloids, including vindesine, vincristine and vinblastine, have been isolated from Catharanthus. These alkaloids possess antineoplastic activity. In addition to alkaloids, monoterpenes, sesquiterpene, indole and indoline glycoside have also been reported.

Uses : Catharanthus is used to cure diabetes and in wasp-sting. Vinblastine sulphate is an antitumor alkaloid employed to cure Hodgkin's disease and chlorionepithelioma. Vincristine sulphate is a cytotoxic compound and used to treat leukaemia in children. Catharanthus alkaloids are antineoplastic in nature.

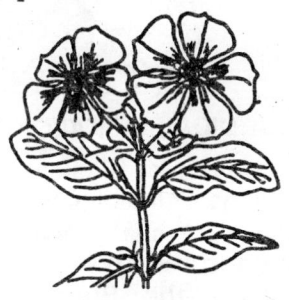

Fig. 13.19. *Catharanthus roseus* flowering part

Lochneridine

Lochnerinine (R=OCH$_3$)
Lochnericine (R=H)

Tetrahydroalstonine

Vinblastine, R$_1$ = CH$_3$, R$_2$ = OCH$_3$, R$_3$ = COCH$_3$
Vincristine, R = CHO, R$_2$ = OCH$_3$, R$_3$ = COCH$_3$
Vindesine, R$_1$ = CH$_3$, R$_2$ = NH$_2$, R$_3$ = H

Vindoline   Catharanthine

STEROIDAL ALKALOIDS

The steroidal alkaloids possess a cyclopentenophenanthrene nucleus. Alkaloids with C_{27} group are known as *Solanum* alkaloids, e.g., solanidine, and tomatidine. The alkaloids found in the Apocynaceae (*Holarrhena* and *Funtumia* species) and in the Buxaceae, possess 21 carbon atoms. The important drugs of this group are Kurchi bark and Veratrums.

KURCHI BARK

Synonyms : Holarrhenna; Kurchi (Hindi).

Biological Source : Kurchi bark consists of dried stem bark of *Holarrhena antidysenterica* Wall. obtained from 8-12 years old tree.

Family : Apocynaceae.

Geographical Source : The plant is found more or less throughout India, ascending to 1250 m in the Himalayas, especially in wet forests.

Collection : Kurchi is a deciduous laticiferous shrub or small tree, 9-10 m high. The bark is collected from the tree by making suitable transverse and longitudinal incisions. The alkaloidal content is high soon after the rains when new shoots are produced which declines during winter months.

Morphology : The pieces of Kurchi bark are small and recurved both longitudinally and transversely. The size and thickness vary from piece to piece. Outer surface is buff to reddish brown and bears numerous prominent circular or transversely elongated horizontal lenticels, longitudinal wrinkles. The thicker pieces are rugose and show numerous yellowish warts; inner surface cinnamon-brown longitudinally striated, frequently with portions of pale yellow wood attached; fracture is brittle. The taste is acrid and bitter while the odour is not distinct.

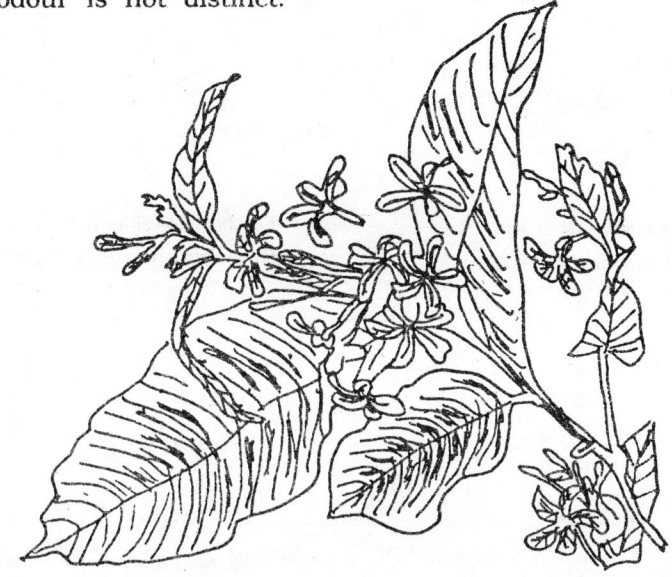

Fig. 13.20. Kurchi flowering shoot

Chemical Constituents : The total alkaloidal constituents of Kurchi bark vary from 1.1 to 4.72 per cent. The main steroidal alkaloid is conessine (20-30%). The other alkaloids isolated include conarrhimine, conimine, conamine, conessimine, isoconessimine, dimethyl conkurchine, 3α-aminocon-5-ene, conkuressine, dihydroisoconessimine, dihydroconessine, 7β- and 7α-hydroxyconessines, kurcholessine, holacine, holacimine, regholarrhenines A, B, C, D, E and F, kurchessine, holarrhimine, holarricine, etc. In addition to alkaloids the bark also contains 5, 20 (29)-lupadien 3β-ol (lupenic triterpene) and sitosta-5, 23-dien-3β-ol (sterol), gum, resin, tannin and lupeol.

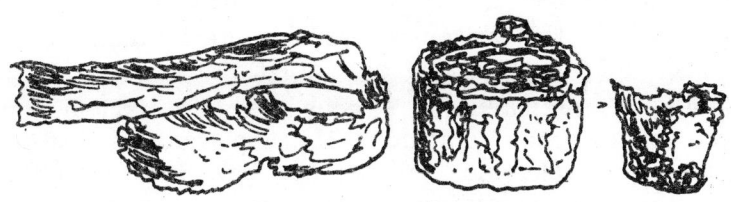

Fig. 13.21. Kurchi bark

Conessine (R = H)
Holarrhenine (R = OH)

Kurcholesine (β-OH)
Regholarrhenine E (α-OH)

Regholarrhenine F

Regholarrhenine A (R = Me)
Regholarrhenine B (R = H)

Uses : The bark is considered to be stomachic, astringent, tonic, antidysenteric, febrifuge and anthelmintic. The dried bark is rubbed over the body in dropsy. Kurchi bark is used to cure amoebic dysentery and diarrhoea.

VERATRUMS

Synonyms : American Hellebore; Green Hellebore; American Veratrum; Indian poke.

Biological Source : Veratrum consists of dried roots and rhizomes of the perennial herbs, *Veratrum viride* Aiton and *Veratrum album* Linn. found in Canada, USA, Carolina, Tennessee, Georgia, etc. The herb is erect, fleshy rhizome. The powdered drug is odourless and bitter and acrid in taste.

Family : Liliaceae.

Collection : The rhizomes are dug in autumn season, cleaned, cut longitudinally and dried.

Chemical Constituents : Various steroidal alkaloids have been isolated from Veratrums. The important alkaloids are jervine, pseudojervine, rubijervine, cevadine, germitrine, germidine, veratralbine, veratroidine, neogermitrine, neoprotoveratrine, protoveratrine and veratridine.

Pseudojervine and veratrosine are glycosides of alkamine. Germine, jervine, rubijervine and veratramine are alkamines.

Uses : Veratrum is used as antihypertensive and insecticides. It is also used for relief in irritation of the nervous system, in convulsions, mania, neuralgia, headache, febrile and inflammatory affections of the respiratory organs and acute tonsillitis. The rhizomes are also used for insecticidal purposes in the form of sprays and in dusts. The alkaloids, especially proveratrines A and B, are effective in reducing blood pressure.

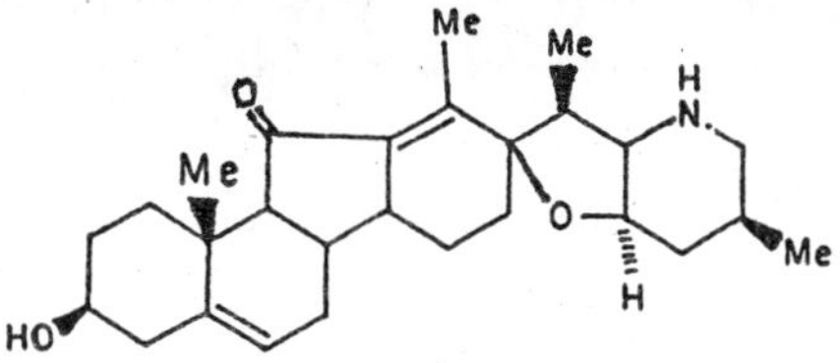

Jervine

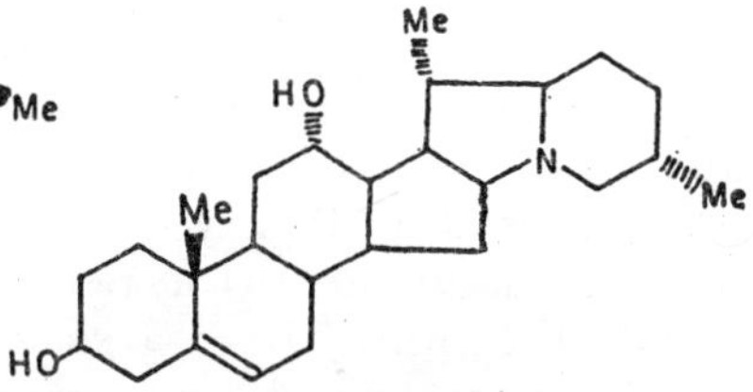

Rubijervine

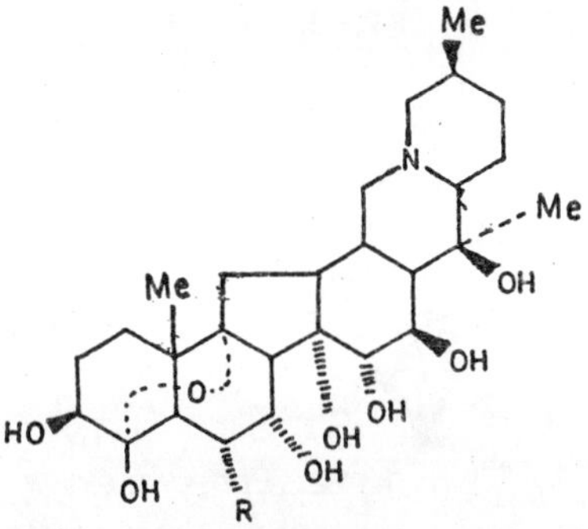

Germine (R = H)
Protoverine (R = OH)

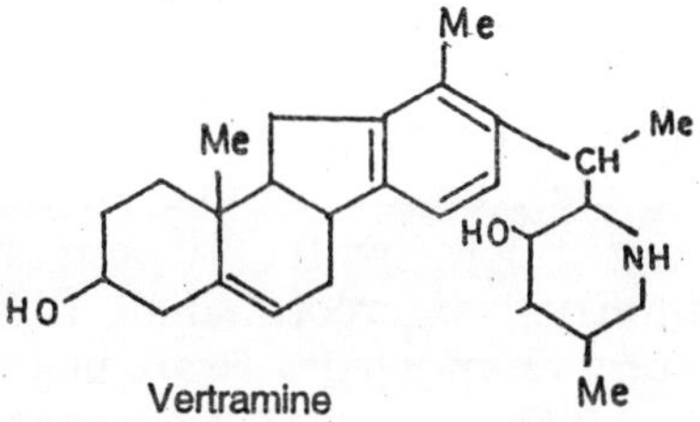

Vertramine

ALKALOIDAL AMINES

The alkaloids of this class do not possess nitrogen in a ring system. Most of them are simple derivatives of phenylethylamine. The important drugs of this group are Ephedra and Colchicum corm.

EPHEDRA

Synonyms : Ma-haung; Tsaopen Ma-huang.

Biological Source : Ephedra consists of whole aerial parts of *Ephedra sinica* Stapf, *E. equisentina* Ma Huang and other species of *Ephedra*

Family : Ephedraceae (Gnetaceae).

Geographical Source : Ephedra is indigenous to China, India and Pakistan. It is most abundantly found near the sea coast in southern China.

Collection : The plant is a low dioecious, usually leafless shrub and 60-90 cm in height. It is collected in the autumn season, dried and packed in bags.

Characters : The stems of Ephedra are slender pieces, containing numerous ridges, nodes and internodes and fine longitudinal ridges on the outer surface. The distance of internodes are nearly 3-6 cm and the diameter of the node is about 1-2 mm. The leaves are small, connate at the base, about 4 mm in length, decussate, in whorls of two, with a subulate recovered apex and a whitish lamina. The characteristic features of Ephedra species are as follows:

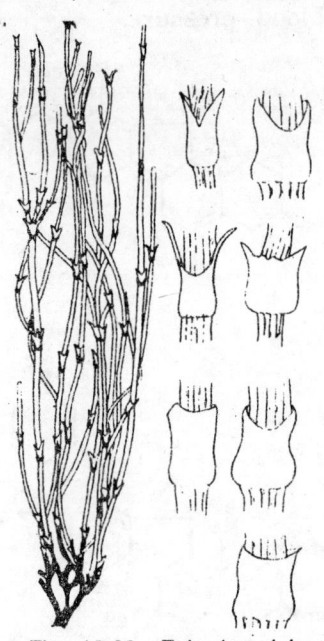

Ephedra sinica : The stems are slender, about 30 cm long, 4-7 mm thick, with 3-6 cm long internodes, erect, small ribbed and channeled. Branches are

Fig. 13.22. *Ephedra sinica*

green, rough with longitudinal ridges. Diameter of lowest green node is 1-2 mm. Leaves are opposite, whitish, 4 mm long with subulate and recurved apex. Lamina is whitish and the base is reddish brown. Small blossoms appear in summer.

Ephedra equisentina : The stems are more woody and branched, 25-200 cm long, yellowish green in colour, internodes are shorter, 1-2.5 cm long. The leaf apex is shorter and it is not recurved. Leaves are brownish-purple colour. Ephedra is odourless and taste is bitter.

Ephedra gerardiana is a small, erect shrub, variable in size, few cm in height. It bears dark green, cylindrical striated, often curved branches arising in whorls; internodes of branchlets, 1-4 cm long and 1-2 cm diameter. Fruit ovoid, red, sweet and edible, containing 1 or 2 seeds, enclosed by succulent bracts. This species is found scattered in the drier regions of temperate and alpine Himalayas.

Ephedra nebrodensis (syn. *E. major*) is an upright, rarely ascending, densely branched shrub, up to 2 meters high. The twigs of this species closely resemble those of *E. gerardiana*.

The plants are propagated by seeds or divisions of the rootstock. The alkaloid content increases with the age of the plant, and the best time to collect the green twigs is when the plants are 4 years old and are in blossom. Rainfall has a marked adverse effect. The alkaloidal content of the green twigs is greater than that of the woody stem. The twigs should be dried in sun. Artificial drying should be avoided. The dried drug must be stored dry. Air-dried drug stored in dry, closed containers, protected from light, retains the activity without loss for a long period. Among the Indian species, *E. major* is the richest source of ephedrine.

Chemical Constituents : Ephedras contain about 0.5 - 2.0% total alkaloid. The chief alkaloid is ephedrine (30-90). The other alkaloids isolated are pseudo-ephedrine, 1-methyl ephedrine, norephedrine and dimethylephedrine.

Chemical Tests

To the drug (10 mg) in water (1 ml) dil. HCl (0.2 ml), copper sulphate solution (0.1 ml) and sodium hydroxide solution (2 ml) are added; the liquid turns violet. On adding solvent ether (2 ml) and shaking vigorously, the ethereal layer turns purple and the aqueous layer becomes blue.

Uses : Liquid extract of Ephedra is used for controlling asthmatic paroxysms. Tincture of Ephedra is useful as cardiac and circulatory stimulant. Decoction of stems and roots is a remedy for rheumatism and syphilis in Russia. Ephedrine is sympathomimetic, has been used to counteract hypotension associated with anaesthesia, as a mydriatic; in

H–C–OH

H–C–NH–R L-Ephedrine (R = CH$_3$)

CH$_3$ Norephedrine (R = H)

HO–C–H

H–C–NHCH$_3$

CH$_3$ D-Pseudoephedrine

allergic reactions and as a CNS stimulant, for the relief of asthma, rhinitis, whooping cough and hay fever. Ephedrine is also a bronchodilator.

COLCHICUM CORM

Synonyms : Meadow Saffron: Autumn Crocus: Wild Saffron; Meadow Crocus; European Colchicum seed; Colchicum root.

Biological Source : Colchicum seed and corm are obtained from *Colchicum autumnale* Linn. Indian drug is obtained from the species *C. luteum* Baker.

Family : Liliaceae.

Geographical Source : The plant is an annual herb found in England, Poland, Czechoslovakia, Yugoslavia, U.S.A. and Holland. In India *C. luteum* is used as a substituent for *C. autumnale.*

Cultivation and Collection : Fresh seeds are sown which germinate up to about 30%. In August-September 2-6 flowers bloom which are identical to Saffron and has liliac or pale purple colour. More than half the length of the flower is below in ground. Leaves and capsular fruit are produced in the next spring. The fruit is a three lobbed, three-celled and septicidal capsule. On expension of leaves in the spring the fruit comes out the ground. It is collected in July or August before its dehiscence and kept in muslin bags. Numerous seeds are liberated on septicidal dehiscence of the fruit into three valves. The matured seeds are dark in colour and surrounded by a sweet saccharine secretion. Before flowering corms are dug out for medicinal use, their outer membraneous scales are removed, cut in transverse or longitudinal pieces and dried up to 65ºC.

Morphology : Seeds are ovoid or globular in shape and 2-3 mm in diameter. The outer surface is dark reddish brown, pitted and very hard. Endosperm is hard and oily. Small embryo is embedded at one end near the surface of the seeds at the opposite side of the hilum. A distinct strophiole is present which extends for about one quarter of the circumference from hilum. The seed is odourless and bitter in taste.

Fresh corm is conical in shape, 4 cm long and 3 cm wide. One side of the corm is convex and the opposite side is flat. At the apex base flowering stem is present. The outer surface is yellow to brown in colour and slightly wrinkled. A cavity having a bud is seen at the base of the flat side.

New stem germinates from this bud. At the base of the corm numerous fibrous roots or their scars are present. Inner surface is fleshy and white and has fibrovascular bundles.

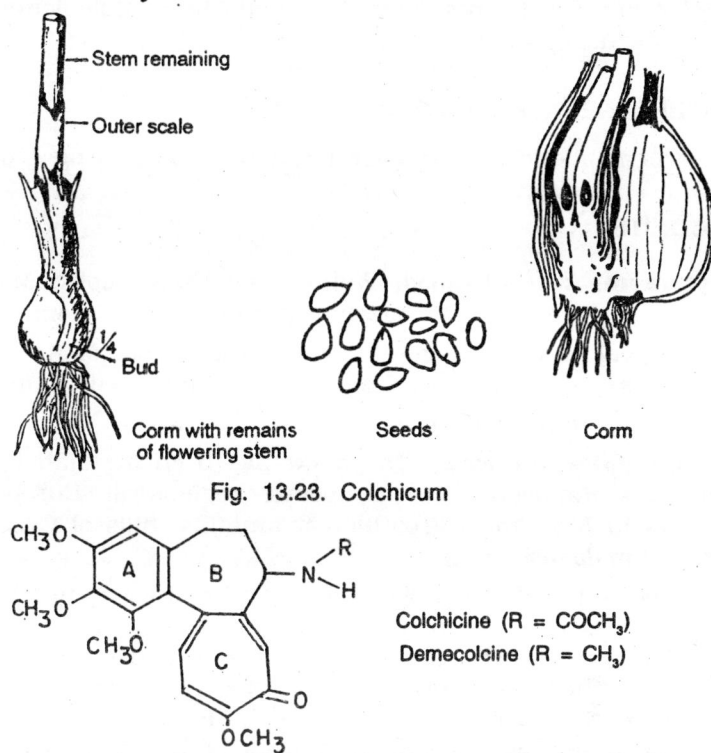

Fig. 13.23. Colchicum

Colchicine (R = COCH₃)

Demecolcine (R = CH₃)

Dried corm consists of transverse or longitudinal slices which are 3 cm long and 2-5 mm thick. The shape is reniform to ovate with a groove on the flat side. Colour is dark brown. Fracture is short and strachy. The corm is almost odourless. Taste is bitter and acrid.

Chemical Constituents : Colchicum contains the alkaloids colchicine (0.3 - 0.8%), colchicein, colchicoresin, demecolcine, starch, etc. Colchicine is an amorphous, yellowish white alkaloid, readily soluble in water, alcohol, or chloroform.

Indian Colchicum corms contain abundant starch and alkaloid. On exposure to UV light, colchicine is changed to lumicolchicine.

Chemical Test : Colchicum corm with sulphuric acid (70%) or conc. HCl produces yellow colour due to colchicine.

Uses : Colchicum corm or colchicine is gout depressant and used to cure gout and rheumatism. Its higher doses cause vomiting and diarrhoea. It is also prescribed to treat myeloid leukaemia. Colchicine is also used to produce polyploidy in biological experiments. Anti-cancer activity of Colchicum has also been reported.

DITERPENE ALKALOIDS

Diterpene alkaloids have been isolated from the drug Aconite.

ACONITE

Synonyms : Monkshood, Wolf's-bane; Friar's cowl; Mouse-bane; Aconite root; Mithazahar (Hindi); Radix aconiti.

Biological Source : Aconite is the dried roots of *Aconitum napellus* Linn. collected from wild or cultivated plants.

Family : Ranunculaceae.

Geographical Source : The plant has been originated from the mountanoeous and temperate regions of Europe. It occurs in Alps and Carpathian mountains, hills of Germany and Himalayas.

Cultivation and Plant Habitat : Aconite is a perennial herb with a fusiform tuberous root. The plant is propagated from the daughter tubers. In the autumn season the aconite root becomes thick. An apical bud on the apex and six lateral buds on its surface are developed. A lateral shoot bearing a thin lateral root is produced from each lateral bud. The lateral roots are called daughter roots and the main root is known as parent root. The daughter root develops gradually, becomes thick in autumn and buds are produced on its apex and surface.

Daughter roots are planted in soil containing leaf mould and some amount of lime. The roots are collected in autumn. Collection of Aconite from wild plants is done during flowering season. Roots are dried at 40-50°. Thus Aconite arises from one or more lateral shoots which develop into conical daughter tubers.

Morphology : Appearance of Aconite varies from season to season. Aconite collected in autum in England is conical in shape and tapering below. Surface is slightly twisted bearing longitudinal ridges. Some Aconites may contain fibrous rootlets or their scars. On the top of parent root some

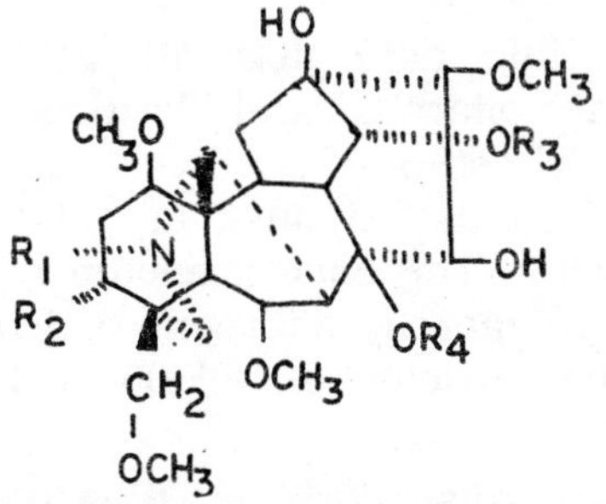

Aconine (R$_1$ = C$_2$H$_5$, R$_2$ = OH, R$_3$ = R$_4$ = H)
Neoline (R$_1$ = Et, R$_2$ = H, R$_3$ = R$_4$ = H)
Benzoylaconine (R$_1$ = C$_2$H$_5$, R$_2$ = OH, R$_3$ = COC$_6$H$_5$, R$_4$ = H)
Aconitine (R$_1$ = C$_2$H$_5$, R$_2$ = OH, R$_3$ = CO C$_6$H$_5$, R$_4$ = COCH$_3$)
Hypaconitine (R$_1$ = Me, R$_2$ = H, R$_3$ = PhCO, R$_4$ = Ac)

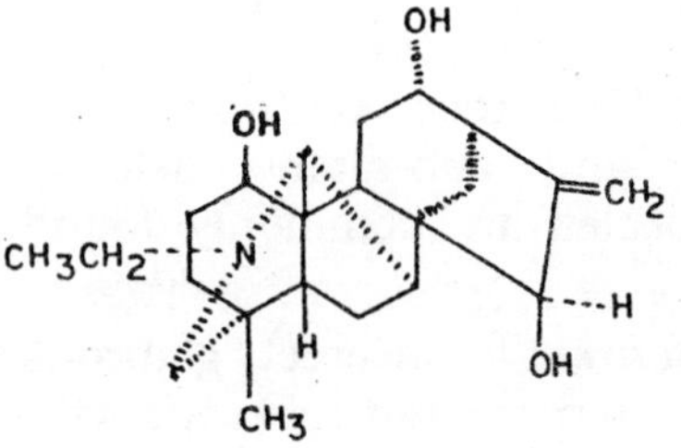

Napelline

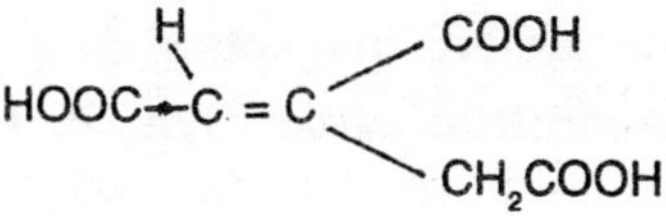

Aconitic acid

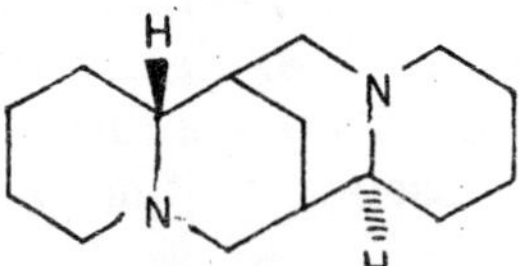

Sharteine

H$_2$C=C(COOH)CH$_2$COOH

Itaconic acid

remains of stem base are present which are more shrivelled. An apical bud is present at the apex. The colour is dark-brown. The root is 4-10 cm in length and 1-3 cm in diameter at the crown. Rootlets may be present. The fracture is short and starchy. The fractured surface is 5-8 angled, contains stellate cambium and a central pith. The odour is slight. Taste is sweet at first followed by tingling and numbness.

Chemical Constituents : Aconite contains aconitine (0.4-0.8%), hypaconiticine, mesaconitine, aconine, napelline (isoaconitine, pseudoaconitine), neoline, ephedrine, sparteine, and are mixed with those *A. spicatum* and *A. ferox.*, *A luridum*, an erect plant, is a potent drug as *A. ferox.*, *A.*

picraconitine, acotinic acid, itaconic acid, succinic acid, malonic acid, fat, starch, and levulose (fructose). The aconitines are diacyl esters of polyhydric amino alcohols and are extremely poisonous. Atisines are also amino alcohols but have low toxicity. The basic skeleton of aconite alkaloid is consisted of a pentacyclic diterpene which is derived from phyllocladene. The toxicity of alkaloids is decreased on hydrolysis.

Uses : Aconite is cardiac effective. It is used externally as a local analgesic in liniments and to treat neuralgia, rheumatism and inflammation. Tincture Aconite is antipyretic in small doses. Aconitine in amount 2-3 mg can lead respiratory failure, heart failure and in the end death.

INDIAN ACONITES

About 28 *Aconitum* species have been reported from India, mostly present in the alpine and sub-alpine belt of Himalayas. The roots of nine species are commonly found in the Indian markets.

Aconitum atrox (Syn. *A. balfourcii)* is an erect, glabrous herb. Roots are biennial, paired; or ternate and tuberous with several attached hardened rootlets. It is a poisonous species and is one of the common constituents of *Aconitum ferox* of commerce. The roots resemble those of *A. deinorrhizum* but are somewhat shorter and thicker. They contains 1.20 - 2.04 % of total alkaloids, of which pseudaconitine is 0.4-0.5 per cent.

Aconitum bisma (syn. A. palmatum) is a biennial herb. Roots are tuberous, paired, the mother root is often dry and cylindrical, the daughter root conical to long-cylindrical, external surface somewhat smooth, light brown. The roots contain five diterpene alkaloids, viz. palmatisine, vakognavine, vakatisine, vakatisinine and vakatidine. Benzamide is also present. The root is intensely bitter like quinine and is used in combination with long pepper for pain in the bowels, for diarrhoea, vomiting, rheumatism, sharp cuts, wounds and as a tonic.

Aconitum chasmanthum is an erect, perennial herb. Roots are biennial, paired and tuberous. This species is identical to *A. napellus.* Its roots are smaller, shorter and thicker; the mother tubers are deeply grooved and wrinkled and are black outside and brown inside. The daughter tubers are conic to conic-cylindrical with a broad base having numerous root fibres. Fracture is cartilaginous, hard and white within the cambium ring and brownish outside. The drug is collected in September. It has the same uses as *A. ferox*. The alkaloid content of the roots ranges from 2.98 to 3.11%. The alkaloids isolated are indaconitine, chasmaconitine, chasmanthinine, chasmanine, and homochasmanine.

Aconitum deinorrhizum is an erect, tall plant with long terete stem. Daughter root is conical, brown externally, mother tubers are more or less similar, but have longer filiform root fibres. *A. atrox* is the principal constituent of the Aconite of commerce. The drug is very hard and horny and its starch is gelatinized during drying. The roots contains 0.9% total alkaloids of which 0.51% is pseudoaconitine.

Aconitum ferox is a perennial herb. Roots are biennial, tuberous, paired, daughter tuber ovoid-oblong to ellipsoid, with filiform root fibres, dark brown, taste indifferent. It is known as Indian Aconite. The total alkaloid content varies from 0.63 to 4.7%. The alkaloids pseudaconitine, chasmaconitine, indaconitine, bikhaconitine, veratroyl pseudaconitine and diacetyl pseudaconitine are present. The roots are used after mitigation to treat neuralgia, muscular rheumatism, inflammatory joint affections, nasal catarrh, tonsillitis, sore throat, gastric disorders, debility and fever.

Aconitum heterophyllum is a tall herb. Root are biennial, tuberous, paired; daughter tuber cylindric or conic. The roots yield 0.79% of total alkaloids like atisine, heteratisine, histidine, heterophyllisine, heterophylline, heterophyllidine, atidine, hetidine, etc. Atisine is much less toxic than aconitine and pseudaconitine. Therefore, this species is often regarded as non-poisonous. It is used as a febrifuge and bitter tonic. The roots are used to treat hysteria and throat diseases.

Aconitum spicatum is a robust and typical species. Roots are biennial, tuberous, paired and brown or blackish. The roots are used as poison. The fresh roots are soft and flexible; dried roots are hard and dark brown. The roots yield 1.75% of alkaloids which contain mainly pseudaconitine and bikhaconitine.

Aconitum falconeri is an erect herb. The biennial, paired roots yield two alkaloids, bishaconite and bishatisine are used to treat disease of nervous and digestive systems, and for rheumatism. *A. laciniatum* biennial roots are slightly bitter

rotundifolium contains two alkaloids in the aerial portion. *A. violaceum* is an erect plant, found mixed with the commercial varieties of Aconites. It contains 1% indaconitine.

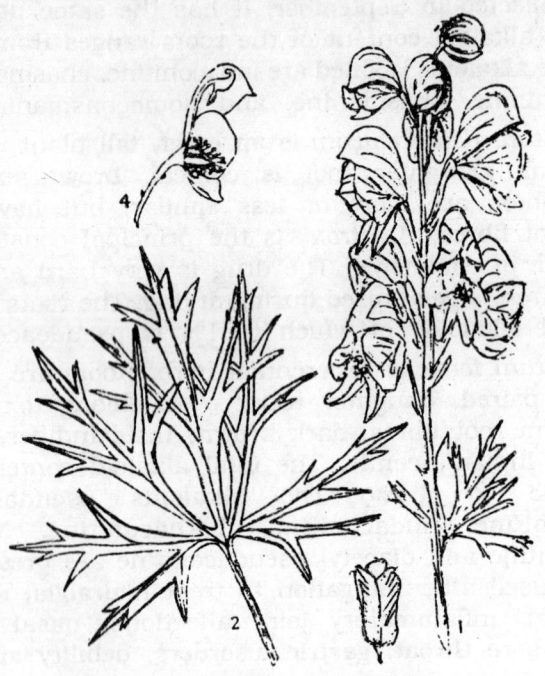

Fig. 13.24. *Aconitum napellus.*

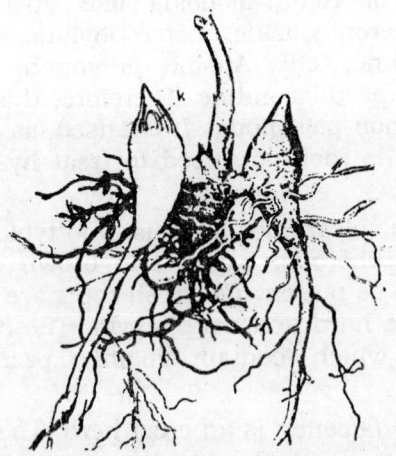

Fig. 13.25. Aconite with a daughter root.

QUESTIONS

1. What are alkaloids ? Write short notes on the following alkaloid containing drugs : (a) Physostigma (b) Opium (c) Ephedra (d) Aconite.

2. Give official source, morphology, chemical constituents and uses of a drug belonging to the following families: (a) Solanaceae (b) Rubiaceae (c) Papaveraceae (d) Loganiaceae (e) Clavicipitaceae (f) Apocynaceae.

3. Write notes on : (a) Opium, (b) Rauwolfia (c) Vinca (d) Nux-vomica.

4. What are Solanaceous drugs ? Give sources, constituents and substitutes of drugs containing tropane alkaloids.

5. Give the official sources, salient morphological characters, chemical constituents and uses of the following : (a) Opium (b) Ergot (c) Ephedra (d) Lobelia.

6. Give the biological source, identification test, chemical nature and therapeutic uses of the following phytoconstituents : (a) Scopolamine (b) Glycyrrhetinic acid (c) Reserpine (d) Quinine (e) Conessine.

7. Discuss the general methods of extraction of alkaloids. Write an account of piperidine alkaloids.

8. Give the distribution and biogenesis of tropane alkaloids. Comment upon the various sources for scopolamine and give a suitable scheme for its isolation.

9. Give distinguishing features of the following :
   (a) Hyoscyamine and Atropine
   (b) *Cinchona succirubra* and *Cinchona officinalis.*
   (c) Nicotine and nornicotine
   (d) *Cephaelis ipecac* and *Cephaelis acuminata*

10. Give the distinguishing features of the following : (a) Quinine and quinidine (b) Codeine and thebaine (c) Arecoline and arecaidine (d) Reserpine and rescinnamine (e) Strychnine and brucine (f) Emetine and cephaeline.

11. Give general methods of extraction and isolation of an alkaloid and suggest suitable scheme for the isolation of antitumor alkaloids of Catharanthus.

12. What is Ergot ? Describe various stages of development of this fungus, its chemical constituents and clinical importance.

14

INDIGENOUS TRADITIONAL DRUGS

Medicinal plants have been playing a significant role in the treatment of various ailments in India. The important traditional methods in our country are Ayurvedic, Homoeopathy, Unani and Sidha systems of medicine. Ayurveda offers traditionally a highly scientific health-care therapy as a divine gift, and as a result, the global interest of the medical profession is nucleated on the Ayurvedic and Unani systems of medicine. A traditional ingredient is fundamentally preventive, protective, nutritive and curative. Therefore, traditional medicines are safe, sure and harmless which treat the patients and does not end at rendering relief.

In spite of phenomenal progress in the area of development of new drugs from synthetic sources and appearance of antibiotics as major therapeutic agents, plants continue to provide basic raw material for some of the most important drugs. An analysis of prescriptions dispensed from community pharmacies in USA was carried out in 1973, and this showed that as many as 41% prescriptions contained one or more products of natural origin as the therapeutic agent. Of these prescriptions, 25% were based on drugs from higher plants, some 13% represented metabolities of microbes and about 7% were of animal origin. Among 200 most frequently prescribed drugs in USA, 25% were of natural origin. The situation would appear to be similar for many other countries including India, Russia, Germany, England, Italy, China and Japan. About three hundred herbal drugs of Indian origin are used in England to treat various diseases. The *Pharmacopoeia of the Peoples Republic of China*, issued in 1978, describes 882 crude drugs of which 637 are of plant origin. *Japanese Pharmacopoëia X* released in 1981, contained 102 plant drugs.

In India there are about 700 naturally occurring drugs used in various formulations. There are about 20 large scale manufacturers of traditional drugs in addition to 1200 small manufacturers and thousands of miniature manufacturing units running by vaids and hakims.

More frequently traditional drugs are used to cure the following ailments :

Cold and Cough : Senega, Ipecac, Squill, Glycyrrhiza and Ginger contain expectorant activity. The leaves of *Angelica archangelica, Pimpinella anisum* (Anise fruit), *Allium sativum* (Garlic), *Thymus vulgaris, Mentha spicata* (Mint), *Ocimum sanctum* (Tulsi), *Viola odorata* (Banafsha) and *Eucalpytus* sp. are used to treat cough, cold and bronchitis. Dried stigma of *Crocus sativus* (Saffron or Kesar) are used in cough preparations. Most of these drugs contain essential oils which are responsible for the biological activity.

Gastrointestinal Disorders : Gastrointestinal disorders include colitis, constipation, diarrhoea, duodenal ulcers, dyspepsia and hyperacidity. Dried extract of *Acacia catechu* and *Geum urbanum*, leaf and bark of *Hamamelis virginiana* and root bark of *Myrica cerifera* are used to treat the inflammation of colon (colitis). Constipation is treated by seed husk of Plantago, leaves of Senna, bark of Cascara, Aloe juice, Rhubarb and Honey. Stomachic drugs include Chirata, Garlic, Kalmegh, Kapur kachari, Saffron, Nux-vomica and Picrorhiza. Agar, Aloe, Cascara, Guar gum, Isapgol, Myrobalan, Rhubarb and Senna. Carminative drugs contain volatile oils and they are Asafoetida, Black pepper, Capsicum, Caraway, Cardamom, Cinnamon, Coriander, Dill, Fennel, Garlic and Mentha oil. The herbal drugs like Ipecac, Isapgol, Kurchi and Sankhpusphi are anti-dysenteric drugs which generally contain mucilage or alkaloids. Diarrhoea is treated with Bael, Isapgol, Kurchi, Pale Catechu and Pectins.

Urinary Disorders

Saxifraga liqulata and *Tribulus terrestris* (Gokhru) are used to break and disintegrate urinary stones. Guargum,

Gurmarbuti and Vijayasar are employed as anti-diabetic drugs. Cholagogue disorder is treated with *Eclipta alba* (Bhringraja), *Phyllanthus fracternus* (Jar-amla), Kalmegh and Picrorhiza. The crude drugs like Gokhru, Arjuna and Punarnava are used to cure diuretic ailments.

Liver Diseases

There are about 33 formulations containing traditional drugs for the treatment of liver ailments. Some of them are Liv 52, Stimulive, Liomyn, Livergen, Livotrit and these formulations are prepared from Kalmegh, Picrorhiza, Bhringraja, Sarponkha *(Tephrosia purpurea)*, *Boerhaavia diffusa* (Punarnava), *Trianthema portulacastrum* and Chirata.

Antiarthritic Agents

Rasna *(Alpinia officinarum, Pluchea lanceolata, Vanda roxburghii,* and *Vitex negundo)* is used as a traditional remedy to cure rheumatism and arthritis. The resin obtained from *Commiphora mukul* (Gugul) and the exudate of *Boswellia serrata* (Sallai gugul) are also employed as antiarthritic agents. *Aconitum napellus* also contains anti-rheumatic activity.

Sedative and Tranquillizers

The sedative traditional drugs include Aswagandha, Belladonna, Brahmi, Datura, Cannabis, Hyoscyamus, Jatamansi, Myrrh, Rauwolfia, Valerian, Vaj and Wild Cherry bark. Most of these drugs are the source of alkaloids. Celery, Chamomile and Valerian exhibit mild sedative effects. Indian Valerian is superior than European one due to higher concentration of active constituents. Valepotriates are more tranquillizers and sedatives than meprobamate. Jatamansi contains safe sedative and spasmolytic agent.

Cardiac Drugs

Cardiovascular diseases are the major cause of mortality all over the world. The most popular drug is digoxin isolated from Digitalis. The cardiotonic glycoside, peruvoside, obtained from an Indian ornamental plant Kaner, *Thevetia peruviana*, (Fam. Apocynaceae) has been introduced in German under the trade name 'Encordin'. Forskolin (Coleonol) is another antihypertensive compound isolated from a fragrant herb *Coleus forskohlii* (fam. Labiatae). Asclepin, obtained from *Asclepias curassavica*, is more potent than digoxin. The popular Ayurvedic drug 'Sarpgandha' *(Rauwolfia serpentina)* shows hypotensive and tranquillizing effect. Strophanthus and Urginea are also used as cardiotonic.

Other Disorders

Cannabis and Opium are used as analgesics and narcotics. Anthelmintic drugs include Artemisia, Chenopodium oil, Kapur kachari, Vidang, Male Fern. Ephedra, Lobelia, and Sankhpushpi,

Vasaka and Tylophora are anti-asthmatic drugs. Turmeric, Punarnava, Aswagandha, Kapur kachari and Colchicum are used as anti-inflammatory drugs. Malaria is treated with Cinchona bark and Artemisia. Balsam Tolu. Benzoin, Camphor, Clove, Neem *(Azadirachta indica),* Eucalyptus, Myrrh, Neem, Mint, Tulsi, Turmeric and Pine oil are used as antiseptic drugs. Antitumor agents are Podophyllum and Vinca. Asafoetida, Belladonna, Caraway, Datura, Fennel, Hyoscyamus, Kapur kachri, Kesor, Aswagandha and Mentha oil show antispasmodic property and some of them possess aphrodisiac action. Amla, Arjuna, Ashoka, Bahera, Black Catechu, Myrobalan and Tannic acid exhibit astringent action. Chirata, Gentian, Kalmegh, Picrorhiza, Orange peel and Quassia are used as bitter tonics. Acacia, Honey, Isapgol, Aswagandha, Linseed, Sesame oil, Starch and Tragacanth have demulcent property while emollient action is exhibited by the drugs such as Arachis oil, Kokum butter, Lanolin, Linseed oil and Sesame. Ergot and Vasaka are reputed as oxytocic drugs. Coffee beans, Cocaine, Coriander, Dill, Ginger, Nux-vomica, Pipal, Rasna and Storax show stimulant action.

KAPUR KACHARI

Synonyms : Spiked ginger lily; Karpur (sans.), Sitruti (Hindi).

Biological Source : Kapur kachari consists of the dried slices of roots and rhizomes of *Hedychium spicatum* Hem ex Smith.

Family : Zingiberaceae.

Habitat : The plant is found in subtropical Himalayas, Nepal and Kumaon at an altitude 1,700-2,000 m.

The plant is a one meter high perennial rhizomatous herb cultivated as an ornamental plant. It bears white ascending flowers growing in terminal spikes.

Characters : The drug occurs as reddish brown flat or spherical slices. The outer surface is rough, rootlets are attached here and there. Odour is intense aromatic and taste is bitter and camphor-like.

Chemical Constituents : The drug contains essential oil (4%), furanoid diterpene, 7-hydroxyhedychinone, organic acids, resinic acids and starch (50%). The principal constituent of the volatile oil is ethyl p-methoxycinnamate (68%); the others being limonene, β-phellandrene, p-cymene, linalool, β-terpineol, β-caryophyllene, ethyl cinnamate (10%), d-sabinene (4%), 1,4-cineole (6%), sesquiterpenes (5.5), and sesquiterpene alcohol (4.7%).

Uses : The drug is used as stomachic, carminative, tonic, stimulant, emmenagogue, expectorant, in liver complaints, vomiting, diarrhoea, inflammation and pains. It is also used as insect-repellent, flavouring agent in tobacco and cosmetic industry, for preserving clothes and in dyspepsia in the form of powder or decoction.

$$RO-\bigcirc-CH=CH-COOC_2H_5$$

Ethyl p-methoxycinnamate (R=CH$_3$)
Ethyl cinnamate (R = H)

PIPAL

Biological Source : Pipal consists of stem bark of *Ficus religiosa* Linn. (Family Urticaceae/Moraceae).

Habitat : Pipal is found in sub-Himalayan forests, Bengal, Central India, Sri Lanka and Burma as wild or cultivated plant.

The plant is a large evergreen deciduous tree up to 35 m in height. The leaves are typically cordate, tapering towards the apex forming a linear lanceolate tail. The fruits are small berries with purple colour on ripening.

Characters : The bark is greyish, occurring as irregular pieces, 2-2.5 cm thick. Young bark is smooth, the old bark is covered with greyish patches of lichens. It is odourless and taste is astringent.

Chemical Constituents : Pipal contains tannins (4%) and other phenolic constituents.

Uses : The bark is astringent and used in gonorrhoea.

PUNARNAVA

Synonyms : Hog weed; Sant; Beshakapori (Hindi).

Biological Source : Punarnava consists of the herb *Boerhaavia diffusa* Linn.

Family : Nyctaginaceae.

Habitat : The plant is a weed found throughout India during rainy season.

Description : Stem is greenish-purple, stiff, slender, cylindrical, thickened at nodes, minutely pubescent or glabrous, prostrate or ascending, divertically branched. Leaves are opposite in unequal pairs; petiolate, ovate-oblong or suborbicular, apex is rounded or slightly pointed; base is subcordate or rounded. Lamina is green and glabrous above and whitish below, margin is entire or subundulate, turned up and pinkish in certain cases. Flowers are very small. Fruit is one-seeded nut, 6 mm long, clavate, 5-ribbed, viscidly glandular.

Chemical Constituents : The active constituent is a mixture of alkaloids 'punarnavine'. Xanthine derivatives, ursolic acid, β-sitosterol, fatty acids such as stearic acid and arachidic acid, have been isolated from the drug. The plant also contains inorganic salts such as potassium nitrate, potassium sulphate and chlorides.

The roots contain alkaloids (0.05%), triacontanol, hentriacontane, β-sitosterol, ursolic acid, 5, 7-dihydroxy-3,4-dimethoxy-6, 8-dimethyl flavone, glucose, fructose, sucrose, ecdysone and hypoxanthine-9-arabinoside.

Recently, a purine nucleoside, identified as hypoxanthine-9-L-arabinofuranoside, a dihydroisofuranoxanthone (borhavine), C-methyl flanone, 6'-O- ester of sitosteryl D-glucose, and rotenoid analgues like boeravinones A, B, C, D, E and F have been isolated from punarnava.

Uses : Punarnava is diuretic, useful in nephrotic syndrome, chronic oedema and liver diseases.

The plant is used as a maintenance drug, in abdominal tumors and cancer. It also possesses anti-inflammatory, antibacterial and cardiotonic properties. The roots are credited with anti-convulsant, analgesic, laxative, diuretic and expectorant properties.

Borhavine

C-Methylflavone

Boeravinone A : R₁=CH₃, R₂=H

Boeravinone B : R₁=R₂=H

Boeravinone A : $R_1=CH_3$, $R_2=H$
Boeravinone B : $R_1=R_2=H$

Adulterant : Punarnava is substituted with *Trianthema portulacastrum* (Family-Ficoidaceae), a prostrate weed, with branches up to 2 m long found in South India, Gujarat, Rajasthan and U.P. Leaves are oblong, elliptic, the opposite pair somewhat unequal, flowers are dense, axillary. *T. portulacastrum* cantains an alkaloid trianthemine and ecdysterone. The leaves are diuretic, used in oedema and dropsy and in cases of ascites especially due to liver, peritoneal and kidney conditions.

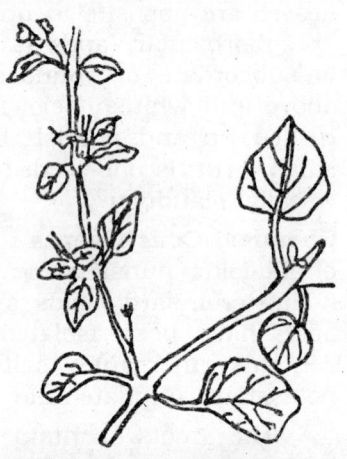

Fig. 14.1. Punarnava (*Boerrhaavia diffusa*).

SHANKHPUSHPI

Biological Source : Shankhpushpi consists of the whole aerial parts of *Convolvulus pluricaulis* Choisy (syn. *Convolvulus microphyllus* Sieb) and *Evolvulus alsinoides* Linn.

Family : Convolvulaceae.

Habitat : Both the plants grow widely in plains of India.

Convolvulus pluricaulis : Plant is a procumbent shrub. Stem is woody at the base, 10-30 cm long, leaves are 2.5-3 cm long linear, oblong, villous on both sides, tapering at base, flowers are small, funnel shaped, light pink or white coloured; fruits are small, up to 2.5 mm long, glabrous, scarcely papillose.

Ursolic acid

$$CH_3(CH_2)_{18}COOH$$

Arachidic acid.

Chemical Constituents : The drug contains an alkaloid known as 'shankhpushpine', volatile oil, n-triacontane, higher fatty alcohols, kaempferol, its 3-D-glucoside, 2, 3-dihydroxycinnamic acid, β-sitostoerol, carbohydrates such as glucose, rhamnose, sucrose, starch and potassium chloride.

Uses : The drug is used as a brain tonic, in hypertension and as tranquillizer.

Evolvulus alsinoides : It is a perennial herb with prostrate branching developing from a small woody rootstock. Stems are numerous, about 30 cm long, prostrate, spreading, slender, wiry with hairs. Leaves are simple sessile, alternate, lanceolate to suborbicular. Flowers are light blue, solitary, peduncles very long, filiform, and axillary. Fruit is a four angled capsule.

Chemical Constituents : The herb contains betain [(CH$_3$) CH$_2$COOH·] and evolvine in addition to proteins, amino acids, and phenolic compounds.

Uses : The plant is used as tonic, febrifuge, vermifuge and in dysentery. Cigarettes containing leaves are smoked in chronic bronchitis and asthma. Oil of the plant is used for promoting growth of hair.

VASAKA

Synonyms : Adhatoda, Vasaka folium, Adulasa (Hindi).

Biological Source : Vasaka consists of the fresh or dried leaves of *Adhatoda vasaka* Nees.

Family : Acanthaceae.

Habitat : The plant is found throughout the plains of India in the sub-Himalayan tracts up to 13,00 m, Sri Lanka, Burma and Malaya.

It is an evergreen, gregarious, stiff, perennial shrub growing on waste lands. It can be raised from seeds or cuttings.

Characters : Leaves are entire when fresh and crumpled or broken when dried. Shape is lanceolate to ovate-lanceolate, margin is slightly crenate to entire; apex is acuminate, base-tapering; petiole 2-8 cm long. The leaves are 10-30 cm long and 3-10 cm broad, venation is pinnate, midrib and 8-10 pairs of lateral veins, surface is glabrous or slightly pubescent, green when fresh, on drying the colour changes from brown to grey. Odour is characteristic and taste is bitter.

Chemical Constituents : Vasaka leaves contains alkaloids (0.25%) which include vasicine, vasicinone, 6-hydroxyvascine, 1-peganine (1-vasicine), betaine and vasakin as well as volatile oil, fat, resin, sugar, mucilage, adhatodic acid, triacontane, β-sitosterol and vitamin C. The oil is golden yellow which contains limonene.

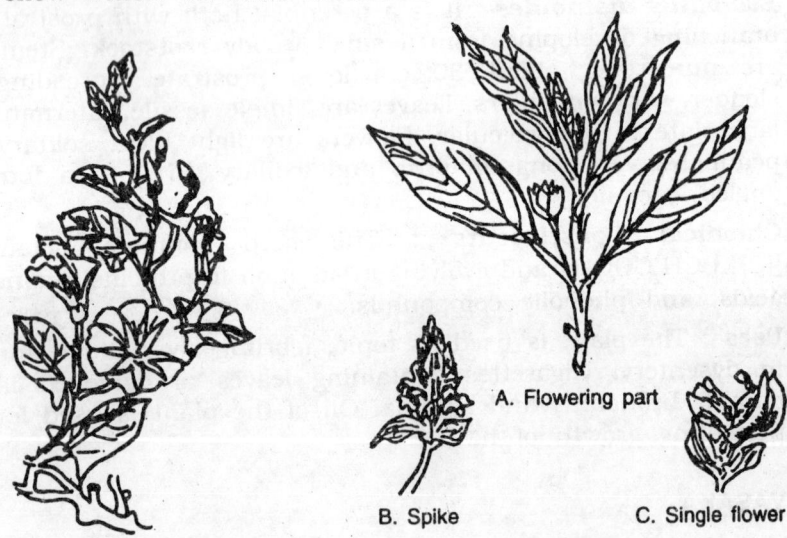

A. Flowering part

B. Spike   C. Single flower

Fig. 14.2. Shankhpushpi :   Fig. 14.3 Vasaka
Convolvulus pluricaulis

Uses : Vasaka is used to treat cold, cough, whooping-cough, chronic bronchitis and asthma, as sedative, expectorant, antispasmodic and as anthelmintic. The drug is employed in different forms, such as fresh juice, decoction, infusion and powder; also given as alcoholic extract and liquid extract or syrup. The dried leaf is smoked as a cigarette. It is also given along with other expectorants, and forms a part of several proprietary compounds. The cough is relieved and the sputum is liquefied and is easily expelled. The leaf-juice cures diarrhoea, dysentery and glandular tumor, and is given as emmenagogue. The powder is used as poultice on rheumatic joints, as counter-irritant on inflammatory swellings, on fresh wounds, urticaria and in neuralgia.

The flowers and fruits are bitter and aromatic and their uses are similar to those of the leaves. The flowers are also given to improve the circulation of blood and in ophthalmia. They contain vasicine, vasicinine, β-sitosterol, an essential oil, colouring compounds luteolin, quercetin and kaempferol, α-amyrin, tritriacontane, etc.

1-Vasicine (1-Peganine)   Vasicinone

PIPER LONGUM

Synonyms : Piplamul, Pippali.

Biological Source : The drug consists of transversely cut pieces of roots or underground stems or of fruits of *Piper longum* Linn.

Family : Piperaceae.

Habitat : The plant is native of Phillipine and found in hotter states of India, Sri Lanka and Malaya.

The plant is a slender aromatic climber with perennial woody roots.

P. longum is cultivated on a larger scale in limestone soil by layering of mature branches or by suckers planted at the beginning of the rainy season. The vines are well manured with cow dung cake and start bearing 3 or 4 years after planting. The spices are harvested in January, while still green and unripe, as they are most pungent at this stage. They are dried in the sun when they turn grey. The roots and thicker parts of stem are cut and dried.

Description : Drug occurs   0.5 to 2.5 cm long and

2-7 mm in diameter; shape is cylindrical, sraight or slightly curved and some with distinct swollen internodes, showing a number of leaf rootlets and scars. Colour is light brown, odour is characteristic, taste is bitter and pungent producing numbness on the tongue.

Fruits are also used as drug. They are small, ovoid, yellowish-orange, sunk in fleshy spikes which is 2.5 - 3.8 cm, ovoid long, erect, blunt, blackish-green; odour is aromatic and taste is pungent.

Chemical Constituents : Both roots and fruits have alkaloids like piperine, piperlonguminine, piplartine and piperlongumine. Fruits also contain volatile oil, resin, a waxy alkaloid N-isobutyl 2, 4-decadienamide, and sesamine.

The other constituents of the drug are triacontane, dihydrostigmasterol, reducing sugars and glycosides.

Uses : Both Piplamul and fruits are used for diseases of respiratory tract like cough, bronchitis, asthma, cold, etc; as counter-irritant and analgesic when applied locally for muscular pain and inflammation; internally as carminative, sedative, and general tonic.

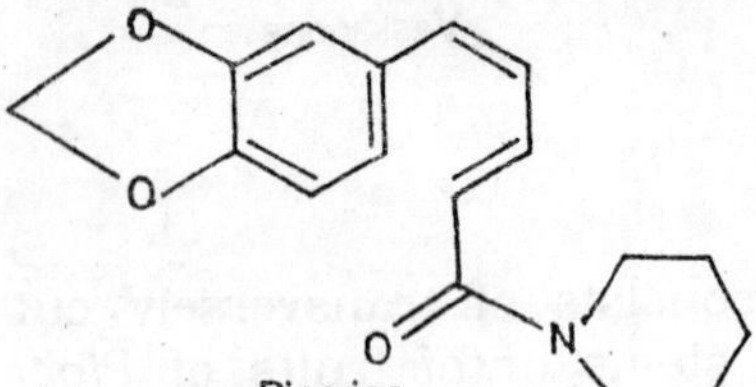

Piperine

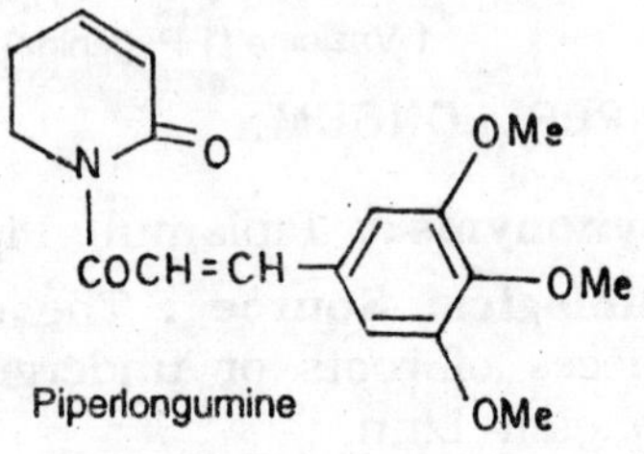

Piperlongumine

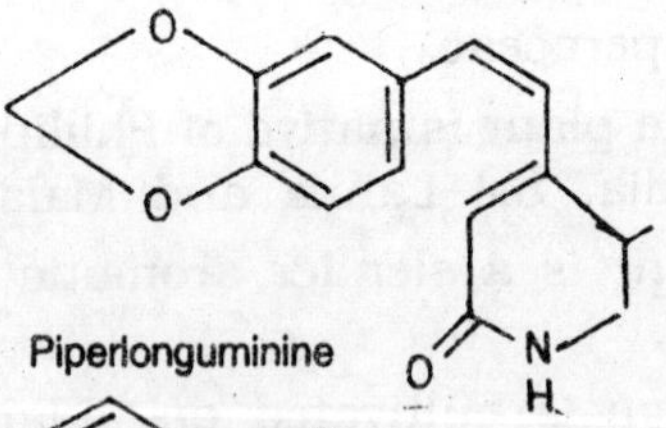

Piperlonguminine

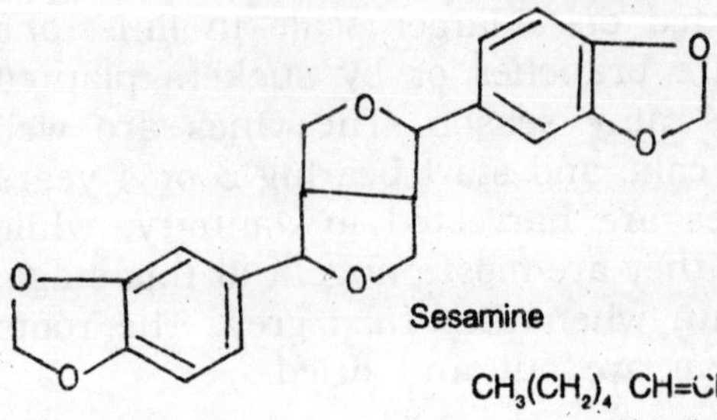

Sesamine

$$CH_3(CH_2)_4 \ CH=CH-CH=CH-CO-NHCH_2 \ CH \ (CH_3)_2$$
N-Isobutyl 2, 4-decadieamide

TYLOPHORA

Synonym : Anantmul.

Biological Source : The drug consists of dried leaves of *Tylophora Indica* (Burm f.) Merr (syn. *T. asthmatica* W. & A.) (Family Asclepiadaceae).

Habitat : The plant is a perennial branching climber with long fleshy roots. It grows widely in planes and hilly places of India up to altitude of 1,000 m in Bengal, Assam, Cachar, Orissa, Konkan, Kanara and Southern India.

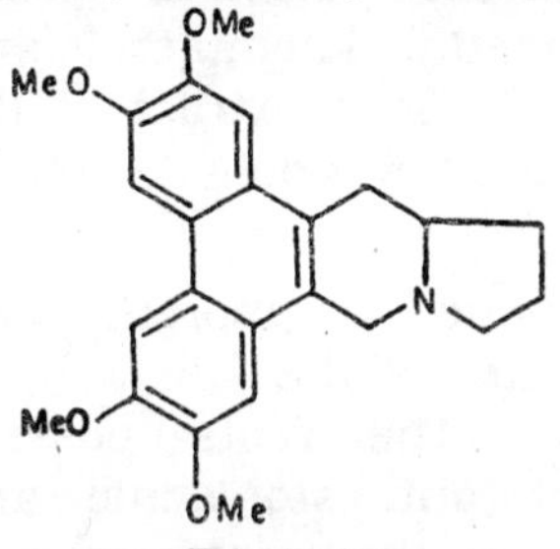

Tylophorine

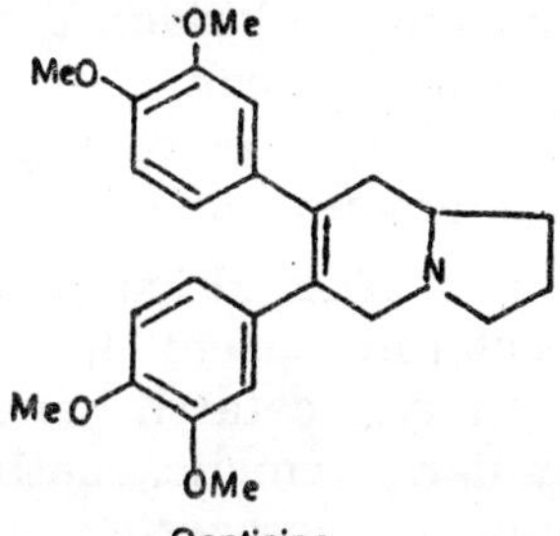

Septicine

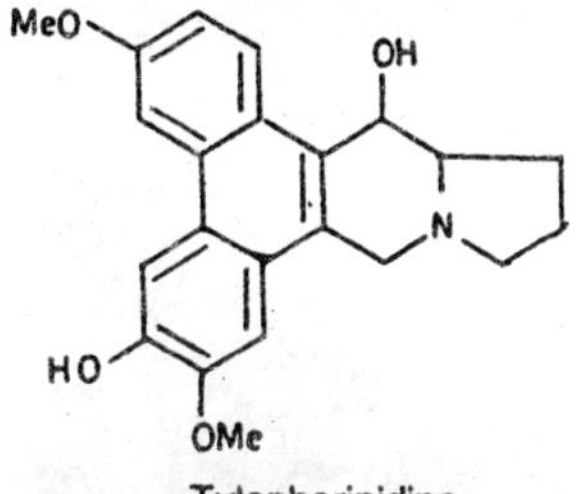

Tylophorinidine

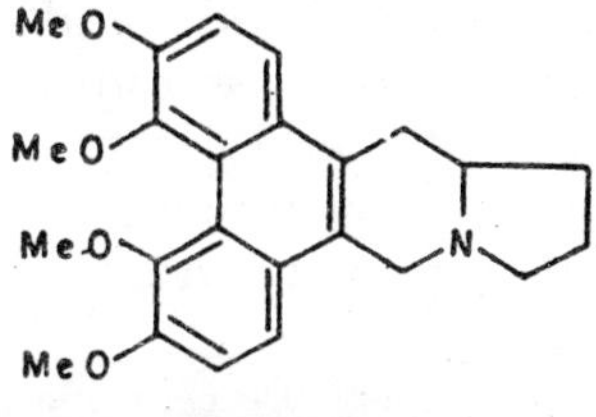

Tyloindicine A

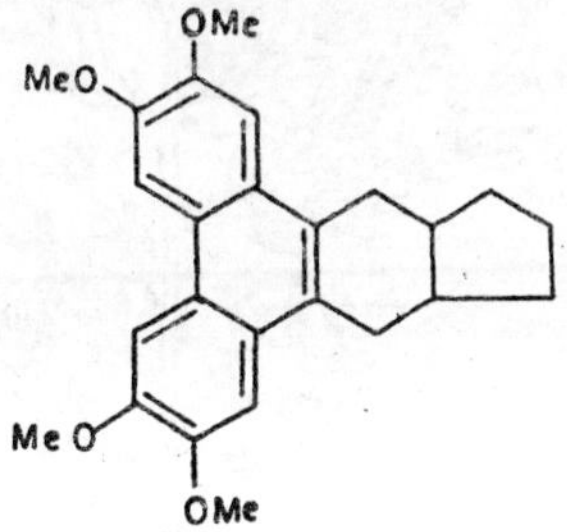

Tyloindane

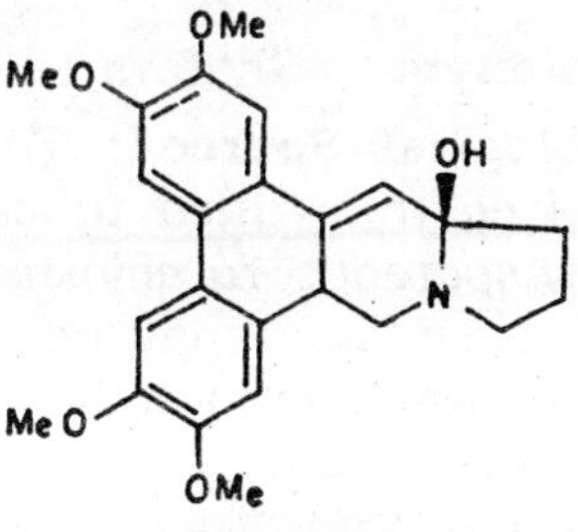

Tyloindicine G

Characters : Leaves are 5-10 cm. long, 2.5-5.7 cm wide, ovate or elliptic-oblong, acute or acuminate, often apiculate, glabrous, pubescent beneath, base usually cordate, petioles

6-13 mm long. The whole plant is of a pale yellow brown colour and has no marked odour but has a sweetish and subsequent acrid taste.

Chemical Constituents : The active constituents of *Tylophora indica* are phenanthroindolizidine alkaloids like tylophorine, tylophorinine, tylophorinidine and septicine. Recently some rare alkaloids, namely tyloindicines A, B, C, D, E, F, G, H, I and J have been isolated from *T. indica* aerial parts by the author. Apart from alkaloids the plant also contains cetyl alcohol, phytosterol, wax, resin, coutchone, pigments, tannin, glucose, calcium salts, potassium chloride, α-amyrin, quercetin, kaempferol and tyloindane. Steam distillation of an alcoholic extract of the air-dried root powder gave p-methoxysalicylaldehyde and a small amount of oil matter.

Uses : The dried leaves are emetic, diaphoretic and expectorant, useful in over-loaded states of the stomach, in dysentery, catarrh and as emetic. The roots possess stimulant, emetic, cathartic, expectorant, stomachic and diaphoretic properties and are used in the treatment of asthma, bronchitis, whooping cough, dysentery and diarrhoea. They are recommended in rheumatic and gouty pains. They possess bacteriostatic properties and are good natural preservative for foods.

SHATAVAR

Synonym : Shatavari.

Biological Source : The drug is derived from dried tuberous roots of *Asparagus racemosus* Willd. It has been found that the commercial 'Shatawar' may not be the root of *A. racemosus*.

Family : Liliaceae.

Habitat : The plant is a climber found all over India, especially in northern region.

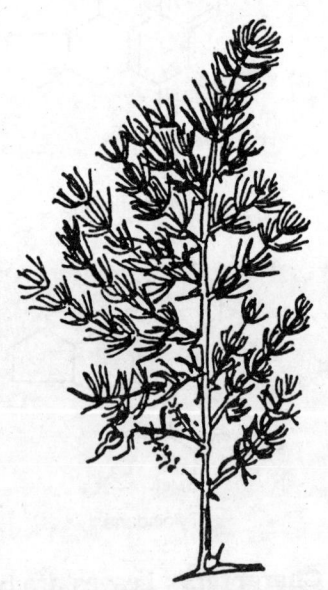

Fig. 14.4. Shatavar, *Asparagus racemosus.*

It is an extensively scandent, much-branched, spinous under-shrub, with tuberous, short rootstock bearing numerous fusiform, succulant tuberous roots. Stem is woody, whitish grey or brown armed with strong, straight or recurved spines.

The plants can be grown successfully in black cotton soil mixed with river sand. They can be propagated from adventitious roots which are dipped in liquid cow dung for 24 hours before planting. The sprouted saplings are transferred to beds. They require hoeing and weeding during the rainy season.

Morphology : The roots of A. *racemosus* are borne in a compact bunch and are fleshy, and spindle shaped. They are silvery white or light ash-coloured externally and white internally, smooth when fresh.

Macroscopy : The roots are peeled, dried, cylinclrical, fleshy tuberous, straight or slightly curved, tapering towards the base and swollen in the middle; white to buff in colour, length 5-10 cm; diameter 1-2 cm; fracture is irregular; longitudinal furrows and minute transverse wrinkles on upper surface. Drug is hard, swells in water; taste is bitter; lack a well-marked odour.

Glu - Glu - Glu - O
|
Rham

Shatavarin I

Chemical Constituents : The active constituents are steroidal saponins, viz. shatavarin I - IV (0.1 - 0.2%). The aglycone unit is sarsapogenin. In shatavarin I three glucose and rhamnose molecules are attached whereas shatavarin IV possesses two glucose and one rhamnose molecules.

Uses : Roots are refrigerant, demulcent, aphrodisiac, antiseptic, alterative, antidysenteric and galactagogue. Shatavarin I has antioxytocic property. In Ayurveda Shatavar is used to cure threatened abortion and safe delivery.

GOKHRU

Biological Source : In Ayurveda two types of Gokhru are used. The smaller or Chhota Gokhru is the dried ripe seeds of *Tribulus terrestris* Linn. (Family : Zygophyllaceae). The large or Bara Gokhru consists of dried ripe fruits of *Pedalium murex* Linn. (Fam. Pedaliaceae).

***Tribulus terrestris* (Chhota Gokhru) :** The plant is an annual, prostrate herb with yellow flowers growing throughout India up to 3600 m in Kashmir.

Morphology : The fruits are yellowish globose, diameter nearly 1.2 cm containing five woody, densely hairy, spiny cocci. Each coccus possesses two large sharp, pointed spines directed towards the apex. The other two smaller shorter spines are directed downwards. Each coccus contain several seeds.

Chemical Constituents : The fruits of *T. terrestris* contain saponins which produce diosgenin, ruscogenin and gitogenin on hydrolysis. The fruits also contain flavone glycosides, viz. kaempferol 3-rhamnoside and kaempferol 6"-p-coumaroyl 3-D-glucoside; traces of alkaloid, fixed oil, potassium nitrate, essential oil and resin.

Uses : The fruit has cooling, diuretic, tonic, aphrodisiac properties and used in painful micturition, calculus affections, urinary discharges and impotency. In the form of infusion it is useful as a diuretic in gout, kidney diseases and gravel.

Pedalium murex (Bara Gokhru)

Pedalium murex is an annual succulent herb found near seacoasts of Kathiawar, Gujarat, Konkan, Southern Peninsula, Sri Lanka and Africa. It is also found in Rajasthan, Punjab and Delhi in autumn session.

The plant is annual, diffuse, succulent herb. The fruits are four-sided, about 2 cm long, pyramid-ovoidal shape and tapering at the base and apex. Each fruit has four spines and it tapers into a hollow cylindrical tube at the base.

The fruits conain mucilage, fatty oil, resin, and an alkaloid.

The fruits have demulcent, diuretic, antiseptic, aphrodisiac and tonic properties and given for incontinence of urine, spermatorrhoea, nocturnal emission, dysuria, gonorrhoea and impotency.

BRAHMI

Synonyms : Indian pennywort; Mandooki.

Biological Source : Brahmi is the fresh or dried herb of *Centella asiatica* (L.) Urban (syn. *Hydrocotyle asiatica* Linn.) (Family Umbelliferae).

Habitat : The plant is found throughout India in marshy places up to 2,000 m; in Pakistan, Sri Lanka and Madagascar.

Morphology : It is herbaceous creeping herb with long prostrate reddish stem possessing long internodes and rooting at the nodes. Leaves are reniform or orbicular arising from each node of the stem, cupped, entire, crenate, glabrous on both sides; petioles are 7.5 - 15 cm long, channelled, glabrous, stipules short, sheathing base. Flowers are pink, sessile, umbel consisting of 3-4 flowers.

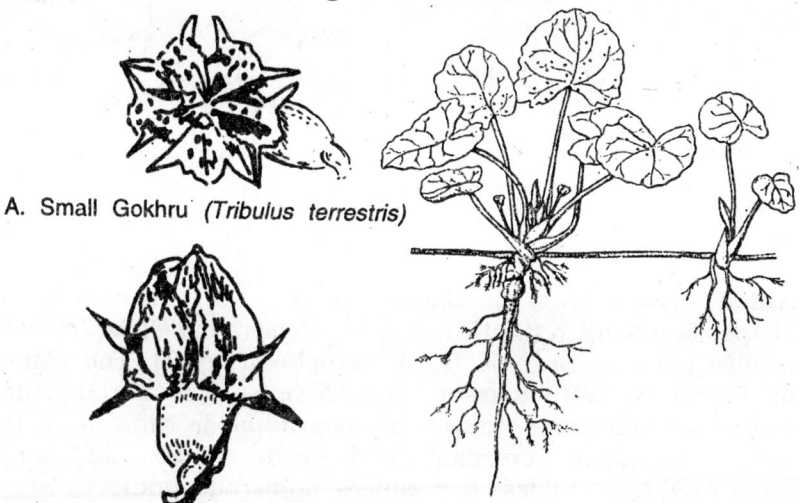

A. Small Gokhru *(Tribulus terrestris)*

B. Large Gokhru *(Pedalium murex)*

Fig. 14.5. Gokhru   Fig. 14.6. *Centella asiatica* (Brahmi)

Chemical Constituents : The drug contains triterpenoid saponin glycosides called asiaticoside, oxyasiaticoside, brahmoside, brahminoside and thankuniside. Sugar moieties are attached at carboxylic group. Hydrolysis of asiaticoside affords two molecules of glucose, one rhamnose and the aglycone asiatic acid. In addition to these the drug contains alkaloids, sterols (β-sitosterol, stigmasterol), tannins, amino acids (aspartic acid, glycine, glutamic acid, α-alanine and phenylalanine), and inorganic salts (chloride, sulphate, phosphate, iron, calcium, magnesium, sodium and potassium). Triterpenes reported in free state are brahmic acid, isobrahmic acid, betullic acid, indocentoic acid and asiatic acid. Mesoinositol and centellose have also been reported. Hydrolysis of thankuniside yields tritrerpenic acid, thankunic acid. A new triterpenic acid, medasiatic acid, isolated from Brahmi, has been identified as 2α, 3β, 6β - trihydroxyurs-12-enoic acid.

Uses : The plant has been used in diseases of skin, nerves and blood. Leaves are taken as tonic and for improving memory and useful in syphilitic skin diseases.

Asiaticoside

Medasistic acid

Allied drug : Herb of *Bacopa monnieri* (L.) Pennell (syn. *Herpestis monniera* (L.) H.B. & K. or *Moniera cuneifolia* Michx) is also used as Brahmi. (Fam. Scrophulariaceae). The plant is found in wet, marshy and damp places throughout India and, therefore, known as Jalbrahmi or Nirbrahmi. It is a succulent, creeping herb with 10-20 cm long stem rooting at nodes. It produces numerous branches and sessile, decussate leaves, 0.6-2.5 cm long, obovate, and oblong.

The drug contains alkaloids brahmine and herpestine, D-mannitol and saponins, bacosides A and B. The saponins on hydrolysis yield the same triterpenoid aglycone bacogenin A and sugars arabinose and glucose.

The plant is used as nervine tonic, diuretic and aperient and to treat asthma, epilepsy, insanity and hoarseness.

ARJUNA BARK

Synonyms : Arjuna (Sans.); Arjun (H).

Biological Source : Arjuna bark is the dried bark of *Terminalia arjuna* W. & A.

Family : Combretaceae.

Habitat : The plant is found throughout India.

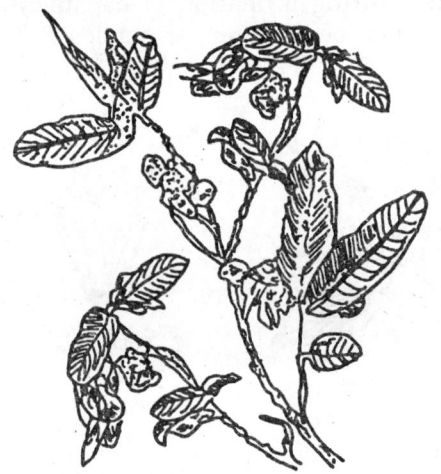

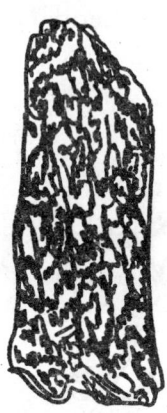

Fig. 14.7. *Terminalia arjuna* branch   Fig. 14.8 Arjuna bark

Arjuna is a large deciduous evergreen tree, 20-30 meters in height. Bark is collected and dried. It occurs in flat pieces of various sizes, 3-15 cm long, 1-10 cm wide, 3 mm - 1 cm thick; outer surface is smooth and grey-coloured; inner surface is striated and brown; fracture is short and fibrous; odourless, taste is astringent.

Chemical Constituents : Arjuna bark contains tannins (12%), β-sitosterol, triterpenoid saponins, arjunine, arjunetin, arjunolic acid, essential oil, reducing sugars, calcium salts and traces of aluminium and magnesium salts.

Uses : Arjuna bark is used as tonic, astringent, in heart diseases as a cardiac tonic, bilious afffections, diuretic, for sores and

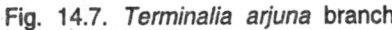

Arjunolic acid

as an antidote to poisons.. It has styptic, tonic, febrifugal and anti-dysenteric properties. The bark gives relief in hypertension.

CHIRATA

Synonyms : Chiretta; Chirayita; Bitter stick; East Indian Balmony.

Biological Source : Chirata is the entire dried plant of *Swertia chirata* Linn. collected during formation of capsules. It should contain about 1.3 per cent bitter principles.

Family : Gentianaceae.

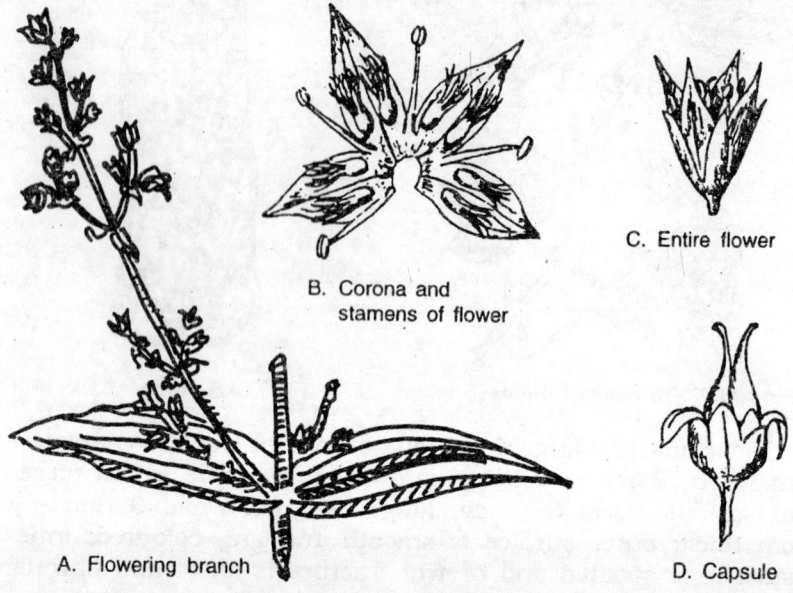

B. Corona and stamens of flower

C. Entire flower

A. Flowering branch

D. Capsule

Fig. 14.9. *Chirata*

The plant spread quickly from seed which is shed during October-November. The herb can be cultivated in suitable localities in the temperate Himalayas. The seeds, which are very small; should be sown in a nursery and the seedlings transplanted later in the field. Flowering occurs from July to October and the plants are collected when the capsules are fully formed. The stem forms the major portion of the drug which are 1 m long, brown or purplish brown, contains a large, continuous and easily separable pith. The drug is odourless, but it has an extremely bitter taste. The whole plant is medicinal but the root is the most powerful part. The root is generally small, 5-10 cm long, light brown, somewhat twisted and gradually tapering.

Habitat : The plant is found in temperate Himalayan region, 1300-3300 m, from Kashmir to Bhutan and Khasia Hills.

Characters : Chirata is a small, hairy, erect, annual herb. The stem is round, purple at the base and angular and yellowish brown at the upper side. The upper part is much branched. Leaves thin, opposite, unequal, sessile, decussatte, ovale oblong with 5-7 veins. Flowers are purple, solitary, calyx and corolla are of the same size. The fruits are ovate capsules. The drug is odourless and taste is very bitter.

Chemical Constituents : Chirata contains a bitter glycoside gentiopicrin; amarogentin, chiratin, ophelic acid and a xanthone, swerchirin.

Gentiopicrin   Amarogentin

Uses : Chirata is used as bitter tonic, ferbrifuge, stomachic and laxative. In excess dose it may cause nausea and oppresses the stomach.

The most important adulterant of Chirata is *Swertia angustifolia* which is distinguished by its inferior bitter tonic properties. The roots of *Rubia cordifolia* are also used as adulterant and distinguished by their purple colour. Green Chiratta *(Andrographis paniculata)* is also used as an adulterant.

PICRORHIZA

Synonyms : Kathi; Kuru (Hindi); Katvee.

Biological Source : It consists of dried rhizome of *Picrorhiza kurroa* Royle·ex Benth., cut into small pieces and freed from attached rootlets.

Family : Scrophulariaceae.

Habitat : The plant is common on the alpine Himalayas, from Kashmir to Sikkim, 3,000 to 5,000 meters.

Characters : It is low, hairy herb with a perennial woody bitter rhizome, 15-25 cm long. covered with dry leaf-bases. It occurs as pieces, 2-4 cm long and 0.3-1.0 cm in diameter. Scales at distant intervals are present; frequently small protuberances, which probably represent accessary buds, are observed both at the rhizomes and the stolones.

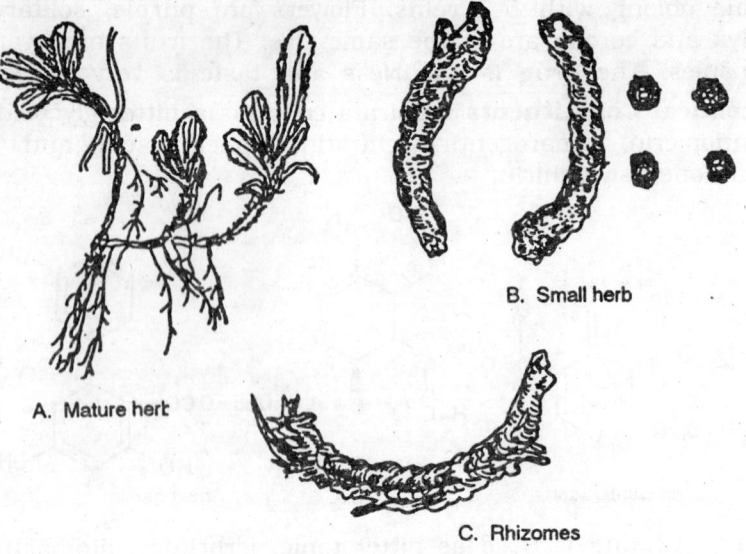

B. Small herb

A. Mature herb

C. Rhizomes

Fig. 14.10. *Picrorhiza kurroa*

The drug consists of small pieces. Colour is greyish-brown, light, cylindrical, straight or slightly curved, often with remains of aerial stem which is very dark brown and wrinkled longitudinally, upper and lower surfaces bear a few small root scars, numerous scale leaves and thin scars; odour-slightly unpleasant, taste-very bitter.

Chemical Constituents : The active constituents of Picrorhiza is picrorhizin, a glucoside which yields picrorhizetin and dextrose on hydrolysis. It also contains kutkin, a glucosidal bitter principle, picroside-I, picroside-II, picroside-III, D-mannitol, vanillic acid, kurrin, kutkiol, kutki-sterol, apocynin, phenolic glycosides picein and androsin, and seven cucurbitacin glycoside.

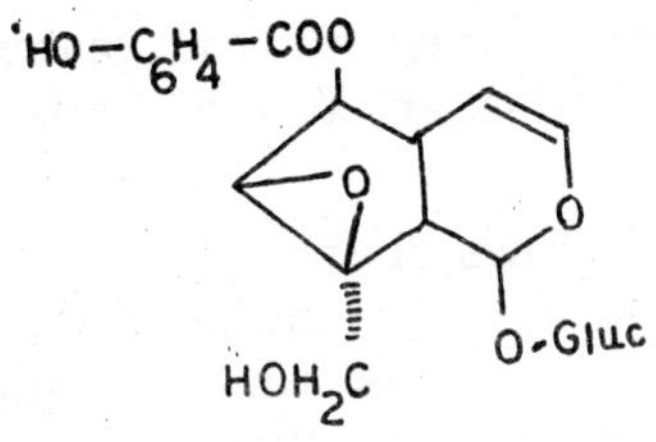

Picroside I

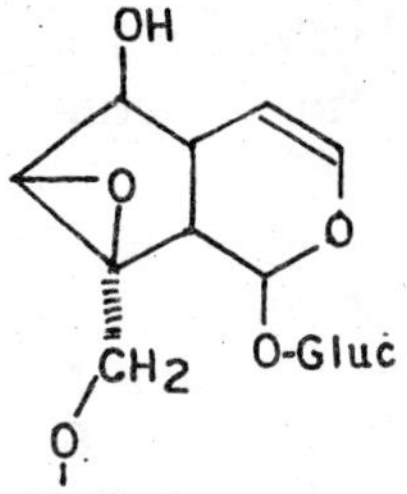

Vaniloyl
Kutoside

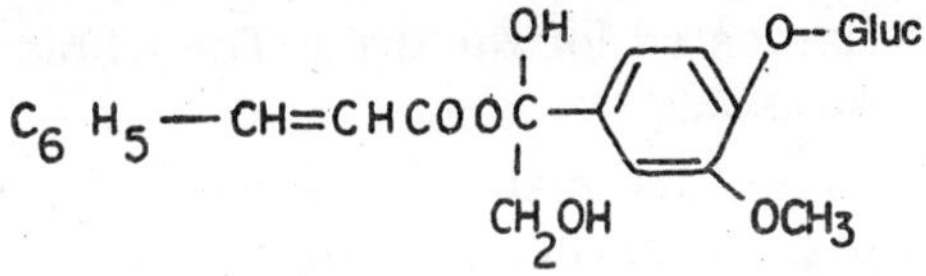

Kutkin

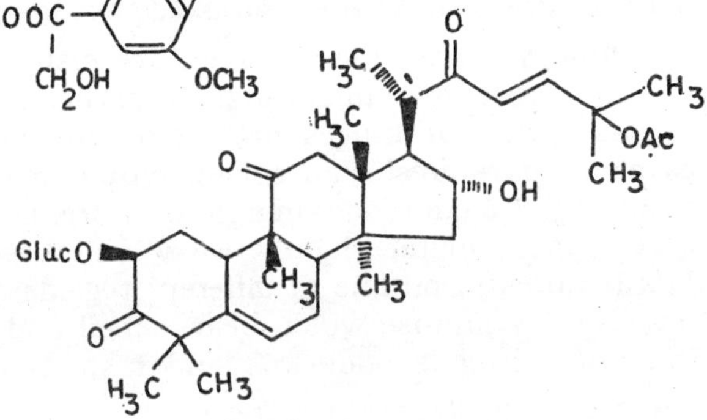

Cucurbitacin β-2-glucoside

Uses : Picrorhiza is bitter, cathartic, stomachic, used in fever and dyspepsia and in purgative preparations. It is reputed as an anti-periodic and cholagogue, as febrifuge including as antimalarial. Different types of jaundice are cured with Picrorhiza. It removes kidney stone, used as emmenagogue, emetic, abortifacient, antidote for dog-bite; externally it is used in skin diseases and improves eye-sight. It is a valuable bitter tonic almost as efficacious as Gentian. It is laxative in small doses and cathartic in large doses.

It is used as an adulterant or substituted for Indian Gentian *(Gentiana kurreo).*

KALMEGH

Synonyms : Andrographis, King of bitters, Chiretta; Bengal Chirata; Green Chirata; Kiryet (Hindi).

Biological Source : Kalmegh consists of leaves or entire aerial part of *Andrographis paniculata* Nees.

Family : Acanthaceae.

Distribution : The plant occurs thoughout the plains of India and sometimes cultivated. It is an annual herb, 1-3 ft in height.

The plant is gregarious and grows abundantly in moist, shady waste grounds. It prefers a sunny situation.The seeds are sown during May-June. The seedlings are transplanted at a distance of 60 cm × 30 cm. Two or three irrigations may be given during the dry period. It flowers during August-November, and the whole plant starts maturing during February-March when it is harvested for the drug. The whole plant is dried in shade and sold.

Morphology : The stem is erect, greenish brown, woody, 1-3 ft in height, and quadrangular particularly in the upper regions with four bulges arising on the four corners. The leaves are dark green, lanceolate, with a small winged petiole, 7 cm long, 2-5 cm broad, margin is entire, lamina is glabrous, apex is acuminate, slightly waxy and base tapering. The midrib varies in outline at different regions of the leaf. Stem branching is profuse which bears small and solitary flowers. The dried drug is odourless and taste is extremely bitter.

Chemical Constituents : The plant possesses kalmeghin, a bitter crystalline diterpene lactone, viz. andrographolide flavonoids and phenols.

The lactones isolated from Kalmegh are andrographolide, 14-deoxy-11-oxo-andrographolide, 14-deoxy-11, 12-didehydroandro-grapholide, 14-deoxyandrographolide and a non-bitter constituent, and neoandrographolide. From the leaves of Bangladesh plant homoandrographolide, andrographosterol, andrographane, andrographone, a wax and two esters have been isolated.

Andrographolide

The roots also contain a monohydroxytrimethylflavone, andrographin, a dihydroxy-dimethoxyflavone, a 5-hydroxy tetramethoxyflavone and panicolin.

Uses : Kalmegh has febrifuge, tonic, alterative, anthelmintic, astringent, anodyne, alexipharmic and cholagogue properties. It is useful in debility, cholera, diabetes, swelling, itches, consumption, influenza, piles, gonorrhea, bronchitis, dysentery, dyspepsia, fever and in weakness. A decoction of the plant is a blood purifier. It is used as a cure for torphid and jaundice. It forms the major constituent of the Ayurvedic drug *SG-I Switradilepa* which is effective in treating vitiligo - a dermatological disease. The pills prepared from macerated leaves and certain spices (e.g. Cardamom, Clove and Cinnamon) are given for stomach ailments of infants. A tincture of root is tonic, stimulant and aperient.

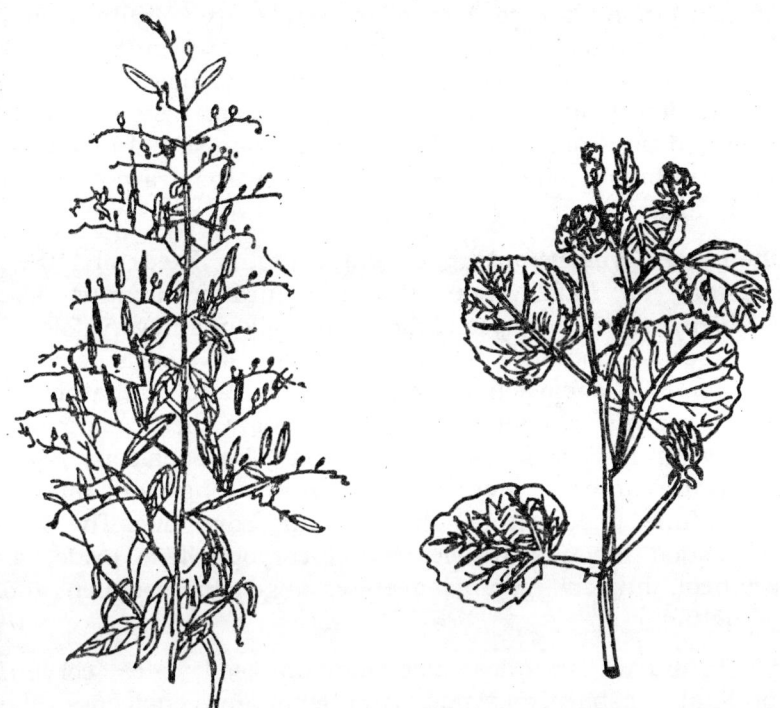

Fig. 14.11. Kalmegh :*Andrographis paniculata*

Fig. 14.12 *Psoralea corylifolia* twig (Bvbchi)

Sometimes, the drug is mixed with the genuine Chirata (*Swertia chirata*) but can be distinguished from the latter by the green colour of its stem, numerous erect, slender, opposite branches and its lanceolate, green leaves.

BAVCHI

Synonyms : Psoralea; Bavachi fruits; Bavachi seeds; Malaya tea.

Biological Source : The drug consists of the dried fruits and seeds of *Psoralea corylifolia* Linn.

Family : Leguminosae.

Natural Distribution : The plant grows widely throughout India.

Morphology : The plant is an annual herb attending a height of 60 cm to 1 m. Prominent groove of glands and white hairs are present on the stem and branches. Bluish purple flowers bloom from August to November. Fruits are minute, ovate, oblong, glabrous, rounded or mucronate and pitted; about 4 mm long, 2-3 mm broad; dark chocolate or black in colour, with pericarp attached to seeds; odourless, taste is bitter, acrid and unpleasant. Seeds are kidney shaped, 2-4 mm long, 2-3 mm broad, smooth exalbuminous with straw coloured hard testa.

Chemical Constituents : Bavchi contains fixed oil (10%), essential oil (0.2), resin and the furanocoumarins like psoralen, isopsoralen, psoralidin, isopsoralidin and corylifolean. The seeds contain flavonoids such as bavachalcone, bavachinin, isobavachalcone, bavachin and isobavachin; monoterpenoid phenol named bakuchiol. Other compounds isolated from the seeds are 4-O-methylbavachalcone, 7-O-methylbavachin, neobavaisoflavone, bavachromene, triacontane, β-sitosterol-D-glucoside and corylidine. The seed oil yielded limonene, α-elemene, β-caryophyllene oxide, 4-terpineol, linalool, geranyl acetate, angelicin, psoralen and bakuchiol.

Fruits of Psoralea also contain isoflavones corylin, corylinal, neobavaisoflavone, psoralenol and chalcones like 5-formyl-2, 4-dihydroxy-4'-methoxychalcone and bavachromanol.

Uses : Bavchi is used to cure leucoderma and other skin diseases. Seeds are used as stomachic, deobstruent, anthelmintic, diuretic, diaphoretic, febrile conditions, billious affections, in leprosy, psoriasis and inflammatory diseases of the skin and leucoderma. The drug in taken orally as well as locally applied in the form of paste or ointment. Psoralen and isopsoralen possess the curative action of Psoralea in leucoderma.

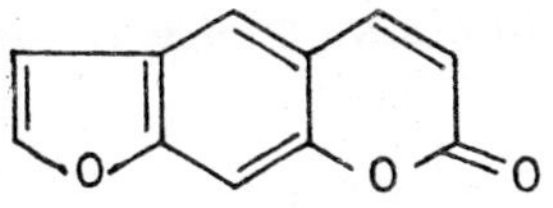

Psoralen

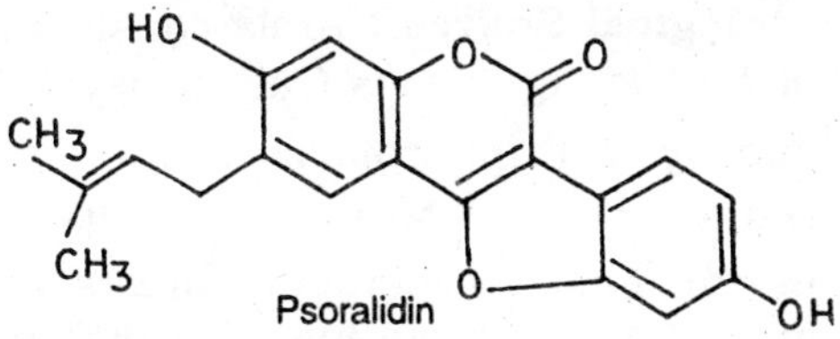

Psoralidin

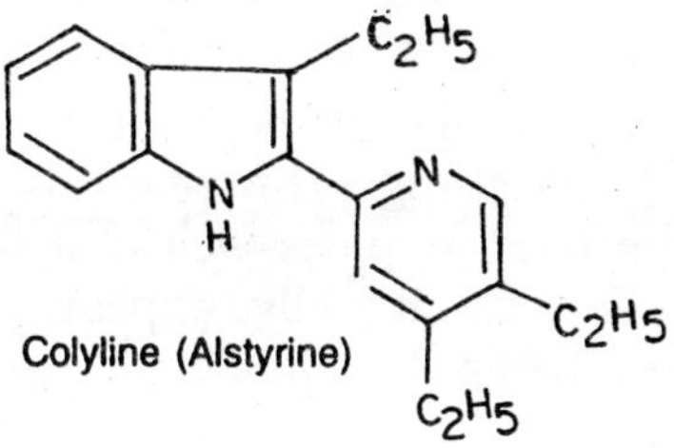

Colyline (Alstyrine)

ASHOKA BARK

Synonyms : Ashoka (Hindi); Asoka (Bengali).

Biological Source : Ashoka is the dried bark of stem of *Saraca indica* Linn.

Family : Leguminosae.

Habitat : Ashoka tree is found in central and eastern Himalayas, eastern Bengal, western Peninsula, Burma, Sri Lanka and Malaya.

Morphology : Ashoka bark is available in channeled pieces, 40 cm long, 4-6 mm wide and 5-8 thick. External surface is yellowish to grey, smooth with circular lenticels, transversly ridged or cracked. Inner surface is reddish-brown, smooth and longitudinally straight. Fracture is short and fibrous; odourless; taste is astringent and bitter.

Chemical Constituents : Ashoka bark contains tannins (6%), catechol, sterol, haemotoxyline, phlobaphenes, organic calcium compound and a ketosterol.

Uses : Ashoka bark is astringent, used in uterine affections, biliousness, dyspepsia, dysentery, colic, piles, ulcers, pimples and in menorrhagia (excessive mensturation) and leucorrhoea.

Adulterant : The bark of *Polyalthia longifolia* (Fam. Anonaceae), known as Asopalava bark, is used in place of Ashoka bark.

AMLA

Synonyms : Embelic myrobalan; Embelica, Indian goose berry.

Biological Source : Amla consists of the fresh or dried fruits of *Emblica officinalis* Gaertn. (syn. *Phyllanthus emblica* Linn).

Family : Euphorbiaceae.

Habitat : The plant is a middle-sized tree commonly found in the mixed deciduous forests of India, Sri Lanka, China and Malaya ascending to 1,500 m on the hills. It is often cultivated in gardens and homeyards.

Amla is usually propagated by seeds or by budding, cutting and inarching. The plant is sensitive to frost and drought. The tree coppices well and the coppice shoots grow vigorously. Flowers usually appear in the hot season and fruits ripen during the following winter.

Morphology : The fruit is drupe, fleshy globose, 1.5-2.5 cm in diameter, smooth, shiny with light coloured specks. It is distinctly marked in six lobes. The fruit is green when tender but the colour changes to light yellow or brick red on maturity. A minute depression is present at one end which is left due to removal of peduncle. The taste is sour and astringent giving feeling of sweetness afterwards.

Chemical Constituents : The principal chemical constituent of Amla is vitamin C (650 - 900 mg/100 g). The fruit juice contains about 20 times more vitamin C than orange juice. It also contains tannins (5%), glucose, pectin, and minerals like iron, phosphorus and calcium. Tannins are the mixture of gallic acid, ellagic acid and phyllembin. The presence of the tannins prevents the oxidation of the vitamin.

Uses : Fruit has acrid, cooling, refrigerant, diuretic and laxative properties. Dried fruit is useful in haemorrhage, diarrhoea, diabetes and dysentery. In combination with iron it is used to treat anaemia, jaundice and dyspepsia. Fermented liquor prepared from the fruit is used in jaundice, dyspepsia and cough. It has antibacterial, antifungal and antiviral activities. Amla is an ingredient of the Ayurvedic formulation 'Triphala' and 'Chyavanprash'. Triphala is a laxative and used to treat headache, biliousness, dyspepsia, constipation, piles, enlarged liver and ascites. Acute bacillary dysentery is cured by drinking a sherbet of Amla with lemon juice. The exudation from incisions on the fruit is used as an external application for inflammation of the eye. The fruits are also used in the preparation of writing inks and hair dyes. The dried fruit is detergent and is used as shampoo for the head. A fixed oil extracted from the fruit is reported to promote hair growth.

BAHERA

Synonyms : Beleric Myrobalan; Bahira (Sanskrit).

Biological Source : Bahera is the dried ripe fruit of *Terminalia belerica* Roxb.

Family : Combretaceae.

Habitat : The plant is found throughout the forests of India, Burma and Sri Lanka below elevations of about 1000 m except in dry and acrid regions of Sind and Rajasthan.

Bahera is a large handsome, deciduous tree, with characteristic bark, 20-35 m high and 2-3 m in girth.

The good seed crop, high germinative capacity of the healthy seeds and their quick and easy germination are favourable for the natural regeneration. The plant can be raised in fields by direct sowing. The tree is not subjected to fungal attack of any consequence.

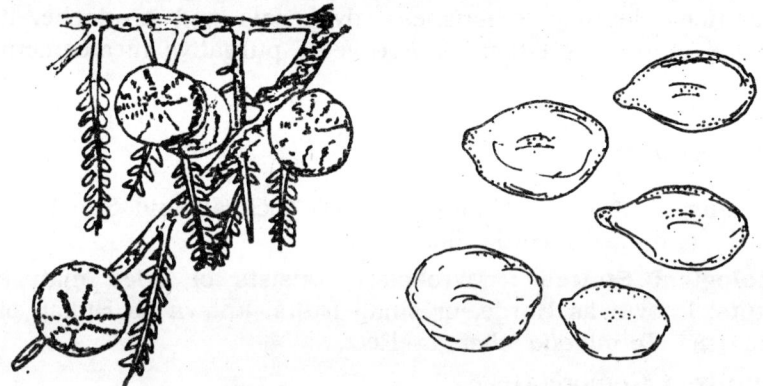

Fig. 14.13. Amla fruits   Fig. 14.14. Bahera fruits

Morphology : Fruits are globular drupe, 1.3-2.5 cm in diameter, obscurely 5-angled, ovoid, suddenly narrowing into a short stalk. Outer surface in velvety, irregularly wrinkled containing five well defined longitudinal ridges. The upper end is depressed and a prominent, sound scar of pedicel is present at one end of the fruit. Fruit is very hard and broken surface is yellow in colour. The fruit is odourless and taste is astringent.

Chemical Constituents : Bahera contains tannins (20-25%), phyllemblin, β-sitosterol, mannitol, glucose, fructose, rhamnose, fixed oil (30-40%) and hydrocarbons such as tetratriacontane, ditriacontane-2-ol, tritriacontan-9-one and n-tritriacontane. Tannin component is the mixture of gallic acid, ellagic acid, ethyl gallate, galloyl glucose and chebulaginic acid. A hexahydroxy-diphenic acid ester has been reported by the author which on hydrolysis yielded two moles of hexahydroxydiphenic acid. The fixed oil contains the esters of palmitic, stearic, oleic and linoleic acids.

Hexahydroxydiphenic acid ester

Uses : The fruit has bitter, astringent, tonic, laxative, antipyretic activity and is used in piles, dropsy, dysentery, diarrhoea, leprosy, biliousness, dyspepsia and headache. It is one of the ingredient of Ayurvedic purgative medicament 'Triphala'.

MYROBALAN

Synonyms : Harar (Hindi), Haritaki (Bengali and Sanskrit), Hirdo (Gujarati); Hirda (Marathi).

Biological Source : Myrobalan consists of dried mature fruits, known as Harde, or small fruits, known as Himaj, of the tree *Terminalia chebula* Retz.

Family : Combretaceae.

Habitat : The plant is found abundantly in north India from Kangra and Kumaon to Bengal and southern region in Madhya Pradesh, Maharastra, Gujarat and Travancore as well as in higher forests of the Bombay Ghats, Satpuras, Belgaum and Kanara.

The fruits ripen from November to March, depending upon the locality, and fall soon after ripening. They are dried and the seeds stored for one year. The germination capacity of the seeds is low due to the presence of hard cover and the seeds require pre-treatment.

Characters : The fruit is a drupe, ellipsoidal, ovoid; yellow to orange brown in colour; 2 - 3.5 cm long, 1.3 - 2.5 cm wide, longitudinally wrinkled; carpel, 5-6 ribbed longitudinally; hard and strong; seeds are light yellow, 1.5 - 2.5 cm long and rough. Odour is slight and taste is astringent and bitter.

Chemical Constituents : Myrobalan contains hydrolysable tannins (30-40%), purgative compounds like anthraquinones, fixed oil containing esters of palmitic, oleic and linoleic acids, astringent compound chebulinic acid; ellagic acid, gallic acid and resin.

The tannins in Myrobalan belong to the pyrogallol type. They are very complex. The hydrolysable tannins, chebulagic acid, chebulinic acid, and corilagin are the major tannin constituents. On hydrolysis they form chebulic acid, 3, 6-digalloylglucose, ellagic acid, gallic acid, and β-glucogallin. The carbohydrates present in Myrobalan are : glucose, sorbitol, fructose, sucrose and gentiobiose. Eighteen typical amino acids are also present in addition to phosphoric, succinic, quinic, shikimic, dihydroshikimic and dehydroshikimic acids. During maturation of the fruits, the amount of tannin decreases whereas the acidity increases.

Uses : Myrobalan is astringent, laxative, and alterative; used externally as a local application to chronic ulcers and wounds and as a gargle in stomatitis. Finely powdered drug is used as a dentifrice and considered useful in carious teeth, bleeding and ulcerations of the gums. Myrobalan

Chebulic acid

in combination with Amla *(Emblica officinalis)* and Bahera *(T. belerica)* forms the well known Ayurvedic preparation 'Triphala', which is used as laxative and stomach disorders.

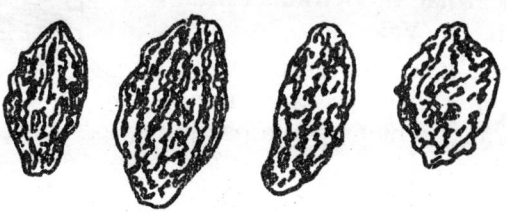

Fig. 14.15. Myrobalan fruit

JATAMANSI

Synonyms : Indian Spike Nard; Nard.

Biological Source : Jatamansi consists of the dried rhizome of *Nardostachys jatamansi* DC.

Family : Valerianaceae.

Geographical Source : The plant is found in the alpine Himalayas, 4,000 - 5,000 meters, extending eastwards and Kumaon to Sikkim and Bhutan.

Characters : Jatamansi is a perennial herb containing a cylindrical rhizome covered with brown to deep greyish fibres, length is 2.5 - 7 cm, diameter 0.5 - 3 cm. Fibres are produced by an accumulation of skeletons of the leaf bases. Removal of the leaf bases, aerial parts and adventitious roots show the presence of rough surface with transverse rings. The rings indicate the scars of nodes, leaf bases and the adventitious roots. Internal colour is reddish brown. Fracture is easy and splintery. Adventitious roots are thin, branched and red to brown in colour. Odour is slight and aromatic and taste is acrid, slightly bitter and aromatic.

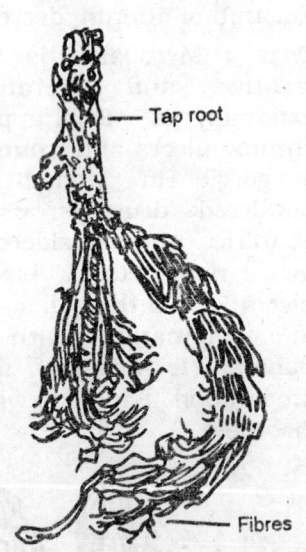

Chemical Constituents : Volatile oil of Jatamansi possesses an alcohol and its isovaleric ester, a saturated bicyclic sesquiterpene ketone, named jatamansone, and jatamansic acid.

Uses : Jatamansi has aromatic, bitter, tonic, stimulant, spasmolytic, and antiseptic properties. It is employed for the treatment of epilepsy, hysteria, convulsive affections, in intestinal colic, palpitation of heart, high blood pressure, cardiac arrhythmias and substituted for Valerian.

Adulterant : It is adulterated with rhizome of *Selinum vaginatum* (Umbelliferae), which contains a volatile oil.

— Tap root

— Fibres

Fig. 14.16. Jatamansi

BANAFSHA

Biological Source : Banafsha consists of dried flowers or aerial parts with or without flowers of *Viola odorata* Linn.

Family : Violaceae.

Geographical Distribution : The plant is a herb, 30 cm in height found in Kashmir up to 1,700 - 2,000 meters height. It is planted in many hill stations.

It arises from a rootstock. The plant is very variable, and several single and double-flowered types are grown for ornament. It can easily be cultivated in the hilly areas of North India; in the plains, the plants do not flower freely and are grown only in winter. The plant grows well in a cool and moist climate, but exposure to heavy rain is fatal to blooming. Propagation is by division, cuttings or seeds. The plants are repotted once or twice a year. The old plants are removed once in 4-5 years.

The drug, Banafshah, is available in commerce in three forms : (1) the dried aerial parts of the herb, viz. the stems, leaves and flowers *(Kashmiri Banafshah)*, (ii) only the dried flowers *(Gul-i-Banafshah)* and (iii) the aerial parts without flowers *(Berg-Banafshah)*.

Morphology : Herb is glabrous or pubescent; leaves tufted, broadly ovate-cordate, crenate, stalked, stipulses persistent. Flowers irregular, 2-sexual, noding, on axillary stalk, usually solitary, deep violet with a white base, sweet scented. Capsules ovoid, opening horizontally by 3 boat-shaped valves, often purple.

Chemical Constituents : Flowers contain a volatile oil, rutin, cyanin, glycoside of methyl salicylate and an emetic principle, called violin, which is acrid and bitter. The main components of the essential oil are α- and β-irones and α- and β-ionones. The ketones are responsible for the typical odour of the flower. Leaves possess a delightful volatile oil, an alkaloid, colouring matter, friedelin, β-sitosterol and a straight chain alcohol.

The presence of methyl salicylate, alkaloid violine, a glycoside violaquercitrin and a saponin has been reported in the roots.

The stem-violatile oil (4-12%) consists of 2, 6-nonadien-1-al as the major component (30-50%), 2, 6-nonadien-1-ol, n-hexanol, n-hexenol, n-heptenol, n-octenol, eugenol, benzyl alcohol, acids like propionic, enanthic (heptanoic), palmitic, salicylic, octanoic and octenoic acids.

Adulteration : Banafsha is adulterated with other *Viola* species, viz. *V. biflora, V. canescens, V. cinerea, V. pilosa* and *V. sylvestris.*

Uses : Banafsha is valued as an expectorant, diaphoretic, febrifuge, antipyretic and diuretic and as a laxative in bilious affections. The flowers are credited with emollient and demulcent properties and are used to treat coughs, sore throat, hoarseness, and ailments of infants. Petals are made into a syrup and used as a remedy for infantile disorders. The herb is used in homoeopathy to treat diseases of skin and eyes and for relief from pain in the ear. In folk medicine, it is used as a blood-purifier.

TULSI

Biological Source : Tulsi is the dried leaves of *Ocimum sanctum* Linn.

Family : Labiatae.

Geographical Distribution : The plant is cultivated throughout India especially in Hindu houses and temples for worship.

Macroscopy : Tulsi is an annual herb, 30-60 cm high, with much branched stems. The branches are generally purplish, sub-quadrangular and covered with soft hairs.

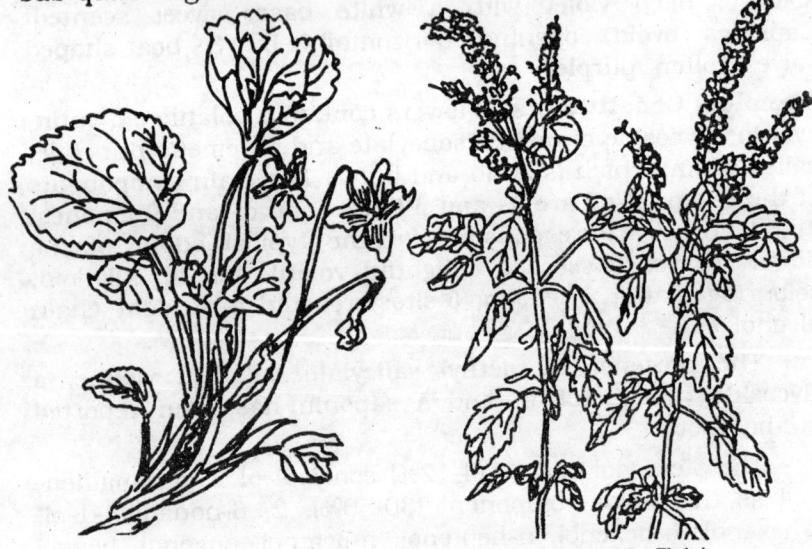

Fig. 14.17. Banaisha : *Viola odorata*   Fig. 14.18. Tulsi : *Ocimum sanctum*

Leaves are simple, elliptical, oblong obtuse or acute, 2-5 cm long 1.5-3.2 cm wide, margin entire or serrate, base obtuse or acute; petiole slender, 1.3-2.5 cm long, hairy surface, pubscent on both sides. Flowers are verticillate, in racemes, 15-20 cm long in close whorls. Odour and taste are aromatic and sharp.

Chemical Constituents : Leaves contain 0.7% of volatile oil. The prominent constituents of the essential oil are eugenol (71%), methyleugenol (20%), carvacrol (3%), and caryophyllene (1.7%). The oil of species grown in Phillipines contains methyl chavicol, cineole and linalool.

Uses : Leaves have expectorant, diaphoretic, antiperiodic, anticatarrhal, antiseptic and spasmolytic properties and are used in catarrh, bronchitis, cold, cough, fever and gastric disorders. The leaves have been employed as aromatic, carminative, stimulant and flavouring agent. Infusion of leaves is used as stomachic in gastric disorders of children and in hepatic affections. Dried powdered leaves are taken as snuff in ozena. Seeds are demulcent and given in disorders of the genito-urinary system. The plant is also used in snake-bite and scorpion-sting.

Methyl eugenol

Carvacrol

NEEM

Synonyms : Nim; Nimba (Sans.); Limba (Marathi, Gujarati); Vepa (Telgu).

Botanical Source : Neem is the fresh or dry leaves and seed oil of *Azadirachta indica* J. Juss. (syn. *Melia indica* Bran. or *M. azadirachta* Linn).

Family : Meliaceae.

Habitat : Neem tree is habitated in south-east Asia, India, Andamans, Pakistan, Sri Lanka, Burma, Malaya, Indonesia, Japan, tropical regions of Australia and Africa.

Characters : Neem is a large glabrous tree, 10-20 m high with a straight trunk and long spreading branches. Leaves are imparipinnate, alternate, existipulate, 3-6 cm long on long slender petioles; leaflets 7-17; alternate or opposite, very shortly stalked, 1-1.5 cm long, ovate-lanceolate, attenuate at the apex, unequal at the base, the upper half much longer than the lower and the leaflet in consequence more or less falcate, coarsely and bluntly serrate, smooth and dark green. Odour is typical and taste is bitter.

The fruit is an ovoid, bluntly pointed, smooth drupe, green when young and unripe, yellow to brown when mature and ripe, with a very scanty pulp and a hard bony endocarp. The seed is solitary with a thick testa and embryo with foliaceous cotyledons in the axis of scanty endosperm.

The seeds contain fixed acrid bitter oil (23-31%), deep greenish-yellow to brown in colour, extracted from the seeds by pressure; sp. gr. 0.91; soluble in ether, chloroform; practically insoluble in alcohol and water, odour of garlic, bitter taste.

Chemical Constituents : The leaves contain nimbin, nimbinene, 6-desacetylnimbinene, nimbandiol, nimbolide, quercetin, β-sitosterol, ascorbic acid, n-hexacosanol, nonacosane and amino acids.

The fruits contain gedunin, 7-deacetoxy-7α-hydroxygedunin, azadiradione, azadirone, 17β-hydroxyazadiradione, 17-epiazadiradione and nimbiol.

The seeds contain six tetranortriterpenoids, viz 1-methoxy-1, 2-dihydroepoxyazadirone, 1, 2-diepoxyazadiradione, 7-acetylneotrichilenone, 7-desacetyl-7-benzoylazadiradione, 7-desacetyl-7-benzoylepoxyazadiradione and 7-desacetyl-7-benzoylgedunin. They also contain azadirachtin.

Kernels yield a greenish yellow to brown, acrid, bitter fixed oil (23.5%) having a strong, disagreeable odour resembling garlic. The fatty acid composition of the oil is as : myristic (0.2%), palmitic (16.2), stearic (14.6), arachidic

Nimbin

Nimbidinin

(3.4), oleic (56.6) and linoleic (9%). The component glycerides are : palmitodistearin, oleopalmitostearin, óleodistearin, palmito-oleolinolein, palmitodiolein, stearo-oleolinolein, stearodiolein and linoleodiolein. The oil also contains 2% bitter principles which include nimbidin, nimbidinin, nimbin, nimbinin and nimbidol.

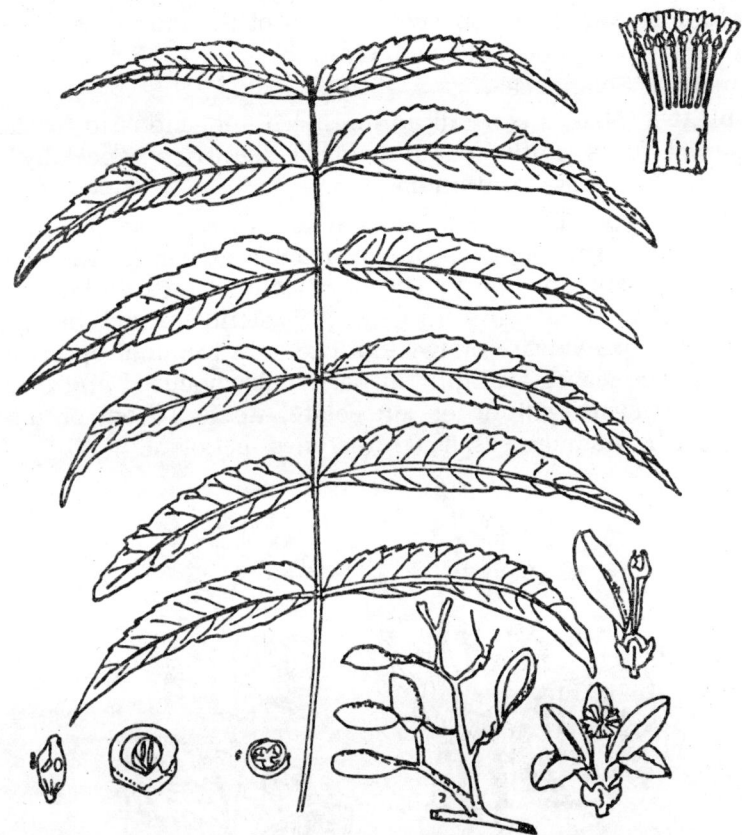

Fig. 14.19. Neem : *Azadirachta indica.*

Uses : Neem oil is stimulant, antiseptic, alterative and used in rheumatism and skin diseases. Leaves as poultice are applied to boils. Neem oil is also used in the manufacture of oleic and stearic acids. Leaf juice is given in worms, jaundice and in skin diseases. Paste of the leaves is used externally in cases of small-pox.

The tender leaves along with *Piper nigrum* are used in intestinal helminthiasis. The paste of leaves is useful in ulceration of cow-pox. Fresh, mature leaves along with the seeds of *Psoralea corylifolia* and *Cicer arietinum* are used to prepare an effective medicine for leueoderma. The leaves are used as insect-repellent, anti-viral and antifungal.

TOBACCO

Synonyms : Leaf Tobacco: Tamaku (Hindi).

Biological Source : Tobacco consists of the cured and dried leaves of *Nicotiana tabacum* Linn.

Family : Solanaceae.

Habitat : Tobacco is a tall annual herb indigenous to tropical America. It is cultivated in tropical countries especially in Brazil, Sri Lanka and India.

Characters : The stem is · simple, giving rise to large, pubescent, ovate, entire, simple, decurrent leaves; the veins are prominent and hairy. The flowers are long tubular, pink or reddish, sepals (5), united, persistent, funnel or cup-shaped, lobes valvate or twisted, occur in terminal spreading cymes. The leaves are hung in barns, slowly cured and dried. They are ovate, elliptic or lanceolate, up to 10 cm or more in length, usually sessile, sometimes petiolate.

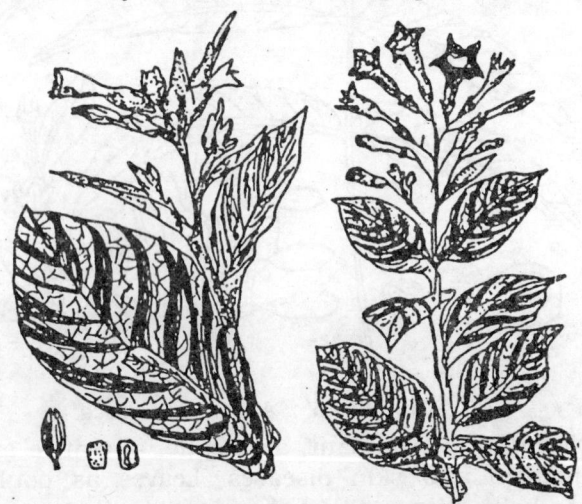

Fig. 12.20. *Nicotiana tabacum* flowering branches.

Cultivation : Tobacco, introduced into India by Portuguese in 17th century, is propagated by seeds raised in nursery beds. Transplanting to the fields is done by hand on a rainy day or after irrigating the field. Tobacco is sensitive to the physical and chemical properties of the soil. The best soil is open, well drained and aerated. It requires 100-120 frost-free days with an average temperature of 27° to mature. Nitrogen is required for the development of leaves. Phosphate application improves the size of leaf and promotes uniform ripening. Plants are topped when they are 90-100 cm high or 5-6 weeks old. Tobacco is cured in the sun.

Chemical Composition : Tobacco contains several pyridine alkaloids (4-6%) of which nicotine (0.6-9%) is the most important. The other basic components are nicotyrine, nicotimine, 1-nornicotine, d-nornicotine, piperidine, pyrrolidine, anabasine, anatabine, etc. Tobacco contains 25-50% carbohydrates, mainly sucrose, starch, pectins, cellulose, and lignin. Dextrin, maltose, stachyose, raffinose, rhamnose, ribose, inositol and sorbitol have been identified. Tobacco contains a high percentage of organic acids (~20%), mainly malic, citric acid and oxalic acids. Other acids identified are maleic, fumaric, lactic, malonic, terephthalic, succinic, acetic, methylvaleric, glyceric, crotonic, propionic, methyl ethyl acetic, benzoic and 2-furoic acids. Palmitic, oleic, linoleic and linolenic acids are also reported. Polyphenolic compounds like rutin, chlorogenic acid, quinic acid, shikimic acid, quercitrin, iso-quercitrin and its 7-glucoside, scopolin, aesculetin and its 7-glucoside, and kaempferol glycosides are present. The phenolic compounds reported are caffeic acid, melilotic acid, phenol, guaiacol, eugenol, iso-eugenol, p-allylcatechol, m-cresol and o-hydroxyacetophenone. Nearly sixty phenolic compounds have been distinguished in the extract of flue cured leaf. In addition to these, Tobacco contains resins, paraffins, amino acids, enzymes mineral contents, vitamins, sterols and some other compounds.

Uses : Tobacco is sedative, narcotic, emetic, antiseptic, used in rheumatic swelling, skin diseases and for insect poisoning. It is widely used for smoking and as agricultural insecticide. Tobacco snuff is useful in nasal polypi, nasal catarrh, headache, chronic giddiness and fainting. Its excessive use produces dispepsia, chronic inflammation of bronchial mucous membrane, nervous depression, diseases of liver, sleeplessness, general anaemia, loss of vision or blindness, weakness, cancer, throat troubles, mental fatigue and cardiac diseases.

GUGGAL

Synonyms : Indian bdellium, Salai-gogil.

Biological Source : Guggal is a gum-resin obtained by incision of the bark of *Commiphora mukul* (H. & S.) Engl. (syn. *Balsamodendron mukul* Hook. ex Stocks).

Family : Burseraceae.

Geographical Source : The tree grows in Sind, Rajasthan, Bengal, South India, Maysore and Baluchistan.

Collection : Guggal tree is small, 1.2-1.8 m high, branches slightly ascending. It is sometimes planted in hedges. The ash coloured bark comes off in rough flakes exposing the underbark. Each plant yields about one kilogram of the product which is collected in cold season.

Characters : Guggal occurs as yellowish viscid, brown tears; or in fragment pieces, mixed with hairy stem, pieces of bark; colour brownish dark to golden yellow. It hardens very slowly. With water it forms a milky emulsion with terebinthinate odour, but fainter. Taste is bitter aromatic.

Chemical Constituents : Oleo-gum resin of guggal contains gum (32%) and essential oil (1.45%). The drug also contains sterols (guggulsterols I, II and III, guggulsterone), sugars (sucrose, fructose), amino acids, camphorene, cembrene, allylcembrol, and flavonoids (viz. quercetrin and its glycosides) and ellagic acid.

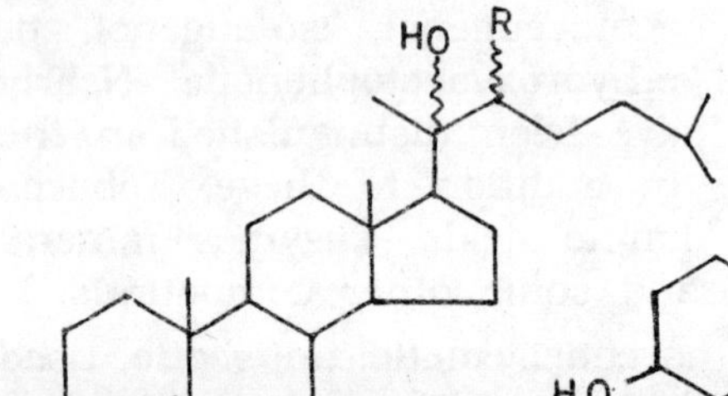

Guggulsterol I (R = OH)
Guggulsterol III (R = H)

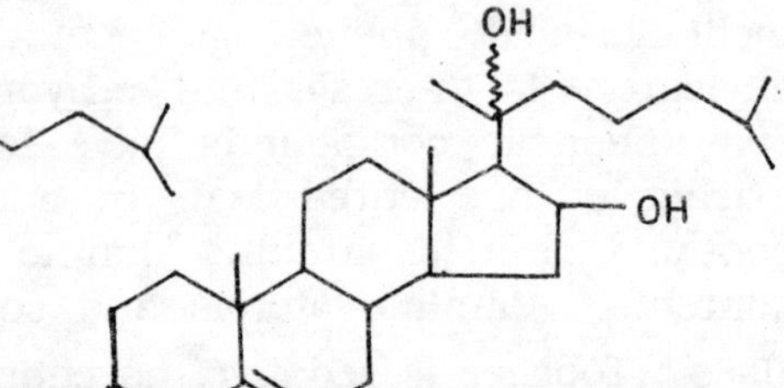

Guggulsterol II

Uses : The gum resin in astringent, antirheumatic, antiseptic, expectorant, aphrodisiac, enriches the blood, demulcent, aperient, and emmenagogue. It is used in the form of a lotion for indolent, as a gargle in teeth diseases, chronic tonsilitis and ulcerated throat; as a stomachic, intestinal disinfectant in chronic

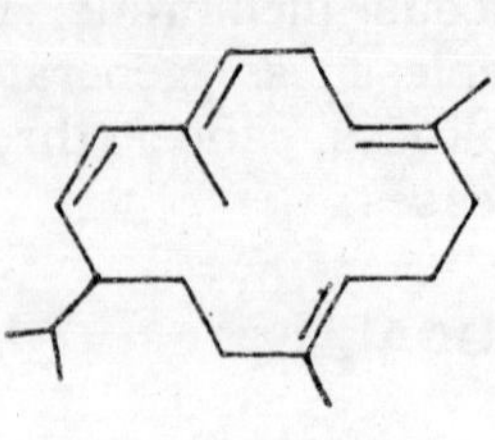

Guggulsterol II

catarrh of the diarrhoea. It is believed to stimulate the appetite, improves the general condition, reduces fever and secretion from diseased surfaces. It is a valuable aphrodisiac and has marked antisuppurative properties. Like all oleoresin it causes an increase of leucocytes in the blood and stimulates phagocytosis. It acts as a diaphoretic, expectorant, diuretic and a uterine stimulant. The resin is usd in the form of a lotion for indolent ulcers and as a gargle in caries of the teeth, weak and spongy gums, pyorrhoea alveolaris, chronic tonsiltis and pharyngitis and ulcerated throat.

PTEROCARPUS

Synonyms : Malabar kino tree; Bijasal.

Biological Source : Pterocarpus consists of an aqueous extract of the wood and other parts of *Pterocarpus marsupium* Roxb.

Family : Leguminosae, Papilionaceae.

Habitat : The tree is found commonly in hilly regions throughout the Deccan Peninsula, and extending to Gujarat, Madhya Pradesh, Utter Pradesh, Bihar and Orissa.

Characters : It is a moderate-sized to large deciduous tree, up to 30 m high and a girth of 2.5 m with a straight clean bole. Bark grey, rough, longitudinally fissured and scaly; blaze pink and whitish markings, older tree exuding a blood red gum-resin, leaves imparipinnate, leaflets usually 5-7, oblong; flowers in large panicles, yellowish fragrant, pods orbicular, flat, winged, up to 5 cm in diameter, seeds 1-2, convex and bony.

The tree is found in deciduous forests both on undulating and flat ground and grows on a variety of formations, provided the drainage is good. It prefers a soil with a fair proportion of sand, though it is often found on red loam with a certain amount of clay. The normal rainfall in its natural habitat ranges from 75 to 200 cm. It produces root suckers sparingly. It is planted as a shade tree in coffee estates in South India.

Natural reproduction is through seeds. The early development of seedlings is favoured by shelter from the sun and a loose soil clear of weeds. Seedlings may show little stem development or may die back annually for several years but ultimately shoot up after they have developed a long stout tap root. Whole pods are sown and germination can be hastened by cutting across their ends and then soaking them in water for a few days prior to sowing. Stump planting of one-year old plants raised in nursery gives good results. Seedlings may also be raised in bamboo baskets for planting out. The tree is attacked by a number of insects, mostly defoliators, and some fungi which cause rotting of the wood.

The tree yields a gum kino which exudes when an incision is made through the bark up to the cambium. The exudate is collected and dried in the sun or shade to give 340 g dried gum per tree. Kino occurs in small (3-5 mm), angular, glistering, brittle fragments, appearing almost black in colour. The edges looked ruby-red and transparent when viewed by transmitted light. It is odourless and bitter with astringent taste and colours saliva pink when masticated.

Chemical Constituents : The bark contains l-epicatechin and a reddish brown colouring matter. The heartwood yields liquirigenin, isoliquiritigenin, a neutral unidentified compound (mp 160), alkaloid (0.017%) and resin (0.9%). The wood also contains a yellow colouring matter, an essential oil and a semidrying fixed oil (0.52%). Kino contains a non-glucosidal tannin kinotannic acid (25-80%), kinoin and kino-red in addition to small quantities of catechol (pyrocatechin), protocatechuic acid, resin, pectin and gallic acid. Kino-red is the anhydride of kinoin, which is a phlobaphene produced from kinotannic acid by the action of an oxidase enzyme present in the kino.

Uses : An aqueous infusion of the wood is used in diabetes. The bark is used as an astringent and in toothache. The flowers are antipyretic. The leaves are employed as an external application for boils, sores and skin diseases. Kino is a powerful astringent and used in the treatment of diarrhoea and dysentery. It is locally applied in leucorrhoea and in passive haemorrhage and in toothache. Kino finds application in dying, tanning and printing and is of potential use for the paper industry.

GYMNEMA SYLVESTRE

Synonym : Gur-mar (Hindi).

Biological Source : The drug consists of leaves of *Gymnema sylvestre* R.Br. (Fam. Asclepidaceae).

It is a large, more or less pubescent, woody climber found in southern India, occassionally cultivated as a medicinal plant. The leaves are opposite, usually elliptic or ovate; flowers small, yellow, in umbellate cymes; follicles terete, lanceolate, up to 7-8 cm in length.

The leaves contain albumin, organic acids, pararabin, hentriacontane, pentatriacontane, α- and β-chlorophylls, phytin, resins, tartaric acid, formic acid, butyric acid, anthraquinone derivatives, inositol, d-quercitol and "gymnemic acid" which is an impure complex mixture. The leaves give positive tests for alkaloids.

The plant is stomachic, stimulant, laxative and diuretic. It is used in cough, biliousness and sore eyes. The leaves have been, sometimes used as a remedy for diabetes. However, the alcoholic extract or leaf powder does not show any effect on the concentration of sugar in the blood or in the urine of patients suffering from diabetes. But they cause hypoglycaemia in experimental animals when administered. This effect is not due to any direct influence on the carbohydrate metabolism but to indirect stimulation of insulin secretion by pancreas.

The leaf powder is tasteless with faint pleasant aromatic odour. It stimulates the heart and the circulatory system, increases the secretion of urine and activates the uterus. The laxative property is attributed to the presence of anthraquinone derivatives. The drug is used as an errhine and for parageusia and furunculosis.

VIDANG

Synonyms : Embelia; Black Vidang; Baberang (Hindi).

Biological Source : Vidang consists of dried ripe fruits of *Embelia ribes* Burm. f. containing 2 per cent of embelin.

Family : Myrsinaceae.

Geographical Distribution : Vidang is common in the mixed deciduous forests of India ascending to 1500 m in Sri Lanka, Burma and South China. It is often cultivated in gardens and homeyards.

Characters : The plant is a large scandent shrub with slender branches and elliptic-lanceolate, gland-dotted leaves. Vidang is a globular brownish-black fruit, 2-4 mm in diameter, warty with beak like projection at the apex, about 1.2 mm long pedicel may be present in some fruits. A presistent calyx with 3-5 sepals is present. When pedicel is not present a circular scar is observed at its place. Each fruit contains a single seed covered with thin membrane. The seed is covered with a small yellow spots of crystalline embelin. Vidang contains an aromatic odour and hot astringent taste.

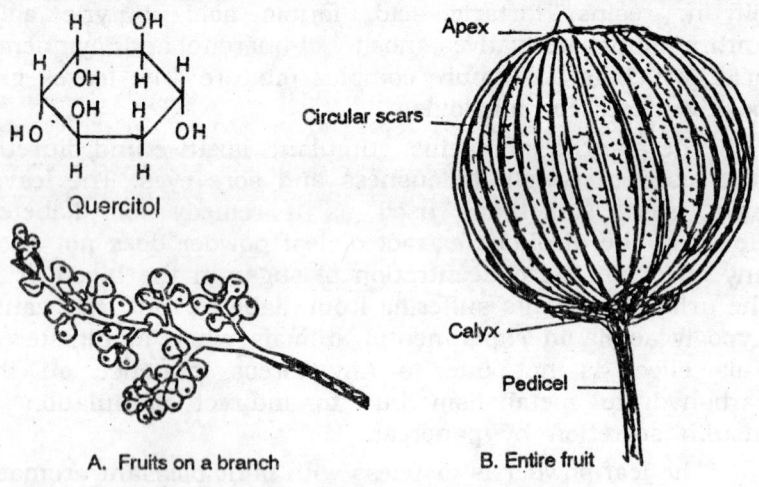

A. Fruits on a branch   B. Entire fruit

Fig. 14.21. Vidang

Chemical Constituents : Vidang contains 2-3% hydroquinone embelin (2, 5-dihydroxy-3-lauryl-p-benzoquinone), a dimer of embelin known as vilangin, an alkaloid christembine, tannins, quercitol, and minute amount of volatile oil. Embelin occurs in golden yellow needles, is insoluble in water but soluble in alcohol, chloroform and benzene. Fatty ingredients are also present in the fruits.

Tests for Identification

1. A mixture of ethereal extract of Vidang powder and aqueous sodium hydroxide gives deep violet colour in aqueous layer. With dilute ammonia solution a bluish violet precipitate is formed (Test for embelin).

2. Alcoholic extract (10 ml) of powdered drug (2 g) with lead acetate solution produces green precipitate.

3. Alcoholic extract of the drug gives reddish brown precipitate with ferric chloride.

Uses : Vidang is anthelmintic especially against tapeworm. The fruit has astringent, carminative, stimulant, alternative and tonic properties. It is used to cure fevers, coughs and diarrhoea. Children suffering from tape-worms are treated by giving milk boiled with the drug. It has no activity against roundworms or threadworms.

Embelin   Vilangin

Substituents - Red Vidang : In commercial supply of Vidang sometimes Red Vidang is mixed which is dried ripe fruits of *Embelia robusta* Roxb. (syn. *E. tsjeriam-cottam* DC.) (Fam. Myrsinaceae). The plant occurs on the Malabar coasts of India,. Sri Lanka and Sylhet. The fruits are relatively larger in size (4-5 mm in diameter) and possess distinctly reddish wrinkled surface. The persistent calyx is more prominent with 5 distinct sepals. It contains embelin (1.5%) and minute amount of volatile oil.

ACHYRANTHES

Achyranthes consists of the entire plant of *Achyranthes aspera* Linn. (Family Amaranthaceae).

The plant is an erect or procumbent, annual or perennial herb, 1-2 m in height, often with a woody base, commonly found as a weed of waysides and waste places throughout India up to an altitude of 2,100 m. Stems are angular, ribbed, simple or branched from the base, often tinged with reddish purple colour, leaves thick, ovate-elliptic or obovate-rounded, but variable in shape and size, flowers greenish white, numerous in axilary or terminal spikes, up to 75 cm long, seeds sub-cylindric, turncate at the apex, rounded at the base, reddish brown.

The plant is very variable, and a few varieties have been recorded. The plant thrives best in the community of *Cassia tora* and is commonly found in shady places as a weed. It also grows in drier situations but does not tolerate waterlogging.

The seeds contain saponins, pentatriacontane, 6-pentatriacontanone; hexatriacontane and triacontane.

The presence of hentriacontane and ecdysterone is also reported. The whole plant contains the alkaloids, achyranthine and betain. Achyranthine, a water-soluble alkaloid, dilates the blood vessels, lowers the blood-pressure, depresses the heart, and increases the rate and amphitude of respiration. Ecdysterone is also present in stem and leaves.

Uses : The plant is pungent, astringent, pectoral and diuretic. It is used as an emmenagogue, and in piles and skin eruptions. A decoction of the plant is useful in pneumonia and renal dropsy. The juice of the plant is used in ophthalmia, toothache and dysentery. The benzene extract of stem bark showed significant abortifacient activity.

The leaves are used as a cure for gonorrhoea, and excessive perspiration. Their extracts showed antibiotic action. The roots are astringent; their paste is applied to clear opacity of cornea, and to wounds as an haemostatic. A decoction of the roots is used for stomach troubles, and an aqueous extract for stones in bladder. The flowers are used for menorrhagia and to treat rabies. Seeds are emetic and given for biliousness. A medicated oil is dropped into the ear in deafness and noise in the ears.

QUESTIONS

1. Give the botanical sources, chemical constituents and uses of the following drugs : (a) Brahmi (b) Punarnava (c) Chirata (d) Aswagandha (Jamia Hamdard, 1994).

2. Discuss the biological source, active constituents and uses of the following : (a) Shankhpushpi (b) Amla (c) Brahmi (d) Satavari.

3. Write short notes on any four of the following drugs: (a) Gokhru (b) Brahmi (c) Pipal (d) Vaj (e) Tulsi

4. Discuss the source, chemical constituents, authentication and clinical uses of (a) *Tylophora indica* (b) *Centella asiatica* (c) *Achyranthes aspera* (d) *Convolvoulus microphyllus*.

15

PHARMACEUTICAL AIDS AND TECHNICAL PRODUCTS

A number of natural products find use in various fields in addition to medicine and pharmacy. These products are called as technical products which are used in beverages, condiments, flavouring agents, spices, paints, varnishes, confectionaries, textiles and cosmetics.

Pharmaceutical Aids

For the production of drugs various techniques such as purification, filtration, adsorption, solubilization, absorption, suspension, emulsification, etc. are employed. A number of natural products are used in these techniques. Flavouring, colouring, coating and perfuming agents are used in drug industries. These agents possess little or no therapeutic value, but they are used in the preparation of many pharmaceutical products. These agents are called as pharmaceutical aids which may be of plant, animal, mineral or synthetic origin.

In pharmaceutical industry Starch and Guar gum are used as a disintegrating agent. Sodium alginate acts as stabilizing, thickening, emulsifying, defloculating, gelling and filming agent. Glucose and sucrose are sweetening and coating products. Agar is used as emulsifying agent and for cultural media. Acacia and Tragacanth are employed as binding, suspending and emulsifying agents. Mucilages like Ispaghol and Linseed act as demulcent and soothing agents.

Quillaia contains saponins and is used in coal tar emulsion. Most of the volatile oils are flavouring products. Fixed oils like Olive, Seasame, Cottonseed, Almond and Castor oils act as emollients and vehicles for drugs. Beeswax, Spermaceti, Wool fat, Lanolin and Lard are the ointment bases. Chlorophyll, Cochineal and Saffron are the natural dyes used as colouring agents. Gelatin is a suspending agent and used for making capsules. Pyrethrum, Derris, Lonchocarpus, Cevadilla seed and Ryania are the natural insecticides. Absorbent Cotton, Jute, Hemp, Flax, Wool, Silk, Viscose, Alginate, etc. are used to prepare fibres for filtering and surgical dressings. Shellac is used for coating confections and medicinal tablets. Kaolin is employed externally as dusting powder, filtering and cleaning agent.

Technical Products

In perfumery the natural substances Lavender, Sandalwood, Citronella, Balsam of Peru, Balsam of Tolu and Storax are used as technical products. Soaps are prepared from fatty acids of Castor oil, Cottonseed oil, and Peanut oil. Myrrh and Quillaia are used in incense and shampoos, respectively. Wool fat, Spermaceti and White wax are the ingredients of creams. Coconut oil, Castor oil and Henna find use in hair dressings. Benzoin is added in lotions.

In food industry Acacia, Agar, Alginates, Starches and Sterculia gum are used in confection and bakery products. Citrus fruits and Ginger are employed in soft drinks (beverages). The vegetable oils used as food are Coconut, Seasame, Cottonseed, Peanut and Mustard. The fruits and other parts of Capsicum, Nutmeg, Cardamom, Clove, Coriander, Caraway and Dill are used as spices and condiments.

In Tobacco industry Glycyrrhiza and Vanilla are used in cigarettes, cigars, snuffs and other products. Hops, Yeast and Malt find use in the manufacture of bear. From Linseed oil, Castor oil, Copaiba and Colophony, paints and varnishes are manufactured. Black Catechu is applied on chewing betel leaf. In textile industry Acacia, Agar, Alginates, Catechu, Cotton, Gambir, Rosin, Starch and Sterculia gum are employed.

SPERMACETI

Synonyms : Cetaceum; Spermwax.

Biological Source : Spermaceti is a solid waxy substance obtained from the oil derived from the head and blubber of the sperm whale, *Physeter macrocephalus* (Fam. Physteridae).

Geographical Distribution : The whales are found in the Pacific, Indian and Atlantic oceans. They attend a length of 20 meters and up to 6-9 meters in circumference.

Collection and Preparation : The whales are killed with torpedo harpoons that explode upon striking the animal. In front of the cranium there is a large cavity which contains an oily fluid. The cranial cavity is opened and the oily liquid removed by buckets or by pumping. A single whale yields 10-12 barrels of oil. On cooling about 11% Spermaceti separates out. The crude material is pressed, melted and strained, and treated with boiling aqueous caustic soda to remove free acids in the form of soap. The purified Spermaceti is cooled to form cakes.

Characters : Spermaceti is white, somewhat transparent slightly unctuous masses with crystalline fracture and pearly luster.. It is almost odourless and tasteless but becomes yellow and rancid on long exposure to air; density 0.93 - 0.94; m.p. 42-50°; viscosity 1.433, saponification number 120 - 136, iodine number 3-4.4. It is insoluble in water and cold alcohol, soluble in chloroform, ether, carbon disulphide, oils, boiling alcohol; slightly soluble in petroleum ether.

Chemical Constituents : Spermaceti consists of chiefly cetyl palmitate $(C_{15}H_{31}$ OCO C_{16} $H_{33})$, cetyl myristate $(C_{15}H_{31}$ OCOC$_{13}H_{27})$, cetyl laurate, acetyl laurate and cetyl stearate; the total ester constituents are about 85%. Free cetyl alcohol is present in appreciable amounts. The esters of higher alcohols are also present. On saponification of esters with alcoholic potassium hydroxide, cetyl alcohol, $(C_{16}$ H_{33} OH), m.p. 49.5°, is formed.

Uses : Spermaceti is used as a pharmaceutical aid for cold creams, as a base for ointments, cerates, etc. and as emulsion with egg yolk or expressed almond oil. It is also used in manufacture of candles, soaps, cosmetics, laundry wax; finishing and lustering linens. It possesses emollient properties.

KAOLINS

Synonyms : Bolus alba; China clay; Porcelain clay; White bole; Argilla.

Kaolins or China clays (white or high-cream burning) are derived from pegmatites or from hydrothermal alterations along fractures.They may also occur as blanket deposits in extensive areas of igneous of metamorphic rocks, bedded deposits derived from feelspathic, sandstones or as pockets in limestones.

Distribution

Kaolins are found in the Garo hills of Assam, banks of Dora river in Lakhimpur districts, Makkiari near Ranjiganj, Birbhum districts, Rajmahal hills in Bhagalpur (Bihar); Begaum, Ratnagiri, Kanera, Thana districts of Maharastra and in some parts of M.P., Delhi, Madras, Kerala and other states.

Chemical Constituents : Clays are made up of mineral grains, some of which may be of very small size. Kaolin group contains kaolinite, nacrite, dickite, annauxite and hallosysite, all Al_2O_3 $2SiO_2$. $2H_2O$ and allophane, Al_2O_3. $nSiO_2$. H_2O. It contains traces of magnesium, calcium and iron.

Preparation

Kaolin is prepared when the rock in mined, excavated and the impurities are washed with water and then powdered. The rock is elutriated with water and large-sized particles are separated. On allowing the turbid liquid to settle, heavy Kaolin containing particles of large size and colloidal Kaolin containing particles of small size are separated and then dried.

Description

Kaolin, Al_2O_3. $2SiO_2$. $2H_2O$ (Al_2O_3 39.3%, SiO_2 46.8%, H_2O, 13.9%, sp. gr. 2.6), is an important member of the family of clay material. It is slightly plastic like and is normally white but is often tinged grey, yellow brown, blue or red by impurities. Its softness is very characteristic. It is unctuous and soapy to touch. On rubbing with a piece of bone, it takes a high polish. It is highly refractory. Its fusion point is in between 1700-1800°. When heated in a closed tube, it gives out water. On heating on charcoal black with cobalt nitrate, it gives a blue mass due to the alumina present. It is not affected by dilute hydrochloric or nitric acid, but is decomposed by prolonged boiling or treatment with concentrated sulphuric acid. It becomes more resistant to acids if it is first heated to white heat.

The particles of heavy Kaolin are 20 μm in diameter, flat and irregularly arranged. With water plastic-like form is obtained which is less sticky. When the aqueous suspension is kept for some time, the whole Kaolin settles below leaving a clear supernatant liquid. Heavy Kaolin polarizes light brightly.

The particles of fine or colloidal Kaolin are small, less than 2 μ in diameter and have various shapes and sizes. They do not polarize light. A sticky mass is obtained with water. Its aqueous suspension remains turbid permanantly and only a small fraction is deposited.

Uses : Heavy Kaolin is used externally as a dusting powder, poultice, carrier of heat, filtering and cleaning agent. Fine Kaolin is used internally as an adsorbent and to coat irritated intestinal mucosa in case of diarrhoea, dysentery and intestinal fermentation. They are also used to manufacture porcelain, pottery, bricks, portlant cement, ultramarine, colour lakes, refractory mortar, plaster material, filler for paper, electric and heat insulators; clarifying liquids, drying and emollient agents.

COCHINEAL

Biological Source : It consists of the dried female insects *Coccus cacti (Dactylopius coccus)* containing eggs and larvae.

Habitat : Cochineal insects are indigenous to Central America. Commercially they are grown in Peru, Mexico, Canary Islands, Algiers, Honduras, East and West Indies, Spain, Florida and California.

Eggs from the previous crop are hatched on the Cacti or Nopal tree *(Nopalea cochenillifer,* Family Cactaceae). Both male and female insects emerge. The males are about 1 mm long and possess wings, while the females are about 2 mm long and without wings. After a time fecundation takes place and the females attach themselves to the Nopal tree by means of their probosces. The males then die. The female insects grow faster and becomes to about twice their original size. The larvae mature in about 14 days.

Collection and Preparation : The insects are separated from the tree, killed with hot water, stove heat or by exposure to the fumes of burning sulphur or charcoal. If heat is used, the colour of insects becomes purplish-black and they are called as *'black grain'*. The fumed-killed purplish-grey insects are known as *'silver grain'*. Small immature insects and larvae are separated by sieves and known as *'granilla'*. About 70,000 insects produce 450 g (1 lbs) of the Cochineal drug.

Characters : Cochineal insects are about 4 mm long and oval in shape. The convex dorsal surface shows from 9 to 11 segments without constrictions between head, thorax and abdomen. The insect has a pair of antennae with 7-joints and three pairs of very incospicuous legs. The surface contains tubular glands which secrete wax.

Chemical Constituents : Cochineal contains a water soluble glycosidic colouring matter known as carminic acid or carmine red (10%) which is a C-glycoside of anthraquinone. The insect also contains fat (10%) and a wax known as coccerin (2%). Carmine is an alkaline preparation of Cochineal containing about 50 per cent of carminic acid.

Uses : Cochineal is used as a colouring agent for food products, drugs and toilet preparations. Carmine and carminic acid are used for manufacture of red and pink inks and lakes. Several grades of cochineal are available such as Silver grain, Black grain, Grannilla, Rosy-black and Red foxy.

Adulteration : The weight of cochineal is increased by adding inorganic matter.

Carminic acid

Shelloic acid

SHELLAC

Synonyms : Lacca; Lac.

Biological Source : Shellac is a resinous substance prepared from the excretion of scale insects, *Laccifer lacca* (Family Coccidae).

Habitat : Shellac is produced in Burma, Assam and India. Most Shellac is produced in Madhya Pradesh, Uttar Pradesh, Bihar and Orissa states of India.

Preparation : The insects live on the juices of various trees such as *Acacia* species, *Butea frondosa* (Leguminosae), *Aleurites laccifera* (Euphorbiaceae), *Ficus* species (Moraceae), *Cajanus indicus, Shorea talura* (Dipterocarpaceae), *Schleichera trijuga* (Sapindaceae), and *Zizyphus jujuba* (Rhamnaceae).

The insects suck the juice of the tree and excrete "stick-lac" almost continuously. Whitest Shellac is produced when the Kusum tree *(Schleichera trijuga)* is the host. The structure and life history of the scale insect are identical to those of Cochineal.

Preparation : Shellac is found most abundantly on the smaller branches and twigs. These are broken off and the excretion is scraped from the twigs with the help of curved knives. It is ground and the colouring matter exctracted with water or dilute alkali solution. The exhausted Shellac in dried form is known as *Seed lac*. The alkaline extract on dryness gives *Lac dye*. The *seed lac* is melted in a long sausage-shaped bag suspended over a charcoal fire and the lac is squeezed out. It is cooled and then stretched into a large sheet. It is broken up to give flake Shellac of commerce. Sometimes the Shellac is poured into circular moulds and, on cooling, stamped with the maker's name. This form of Shellac is known as *Button lac.* When the Shellac is dissolved in hot alkaline solution, bleached with chlorine or sulphurous acid, precipitated with acid, collected by filtration and pulled under water into sticks, it is known as *Bleached Shellac.* When the Shellac is kept under water, it is soluble in alcohol, but the solubility decreases on exposure.

Characters : Shellac occurs in thin, very brittle, yellowish, translucent sheets or powder; m.p. 115-120, saponification no. 185-210°, iodine no. 10-18. It is soluble in alcohol, ether, benzene and petroleum ether; sparingly soluble in oil of terpentine and insoluble in water.

$$\text{HOCH}_2 \, (\text{CH}_2)_5 \, \underset{|}{\text{CH}} - \underset{|}{\text{CH}} - (\text{CH}_2)_7 - \text{COOH}$$
$$\phantom{\text{HOCH}_2 \, (\text{CH}_2)_5 \,\,} \text{OH} \quad \text{OH}$$

Aleuritic acid

It is soluble in aqueous solutions of ethanolamines, alkalies and borax with slightly purple colour.

Various grades and colours are used for particular purposes. Shellac containing brownish-yellow colour is known as *orange Shellac* and the reddish-brown varieties are called *ruby* or *garnet Shellac.*

Chemical Constituents : Shellac contains wax (6%), red colouring matter (6.5%), laccaic acid, resin (70-85%) and few insect remains and vegetable debris. Hydrolysis of the resin gives a complex mixture of aliphatic and alicyclic hydroxy acids and their polyesters. The composition of the hydrolysate depends on the Shellac source and the time of collection. The major component of the aliphatic fraction is aleuritic acid.

Uses : Shellac is used for coating confections and medicinal tablets; finishing leather, in lacquers and varnishes, to manufacture buttons, grinding wheels, sealing wax, cements, inks, phonographs, records, paper; for stiffening hats; in electrical machines; and in polishes.

LARD

Biological Source : Lard is the purified internal fat obtained from the abdomen of the hog, Sus scofa, var. domesticus (Family Suidae).

The abdominal fat, known as *flare,* is obtained by treatment with hot water at a temperature not exceeding 57°C.

Characters : Lard is a soft, white fat, m.p. 34-41°, iodine value 52-66, saponification value 192-198. It has non-rancid odour. It is insoluble in water, very slightly soluble in alcohol and freely soluble in benzene, chloroform, solvent and petroleum ethers and in carbon disulphide. It should be free from moisture, alkalies and chlorides. It is adulterated with beef-fat, Seasame oil and Cottonseed oil.

Lard oil is colourless, pale yellow liquid, density 0.90 0.91, viscosity 1.47. It solidifies in between −2 to +4° C.

Chemical Constituents : Lard contains solid glycerides (40%) such as myristin, stearin and palmitin; and mixed liquid glycerides (60%) such as olein. The fractions are separated by pressure at 0°C into solid fat 'stearin' and liquid 'lard oil'. Hydrolysis of Lard yields oleic acid (48%), palmitic acid (28%), octadecadienic acid (11%), stearic acid (9%) and myristic acid (3%).

Uses : Lard is an emollient and used as a base for ointments and cerates. It has a tendency to become rancid; this can be retarded by combining lard with 1% Siam Benzoin or Sumatra Benzoin to prepare Benzoinated Lard. Lard oil is used as an antifoaming agent in the fermentations and as a tablet lubricant, illuminant, oiling wool and to manufacture soap.

DIATOMITE (KIESELGUHR)

It occurs as large deposits in California, Germany, North Africa and Virginia.

The material is dried, powdered, ignited to remove organic matter, boiled with dilute hydrochloric acid to remove iron and other impurities, washed with water and dried. Purified form occurs as fine, white, odourless powder. The diatoms consist of two halves or valves fitted together. The valves vary in shape. Many diatoms contain a median cleft in the valves, called as the raphe. The valves also show dots, lines and minute cavities in the walls. It is insoluble in all acids except hydrofluoric acid. After fusion with alkalies, it is soluble in acids.

The crude product contains silica (68-87%), organic matter, clay, iron oxide and water (5-15%). Diatomite is used for the filtration of oils, fats, syrups, for sterilization; as an inactive support in column, gas and thin layer chromatography; in face powders, pills, polishing powders, soaps and to absorb nitroglycerine in the manufacture of dynamite.

QUESTIONS

1. What are pharmaceutical aids and technical products? Write biological sources, preparation, characters, chemical constituents and uses of any two such products studied by you.
2. Write notes on :
   (a) Spermaceti,
   (b) Kaolins,
   (c) Cochineal,
   (d) Shellac.

16

FIBRES, SURGICAL DRESSINGS AND SUTURES

Natural and artificial fibres are used in surgical dressings. The natural fibres are obtained from vegetable sources (e.g., Cotton, Flax, Hemp, Jute, etc.) or from animal sources (e.g. Wool and Silk). These fibres are made up of long-chain molecules which may be a carbohydrate or a protein molecule. Some fibres, e.g., Nylon and Terylene, are synthetic fibres prepared from long-chain molecules of polymers. Regenerated carbohydrate materials and chemically modified fibres are Viscose, Acetate Rayons, Alginate yarn and Oxidized Cellulose. Asbestos and glass are obtained from mineral sources.

Fibres can be distinguished by chemical test and by studying their microscopic structures. Vegetable and regenerated carbohydrate materials are composed of cellulose units and respond to the following tests :

Tests of Vegetable and Regenerated Carbohydrate Fibres :

1. With Molisch reagent they produce violet colour.
2. On heating with aqueous picric acid solution they are not stained permanently.
3. With chlor-zinc iodine or a mixture of iodine and sulphuric acid they yield blue colour.
4. On ignition as such or boiling with sodalime they do not produce foul smell.
5. Vegetable fibres are soluble in copper oxide ammonia solution (cuoxam) forming a blue colour.

6. On boiling with Millon's reagent they do not produce red colour.

Tests of Animal Fibres : Animal fibres and regenerated protein fibres are proteinous compounds containing peptide linkage. They show the following tests :

1. On ignition they produce disagreeable odour.
2. They are dissolved in 5% aqueous potassium hydroxide solution.
3. They respond positively with Millon's test.
4. They are stained permanently with picric acid.

Synthetic and mineral fibres give negative tests of vegetable and animal fibres. Glass fibres melt on heating and form beads. There is no effect of heat on asbestos fibres.

ABSORBENT COTTON

Synonyms : Absorbent Wool; Purified Cotton; Kapas (Hindi).

Biological Source : Absorbent cotton consists of epidermal hairs of the seeds of *Gossypium herbaceum* Linn. and other species of *Gossypium* like *G. hirsutum*, Linn., *G. arboreum* Linn. and *G. barbadense* Linn. which are freed from adhering impurities, deprived of fatty matters, bleached and sterilized.

Family : Malvaceae.

Habitat : Cotton is cultivated in Egypt, India, South America, U.S.A., South Africa and Pakistan.

Preparation : The plants are shrubs or small trees which produce 3 to 5 celled capsules possessing numerous seeds. The capsules open on ripening along longitudinal sutures and a mass of white hair attached to the brownish seeds is visible. The cotton fibres are collected, dried and ginned to remove the hair from the seeds. The gin may be a roller or pneumatic type which is designed to pull the hair through a narrow space. For preparing Absorbent Cotton, the cotton is first carded to remove impurities such as immature and broken seeds, fragments of leaves and short hairs called as 'linters'. The linters are used to prepare the lower grades of cotton wool and rayons. It is subjected to cotton-combing machine which separates all the shorter fibres and a thread is spun consisting of long paralleled, uniform fibres. The short fibres of comber waste are used to prepare the best grades of cotton wool.

The comber waste is loosened and heated with dilute sodium hydroxide solution and soda ash solution at 1-3 atmospheric pressure for 10-15 hours. Most of the fatty cuticle is removed and trichome wall becomes absorbent in this process. It is washed with water, decolourized with sodium hypochlorite solution and treated with dilute hydrochloric acid. The dried fibres are in matted conditions and opened up by machines. It is converted into a continuous flat sheet, packed and sterilized.

Characters : Absorbent Cotton occurs as white, soft, fine hairy filament. Microscopically the filament consists, of unicellular hair appearing like empty-twisted five-hoses, 2.5-5 cm in length, 9-24 μm in diameter. The number of twists varies from 75 per cm in Indian variety to 150 per cm in the Sea Island variety. The Cotton hair is cylindrical when young and becomes flattened and twisted on maturing. The Cotton is almost odourless and tasteless.

Chemical Nature : Absorbent Cotton consists of cellulose which is composed of glucose units linked by 1,4 β-linear glucoside bonds.

Uses : Absorbent Cotton is used for surgical dressings. It serves for mechanical support to absorb blood, mucus, pus, etc. It protects the wound from bacteria. Cotton is also used in textile industry; for manufacturing explosives, cellulose acetate, other cellulose derivatives like carbomethyl cellulose, cellulose acetate phthalate, ethyl cellulose, hydroxypropyl methyl cellulose, methyl cellulose, oxidized cellulose and pyroxilin.

CELLOBIOSE UNIT ⟶ n

1.03 nm

JUTE

Synonym : Gunny.

Biological Source : Jute consists of the strands of phloem fibres obtained from the stem bark of *Corchorus capsularis*,

Linn., *C. olitoritus* Linn. and other species of *Corchorus.*

Family : Tiliaceae.

Habitat : It is cultivated throughout the hotter parts of India in Bengal, Assam, Bihar and Orissa as well as in most tropical countries.

Jute is a rainy season crop. The maximum temperature during the crop season rarely exceeds 38°C. The seeds are sown from March to May. The crop is cultivated on alluvial soil. Jute seed is sown broadcast early from mid-February to mid-March. Germination takes place within 2 or 3 days. Jute plants respond quickly to early weeding, thinning and mulching. The plant harvests between June and September.

Preparation : Jute is an annual plant 3-4 m in height. The straight stems are cut in July during flowering stage. The leaves are removed and the stems are submerged into water tank in bundles for retting. The bundles are covered with straw to protect them from direct sunlight which would make the fibres specky. After 3 weeks the bark from the wood and the strands of phloem fibres from the surrounding softer tissues are removed. The ends of stems are beaten with a mallet to separate the wood from the fibres. The fibres so obtained are cleaned by jerking them backwards and forwards on the surface of the water. They are hanged in the sun to dry and bleach for few days. The fibres are graded on the basis of length, colour and glossiness.

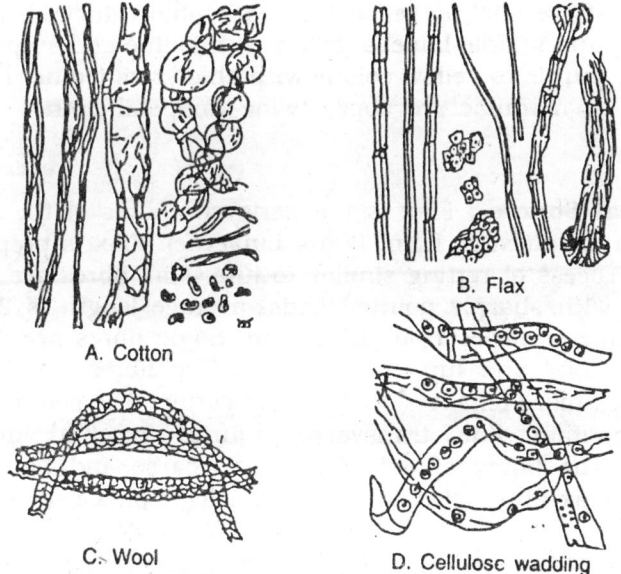

A. Cotton

B. Flax

C. Wool

D. Cellulosc wadding

Fig. 16.1. Fibres

Characters : Jute is a yellowish-brown in colour, 1-3 m long and 30-140 μm in diameter. The individual fibres are 0.8-5 mm long and 10-25 μm in diameter. The apex is bluntly pointed and rounded wall is without markings and lumen is varying in size. They give deep red colour with phloroglucinol, yellow with iodine and sulphuric acid and with chlor-zinc-iodine.

Chemical Composition : Jute contains liganocellulose. The middle lamella is extensively lignified and is destroyed by oxidizing agent (a mixture of nitric acid and potassium chlorate).

Uses : Jute is used to prepare medicated tows, as a filtering and straining medium and to make gunny bags, yarns and ropes.

HEMP

Biological Source : Hemp is prepared from the pericyclic fibres of the stem of *Cannabis sativa* (Fam. Cannabinaceae). Plant is grown for fibres in Russia, Italy, France and America. The fibres are prepared by retting process as in case of jute. The individual fibre are about 22 μm in diameter and 35-40 mm in length. The fibre ends are bluntly rounded, some ends are bifurcated like fork due to injuries to the stem. The lumen of the hemp fibre is large, uniform and flattened. The wall is thick with fine cross lines, some are intersecting. The fibres give slightly red colour with phloroglucinol, inner wall blue and middle lamella yellow with iodine and sulphuric acid and purple to yellow colour with chlor-zinc iodine. Hemp is used to manufacture rope, twine and sail-cloth.

FLAX

Biological Source : Flax is the pericyclic fibres of the stem of *Linum usitatissium* Linn. (Fam. Linaceae). Flax is prepared by the process of retting similar to jute. Flax fibres are non-lignified with sharply pointed ends, average length is 25-30 mm, diameter varies from 12-25 μm. Some fibres are up to 120 mm long and lumen is narrow. The fibres have good lustre and more tensile strength than cotton. The commercial fibres contain fine transverse injuries received during beating. The fibres of old plants are coarse and harsh in texture. Flax fibres give colourless or slight pink colour with phloroglucinol, blue or violet with iodine and sulphuric acid and purple to yellow with chlor-zine iodine. Flax consists of pectocellulose. It is used as a filtering medium.

WOOL

Synonyms : Animal wool; Sheep's wool.

Biological Source : Wool is obtained from the protective covering or fleece of the sheep, *Ovis arries* Linn.

Family : Bovidae, Order - Ungulata.

Geographical Source : Wool producing countries are Australia, Russia, Argentina, India and America.

Preparation : Wool obtained from the animal is spreaded on a frame covered with wire netting to separate it into wool of different sizes and qualities. Simultaneously it is beaten over the netting to remove dust and dirt. The burrs and straw pieces are picked up. The wool is washed in tanks containing warm, soft, soapy water to remove wool greese. The wool is squeezed between rollers, dried and the fibres are mechanically loosened. Then it is carded and spun into yarns.

'Wool grease' from the washing process may be removed by meachanical means or by using organic solvents. Purified 'wool grease' is known as wool fat or anhydrous lanolin. It is employed in cosmetics and ointments.

Characters : Wool consists of elastic, lustrous and smooth hair. The hair are loosely fitted and slippery to touch. The outer most surface, cuticle, consists of imbricated, flattened, translucent epithelial scales. Wool is insoluble in warm hydrochloric acid and in cold concentrated sulphuric acid. Single wool fibre can resist breakage when subjected to weights of 15-30 g 'and when stretched as much as 25-30% of their lengths. Wool fibre has good to excellent affinity for dyestuffs. It may retain about 17% of moisture of its weight.

Wool fibre is deteriorated by ageing, larval attack such as by cloth moths and carpet beetles, exposure to sunlight and charing at 300ºC. It does not continue to burn when removed from a flame. It has good resistance to dry-cleaning solvents, strong alkalies and high temperature.

Chemical Nautre : Raw wool consists of wool fibres (31%), 'wool sweat' or 'suint' composed of potassium salts of fatty acids (32%), dirt and dust (25%) and wool grease (lanolin).

Wool fibres are composed of the protein keratin, which is more easily damaged in unfavourable conditions than the cellulose fibres. Keratin is rich in the amino acid cystine. A cystine bridge, joining adjacent polypeptide chains, can be represented as :

$$S - CH_2 \; CH \; (NH_2). \; COOH$$
$$S - CH_2 - CH \; (NH_2). \; COOH$$

Cystine

Stability of the protein is due to frequent primary valence cross-links (disulphide bonds) and secondary valence cross-links (hydrogen bonds) between neighbouring polypeptide chains. The unstable form of keratin is known as β-keratin, the stable form is called as α-keratin.

Uses : Wool is used to prepare crepe bandages and dressings and as a medium for filtration and staining.

SILK

Biological Source : Silk is obtained in the fibre-form from the cocoons of *Bombyx mori* Linn. commonly known as silk worm or mulberry silk worm, and other species of *Bombyx* and of *Antheraea* such as *A. mylitta, A. assama, A. pernyi* and *A. yama-mai.*

Odour : Lepidoptera.

Geographical Source : Silk is produced in China, Japan, India, Asia Minor, Italy, France and some other countries.

Preparation : Cultivation of domesticated silk is called sericulture in which the care of the domesticated silk worm from the egg stage through completion of the cocoon, and also production of mulberry trees for worm food are involved. Before the silk worm passes from the larval or caterpillar to pupal (chrysalis) stage, it secretes an oval cocoon around itself. The cocoon is about 2.5 cm in length and consists of a filament up to 1200 m long. The thread is composed of two silk fibres joined together by a layer of silk glue known as sericin. If pupal or chrysalis are allowed to mature stage, the insect will escape damaging the cocoon. Therefore, the cacoon are collected at the chrysalis stage and heated at 60-80° for few hours or exposed to steam for a short period to kill the pupae. The cocoons are graded and kept in hot water to soften the silk glue and loosen the fibres. The ends of the fibres from 2-15 cocoons are woven into a single thread by twisting and reeling.

The double fibre in the coccon is called as a *bave* and its constituent fibres are known as *brine*. Silk containing sericin is called as raw silk. It is cleaned out by treatment with hot soap solution to remove sericin. This process is known as stripping or degumming. The degumming process leaves silk lustrous and semitransparent with a smooth surface. The silk is sometimes treated with a finishing substance, such as metallic salt, to increase its weight, density and improve draping quality.

Characters : Silk is a continuous filament, 600-1200 $m_k$long. Silk fibres are soft, smooth and possess remarkable tensile strength. A silk filament can be streched about 20% beyond its original length before breaking but does not immediately resume its original length when stretched more than 2%. Silk is soluble in ammonical copper oxide solution, ammonical nickel oxide solution, concentrated alkalies, and in concentrated hydrochloric acid. It is insoluble in water, alcohol, ether and dilute alkalies.

Chemical Nature : Silk is consisted of the protein fibroin which on hydrolysis yields mainly glycine and alanine.

Uses : Silk is used for making ligatures and sieves.

REGENERATED FIBRES

Regenerated fibres are prepared from naturally occurring polysaccharides. These compounds are modified to yield a suitable fibre form. Viscose, cellulose acetate, oxidized cellulose, nitrocellulose, etc. are the regenerated fibres.

VISCOSE

Synonyms : Rayon; Regenerated cellulose.

Viscose is a viscous orange-red aqueous solution of sodium cellulose xanthogenate obtained by dissolving wood pulp cellulose in sodium hydroxide solution and treating with carbon disulphide.

Preparation : Cellulose, obtained from Coniferous wood or cotton linters, is delignified to produce white pulp containing cellulose (80-90%) and hemicellulose. Hemicellulose is removed by treating the product with sodium hydroxide. The remaining alkali-cellulose (sodium cellulosate) is dissolved in a mixture of carbon disulphide and sodium hydroxide solution to afford a viscous solution of sodium cellulose xanthate. This solution is allowed to ripen, filtered and the filtrate is forced through a spinneret equipped with fine nozzles. It is immersed in a bath containing dilute sulphuric acid and sodium sulphate. The cellulose is regenerated as continuous filaments in the bath. The yarns are combined, twisted to strengthen, treated with sodium sulphide to remove free sulphur, bleached, washed, dried and a 10% moisture content is adjusted. Surgical dressings are prepared from the Viscose yarns.

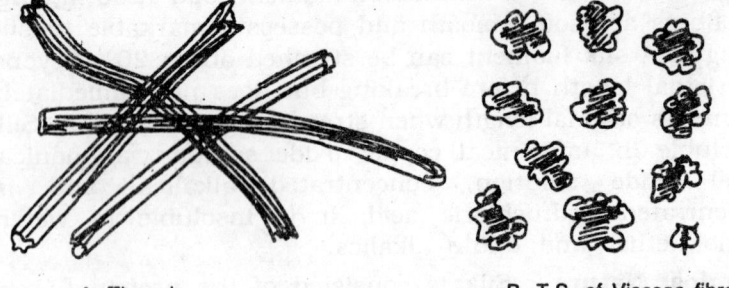

A. Threads   B. T.S. of Viscose fibres

Fig. 16.2. Viscose rayon

Characters : Viscose is a white, highly lustrous, pure form of cellulose. The molecules contain 450 glucose residue units as compared to 9000 glucose units in wood cellulose. Tensile strength is from two-third to one-and a half times that of Cotton. Viscose fibres are solid, transparent, 15-20 μm in diameter, slightly twisted, and contain grooves. Fibre-ends are abrupt and peculiar. The fibres give general tests of vegetable fibres. They can be delustred by addition of white pigment titanium oxide to the solution before preparation of the yarns. The *delustred viscose rayon* or *matt viscose* is used to manufacture surgical dressings. The filaments are identical to Cotton filaments, but they are matted white. The amount of pigment is controlled by assaying ash value.

When viscose solution is allowed to pass through long narrow slits into a regenerating bath, sheets of Viscose are formed. These sheets are washed, bleached, treated with a glycerin solution and dried to produce cellophane, Cellophane is heat-sealable packing material and is also used as a dialysing membrane, as a protective dressing and as a substituent of oiled silk.

$$CH_2OC\overset{\overset{\textstyle S}{\|}}{C}SNa$$

Viscose Unit

Uses : Viscose rayon is used to manufacture fabrics, surgical dressings, absorbent wool, enzyme and cellophane.

METHYLCELLULOSE

Synonyms : Cellulose methyl ether; Methocel, Cellothyl; Syncelose; Bagolax; Cethyplose; Cethytin; Cologel; Cellumeth; Hydrolose; Nicel; Tearisol; Tylose.

Methylcellulose is prepared from wood pulp or chemical cotton by treatment with alkali and methylation of the alkali cellulose with methyl chloride under pressure; to convert hydroxyl groups into methyl ether groups. The molecules containing two of the three hydroxyl methylated groups of the glucose residue units of the cellulose chain are considered of high quality.

Methylcellulose occurs as white, fibrous powder, odourless, tasteless; swells in water and forms a clear to opalescent, viscous, colloidal solution in cold water. It is insoluble in hot water, alcohol and ether. An aqueous solution is best prepared by dispersing the granules in hot water with stirring and chilling to +5°C. The solution is then stable at room temperature. Presence of inorganic salts increases the viscosity. The solubility is dependent upon the degree of substitution. Commercial methylcellulose has a methoxyl content of 29%. Clear film may be casted from the aqueous solution.

Uses : In pharmacy Methylcellulose is used to increase the viscosity and to stabilize lotions, suspensions, pastes, ophthalmic preparations and some ointments. In medicine it is used as a hydrophilic colloid, laxative in chronic constipation and to curb appetite in obese persons as it gives a feeling of fullness. It is also used as a substitute for water-soluble gums; to render paper grease proof, in adhesives, as thickening agent in cosmetics, as protective colloid in emulsions, as binder and stabilizer in foods and as a bulk producer in the formulation of dietetic foods.

CELLULOSE ACETATE

Synonyms : Acetate rayon; Partially acetylated cellulose.

Several acetates of cellulose are known, which differ from one another only in the degree of acetylation. In triacetates, not less than 92% of the hydroxyl groups are acetylated. In characterizing the degree of acetylation, per cent acetyl value and per cent combined acetic acid are used.

All cellulose acetates are obtained by treating cellulose with acetic anhydride at various temperatures for different length of time to produce amorphous white solid material in granular, flake or powder form from which fibres may be produced by extrusion. Acetate rayon is prepared by treating cotton linters or wood cellulose with acetic acid and acetic anhydride in the presence of sulphuric acid as a catalyst to yield acetone-insoluble fully acetylated cellulose (primary acetate). Primary acetylated group is hydrolyzed by addition of water and an acetone-soluble secondary acetate is produced. The acetone solution is forced through a spinneret into a warm air chamber. On evaporation of the solvent filament of Cellulose acetate rayon is obtained.

Characters : Cellulose acetate resembles with Viscose rayon in its appearance. Commercial products do not have sharp melting points. Solubility is affected by the acetyl value; the triacetate is insoluble in water, alcohol, ether, but soluble in glacial acetic acid. The penta acetate is insoluble in water, but soluble in alcohol. The filaments are highly lustrous, grooved and slightly twisted.

Uses : Cellulose acetate rayon is used to manufacture rubber and celluloid substitutes, nonflammable photographic and cinema films, airplane dopes, varnishes and lacquers, filaments, phonograph records; water-proofing fabrics and rendering balloons gas-tight; sizing and finishing fabrics, coating skins, insulating electric wires; and tow for cigarette smoke filters. Acetate rayon is much less absorbent than viscose rayon. It is, therefore, unsuitable for manufacturing surgical dressings.

OXIDIZED CELLULOSE

Synonyms : Absorable cellulose; Cellulosic acid; Polyanhydroglucuronic acid; Oxycel; Hemo-Pak.

It is a cellulose of varied carboxyl content retaining the fibrous structure. It is prepared by oxidizing cotton wool or gauze with nitrogen dioxide until the number of carboxylic groups formed by the oxidation of the primary alcohol groups of the glucose moieties of the cellulose molecules reaches 16-22 per cent. After reaction the cellulose molecule contains glucuronic acid residue units and some glucose residue units.

Characters : Oxidized cellulose is identical with the normal cotton in appearance. It has dull colour, a harsher texture, charred odour and a sour taste. It tends to disintegrate on handling and does not turn into pasty on chewing. The degree of oxidation is sufficiently high to make the product soluble in dilute alkaline solutions. It is insoluble in water or acidic solutions.

Uses : It is used as local absorable haemostatic in surgery and in chromatography. But it delays bone repair and can not be sterilized by heat.

ALGINATE FIBRES

Alginate fibres are composed of calcium alginate. An aqueous solution of sodium alginate is pumped through a spinneret which is immersed in a bath containing acidic calcium chloride solution. In the bath sodium cations are substituted with calcium cations and the insoluble calcium alginate is precipitated as continuous filaments. The filaments are collected, washed and dried for surgical purposes, the filaments are cut up to give stable form of length 1 to 8 inches for preparing calcium alginate wool or a fabric. Trace amounts of substances are added to the calcium alginate to inhibit mould and bacterial growth.

Alginate fibres are fairly lustrous and pale cream coloured. The fibres may be processed into absorable haemostatic dressings. They give general tests for vegetable fibres. They are soluble in ammonical copper nitrate and 5% sodium citrate solution.

Uses : Alginate fibres are used as absorable haemostatic dressings; in neurosurgery, endaural and dental surgery; internally to arrest bleeding and form protective dressing for burns or sites from which skin grafts have been taken. Alginate fibres are compatible with antibiotics like penicillin. Calcium alginate wool is used as a swab for pathological work or bacterial study.

SYNTHETIC FIBRES

Synthetic fibres are produced by polycondensation of organic molecules which are more stronger than the natural fibres. Nylon, terylene, orlon and polyethylene are the polymers used as pharmaceutical aid.

NYLON

Synonyms : Caprolan; Enkalon; Grilon; Kabron; Mirlon; Perlon; Phrilon; Amilon.

Nylon is a manufactured fibre in which fibre forming substances are long-chain synthetic polyamide having recurring polyamide groups ($-CONH_2-$) as an integral part of the polymer chain. Nylon is usually prepared by condensing adipic acid with hexamethylene diamine. The molted polymer is pumped through a spinneret to produce filaments.

The filaments are smooth, solid cylinders, softens at $210°$ and melts at $223°$; moisture regain is about 4%. Swelling is low. They are immune to microbiological attack; resistant to most organic chemicals, but dissolves in phenol, cresol and strong acids. They may be highly lustrous to dull white or coloured. On ignition the fibres melt and form a hard bead. They are soluble in 5 M hydrochloric acid, 90% formic acid, 90% phenol and insoluble in acetone. Chemically, nylon is represented as :

$$H - [NH (CH_2)_5 CO]_n OH; n = approx\ 200.$$

Uses : Nylon is used to prepare filter cloth, sieves, non-absorbable sutures, nylon syringes, film, textile fibres, monofilament, tire cord. fishing lines, tow ropes, etc.

TERYLENE (DACRON)

Terylene is a polyester fibre produced by condensating ethylene glycol with terephthalic acid. Its chemical formula may be represented as $H[OCH_2 CH_2 OOC C_6 H_4 CO]_n OH$. Terylene fibres are prepared by an identical process to that for nylon. On heating the fibres with phosphoric acid (90%) for 1 minute, it retain its form. This test is negative in case of nylon. Terylene is used in the same way as nylon.

ORLON

Synonyms : Polyacrylonitrile; Fiber A.

Orlon is obtained by polymerizing acrylonitrile. It is represented as $[CH_2 CN (CN)]_n$. It is a white fibre; sticks at 235°; ironing temperatures above 160° may cause yellowing; sp. gr. is 1.17. Its flammability is similar to that of rayon and cotton. Generally it has very good resistance to mineral acids; excellent resistance to common solvents, oils, greases, neutral salts, sunlight but it is degraded by strong alkalies. It resists attack by molds, mildew and insects. The 100% polyacrylonitrile fibres are rarely used commercially due to difficulty in dyeing.

Orlon fibre is suitable for furnishing (awnings, tents, furniture), anode bags in electro-plating, knitwear, rugs, dressings, etc.

POLYETHYLENE

Synonyms : Polythene; Ethene homopolymer; Agilene; Alathon; Alkathene; Courlene; Lupolen; Platilon.

Polyethylene is prepared by polymerization of liquid ethylene at high temperature and under pressure. The polymer is a plastic solid of milky transparency, tough and flexible at room temperature, m.p. 85-110°.

It is a good electrical insulator. It burns but hardly supports combustion. It is stable to water, non-oxidizing acids and alkalies, alcohols, ethers, ketones and esters at ordinary temperature. It is attacked by oxidizing acids such as nitric acid, perchloric acid, free halogens, benzene, petroleum ether, gasoline and lubricating oils, aromatic and chlorinated hydrocarbons. It has flexibility over a wide range of temperature.

The polymer $[CH_2 - CH_2]_n$ is transformed into filaments by melt spinning and heat sealable packing film by the similar process as adopted in nylon.

Uses : Polyethylene is used as laboratory tubing, in making protheses, electrical insulation; packing materials, kitchenwire; tank and pipe linings; paper coatings and textile. As fibres are resistant to acid, alkali and most solvents, they are used in filtering fabrics. An outstanding property of polyethylene, both as resin and filament, is its low specific gravity (0.92). A low softening point (110°) limits it application in wearing apparel uses.

SURGICAL DRESSINGS

A material used to protect a wound and to heal is called a surgical dressing. They serve various function for the injured site. They remove wound exudates from the site, prevent infection, give physical protection to the healing wound and mechanical support to the supporting tissues. A good quality of dressing should be durable, easy to handle, sterilized, formed from loose threads and fibres and it should not adhere to the granulating surface.

Surgical dressings are classified as :
1. Primary wound dressings
2. Absorbents
3. Bandages,
4. Adhesive tapes and
5. Protectives.

1. **Primary Wound Dressings :** Primary wound dressings are applied over the wound surface to absorb pus, mucus, blood, etc. They minimize maceration. Some dressings adhere to the wound surface and cause pain on removing them. Now nonadherent dressings are available such as petrolatum-impregnated gauge, viscose gauze impregnated with a bland, hydrophilic oil-in-water emulsion or an absorbent pad faced with a soft plastic film having openings, etc.

2. **Absorbents :** Absorbent cotton is widely used to absorb wound secretions. Other absorbent materials are rayon wool, cotton wool, gauze pads, laparotomy sponges, sanitary napkins, disposable cleaners, eye pads, nursing pads, cotton tip applications, etc. They are used in the shape of balls or pads.

3. **Bandages :** A bandage is a material which holds dressing at the required site, applies pressure or supports an injured part or checks haemorrhage. The

bandages may be elastic or non-elastic in nature. Common gauze roller bandage and muslin bandage rolls are employed most frequently. Elastic bandages may be woven to form elastic bandage, crepe bandage and conforming bandage.

4. **Adhesive Tapes** : Surgical adhesive tapes may be a rubber-based adhesive or an acrylate adhesive. Rubber adhesive tapes are cheap, superior and provide strength of backing. In case of operation or post-operation acrylate, adhesive tapes are used to reduce skin trauma.

5. **Protectives** : Protectives are employed to cover wet dressings, poultices and for retention of heat. They prevent the escape of moisture from the dressing. Some protectives are plastic sheeting, rubber sheeting, waxed or oil-coated papers and plastic-coated papers.

SUTURES AND LIGATURES

A surgical suture is a thread or sting used for sewing or stiching together tissues, muscles and tendons with the help of a needle. It these threads or fibres are used to tie a blood vessel to stop bleeding without the use of a needles, then they are called ligatures. Sutures may be absorable which are digested in animal tissues, e.g. catgut, kangaroo tendon and synthetic polyesters. If the sutures are not absorbed in the body, they are called nonabsorbable sutures, e.g. Silk, Cotton, Nylon, Synthetic Polyester fibres and Stainless Steel wire. A good quality of suture should be well-sterilized, non-irritant; having well-mechanical strength, fine gauze and with minimum time of absorption.

Absorable sutures

Surgical Catgut : Catgut is a sterilized fibre or strand prepared from collagen of connective tissues obtained from healthy animals like sheep and cattle.

Preparation : The submucosal layer of small intestine of a freshly killed animal is used for the preparation of catgut. About 7.5 meter long intestine is cleaned and split longitudinally into ribbons. The inner most mucosa and two outer layers of submucosa, muscularis and serosal layers, are removed with the help of a machine leaving behind the submucosa. Up to six such ribbons are stretched, spun and dried to form a uniform strand. These fibres are polished to get smooth strings, gauzed for their diameter, cut into suitable lengths and sterilized by placing the catgut in glass tubes filled with anhydrous high-boiling liquids like toluene or xylene and then heating in an autoclave. Sterilization may be done by irradiating the suture by electron particles or by gamma rays from cobalt-60.

Kangaroo tendons, used in hernia and bone repairs, are prepared from the tails of kangaroo by the identical method adopted for the preparation of catgut. Chromicized surgical catguts are prepared by soaking the ribbons in solutions of chromium salts for tanning the tissues. These fibres are not affected by proteolytic enzymes in the body and they are not absorbed rapidly in the body.

Synthetic Polyesters : The polymers obtained by condensation of cyclic derivatives of glycolic acid (glycolide) with cyclic derivatives of lactic acid (lacticide) are used to prepare synthetic absorbable sutures. These sutures have high tensile strength and degradated by hydrolysis and absorbed in the tissue.

Non-absorbable sutures

Non-absorbable sutures are not affected by the body fluid and remained unchange for a long period. They are removed after healing of the wounds. Silk, cotton, nylon and metallic sutures are classified as non-absorbable sutures.

Silk Sutures : Silk sutures are prepared by spinning or twisting silk fibres into a single strand of varying diameters. The sutures are smooth and strong and braided by combining several twisted yarns into a compact mass. The strands are sterilized and boiled with water to soften them.

Cotton Sutures : Cotton sutures have uniform size and recommended in critical parts where strength of the sutures is required for long time.

Nylon Sutures : The microfilaments of nylon are braided into strands of required diameter. These sutures are strong, water resistant and used in skin and plastic surgery.

Linen Suture: A linen suture is cheap, very strong under moist condition but not uniform in diameter.

Metallic Sutures : Metallic wires of silver or stainless steel are used as surgical aid. These wires are available as monofilaments, twists and braids.

QUESTIONS

1. Give preparation and microscopical characters of Silk and Wool. What chemical tests will differentiate these fibres from other fibres ?

2. What are absorbable haemostatic dressings ? Give details of any one material used in the manufacture of these dressings.

3. Define dressing, bandage, sutures and ligatures. What are functions and properties of surgical dressings ? How will you differentiate absorbent and non-absorbent cotton fibres ?

4. Give an account of preparation of Absorbent Cotton. How does Cotton fibre differ from Wool in microscopic characters. What chemical tests will you perform to characterize the two fibres ?

5. Enumerate the various fibres used for surgical dressings. Give the microscopical characters and microchemical tests to distinguish the following : (a) Wool from nonabsorbent cotton (b) Absorbent cotton from nonabsorbent cotton (c) Cotton from silk.

6. Give the method of collection and preparation of silk. How are cotton, rayon and alginate fibres differentiated from one another by chemical tests ?

7. Give the source, preparation, microscopy, test of identification and constituents of animal wool.

17

PLANT ANATOMY

Cell is a fundamental unit of a living organism. The cell contains a cell wall and consists of the protoplasmic components and nonprotoplasmic materials.

A group of cells with the identical form and function is knwon a *tissue* in which the cell membranes are connected with a pectin layer called middle lamella. The cytoplasmic threads, called *plasmodesmata*, are consisted of cell wall, cell membrane, protoplasm and middle lamella. They interconnect the protoplasm of different cells and assist to conduct food and communicate stimuli. Plant tissues are divided into three main groups :

1. Dermal tissues,
2. Fundamental or group tissues, and
3. Vascular tissues.

1. Dermal Tissues

These tissues consist of outer protective coverings such as epidermis, periderm, trichomes, stomata, etc.

(i) **Epidermis :** Epidermis is the outermost protective single layer of young plant body. The epidermal cells are narrowly placed with no intercellular spaces. They show wide variation in shape, size and arrangement. A cuticle layer, containing cutin, is usually present on the outer surface. The cuticle layer is not present in root epidermal tissues.

Suberin, found in cork cells, and cutin consist of mixtures of polymerized fatty acids such as suberic acid, COOH [CH$_2$]$_6$ COOH. These compounds give yellow to brown colour with chlor-zinc iodine; red colour with Soudan glycerin and yellow colour with potash solution.

The structures of the epidermis and stomata are helpful in the identification of leaves. Straight-walled epidermal cells are present in Coca and Senna leaves, wavy-walled epidermal cells in Stramonium, Hyoscyamus and Belladonna; beaded walls in Lobelia and Digitalis species; a papillose epidermis in Coca Leaf.

(ii) **Stomata :** A stomata is made of a pair of similar cells, called guards cells, placed parallel to each other. It contains a pore in the centre through which gaseous exchange takes place. The epidermal cells surrounding the stomata are called subsidiary cells and they are different in shape. On the basis of arrangement with the subsidiary cells, the stomata are divided into four different classes :

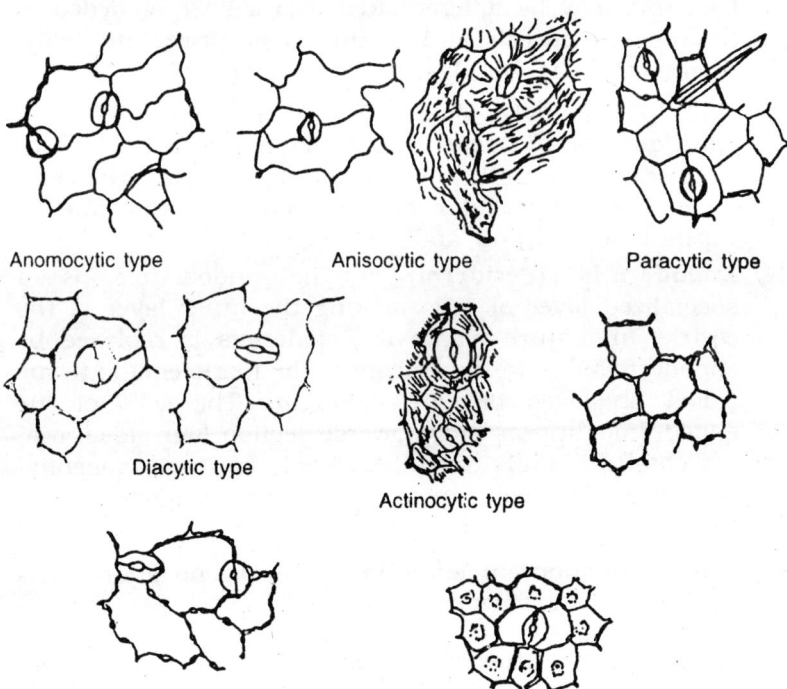

Anomocytic type   Anisocytic type   Paracytic type

Diacytic type

Actinocytic type

Fig. 17.1. Different kinds of stomata

(a) *Anomocytic or Ranunculaceous* type (Irregular type): The cells surrounding the stomal pore are irregularly arranged and cannot be distinguished from the other epidermal cells, e.g. Lobelia, Digitalis, Buchu.

(b) *Cruciferous or Anisocytic* (Unequal celled) : The stomal pore is surrounded by three or four subsidiary cells, one of which is markedly smaller than the others, e.g. Belladonna, Stramonium.

(c) *Rubiaceous or Paracytic* type (Paralled-celled) : Two subsidiary cells with their long axis are parallel to the pore, e.g. Senna, Coca.

(d) *Diacytic or Caryophyllaceous* type (Crossed celled) : The stoma is accompanied by two subsidiary cells, with their long axis at right angles to the pore of the stomata, e.g. Spearmint, Peppermint, Thyme, etc.

(e) *Actinocytic* (radiate-called) : This stoma is surrounded by a circle of radiating cells, e.g. Ursi.

(iii) **Epidermal Trichomes :** Trichomes are present on many leaves, herbaceous stems, flowers, fruits and seeds. A trichome may be differentiated into a base embeded in the epidermal cell and a tube like projecting body. Trichomes may be classified into two groups :

(a) *Covering trichomes :* They have protective function.

(b) *Glandular trichomes :* They secrete essential oils or oleo-resins. Both covering and glandular trichomes may be unicellular or multicellular, uniseriate or multiseriate and stalk or sessile.

(iv) **Endodermis (Periderm) :** The endodermis is a specialized layer of cells making the inner layer of the cortex. In mature plants the epidermis is replaced by endodermis due to the activity of the meristematic tissue called phellogen or cork cambium. The cells of the endodermis appear in transverse section four sided, oval or elliptical and often extended in the tangenital direction. The cells are longitudinally elongated.

In periderm lenticels are present which are pores identical in function. In lenticels, there are no guard cells and they remain always open.

2. Fundamental or Ground Tissues

Fundamental tissues include hypodermis, cortex, pith, mesophyll and midrib region.

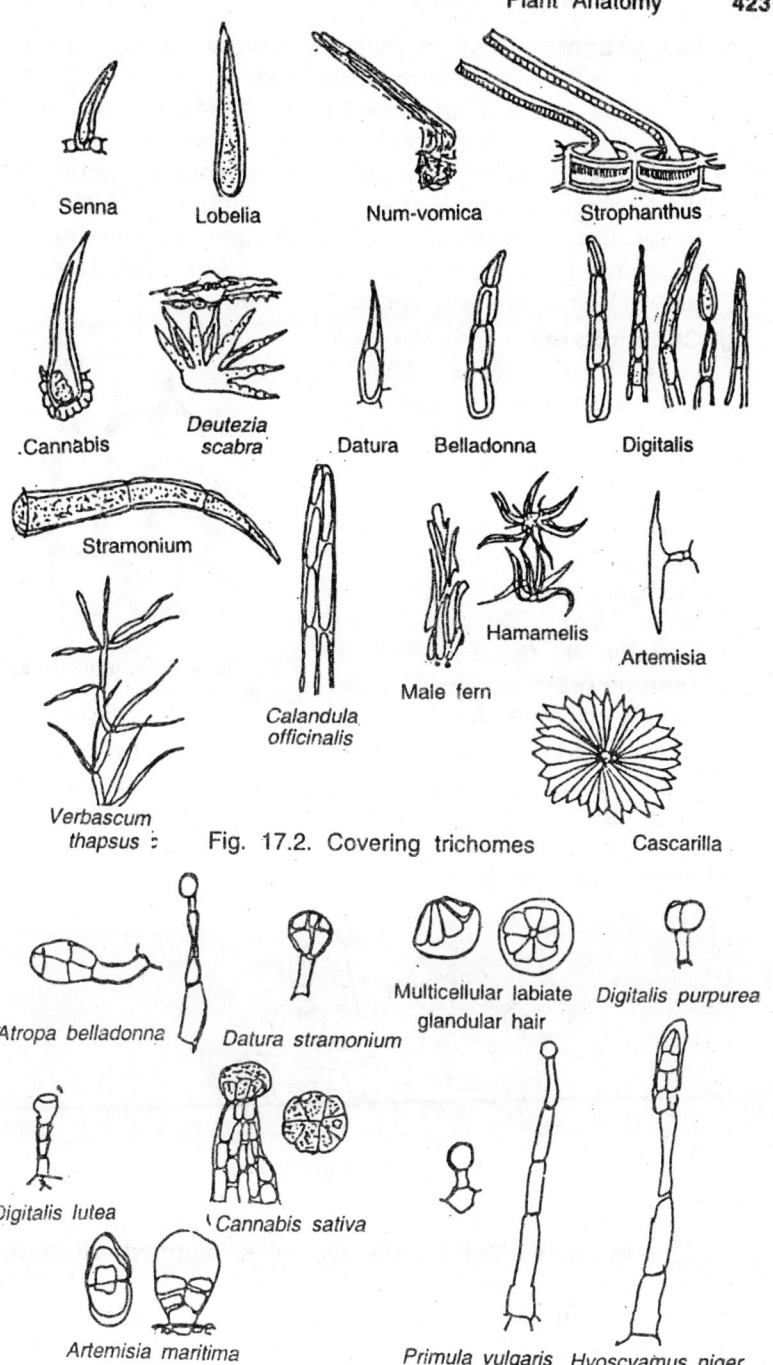

Senna   Lobelia   Num-vomica   Strophanthus

.Cannabis   Deutezia scabra   Datura   Belladonna   Digitalis

Stramonium

Hamamelis

Artemisia

Male fern

Calandula officinalis

Verbascum thapsus ;   Fig. 17.2. Covering trichomes   Cascarilla

Atropa belladonna   Datura stramonium   Multicellular labiate glandular hair   Digitalis purpurea

Digitalis lutea   Cannabis sativa

Artemisia maritima   Primula vulgaris Hyoscyamus niger

Fig. 17.3. Grandular hairs

(i) **Parenchyma** : Parenchyma contains living and thin walled cells with intercellular spaces. These cells vary in shape and are present in the cortex of root, cortex and pith of stem and mesophyll of leaves. Some parenchyma cells are pitted and contain reticulated thickening. Aerenchyma is parenchyma with large intercellular spaces. Chlorenchyma is parenchyma containing chloroplasts. The main functions of parenchyma are storage and photosynthesis.

(ii) **Collenchyma** : Collenchyma is a living tissue derived from parenchyma and has greater mechanical strength. The walls are thickened due to deposition of cellulose. These cells are usually present in cortical region of stem, petiole, bark and midrib of a leaf. The cells are usually 4 to 6 sided in transverse section, and axially elongated.

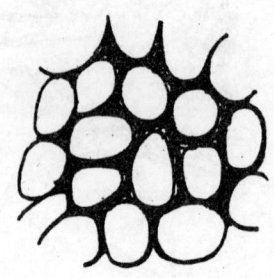

Fig. 17.4. Collenchymatous tissue

(iii) **Sclerenchyma** : Sclerenchyma cells are the dead and lignified tissues. The cell walls are heavily thickened with lignin. They occur in all parts of the plant body and give mechanical strength. These cells may occur as stone cells or fibres.

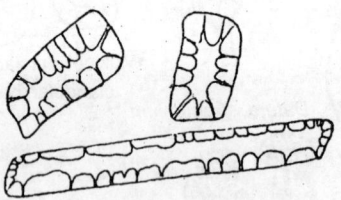

Fig. 17.5. Stone Cells

The stone cells or sclereids are isodiametrical or irregular in shape. Their walls are thick, lignified, often show well-marked stratification and traversed by pit-canals which are usually funnel-shaped or branched. The cell lumen is small and cell contents of diagnostic significance may be present. Stone cells are present in the hard outer coats of seeds and fruits and in the bark and pericyclic regions of woody stems. They occur singly or in groups.

Sclerenchymatous fibres are narrow, usually elongated with pointed ends. The tissue is composed of spindle-shaped or elongated cells with pointed ends and known as prosenchyma. The cell wall may be composed of pure cellulose and is usually lignified. Most mature fibres are unicellular and give mechanical support to the plant.

Isolated groups of pericyclic fibres occur in Lobelia and Cinnamon bark. Xylem fibres are derived from tracheids and have smaller pits, thicker walls and tapering ends. Phloem fibres may be lignified or unlignified.

3. Vascular Tissues

Vascular tissue system conducts food material and water. Phleom is a living tissue and conducts food material from leaves to the different parts of the plant. Xylem is a dead tissue and conducts water from roots to the leaves.

(i) **Phloem** : Phloem consists of sieve-tubes, companion cells, phloem parenchyma and secretory cells. It contains a vertical series of elongated cells and interconnected by perforations in their walls in areas known as sieve plates. Laticiferous tissues may also occur in the phloem.

(ii) **Xylem** : The structural elements of xylem are tracheids, vessels or tracheae, xylem fibres, xylem parenchyma and rays.

Tracheids are elongated tubes pointed at both ends. Their cell walls are lignified and pitted. Vessels or tracheae constitute of elongated tubes but without any oblique perforated walls. The vessels of the protoxylem show annular or spiral thickenings. The later-formed xylem contains sclariform and reticulate thickenings. The secondary wall thickening is composed of lignocellulose.

The living meshwork of a secondary xylem is composed of rays and xylem parenchyma. The xylem parenchyma cells are often axilly elongated, sometimes thin-walled but usually are thick and lignified. The formation of concentric zones of xylem parenchyma may give rise to 'false annular rings'.

According to the mode of presence of the xylem and phloem the vascular bundles may be collateral, bicollateral, concentric, and radial.

(a) **Collateral** : This is the most common type of vascular bundle found in stems and leaves. In this system the xylem and phloem remain side by side arranged on the same radius, phloem on the outer side and xylem on the inner side. Collateral bundles may be open when cambium is present in between phloem and xylem or closed when cambium is absent.

(b) **Bicollateral** : When another patch of phloem is present on the inner side of the external phloem, then the vascular bundle is called as bicollateral.

(c) **Concentric** : In this system one kind of vascular tissue surrounds the other.

(d) **Radial** : Here the xylem and phloem occur in separate patches on alternate radii on the axis. Radial vascular bundles are characteristic of roots.

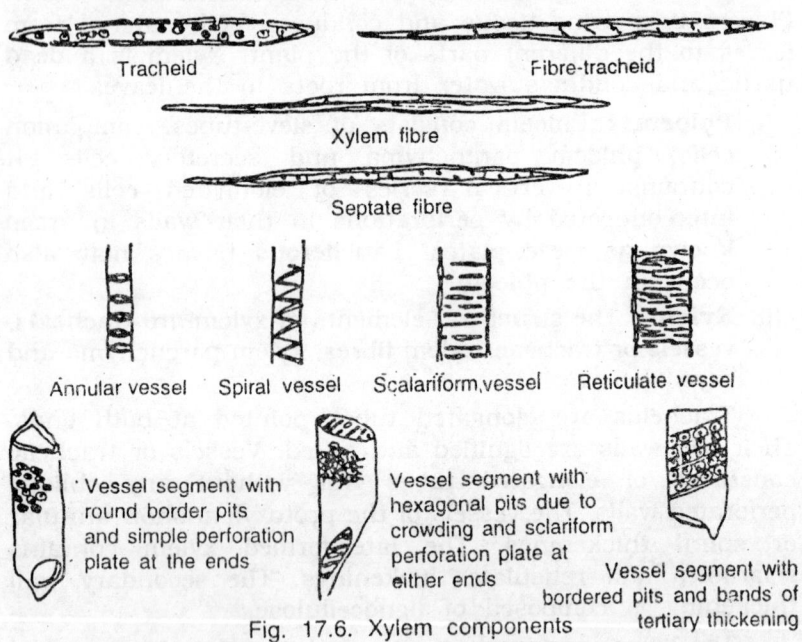

Tracheid   Fibre-tracheid

Xylem fibre

Septate fibre

Annular vessel   Spiral vessel   Scalariform vessel   Reticulate vessel

Vessel segment with round border pits and simple perforation plate at the ends

Vessel segment with hexagonal pits due to crowding and sclariform perforation plate at either ends

Vessel segment with bordered pits and bands of tertiary thickening

Fig. 17.6. Xylem components

In dicot stems the vascular bundles are arranged in the form of a ring and in monocot, the bundles are scattered.

Cambium : Cambium is a meristematic tissue present between the phloem and xylem in dicot stems. It is absent in young roots, but appears on maturing the plant between the radially placed phloem and xylem. Then it forms a zig-zag ring giving out secondary xylem on the inner side and secondary phloem on the outer side. The delicate primary structures are either crushed or poorly represented in developed plant parts.

Medullary rays are composed of parenchymatous cells, run diagonally and extend from pith (medulla) to the cortex through the secondary xylem and secondary phloem.

Secretory Tissues : Secretory cells, secretory cavities or sacs, secretory ducts or canals and latex tissue are the secretory tissues. Cells containing oils, resins, oleoresins and mucilage are present. The vittae of Umbelliferae are schizogenous oleoresin canals and they are found in the stem, roots and leaves. Latex (laticiferous) tissue consists of cells or tubes which contains a milky fluid.

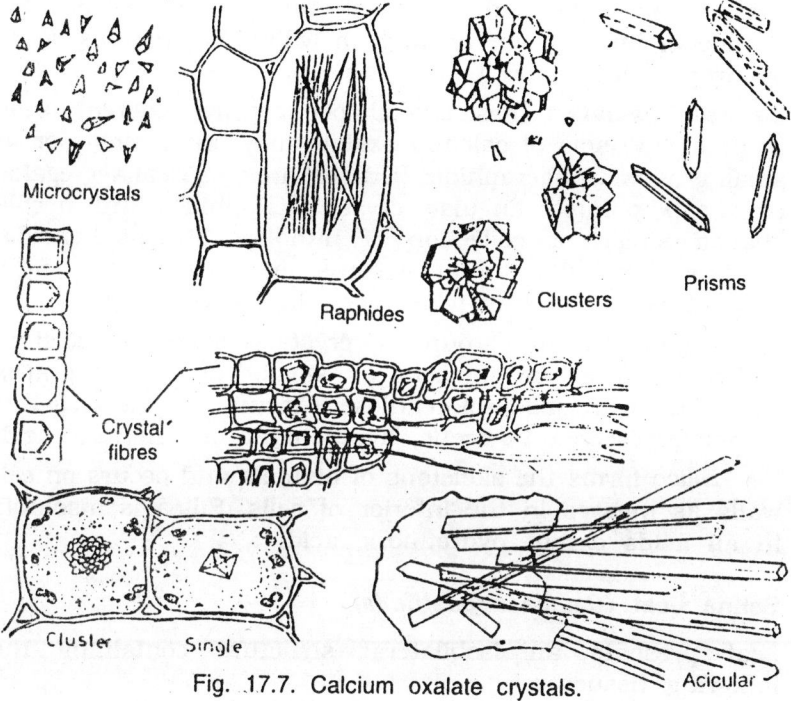

Fig. 17.7. Calcium oxalate crystals.

Three types of secretory cavities are known : *Schizogenous* cavity which is formed due to splitting of the epithelial cells; *Lysigenous* cavity - formed due to dissolution of cells and *Schizo-lysigenous* cavity - formed by both the operations.

Ergastic Cell Contents : These cell contents are identified by microscopical examination or by physical and chemical tests. They include carbohydrates, proteins, fixed oil, fats, alkaloids, volatile oils, resins, gums, calcium oxalate, silica, etc.

Starch : Starch occurs as granules in roots, rhizomes, fruits and seeds. Starch of various sources differs in shape and size.

Proteins : Protein is found in the form of aleurone grains surrounded by thin membrane. The ground mass of protein encloses one or more rounded bodies and an angular body known as the crystolloid.

Fixed Oils and Fats : They are usually present in seeds.

Gum, mucilage and pectins are polysaccharide complexes formed from sugar and uronic acid units. They are insoluble in alcohol but dissolve or swell in water. Volatile oils occur as droplets in the cell.

Calcium Oxalate : These crystals occur in five different forms in plants. Prisms of calcium oxalate may occur singly or in small groups. Sphaeraphides (Druses) are spherical aggregates of sharp pointed angular crystals. Raphides are needle shaped single or collection of bundles. Micro-sphenoidal crystals occur like an amorphous mass in a cell. These crystals shine brightly when seen in polarized light.

Crystoliths are group of crystals made of calcium carbonate. They are present as small bunches of grapes whose stalk are made of cellulose. Calcium oxalate dissolves with effervescence in acetic, hydrochloric or sulphuric acid.

Silica forms the skeletons of diatoms and occurs on cell walls as masses in the interior of cells. Silica is insoluble in all acids except hydrofluoric acid.

Senna Leaf *(Cassia angustifolia)*

Leaf presents an isobilateral structure containing the following tissues :

Epidermis : Epidermal cells are tabular with straight anticlinical walls and frequently containing mucilage. Upper epidermis is single-layered with a thick layer of cuticle on outerside. Covering trichomes, present on both sides, are unicellular, with thick warty walls, usually curved near the base and pointed in the direction of the limb; the base surrounded by radial epidermal cells. Two-celled paracylic stomata are present on both sides in equal numbers.

Mesophyll : Palisade layers, cluster crystals and spongy mesophyll are the part of mesophyll. Upper palisade layer is compact, single-layered, with elongated, narrow, columnar cells present over the midrib portion. The cells of lower palisade are smaller than that of upper palisade, loosely arranged with warty walls and present at lamina. The parenchymatous cells of spongy mesophyll are narrow, thin, loosely arranged and present between upper and lower palisade. Occasional cluster crystals of calcium oxalate are present in the mesophyll.

Midrib : The midrib is biconvex and its lower part contains collenchymatous cells. The cells of the upper palisade are smaller. Collateral vascular bundles are incompletely surrounded by sclerenchymatous fibres with a crystal sheath of calcium oxalate crystals and present on the central part of the midrib. Xylem is towards the ventral surface and phloem towards the dorsal surface.

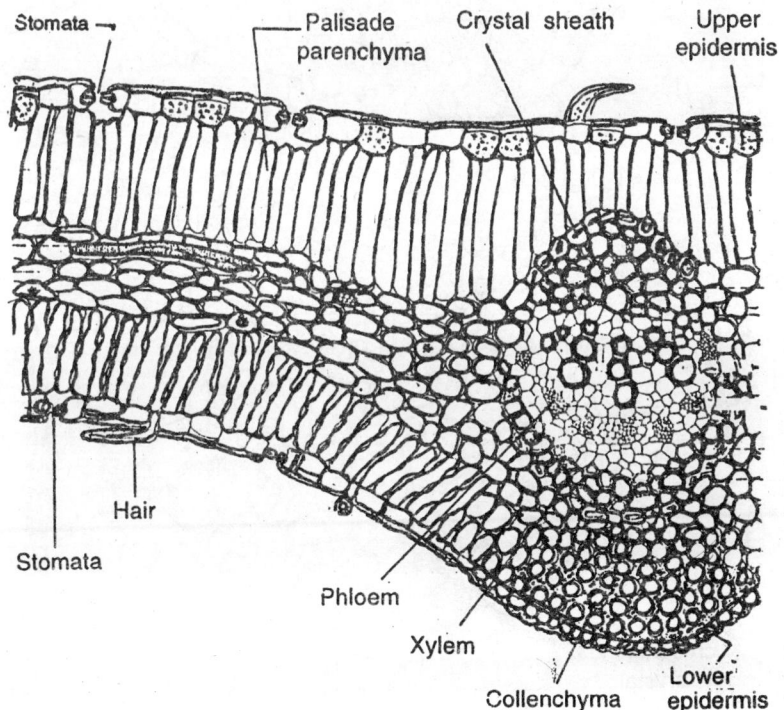

Fig. 17.8. Transverse section of Senna Leaflet

Datura Leaf *(Datura stramonium)*

A transverse section of Datura leaf shows a bifacial structure. The important tissues of epidermis, mesophyll and midrib region are :

Epidermis : The cells of upper epidermis are single layered and rectangular. The lower epidermal cells have wavy walls. Both surfaces are covered with smooth cuticle. Covering and glandular trichomes are present, being more numerous in young leaves. The covering trichomes are uniseriate, conical, composed of three to five cells with warty walls; blunt at the apex. The glandular trichomes are short and clavate, with two to seven cells in the head. Stomata are anisocytic and more frequent on the lower epidermis.

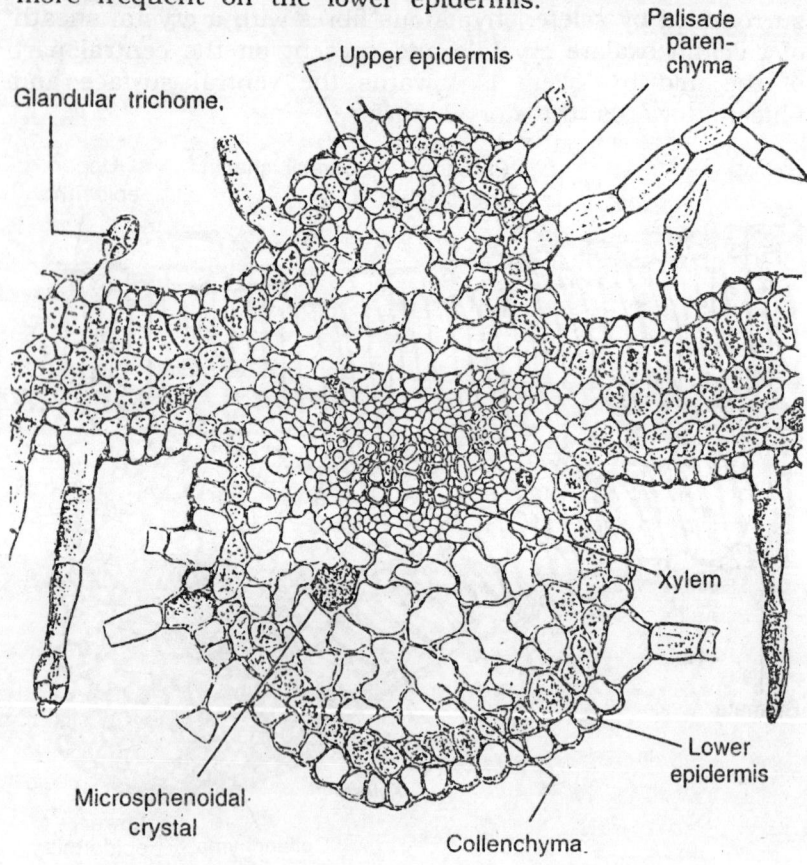

Fig. 17.9. Transverse section of Datura Leaf

Mesophyll : Mesophyll is dorsiventral with single palisade layer containing compact and radially elongated cells. Under palisade layer there is a crystal layer with each cell containing cluster crystals of calcium oxalate, long, or occasional prisms of microsphenoidal crystals. No crystals are present in cells adjoining the veins. Spongy parenchyma of mesophyll is multilayered and loosely arranged with intercellular spaces.

Midrib : The midrib shows a bicollateral structure. Typical subepidermal cells of collenchyma are present on both surfaces. The epidermal layers of lamina are continuous in the midrib region. Collenchymatous layer is followed by cortical parenchyma containing prisms of calcium oxalate and microsphenoidal crystals.

Cinchona Bark *(Cinchona succirubra)*

Transverse section of the bark shows periderm, cortex and secondary phloem.

Periderm : It is composed of multi-layered thin-walled cork cells, arranged in a regular radial rows and appearing polygonal. The contents of the cells are thin-walled and dark reddish in colour. The cork cells are impregnated with suberin. There are 3-4 layers of thin walled rectangular cells of phellogen without any cellular contents. There are 6-8 layers of thin rectangular cells without any cellular contents near the phellogen and arranged in radial rows.

Cortex : The cortex is composed of thin-walled, tangentially elongated, pitted and multi-layered cells. They contain starch granules, or amorphous reddish brown matter, with scattered idioblasts, possessing microprisms of calcium oxalate and large secretory cells, spaced at intervals near the inner part.

Phloem : It consists of narrow sieve tubes, sieve plates, phloem parenchyma which resembles that of the cortex and with large characteristic spindle shaped phloem fibres. The fibres occur with thick, conspicuously striated walls transversed by funnel-shaped pits, with isolated or in irregular radial rows.

Medullary rays are two to three cells wide, with thin-walled, somewhat radially elongated cells. The fibres are present with phloem parenchyma and in between medullary rays. Phloem fibres are numerous, fusiform, mostly isolated, rounded to oval, in different sizes, yellow in colour, thick-walled, heavily lignified with a small lumen and stratification. The distribution and size of the phloem fibres differ in various species. Sclereids are rare.

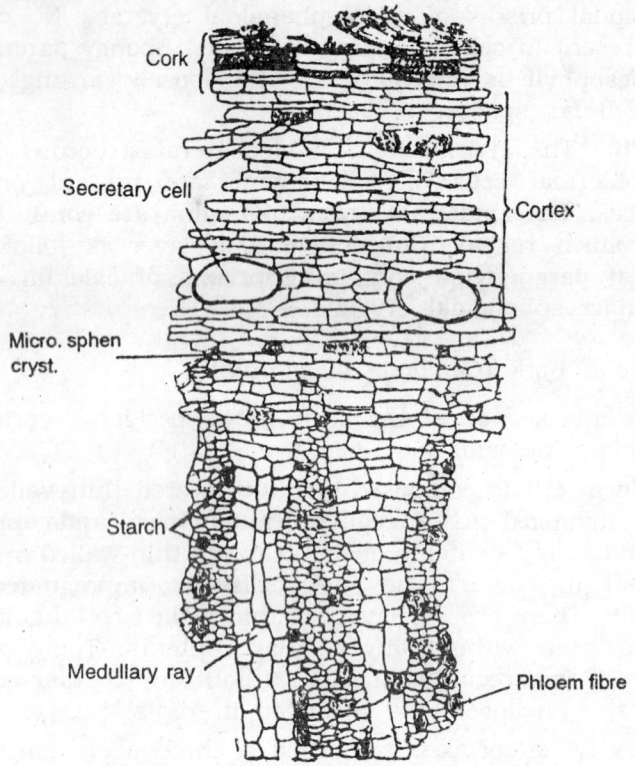

Fig. 17.10. Transverse Section of Cinchona bark

Fennel *(Foeniculum vulgare)*

Transverse section of Fennel mericarp shows commisural and dorsal surfaces. The commisural surface is flat containing two pronounced ridges and carpophore in the middle. The dorsal surface has five ridges. Mericarp is divided into pericarp, testa and bulky endosperm. The epicarp (exocarp) of the pericarp encircles the entire mericarp and consists of a layer of polygonal, tangentially elongated cells with smooth cuticle.

The mesocarp is made of parenchyma and bicollateral vascular bundles below the primary ridges. Vascular bundles are surrounded by reticulate and lignified parenchyma. Yellowish brown and elliptical vittae (schizogenous ducts), four on the dorsal surface and two on the commissural surface, are present in the mesocarp.

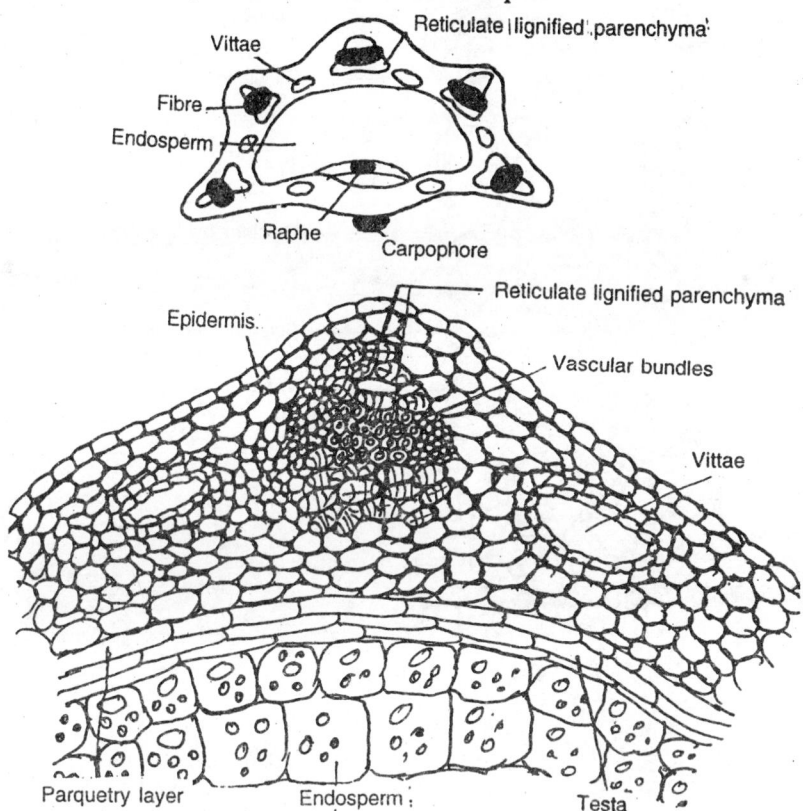

Fig. 17.11. Transverse section of Fennel fruit (A) Mericarp (diagramatic) (B) Cellular

Endocarp contains cells in a single layer between mesocarp and testa. The testa is single layered and yellowish brown in colour.

Endosperm consists of thick-walled, polygonal, colourless parenchyma. It contains aleurone grains and oil globules. A crescent shaped embryo is seen in sections through the apical region of mesocarp. Raphae is present in the middle of commissural surface in front of carpophore.

Clove Flower Bud (Syzygium aromaticum)

Transverse section of Clove hypanthium below the ovary shows epidermis, cortex and columella.

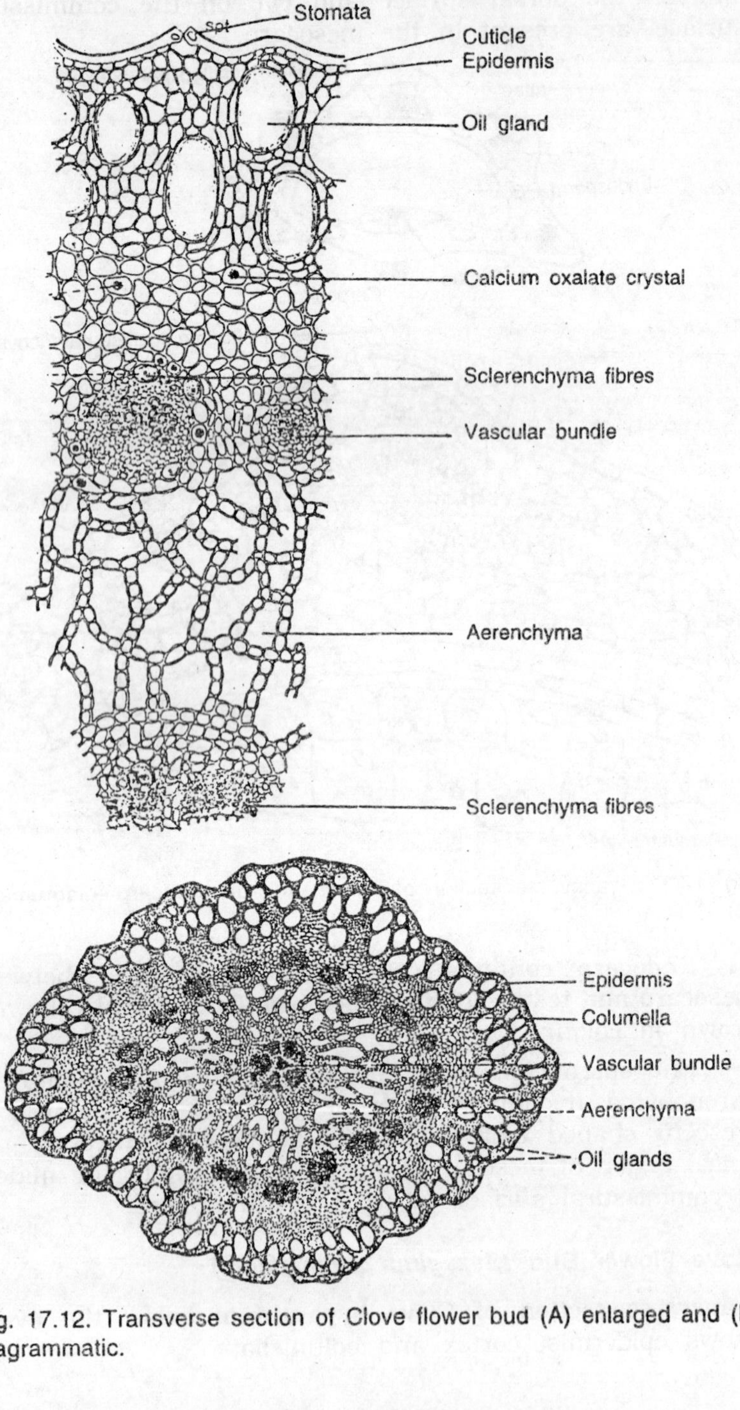

Fig. 17.12. Transverse section of Clove flower bud (A) enlarged and (B) diagrammatic.

Epidermis is heavily cuticularized with straight walls in which occur ranunculaceous stomata.

There are three different regions in the cortex. The peripheral region is composed of 2-3 layers of large, ellipsoidal, schizolysigenous oil glands arranged in two or three intermixed layers. The oil glands are ellipsoidal in shape, with the long axis radial and show an epithelium composed of two or three layers of flattened cells. Clusters of crystals of calcium oxalate occur in many of the parenchymatous cells. Within the oil gland layer there is a zone of cells with somewhat thickened walls embedding a ring of bicollateral vascular bundles. The ground tissue of this zone contains cluster crystals of calcium oxalate. The meristeles are enclosed in an incomplete ring of lignified fibres.

The middle region contains one or two rings of bicollateral vascular bundles with few pericyclic fibres. The xylem is composed of 3-5 lignified spiral vessels. Within the ring of vascular bundles is a zone of aerenchyma, composed of air spaces and columella. The ground tissue of the columella is parenchymatous and rich in calcium oxalate clusters. In the outer region of the columella is a ring of some 17 small vascular bundles. Numerous sphaeraphides are present scattered throughout the columella.

The hypanthium, in the region of the ovary, shows epidermis, oil gland layer and ring of bicollateral bundles. Within this is a zone of cells with strongly thickened cellulose wall. The dissepiment of the ovary is parenchymatous; the placentae are rich in cluster crystals and contains vascular bundles.

Ginger Rhizome *(Zingiber Officinale)*

A transverse section of unpeeled Ginger rhizome shows a zone of cork cells, cortex, endodermis and ground tissues.

Outer zone of cork tissue consists of irregularly arranged cells. The cork cambium is differentiated. Within the cork is a broad cortex, differentiated into an outer zone of flattened parenchyma and an inner zone of normal parenchyma. The cortical cells contain abundant starch grains. These are almost entirely simple, ovoid or sack-shaped and have a markedly eccentric hilum. Numerous oil cells, with suberized walls enclosing yellowish-brown oleoresin, are scattered in the cortex. The inner cortical zone usually contains about three rings of collateral, closed vascular bundles. The larger bundles are enclosed in a sheath of septate, non-lignified fibres. Each vascular bundle contains phloem, showing well-marked sieve-tubes and a xylem composed of 1-14 vessels with annular spiral or reticulate thickening. The inner part of the cortex is marked by a single-layered endodermis free from starch. The outermost layer of the stele is marked by a single layered pericycle. The vascular bundles of stele resemble those of the cortex, and are scattered as in monocotyledonous stems.

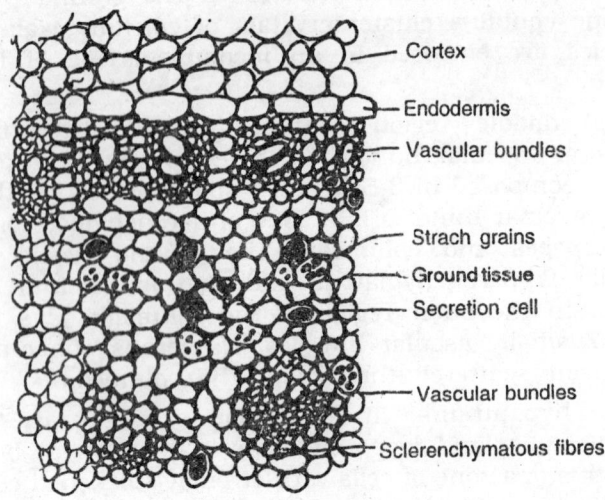

Cortex
Endodermis
Vascular bundles

Strach grains
Ground tissue
Secretion cell

Vascular bundles
Sclerenchymatous fibres

Fig. 17.13. Transverse section of Ginger rhizome (cellular)

Ground tissue contains large parenchymatous, rounded, polygonal cells containing excess of starch, oleo-resin and vascular bundles. Starch occurs as flattened, oval or subrectangular, transversely striated, simple granules, each with a hilum in a projection towards one end. Oleo-resin cells contains suberized cell walls and yellow contents. Pigment cells contain dark, reddish brown contents and occur either singly in ground tissue or in axial rows accompanying the vascular bundles. Sclereids and calcium oxalate crystals are absent.

Nux-Vomica Seed *(Strychnos nux-vomica)*

The transverse section shows hairy thin testa and a bulky endosperm.

The testa consists of collapsed parenchyma and a single epidermal layer of very typical lignified hair. Each hairy epidermal cell has a very large, thick-walled base with slit-like pits. The upper portions of each hair are set at almost a right angle to the bases and all radiate out towards the margin of the seed giving the testa a silky appearance. The upper part of the wall of the hair is composed of about ten longitudinal ridge-like thickenings united by a thin wall. The lumen is circular in the upper part but in the base has branches.

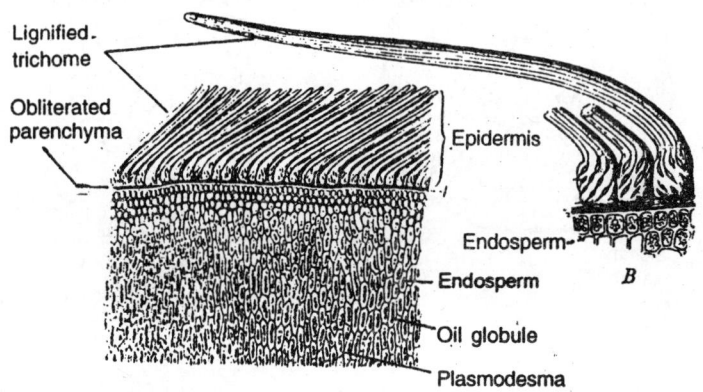

Fig. 17.14. Transverse section of Nux-vomica seed (cellular)

The endosperm consists of a large, thick-walled cellulosic parenchyma. The walls are non-lignified, composed mainly of hemicellulose and swell considerably in water; the lumen is polygonal. Outermost layers of the endosperm appear palisade like whereas polyhedral, unlignified, parenchymatous cells are present in the inner layer. Well-marked interconnected plasmodesma (protoplasmic threads) is observed by staining the section with dilute iodine. Aleurone grains and fixed oil droplets are also present in endosperm. Strychnine is most abundant in the inner layer of the endosperm and brucine in the outer layers. The epidermis of the endosperm is formed of smaller cells.

Ipecac Root (Cephaelis ipecacuanha)

A transverse section of the root shows a thin brown cork, wide secondary cortex (phelloderm) and vascular bundles.

The cork layer is composed of thin-walled polyhedral, tabular cells. The cells of phelloderm are parenchymatous and contain starch, usually in compound grains with from two to eight components or raphides of calcium oxalate. The individual starch granules are oval, rounded or roughly hemispherical.

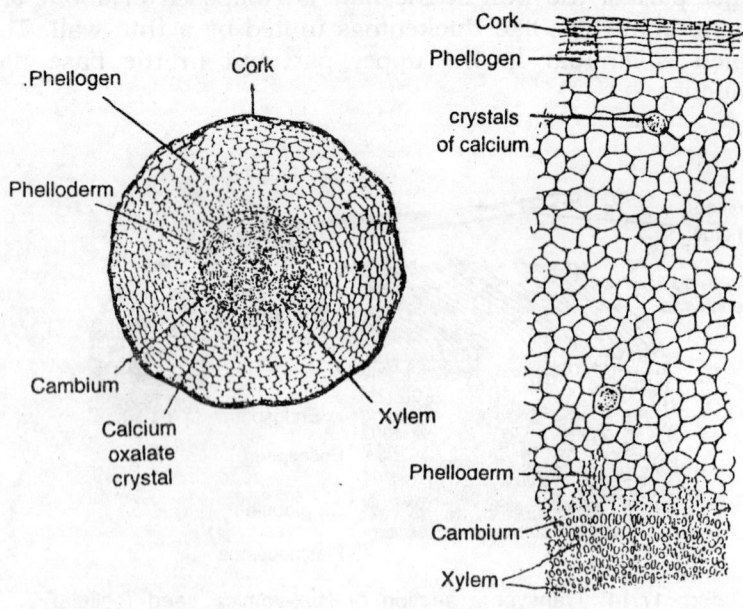

Fig. 17.15. Transverse section of Ipecacunha root.

The secondary xylem consists of narrow tracheidal-vessels and tracheids, both having bordered pits in their lateral walls, associated with xylem parenchyma. The segments of the tracheidal-vessels usually have the communicating opening on the side walls near the ends. The cells of the xylem parenchyma have simple pits. The vessel elements have simple and circular perforations. Cells of xylem parenchyma and medullary rays contain abundant starch consisting of simple granules. The medullary rays are one or two and their cells are wide.

The phloem occurs as small groups of sieve tissue embedded in parenchyma. The phloem is entirely parenchymatous, containing no sclerenchymatous cells or fibres.

Coriander Fruit *(Coriandrum sativum)*

A transverse section of a fully ripe fruit shows only two mature vittae in each mericarp, pericarp, mesocarp and endosperm.

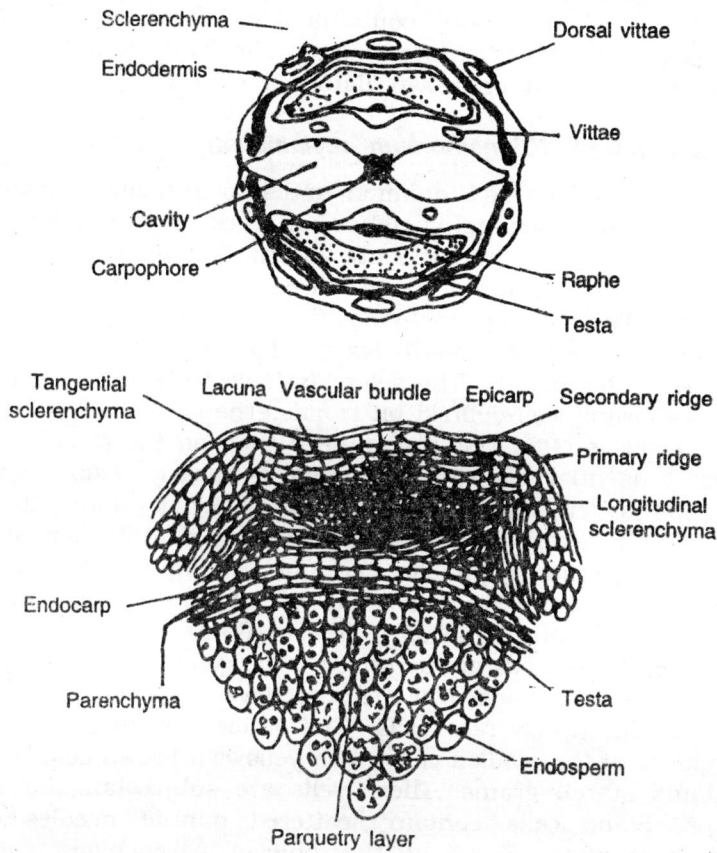

Fig. 17.16. Transverse section of Coriander fruit (A) Outline diagram (B) Cellular x 150

Vittae are present on the commissural surface. Mesocarp is differentiated into outer, middle and inner zones. Outer zone is parenchymatous, containing degenerated vittae as tangentially flattened cavities. Middle zone is sclarenchymatous, composed of sinuous rows of pitted, fusiform lignified cells often crossing one another at right angles and forming definite longitudinal strands in the primary ridges and tangentially directed in the secondary ridges. Inner mesocarp is partially composed of thin-walled hexagonal sclereids. The inner epidermis of mesocarp consists of cells showing parquetry arrangement and the hypodermis of large, slightly thickened, flattened hexagonal sclerenchyma. Endosperm is parenchymatous, made up of thickened cellulose walls, contains fixed oil and numerous aleurone grains with minute rosettes of calcium oxalate. The testa is composed of brown flattened cells.

Cinnamon Bark *(Cinnamomum zeylanicum)*

Transverse section of Cinnamon under microscope indicates that except occasional patches of cork and underlying parenchyma, cork and cortex are absent. The outermost layer consists of a continuous band, three or four cells wide, of pericyclic lignified sclerenchyma. On the outer margin there are small group of about six to fifteen *pericyclic fibres* occurring at intervals. The sclereids have thickened lignified walls, showing well-defined pit canals. The thickening on the outer walls is often less pronounced than on the radial and inner tangential walls. The lumen is clearly visible and contains a few starch grains. The pericyclic fibres have strongly thickened lignified walls showing stratification and pit canals. Primary phloem can not be differentiated. The secondary phloem is consisted of phloem parenchyma, containing oil and mucliage; phloem fibres and medullary rays. The *sieve-tubes* are arranged in tangenital bands which are completely collapsed in the outer layers. The sieve plates are on the transverse walls. The phloem parenchyma is composed of thin-walled cells, with yellowish-brown cells and contains starch grains. These cells are sub-rectangular in shape. Some cells contain scattered minute needles of calcium oxalate. Some of the phloem parenchyma cells contain tannins. The secretary cells, containing volatile oil or mucilage, are two or three times the diameter of the phloem fibres, and are axially elongated. The phloem fibres, which occur isolated or in tangential rows, are more abundant towards the inner part of the bark. The secondary phloem is divided up by the radial medullary rays, which are uni- or biseriate near the cambium but become broader towards the outside by tangenital growth the the cells. The rays are 7-14 cells in height. The medullary ray cells are radially elongated, thin walled with yellow-brown cell contents possessing numerous acicular crystals of calcium oxalate.

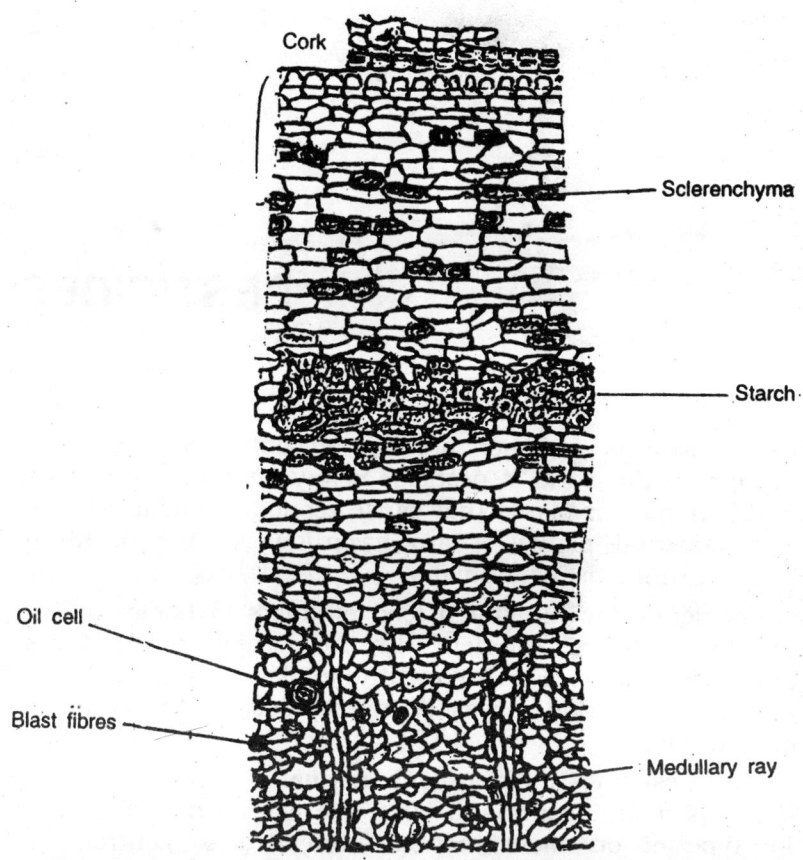

Fig. 17.17. Transverse section of Cinnamon bark.

QUESTIONS

1. Describe various plant tissues with suitable examples? How do these tissues assist in authentication of a drug ?

2. Discuss different types of stomata, secretary tissues and calcium oxalate crystals.

3. Draw cellular diagrames of any two of the following : (a) Clove, (b) Senna (c) Fennel.

18

PESTICIDES

Pest control is a major problem in cultivation of plants throughout the world. A pesticide is any toxic substance used to kill animals or plants that cause economic damage to crop or ornamental plants or are hazardous to the health of domestic animals or humans.

Rodents damage stored food products in homes and in warehouses. Weeds interfere with the normal growth of crop and garden plants. Fungi growth take place on vegetable and fruit plants. Various types of insects destroy the crop and food articles.

All pesticides interfere with normal metabolic processes in the pest organisms and often are classified according to the type of organism they are intended to control, *viz.* fungicides, herbicides, insecticides, rodenticides, molluscacides, nematocides and fumigants. Methods of these pesticides employ similar toxic substances. The means of application, chemical nature, types of products, precautions to be taken, symptions of accidental poisoning and immediate means of treatment are part of knowledge which must be known to the distributors and customers. The manufacturer must provide the efficacy of the product, its safety toward human beings, crops, livestock, wildlife and the general environment. The pesticide should not be deposited as residue on food which causes such a hazard.

Types of Pests

Rodents and arthropods are the most destructive animal

pests. The plant pests include weeds and the fungi pathogenic to cultivated plants.

Rodents : Rodents are mammals like rat, mouse, rabbit and monkey, which have sharp gnawing incisor teeth. In some stores the crude drugs are often contaminated due to fecal pallets and hair from the fur of rats and mice. Rodents are responsible for transmitting diseases from which they are suffering. Biting of a rat causes rat-bite fever, an infectious disease caused by microorganisms. A large number of lice infected rodents transmit typhus fever, bubonic plague, and rat leprosy. Rats carry ticks and mites which carry tularemia, Rocky Mountain spotted fever, and undulant fever producing microorganisms.

Arthropods

Arthropods are the insects, spiders, ticks, mites, and lice. Some of these cause discomfort only, while others cause fatal diseases. Insects represent the class of the phylum Arthropoda and according to their mouth parts they are divided into two morphologic groups :

1. biting and chewing, and
2. piercing and sucking.

The insects of the first category are dependant on the leaves and stems of plants. They are present in excess number to strip a cultivated field. Grasshoppers and locusts destroy the crop during the developmental process and after maturity stage. Tomato horn worms and army worms cause destruction during larva or caterpiller stage.

Most of the insects possess a piercing-sucking modification of mouth parts with which they penetrate into the epidermal tissues of plant organs and suck the juice from the soft tissues. The examples are aphids (plant lice), San Jose scale, Chinch bugs, squash bugs, cabbage bugs and leafhoppers.

Cockroaches, termites, silverfish, cloth moths, carpet beetles, flies, bedbugs, fleas, and mosquitoes are house hold insects which have either chewing jaws or possess a piercing sucking mechanism. Mosquitoes and deerflies bite human beings and animals. The malarial mosquito exples some of its protozoan-laden saliva during penetration of the human epithelium. The microorganisms enter the blood stream when the long hollow tube, called probocis, contacts the capillaries to obtain the drop of blood. Malaria, yellow fever, sleeping sickness, dengue fever, and other infectious diseases are spread by this process. The destruction of mosquitoes, flies, ticks and related arthropods stop spreading of these disastrous diseases for ever.

Piercing-sucking mouth parts are present in lice, fleas, mites,ticks and spiders. Rocky Mountain spotted fever is spread by the wood tick, *Dermacentor andersoni* and the dog tick *D.variabilis*. The rat flea, *Xenopsylla cheopsis*, is responsible for the spread of endemic typhus fever, and the body mouse, *Pediculis corporis*, causes typhus. Mites like *Sarcoptes scabiei* produce scabies. The hairy spiders bite can kill birds and small mammals. The black widow spider, *Latrodectus mactans*, bite is painful. A bacterium transmitted to human beings by the bite of a deer tick, *Ixodes ricinus*, causes lyme disease in U.S.A. which is an affliction of summer.

Weeds

Any undesirable plant is known as weed. A weed may be a dandelion in a lawn, a thistle plant (Gokhru) in a vegetable garden, or mustard in a clove field. Undesirable plants in gardens interfere in the growth of cultivated plants by consuming most of the available water contents and minerals of the soil. Weeds grow and flourish in the conditions of much sunshine, ample moisture and well-fertilized soil which are provided for cultivation of some ornamental plants and vegetables. If weeds are allowed to grow, they will soon acquire possession of the garden and gradually destroy the more dilicate, cultivated plants. Similarly, the quality of the field crops, specially grains, become poor due to presence of weed seeds.

A considerable number of weeds are toxic in nature. Corn cockle, *Agostemma githago*, contains a cyanophore type of glycoside, and its seeds cause death when they are present in excessive quantities in wheat flour. A large number of plants give rise to allergic reactions in certain individuals. Once a person has been sensitized to a particular allergen, subsequent exposure to the materials produces an antigen-antibody reaction which results in the liberation of histamine or identical compounds causing allergic symptoms. Allergies are commonly asthma and dermatitis. Pollens of grasses like timothy (*Phleum pratense*), cocks foot (*Dactylis glomerata*) and perennial rye (*Lolium perenne*) as well as that of nettle (*Urtica dioica*), Plantain (*Plantogo* spp.) and ragweeds (*Ambrosia* spp.) are responsible for seasonal hay fever. A number of common moulds produce spores which cause rhinitis and asthma in sensitive individuals. *Rhus* spp.like *R. radicans* (poison ivy), *R. toxicodendron* (poison oak), *R. deversiloba* (Pacific poison oak) and *R. vernix* (poison elder) (fam. Anacardiaceae) contain contactant allergens which produce severe dermatitis associated with watery blisters. Sesquiterpene lactones from the species of Compositae, Lauraceae and Magnoliaceae and from the Liverwort *Frullania* (Fam. Jubulaceae) are a major class of compounds causing allergic contact dermatitis in human. The fruits and seeds of *Menispermum canadense* and *Datura stramonium* are poisonous when swallowed.

Some of the poisonous fungi when taken orally produce hallucinations. The examples are *Amanita*, *Psilocybe* and *Conocybe*. Certain cacti contain protoalkaloids, some of which have marked hallucinogenic properties.

Fungi Parasitic on Plants

Various type of fungi growing on plants produce many diseases such as wheat rust, white pine blister rust, Dutch elm disease, hollyhock rust, orange leaf rust of black berries and raspberries, asparagus rust and rose rust. Various fungicides and chemical agents are available for the control of fungus disease. Precaution is taken from the beginning of cultivation of a crop. The seeds should be freed of adhering fungus spores before being planted. It is treated with a suitable fungicide such as Thiram (tetramethylthiuram disulphide). Different type of windborne bacteria and fungi grow on tender shoots. They contaminate young seedlings and plants growing near these infected plants. In such cases, sprays or fungicidal dusts are applied to prevent germination of the parasitic species.

Different types of microorganisms produce a number of plant diseases. Viral diseases are caused by tobacco mosaic and the bean mosaic. Bacteria are responsible for the diseases like carrot rot, 'fire blight' of pear and apple and the wilt of cucumber, squash and melon. Physmycetes cause damping off fungus, downy mildew of grapes and 'late blight' of potatoes. The diseases such as powdery mildew of lilac, American chestnut blight and Dutch elm disease are produced by Ascomycetes. The microorganisms Ascomycetes cause the corn smut, 'loose smut' of oats, wheat rust, apple rust and other rusts.

Methods of Control of Pests

The following methods are adopted for pest control.

Mechanical Methods : Mechanical methods include hand-picking, burning, trapping and pruning. Large caterpillers, e.g. a large, green tomato hornworm larva, can be located rapidly and removed by hand. Weeds are removed by hand-picking. The tent caterpillers gather on branches of trees and shrubs. By pruning or cutting out such branches is an effective measure. If the insect's tent is located near the trunk where cutting is difficult, then this part is burnt by a torch of burning oil-soaked rags at the end of a long pole. Burning helps in destruction of both animal and plant pests removed by hand-picking or pruning.

For determining the spread of certain flying insects in an infected area, they are trapped by a pleasantly flavoured attractant placed in funnel-shaped containers. Anise oil, Rose oil or other attractants are mixed with sawdust and placed in glass containers over which a funnel-shaped entrance has been fitted. The insects fly or crawl through the opening into the jar. Japanese beetles, gypsy moth, codling moth, etc. are located by this method.

Special traps are used to catch larger field insects, rats and mice. Metal reinforcement corners on window frames and door sills are used to prevent the access of rodents to storage sheds and barns. Modern concrete warehouses are helpful to control rodents. Window screens, electrified screens, specially coloured lights and other devices are also employed for controlling insects.

Biological Methods : Some animals or insects feed upon smaller forms which destroy the plants. Some insects have a short life cycle which parasitize larger insects. For examples, rabbits are helpful in destroying certain type of weeds. Cats, owls, kites and hawks are enemies of mice and rats. Insects are eaten by birds.

Certain flies and wasps lay eggs on the body of large destructive insects like slow-moving larvae. The eggs of the parasitic insects hatch rapidly into small larvae which consume the body tissues of the larger species. Ultimately, the larger forms die and the parasitized organism is developed into cocoon stage. It is emerged as adult fly and begins the cycle once again.

Environmental Methods: The environmental conditions surrounding the pest are changed either by removing its food supply or by interfering the completion of its life cycle. Mosquito larvae in water are killed by spreading a layer of oil.

Agricultural Methods : A more select crop plant is developed that will resist attack by pests like fungus and bacterial attack. Plants can absorb sufficient organic phosphorus compounds through the roots and foliage to cause the death of insects eating the leaves. Crop rotation is another useful agricultural method. If the chief source of food of a particular insect is withheld for one or more seasons, insects are controlled dramatically. The development of varieties of winter wheat, grown when insect pests are inactive, is important. Grub stage of some insects is unearth by deep ploughing rather than shallow furrowing.

Chemical Methods : Chemicals are designated to be effective as rodenticide (against rats, mice, moles, etc), insecitides (against various insects and arthropods), herbicides (against weeds and undesirable plants) and fungicides (against all types of fungi).

Particular chemical agents are used as poison baits, spray solutions, suspensions for spraying, aerosols, fumigants, residual poisons, stomach poisons, and repellents. They may be inorganic, or organic compounds obtained from natural sources, or synthetic organic complexes.

Pest Control by Chemicals

The choice of chemicals is dependent on the type of pest. If the pest is a rat or mouse, the chemical used will differ according to the locating conditions of the pest. An insect pest may be a chewing or sucking type, a running or flying type, an indoor or outdoor type. Similarly, chemicals are selected properly to control weeds and parasitic fungi, herbicide or fungicide.

Rodenticides

Poisonous chemicals are put into poison baits to control rats and mice. The chemicals must be sufficiently toxic to kill in reasonably small amounts. A chemical known as Norbormide, is the most effective rodenticide. Norbormide consistently kills the laboratory rats but has no effect upon other test animals. The other most effective synthetic rodenticide is Warfarin, 3-(α-acetonylbenzyl)-4-hydroxy-coumarin. It does not kill all rodents. Other chemicals are sodium fluoroacetate also known as 1080, 2-pivalyl-1, 3-indandione or Pival, α-naphthyl-thiourea or ANTU, thallium sulphate, zinc phosphide, arsenic trioxide and barium carbonate. Precautions must be taken that animal pets and small childern should not swallow any of these poisonous chemicals.

Two natural plant products are used as rodenticides which are Red Squill and strychnine. Red Squill and White Squill are both varieties of Drimia maritima (Fam. Liliaceae). The Red Squill has reddish-brown outer scales while deep purple inner ones are present in white variety. In addtion to other cardio-active glycosides, the bulb of the Red Squill also contains the glucosides scilliroside and scillirubroside. Unlike other mammals, rodents do not regurgitate the Squill bulb, and death follows convulsions and respiratory failure.

Salts of the alkaloid strychnine are used to control rodents. Such products are effective for small rodents, they are not commonly employed as rat poison. The toxicity of strychnine to other animals and its painful poisonous action do not make it a poison of choice.

Some fumigants have been used either to kill rodents or to drive them from their nesting place. These include calcium cyanide, methyl bromide, and carbon monoxide.

Insecticides

Insecticides are classified according to the life cycle of insects which they affect; e.g., Ovicides, against the egg stage; Larvicides, against the larvae, caterpillares, and maggots; Muscicides, aganist the house fly (Mosca domestica); Pediculicides, against the body louse (Pediculus corporis); and Miticides or Scabicides, against the scabies mite (Sarcoptes scabiei). Insecticides may be stomach poisons or contact poisons. They may be obtained from a natural source or synthesized by chemical reactions.

Systemic Poisons

A systemic poison is ingested by the insect and distributed from the alimentary canal throughout its tissues.

Stomach poisoning chemicals are used to control chewing insects. The death of the insect is caused upon ingestion by interfering with respiratory system, depression of the nervous system, by over stimulation and consequent paralysis of the neuromotor system or by some other mechanism. The poison is sprayed in the form of dust, solution and suspension over the area with the help of power-sprayers or by airoplanes. The chewing insects consume the plants, the poison is taken into the stomach and is absorbed through the gastrointestinal tract. They remain effective till they are not washed away by rain or by sprinkling device or they are not readily oxidized to nontoxic forms.

Lead arsenate in acid or basic form, calcium arsenate, Paris green, and arsenic trioxide are some important poisons. Calcium arsenate is used on cotton, tomatoes, and potatoes. Use of calcium arsenate damages the leaves of many other plants. Paris green is a complex salt of copper and arsenic. In addition to these, a number of phosphorus containing compounds have been synthesized as insecticides. For example, Schradan, (Octamethylpyrophosphoamide), Demeton, Methyl Demeton, Thimet and Di-Syston are the synthetic insecticides. They are readily absorbed through both the roots and the foliage of plants. They remain within the plants tissues and protect the plants. against insects for a long time. These compounds are toxic to mammals and, therefore, are used to treat nonedible crops.

For household pests there are a number of stomach poisons for chewing insects. Cockroaches are killed by sodium fluoride and sodium fluorosilicate. The powdered chemical adhering to the antennae, leg bristles and other body hairs do not enter into the body until the insects clean themselves. During the cleaning process the poison is swallowed and then absorbed. If the powder is carried into the nesting places, other insects may be affected. Sodium arsenite or sodium arsenate in the form of sweetened baits or sodium fluoride as a dust are used to control the ants in the house.

Contact Poisons

Contact poisons come into direct contact with the pests

which are applied as dusts, sprays or aerosols. Insects gathering to the underside of leaves will not be effected if the poison is spread only at the upper side. Insect like flies and mosquitoes will be effected only when they come into contact with the spray or the atmosphere in the particular area is heavily saturated with the aerosol. Sometimes the insects develop resistance to the contact poison and then they are controlled with difficulty. Organic contact insecticides may be of natural origin or synthetic type. The important natural plant insecticides are white hellebore, sabadilla, rotenoids, rotenone, cinerins, pyrethrins, phyrethrum flowers, nicotine and its salts and powdered tobacco leaves.

The examples of synthetic insecticides are DDT, methoxychlor, TDE, benzene hexachloride and its isomer, lindane, chlordane, aldrin, dieldrin, heptachlor, toxaphene, the organic phosphorus insecticides such as parathion, malathion, and fluorophosphates and the organic nitrogen compounds.

Natural Contact Insecticides

Leaf Tobacco : It consists of the cured and dried leaves of the Virginia tobacco plant, *Nicotiana tabacum* (Fam. Solanaceae). The genus *Nicotiana* is comprised of about 100 species. *Nicotiana tabacum* is a tall annual herb indigenous to tropical America and widely cultivated. The stem is simple, bearing large, pubescent, ovate, entire, decurrent leaves, the veins of which are prominent and more or less hairy.

Nicotine (0.6-9%) is the characteristic alkaloid of the genus and is prepared commercially from waste material of the tobacco industry. A lesser amount of nornicotine and an aromatic compound, nicotianin or tobacco comphor are also present in the herb. The characsersitic flavour is due to the nicotianin which is formed during the curing of the leaves. The roots of *N. tabacum* contain about eight pyridine alkaloids, including nicotine, nornicotine, anabasine and anatabine.

Nicotine is a pyridine-type alkaloid which is pale yellow, oily liquid, very hygroscopic; turns brown on exposure to air or light; acrid burning taste; develops odour of pyridine; volatile with steam. It forms salts with almost any acid and double salt with many metals and acids. It is miscible with water below 60°C, very soluble in alcohol, chloroform, ether, petroleum ether, etc. It is poisonous, being a local irritant and paralyzent.

Nicotine is used as insecticide and fumigant. As a contact poison, it is most effective as soap, i.e., as the laurate, oleate, or naphthenate. As a stomach poison a combination with bentonite has come into use. Nicotine sulphate in a 40% solution (Black leaf 40) is quite toxic to aphids; if the solution is alkalised, the toxicity is increased. Soap solution decomposes the sulphate to the free alkaloid which is considerably more poisonous to the insects.

Nicotine is highly toxic. The symptoms include extreme nausea, vomiting, evacuation of bowel and bladder, mental confusion, twitching and convulsions. The base is readily absorbed through mucous membranes and intact skin, but the salts are not.

Pyrethrum Flowers (Synonyms-Pyrethrum Flower Heads, or Insect Flowers, Dalmation insect powder; Persion insect powder). These are the dried flower heads of *Chrysanthemum cinerariaefolium* or of *C. marschallii* (Fam. Compositae). Pyrethrum contains about 0.5% of total pyrethrins (Pyrethrin I and Pyrethrin II).

Pyrethrum flowers are collected from 2- to 6- years old plants by hand. They are dried and stored. The plant is widely grown in Kenya, Ecuador, Japan, Yugoslavia, east central Africa, Brazil and India.

The insecticidal activity of Pyrethrum arises from four esters, the pyrethrins I and II and the cinerins I and II. They are complex esters of chrysanthemum carboxylic acid and the monomethyl ester of chrysanthemum dicarboxylic acid with pyrethrolones and cinerolones. The pyrethroids (or rethroids) are synthetic compounds of a similar structure of the pyrethrins themselves. The most important pyrethroids are allethrin, furethrin and cyclethrin.

The Pyrethrum flowers are a contact poison for insects. They are largely used in the form of powder, but sprays in which the active principles are dissolved in kerosene or other organic solvent. It can cause severe allergic dermatitis and systemic allergic reactions. Large amounts may cause nausea, vomiting, tinnitus, headaches and other CNS disturbances.

Derris and Lonchocarpus : The roots of many species of *Derris* and *Lonchocarpus* (Fam. Leguminosae) show insecticidal properties. Derris consists of the dried rhizome and roots of *Derris elliptica, D. malaccensis* and possibly other species. Lonchocarpus are the dried roots of *Lanchocarpus utilis, L. urucu* and some other species.

Derris is native of Malaya and cultivated there and in Burma, Thailand, Malaysia, Indonesia and the Philippine Islands. The genus Lonchocarpus is grown mainly in Mexico, Central and South America, England, Africa and Australia.

These roots contain rotenone (3-10%), deguelin, toxicarol, or tephrosin. Rotenone is a colourless crystalline substance which is insoluble in water but soluble in many organic solvents. All these compounds show insecticidal properties. It is an insecticide which is widely used to control both chewing and sucking insects.

Derris and Lonchocarpus roots have been used as fish poisons. For dusting purposes the powdered root is finally ground and diluted with a suitable carrier (talc, clay) to a concentration of 1 per cent. For spray purposes the powdered roots may be mixed with water or preferably with organic solvents such as ethylene dichloride, trichloroethylene or chlorbenzene. Rotenone extracts with oil and emulsifying agents and extracts dissolved in paraffin oil are excellent house-hold and cattle sprays. Rotenone decomposes upon exposure. Inhalation or ingestion of large doses may cause numbers of oral mucous membrane, nausea, vomiting, muscle tremors and tachypnea.

Rotenone

Deguelin (R=H)
Tephrosin (R=OH)

Cevadilla Seed (or Sabadilla) : It consists of the seeds of *Schoenocaulon officinale* (Fam. Liliaceae), a plant found from Mexico to Venezuela. The seeds are dark brown to black, sharply pointed and about 6 mm long. The seeds contain veratrine alkaloids (2-4%) which is a mixture of cevadine, veratridine, sabadilline, sabadine and cevadinine. The powdered seeds and preparations of 'Veratrine' are used as a dust or spray to control thrips and various true bugs which attack vegetables.

Ryania : The roots and stems of *Ryania speciosa* (Fam. Flacourtiaceae) contain 0.16-0.2% of alkaloids having insecticidal properties. Ryanodine, the principal alkaloid, is a complex ester involving 1-pyrrole-carboxylic acid. The plant is used in the control of various lepidopterous larvae which attack fruits and particulary European corn borer, codling moth and sugar cane borer. It may be used as a dust made from a 40% extract. Due to its low toxicity, Ryania has no residue hazard.

Ryanodine

Synthetic Contact Insecticides

The synthetic organic insecticides are classified into four groups:

1. organic sulphur,
2. chlorinated hydrocarbons,
3. non-halogenated organic compounds, and
4. organophosphorus derivatives.

Among the sulphur compounds are the carbamates, thiuram derivatives, mercaptans, thiazines, and organic thiocyanates (rhodanates). Sulphur is the traditional and ancient remedy for scabies. Tetraethylthiuram monosulphide, an organic sulphur compound, is as effective as sulphur.

Among halogenated organic compounds, naphthalene (moth flakes or moth balls) and para-dichlorobenzene (Dichloricide) are used as moth repellents.

A large number of chlorinated hydrocarbons have been employed as *contact poison*. These substances exert their lethal action after they have passed through the insect cuticle. Dicophane (D.D.T) is the best known of all chlorinated compounds. It is also known as chlorophenothane. Dicophane is also used for the eradiction of head lice. Important insecticides related to DDT are methoxychlor or TDE. These compounds may be degraded by living systems into less toxic metabolites. They remain unreacted for many years in soil and marine sediments and, therefore, present a continual threat to animal communities.

Gamma Benzene Hexachloride, the γ-isomer of hexachlorocyclohexane, shows insecticidal properties. It has a strong, disagreeable odour and used as sprays for crop plants, animals and garden plants. It is also used to destroy head lice and to treat scabies. Aldrin, a chlorinated hydrocarbon insecticide, has been used to control grasshoppers. It is stable in alkaline condition. Its epoxy derivative, Dieldrin, shows identical action and retains a longer residual effect. Endrin is a stereo-isomer of Dieldrin and exhibits excellent insect-killing effect. Chlordane insecticide is used to control insects in lawns, gardens, and homes.

Pentachlorophenol, C_6Cl_5OH, protects lumber against termites and wood-rotting fungi when used as a 5% mixture in an organic suspension. Methyl bromide is an excellent fumigant for treating store products and green vegetables. In the form of solution methyl bromide is used as a soil sterilizant for the control of nematodes and certain insects. The simpler chlorinated hydrocarbons such as chloroform, paradichlorobenzene, carbon tetrachloride and trichloroethylene also have insecticidal activity and used as fumigants. The compounds like hydrocyanic acid gas, and carbon disulphide are also employed in destroying insects. The chlorinated hydrocarbons are toxic to man and animals and they should be kept well away from foodstuffs and animal feed.

Certain substituents on the benzene ring (C_2H_5-,CH_3O- F-, Cl-, and Br-) increase the potency of these insecticides either by increasing the lipid solubility of the compounds or by improving the fit on the receptor surface. Other substituents (C_4H_9-, C_6H_8-, NH_2-, NO_2-, -OH and COOH) reduce the potency. All the active compounds are very soluble in lipids and their molecular weights lie within the range 270 to 450.

Gamma benzene hexachloride (Quellada) is used to

destroy head lice and to treat scabies. Dicophane is also employed for the eradication of head lice.

Members of organophosphorus derivatives include the insecticides like tetraethylpyrophosphate (TEPP), parathion, chlorthion, diazinon, trichlorphon (dipterex) and octamethyl-pyrophosphate (OMPA). These compounds are used both as contact poisons and as systemic poisons. A systemic poison is one that is ingested by the insect and distributed from the alimentary tract throughout its tissues. These poisons are applied to plants liable to attack by insects.

The organophosphorous insecticides form stable compounds with a number of esterases including cholinesterase. These insecticides are toxic to man and animals. They are being successfully employed in regions in which insects have developed resistance to the chlorinated hydrocarbons. Malathion (Carbofos; Prioderm) is extensively used as a dusting powder in cases of infestation with body lice.

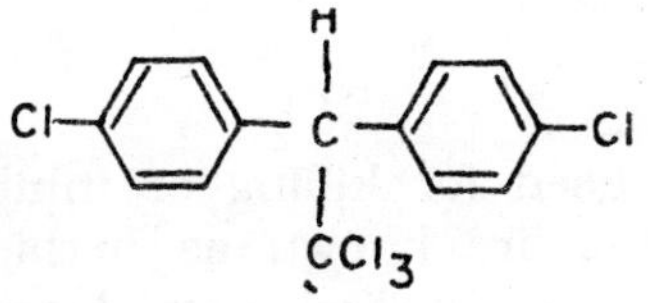

Chlorophenothane (DDT)

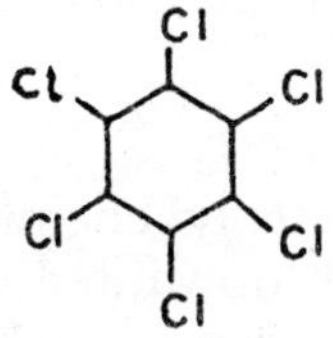

Gamma Benzene
Hexachlorobenzene

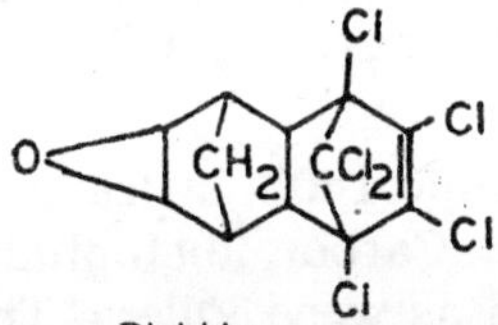

Dieldrin

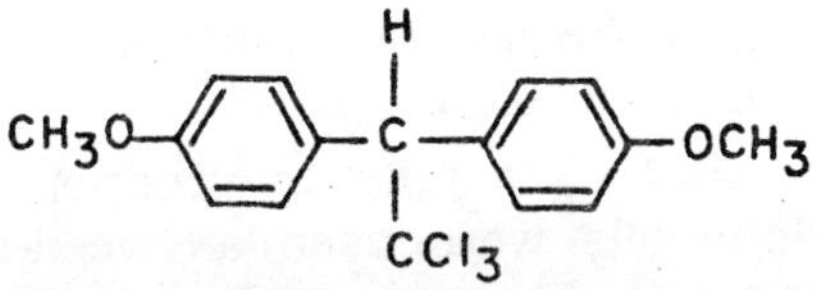

Methoxychlor

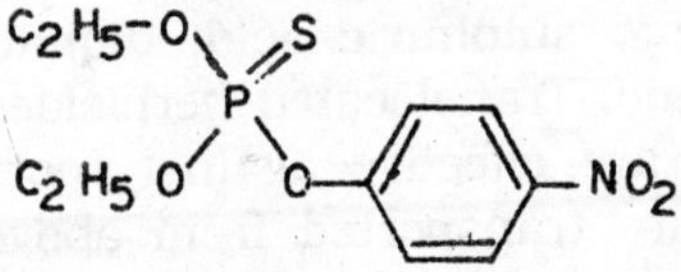

Parathion

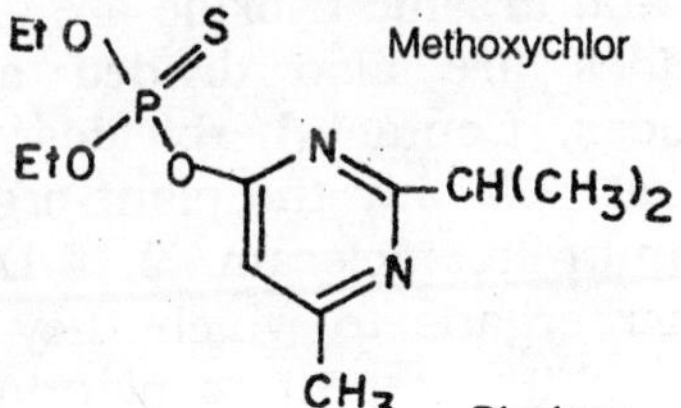

Diazinon

Chlorthion

Dipterex (Trichlorphon)

Malathion

Repellents

The natural product Citronella oil has been used as a mean of preventing insect attack. The synthetic products include dimethyl phthalate, Ethohexadiol (Rutgers 612) and Butopyronoxyl. These compounds are mixed in Dimethyl phthalate in 'ratio of Dimethyl phthalate (6 parts), Ethohexadiol (2 parts) and Butopyronoxyl (2 parts), a synonym for this solution is 622 mixture. Diethyltoluamide is another effective insect repellent.

Herbicides

Any agent, usually chemical, used for killing or inhibiting the growth of unwanted plants, are known as herbicides. They are classified as selective and nonselective depending upon thier destructive properties. Selective herbicides eliminate undesirable species and produce some deleterious effect on the desired plants. Non selective herbicides destroy all types of plant life.

Earlier sea salts, by-products of chemical industries, and various oils were used as weed-killers. Carbon disulphide, borax and arsenic trioxide are also used as weed killers. The herbicides are also divided as foliage applied and soil herbicides. Contact herbicides (e.g. sulphuric acid, diquat, paraquat) kill only the plant organs. Translocated herbicides (e.g. amitrole, picloram, 2, 4-D) are effective against roots or other organs to which they are transported from above ground. With respect to planting times, herbicides are also classified as pre-plant, pre-emergence, or post-emergence weed killers. Pre-plant herbicides may be applied to the soil or to weeds before crop planting.

Weeds and other vegetable grow along railroad sides, highways, around buildings, vacant lands, and playing grounds. They are killed by nonselective chemicals. Calcium cyanamide, potassium and sodium cyanides, ammonium thiocyanate, ammonium sulphamate, sodium chlorate, sodium chloride, arsenic trioxide, sodium arsenate, and sulphuric acid are effective weed-killers.

2,4-Dichlorophenoxyacetic acid (2,4-D) was the first organic herbicide. The compound applied to leaf surface without absorption, penetrates the cuticle and then enters into the vascular system of the plant. The toxic effects of the compound are dependent on its translocation to all parts of the plant.

2,4,5-Trichlorophenoxyacetic acid (2,4,5-T) is a related product which is more effective than 2,4-D. Phenoxyethyl sulphates, 2, 5-D and 3, 4-D have herbicidal properties identical to 2,4-D. Carbomates, urea derivatives, chlorinated acids, phenols, and dinitro .compounds are used as soil sterilizers, floral retarding agents, defoliants and selective herbicides.

The effective synthetic herbicides are 2, 2-dichloropropionic acid (Dalapon), 4-amino-3, 5, 6-trichloropicolinic acid (Tordon) and 3-amino-1, 2, 4-triazole (Aminotriazole). Dalapon is effective against grass-killer, whereas Tordon controls many woody species. Broadleaf weeds and perennial grasses are controlled by aminotriazole.

Plant Growth Regulators

The natural plant growth-promoting substance, gibberellic acid, is obtained from the fungus *Gibberella fugikurai* (Sawada). Six gibberellins, A_1, A_2, A_3, A_4, A_7 and A_9, have been isolated from filtrates of the fungus.

Chemically, gibberellins are the tetracyclic diterpenes. They are more highly functionalized than other groups of terpenoids. These compounds are produced in minute quantities within plants where they act as hormones of various developmental processes. Gibberellin-like compounds occur in higher plants. They are responsible for the development, maturation, budding, flower formation, fruit ripening and various other growth processes. Substances like 2,4-D and 2,4,5-T also possess auxin-like activity, but they are more effective as herbicides.

Fungicides or Antimycotic

Fungicides are any toxic substances which are used to kill or inhibit the growth of fungi, molds, mildews and yeasts that either cause economic damage or endanger the health of domestic animals or humans. Mostly fungicides are applied as sprays or dust. Seed fungicides are applied as a protective covering before germination. Systemic fungicides, or chemotherapeutants are applied to plants, where they become distributed throughout the tissue and act to eradicate existing disease or to protect against possible disease.

Protective fungicides are applied before the disease appears. They are used as sprays or dust to protect leaves and fruits and as seed disinfectants to eliminate the germination of spores simultaneously with seeds. Protectant agents are also used as wood preservatives to prevent dry rot and other fungus attacks on lumber. Eradicant fungicides are applied after the presence of fungi is observed. They kill by direct contact or else prevent the formation of spores. Thus, further spread of the fungus is inhibited.

A chemical combination of copper sulphate, lime and water is known as *Bordeaux mixture*. It is a protective fungicide. Sulphur is also used to control fungus disease. Lime-sulphur mixture is fungicide having both protective and eradicant properties. Its activity is due to calcium polysulphide which are very toxic to the fungus. Sulphur is mixed with nicotine, pyrethrum extracts, and rotenone to get better result. The other useful fungicides are the thiocarbamates, especially the dimethylthiocarbamates and the ethylene bisthiocarbamates; mercury compounds, quaternary ammonium compounds, nitro and heterocyclic nitrogen compounds, antibiotics, chlorophenols and other phenols and formaldehyde.

Fumigant

Fumigant is any volatile, poisonous substance that is used to kill insects, nematodes and other animals or plants that damage stored foods or seeds, human dwellings, clothing and nursery stock. Soil fumigants are sprayed or spread over an area to be cultivated and are worked over an area to be cultivated and into the soil to control disease-causing fungi, nematodes and weeds.

Some chemically simpler chlorinated hydrocarbons such as chloroform, p-dichlorobenzene, carbon tetrachloride and trichloroethylene also have insecticidal activity and they are used as fumigants. They are applied in gaseous form or as an aerosol in enclosed spaces such as rooms, cupboards, boxes, etc. These chlorinated hydrocarbons are highly dangerous to man and they must be used with care.

QUESTIONS

1. What are pesticides ? Classify different type of pests.
2. What are weeds ? Describe fungi parasitic on plants.
3. Discuss pesticides and methods adopted for pest control.
4. Write biological methods for pest control. Discuss different types of rodenticides and insecticides.
5. What are contact poisons ? Describe natural contact insecticides for pest control.
6. Write informative notes on the following :
   (a) Herbicides
   (b) Fungicides
   (c) Fumigant
   (d) Weeds
   (e) Rodenticides
   (f) Insecticides

19

VARIABILITY IN DRUG ACTIVITY

During the development of plants, there is a considerable variation in size, shape, colour and other characters within a given population. There is also a difference in the content of the active constituents in the fresh drug. The content of the active constituents and the ratio between different constituents are not static, but vary continually in the living organisms according to the interaction of factors inside and outside of the organisms. Due to complexity of life processes and as change in one factor affects the influence of another factor, it is generally difficult to ascertain the exact effect of a given factor.

As a rule, there is a greater variation in content of medicinally active components, which are secondary metabolites, than in the contents of normal metabolites and storage products. For example, fat content of bitter almond varies from 40 to 63 per cent, but the amount of amyglalin differs from 0 to 8.5 per cent. The variation of therapeutic components in some drugs are as : atropin in Belladonna leaf (0.3-1.7%), alkaloids in Cinchona (4-14%), glycosides in Digitalis leaf (5.5-21 units), alkaloids in Ergot (0-0.2%), glycyrrhizin in Licorice (3-12%), morphine in Opium (3-12%) and menthol ester in Peppermint oil (2-11%).

The quality of crude drugs is dependent on the amount of active compounds present in it. Variation in the morphology or in concentration of active constituents may be due to several factors which may be due to genetic factors; by differences in the environmental conditions or due to methods used in the collection, preparation and storage of the crude drugs.

EFFECTS OF ENDOGENOUS OR GENETIC FACTORS

Members of a given species are rarely genetically homogenous. When the genetic difference is great, which resides in the genes, the morphology and biochemical diversity for each species are different. They can bring about differences in the amount or the type of chemical constituents produced. Whenever such biochemical variation occurs, each particular type is known as a *physiological variety*. Thus, there is not difference between bitter and sweet almond trees, but the seeds of the former contain a bitter glycoside (amygdalin). *Duboisia myoporoides* of Northern Australia produces mainly scopolamine, while this plant grown in Southern Australia yields chiefly hyoscyamine. *Eucalyptus dives* of Australia yields an essential oil that varies greatly in odour and chemical contents from tree to tree. On the basis of the chemical composition of the oil, four physiological varieties of the tree have been distinguished.

The seeds of *Strophanthus sarmentosus* are biochemically polymorphic. The variety from the Belgian Congo produces sarverogenin; variety from French Sudan yields sarmentogenin; and from French Guiana gives very small amount of either compound. Morphological differences are insignificant. Similar variation is observed in varieties of Comphor trees; in red and white Squills; in Rauwolfia, etc. Some types of *Rheum palmatum* are rich in rhein, other are poor in this compound. There is a little variation in the content of chrysophanol. Among the three forms of diphtheritic organisms known as *gravis, media* and *mitis,* the last causes much less serious infections than the others.

Selection : There is a variation in the intensity of expression of given characteristics in any given population of plants. The plants may be genetically heterogenous to some extent. Genetic differences exist normally from one plant to the other. If a plant having most desirable characteristics is chosen & interbred, a derived second population may have a tendency toward improvement with respect to that particular quality. Continued selection and breeding of the most desirable plants will improve greatly in the particular quality chosen. If the plants are of a 'pure breed' and all variation is due to environmental factors, selection and breeding will have no effect.

Selective breeding of medicinal plants has resulted in plants with increased constancy of quality, increased growth, resistance to disease, winter-hardiness, and other desirable characteristics. It is a tedious and time-consuming task. Selection work on *Cinchona ledgeriana* with about 5% alkaloids has furnished types which yield bark with up to 15% alkaloids. Selection programmes with *Mentha arvensis* have developed drought-resistant and rust-resistant types yielding high amount of menthol. The rotene content of *Derris* (insecticide) has been raised from 3% to 13% in some clones by selective breeding. The average yields of essential oil in several plants have been increased by selective breeding. Selection work is important in the fermentation industries where high-yielding strains suitable for certain economical media are developed. In nature, some strains of a given microbe are active in producing antibiotics, e.g. the strain of *Bacillus subtilis* from the throat of Mary Tracy is used industrially. Careful selection of active strains is important to produce toxins, vaccines, and other pharmaceuticals.

Mutation : Exposure to ionizing radiation (X-ray, gamma rays, radioactive isotopes) or nonionizing radiation (ultraviolet) or some mutagenic chemical agents, sometimes changes the nature of a gene artificially. This change, a mutation, generally may cause the gene to lose its function entirely or in part; or it may cause the gene to do a different job. Mutation may also arise spontaneously in nature. Nothing is known about such changes. The mutant gene is passed from parent to progeny in its changed form. Genes control the morphological characters of an individual and its biochemical nature. Genes determine the presence of enzymes which catalyze the formation of vital biochemical metabolites. The original strain of *Penicillium chrysogenum* used in the production of penicillin yielded about 100 units of penicillin per ml of culture medium. By single-spore isolation, strains were obtained which yielded up to 250 units per ml of medium. X-ray treatment of this strain gave mutants which could produce 500 units per ml, and utraviolet mutants of the latter gave strain which produced about 1,000 units per ml. Similar improvements have been obtained with other antibiotic-producing organisms.

Mutation and selection develop resistance to chemotherapeutic agents by pathogenic microbes. When a microbe is cultured in a medium containing an antibiotic to which it is sensitive, majority of the organisms will be eliminated by the antibiotic, but a few organisms will survive which are mutants resistant to the antibiotic. The resistant organisms are free to multiply and grow, giving rise to a new population which is resistant.

Mutation is a random process occurring at all times. In an industry, the strain of organisms used should be entirely pure and uniform since a change in the strain of organism used in a fermentation process may cause great economic loss and danger to human lives. Therefore, the stock cultures are maintained under very stringent conditions, and constant checks to ensure their uniformity.

Genetic changes in a plant involves multiplication of entire chromosome set to give 3n, 4n, 6n, etc. body cells (polyploidy), addition of one or a few chromosomes (extrachromosomal type), gross structural changes, and submicroscopic changes or point mutations which include alteration in the DNA chromosomal material. Such mutations constantly occur in nature at a slow rate. Many mutations are of recessive type and do not become apparent until, the F_2 generation of a self-pollinated plant.

Polyploidy : Each living cell contains in its nucleus two sets of chromosomes. Since the chromosomes in the nucleus are present in duplicate, the normal cell is referred to as a diploid. If the chromosomes reduplicate within the nucleus, four sets of chromosomes are formed without subsequent division of the cell. In this way a condition arises wherein the nucleus contains more than its normal complement of chromosomes. This condition is called as "polyploidy". Through various mechanisms, a condition arises in which the cell contains three sets of chromosomes (triploidy); four sets (tetraploidy), etc. Polyploidy may develop in a plant through natural means, or by treating the cells, especially the seed, with heat or with colchicine or other specific compound. Various changes take place in the chemical composition of the individual due to the increase in the chromosome component of the nucleus. The most prominent changes brought about are in the size of the plant and its organs along with some physiological changes.

In the presence of colchicine, chromosomes in a cell undergoing mitosis divide without the formation of a mitotic spindle figure. Therefore, sister cells are not formed. A 72 hour treatment of the growing root tips of onion with colchicine solution produces 256 chromosomes. The "C-mitotic" activity of colchicine may arise from its interaction with the disulphide bonds of the spindle protein and by inhibition of the conversion of globular proteins to fibrous proteins. On discontinuation of treatment, the spindle figure again forms in the normal way. Colchicine is 100 time more active than its isomer isocolchicine while colchiceine is almost inactive.

Colchicine   Isocolchicine   Colchiceine

Plant materials are treated with colchicine in various ways. Seeds are soaked in an aqueous solution of colchicine (0.2-2.0%) for 1-4 days before planting. Seedlings are imported on to filter paper soaked in the solution for protection of the growing points. In an other method, the soil around the roots of young seedlings can be moistered with the colchicine solution. Young buds and shoots are also treated by immersion lanolin pastes and agar gels are used in tissue culture technique.

Newly formed polyploids are stabilized themselves in a number of generations. Such type of treatment does not give a uniform plant concerning chromosome number. Typical effects of polyploidy are larger flowers, pollen grains and stomata. With Lobelia, tetraploid plants are smaller than diploid ones. With tetraploid caraway plants, the total volatile oil content was increased by 100 per cent. In opium, the concentration of morphire per unit area increases up to 100 per cent.

In some species polyploidy does not affect the relative proportion of a compound. Solanaceous herbs produce excess amounts of tropane alkaloids in the 4n state and reduced quantities as heploids. The proportion of carvone in oil of caraway obtained from 4 n plants is also unchanged. *Digitalis lanata* in 4 n state contains a relatively high proportion of lanatosides A and B compared with the 2n form. There is also a difference in the sequiterpene lactones of *Ambrosia dumora* in the diploid and polyploid states.

Some medicinal plants have shown an increase in the content of active constituents on induction of polyploidy.

Colchicine-induced tetraploidy of *Datura stramonium* produced two-times more alkaloid than the normal diploids. Double content of an alkaloid is produced in tetraploids of *Atropa belladonna* in comparison to the diploid controls. An increase in alkaloid content has been observed in polyploids of *Lobelia* and *Nicotiana species*. Tetraploids of a *Cinchona* species contained 1.12% of alkaloid, more than twice the amount contained in the diploid plants.

Hybridization : The mating of inherently different individuals to produce hybrid progeny is called hybridization. Some desirable morphological or biochemical characteristics may be developed into the progeny by this process. Genes are introduced by hybridization for resistance to decrease, increased stature, excess production of starch and vitamins, different colour of the flowers, etc. Hybrids of *Cinchona* yield more amount of quinine. A hybrid developed by crossing *C. succirubra* with *C. ledgeriana* yields a bark which contains 11.2% of alkaloid. The parent species produced 3.4% and 5.1% of the alkaloid, respectively.

Each planting must be made with new hybrid seed produced by crossing in original parental species. The seeds will produce progeny which are not uniform, some reverting to the parental types, and others being of intermediate types. When plants of peppermint are allowed to mate at random, the resulting seeds give rise to plants producing oils of varying composition. A gradual change occurred in the flavour of the oil from spearmint hybrid yielding oils of different composition. For maintaining genetic purity of peppermint and spearmint hybrids, the plants must be propagated by planting stolons.

EFFECTS OF EXOGENOUS OR ECOLOGICAL FACTORS

The influence of ecological factors on the activity of drugs is very important. The drug industries pay better prices for drugs of high quality. Many species of medicinal plants grow wild in different parts of the world. The plants are scattered and it becomes difficult to collect and process them. Therefore, there is large demand for certain products and so the necessity to cultivate them on a large scale has become ever more. The following problems should be tackled to obtain an economic yield of good quality.

Climate and Light : Climate, e.g. temperature, rainfall, length of day and altitude, plays an important role in the growth of plants. Different crops require different climatic pattern. In cloudy weather the amount of carbohydrates in leaves is decreased, since photosynthesis is light-dependent. As carbohydrates serve as the initial starting material for biosynthesis, their abundance affect the amount of secondary metabolites. Changes in temperature may also influence plant growth by affecting the rate of chemical reactions. Enzymatic reactions slow down at lower temperatures. Some intermediate may accumulate in the cell and some of them will not produced faster to meet the required demand. It gives rise autointoxication or side reaction products. The contents of alkaloids in Stramonium leaves lower in rainy and cloudy weather. Dry sunny weather and higher temperatures increase the content of essential oil of Lavender, Valerian and Wormwood. Belladonna leaves grown in sunny location contain 3-4 times more alkaloids than plant grown in shade. Similar variations have been observed in case of Opium, Lobelia, Cinchona and Peppermint. The average optimum temperature for nicotine production in *Nicotiana rustica* is 20°C. The fatty acids produced at low temperatures contain a higher content of double bonds than those formed at higher temperatures. The maximum alkaloidal content of Kurchi bark was observed when the atmospheric temperature was around 25°C.

Sudden natural calamities like flood, drought, frost, snow, hail, and wind are unusual features in hilly areas. Preventive measures have to be taken to guard the crops against these natural calamities. Limited crops may be cultivated in these conditions.

Rainfall shows effects on humidity and water-holding properties of the soil. Production of volatile oils varies under different conditions of rainfall. Continuous rain loses water-soluble substances from leaves and roots by leaching and affects the production of some alkaloids in Solanaceous plants, glycoside and volatile oil-producing plants.

Latitude and Altitude : The effect of latitude is important in fat producing plants. Tropical plants (Palm oil, Cocao butter) contain mainly saturated fatty acids, while the subtropical plants give a larger amount of unsaturated acids. The Olive, Almond and Sesame oils are predominant in oleic acid. The plants of temperate zones (Cottonseed, Sunflower) also contain more unsaturated acids. Plants growing at different latitudes produce oils of different saturation.

The coconut palm grows in a maritime climate and the sugar cane is a lowland plant. Elevation is required for tea (100-2000 m), cocoa (100-200 m) coffee (800-1800 m), rhubarb, tragacanth and cinchona. *Cinchona succirubra* grows well at low levels but alkaloids are not produced. The bitter constituents of *Gentiana lutea* are increased with altitude. The alkaloids of *Aconitum napellus* and *Lobellia inflata* and the oil content of Thyme and Peppermint decrease with altitude. Pyrethrum gives the best yields of flower-heads and pyrethrins at high altitudes on Equator (East Africa).

Allelopathy : Living organisms constantly exert an influence, called allelopathy, upon each other. Where different plants are growing side by side, there may be growth promotion or growth suppression. It effects upon leaf development, leaf shedding or maturation of the fruits. Some organisms exists only when living together. They live in *symbiosis*. Allelopathic effect among plants is transmitted by exhalation from leaves or secretions from roots. The flora of the soil changes with the amount of fertilizer, nature of the organic substance, humidity, etc.

Nutrition : Proper nutrition is essential for all living organisms. Suitable media for the microbes is used for the production of drugs. The consistency of Lard depends upon the nature of the hogs food. The content of alkaloids of Ergot shows differences up to 30% according to the variety of the rye host plant. The availability of light of proper intensity and duration is an important factor in plant nutrition. Other factors, such as temperature, humidity, inorganic salts, etc. also affect the efficacy of photosynthesis. Thus, the nutritional status of a plant may have some effect on the formation of secondary constituents such as alkaloids or glycosides.

Sunny weather prior to harvesting of peppermint gives more oil than rainy and overcast weather. Isolated camphor trees give a higher yield of camphor than trees grown in dense stands. The plant of *Fagopyrum esculentum* grown in shade produces less rutine than the plants grown in light. Belladonna leaves contain the most alkaloids in the middle of the summer when there is a maximum of light and growth. The content of glycosides in Digitalis leaves is higher in the afternoon than during the night, due to availability of more sugar.

The density of the plant population is an important factor affecting the availability of light, inorganic nutrient and water. Some species (e.g. Papaver) grow and develop well under the new climatic condition. Sometimes, the ability to elaborate specific substances is lost when the plant is transferred to another climate. The *Astragalus* species, a source of Tragacanth, ceases to produce gum when transferred to northern regions of Mediterranean areas. In some cases; strains of a plant are selected which give rise new plants. *Digitalis purpurea*, Thyme and Peppermint produce less active constituents when grown in lowlands. Aconitum furnishes a drug less active when grown in the mountains than that grown in the lowland. Thus, there is no definite rule to predict the activity of a given species when it is transferred to a new climate.

Minerals, Water and Oxygen : Inorganic ions are essential for growth and biochemical functioning of all living organisms. They serve many functions such as catalysts, cell constituents and proper balance of elements. Their solubility depends upon the pH of the soil. Therefore, one has to study the soil conditions, e.g. the kind of soil, depth, capacity of moisture, its pH, status of macro- and micronutrients.

Different drug plants require specific growth conditions for development and to yield a maximum crop. During transfer of a wild drug plant to cultivation hebitate, it is necessary to provide them with a soil essentially similar to that of their natural habitat. Stramonium gives good yields only on rich soil. Chamomile develops only on an acid soil. The quantity of fertilizer does not affect the content of active principles in plants, if the inorganic elements are present in sufficient amount to prevent deficiency symptoms from developing. An increase of phosphorus or nitrogen increases the production of essential oil in Anise and Coriander and of capsaicin in Capsicum.

Availability of water in the soil affects the activity of some drugs. Valerian produces less essential oil on swampy ground than on dry land. Mucilage content of Althea root is lower in drugs from damp soil. Mucilage acts as a water-absorbing agent, preventing the plant from drying out. Swamy land may cause decreased oxygen tension around roots, affecting in the pH of the soil and the uptake of minerals.

Stage of Development : Aged and young plant organs yield drugs of different activity. The anthelmintic principle, santonin of Levant wormseed, decreases when flower heads increases during growth. In Pyrethrum flowers, the flower buds are more valuable than the expanded flowers, because they contain more active compounds, pyrethrins. The contents of ascorbic acid in rose hips *(Rosa rugosa)* is at its maximum (12%) in the last days of September. The contents of essential oil in American wormseed is highest during pollination. Medicinal Rhubarb contains more anthraquinone in spring and during flowering than during winter. Young leaves of anthraquinone plants contain much more anthraquinone than do fully developed leaves. The Camphor tree accumulates more and more camphor from year to year which is maximum at the age of 40 years. Aconite tuber contains three times more alkaloid in winter time as during summer.

Parasites : Like animals, plants have infectious diseases. Microbes and viruses attack them, creating distrubances of the metabolic processes of the host. Crops are reduced by plant infections. Henbane contains less alkaloid when attacked by rust. Peppermint cultures are affected by *Verticillium.* Valerian, Fennel, Belladonna, Stramonium, etc. are also attacked by mildews and rusts.

Virus infestation of plant changes the leaves and may hinder the development of other organs. Strains of various plants have been developed which are resistant to the more common infectious diseases. *Streptomyces* species, used in the production of antibiotics, are quite susceptible to attack by certain bacteriophages.

Preserving and Processing Procedures : Earlier the drugs were used mostly in fresh form. When the drugs were obtained from far away places, preservation of these products became a necessity. Several drugs lose their effectiveness on drying. *Cochlearia officinalis* on drying destroys its vitamin C content. Spasmolytic properties of Thyme are lost in a dried sample.

Enzyme Activity : Enzymatic processes continue during drying, but gradually the cell loses its control and power to coordinate these processes. Several drugs containing glycosides lose activity during drying due to the action of glycosidases. Normally, enzyme and substrate occur jointly in the cell. In the living cell they are spatially separated.

In some plants, enzyme and substrate are found in different cells, e.g. the glycoside of mustard seed. When the cells are crushed, the enzyme and substrate are united to react each other.

Fresh white Squill bulb contains the cardioactive glycosides scillaren A and B. During preservation of this drug, a large proportion of the glycosides is destroyed.

$$\text{Scillaren A} \xrightarrow[\text{+H}_2\text{O}]{\text{Scillarenase}} \text{Proscillaridin A + Glucose}$$

Proscillaridin A and its anhydride, scillaridin, have weaker cardiac activity than scillaren A. The fresh bark of Cascara sagrada gives no reaction of anthraquinone, but after lying in the air for sometime, it forms red colour with alkali (Borntraeger reaction). Sometimes desirable transformation takes place during drying. For example, vanillin is produced by hydrolysis of a glucoside in a fermentation process in Vanila bean. Cacao beans change in colour and flavour on fermentation process. Caffeine-tannin complex of tea is converted by enzymes into free caffeine and oxidized tannin, phlobaphenes. If the enzymes are destroyed in these materials prior to drying, no changes occur.

Enzymes also cause deterioration in activity of crude drugs. In Opium, a peroxidase is present which can cause a loss of up to 50% of the morphine of aqueous solutions, which can be prevented by heating morphine to 70° to destroy the enzyme. The enzyme present in the fresh latex of the Opium poppy reduces the content of morphine up to 13 per cent.

Browning : Fresh barks of Cinchona, Cascara sagrada and Cinnamon and fresh Cola nuts are white to yellow inside, but darken to brown on drying. Many leaves and fruits become brown on drying and storage. Browning changes the taste, odour and activity. Browning is due to both enzymatic and nonenzymatic reasons and becomes faster in the presence of oxygen and at elevated temperatures. Polyphenol oxidase enzymes cause oxidation of polyphenols (tannins and flavonoids) to relative quinones, which polymerize readily to yield dark-coloured compounds. The reaction is accelerated after damage to the tissue or after physiological injury, such as freezing, thawing or slow drying. This type of browning is inhibited by addition of ascorbic acid which reduces the formation of quinone. The oxidation is highest in powdered drugs as the diffusion of oxygen into the inner portions of the tissues is slow.

Browning also occurs due to interaction of free sugar or dehydroascorbic acid with free amino acids to form dark compounds. Addition of sulphur dioxide prevents browning by eliminating carbonyl groups.

$$R–CHO + SO_2 + H_2O \longrightarrow R–CH(OH)SO_3H$$

Browning of dried leaves is due to transformation of chlorophyll into phaeochlorophyll in the presence of acidic cell sap. Bright green colour is retained in slight acidic conditions.

Oxidation, Evaporation, and Polymerization : Unpleasant odour of Henbane leaves and Coriander fruits disappears on drying due to evaporation or transformation of flavouring substances. Volatile oils evaporate at high temperatures, therefore, drying in sunshine causes greater loss of volatile oil constituents than drying in the shade. Lavender, Peppermint, Sage and Thyme loss about 10% of their oil on drying in the shade, but up to 24% if dried in the sun. Heat created during powdering and artificial heat used in the drying of crude drugs destroy thermolabile constituents.

The oil constituents are first dissolved in water and diffuse through the cell wall in solution. Oxygenated compounds of essential oils, e.g. alcohols, aldehydes and carboxylic acids, are highly soluble in water and evaporated to a greater extent than the hydrocarbons. The drugs which carry oil glands on the surface lose oil faster than thicker organs. Peppermint with oil glands on the leaf surface, loses about 40% of its oil in dried leaves.

Effect of Storage : Chemical changes in drugs occur most readily during storage and the process is known as aging. In the presence of lipases, fats in seeds are hydrolyzed to glycerol and fatty acids. In living cells, the consumption of glycerol and fatty acids is continued to prevent the accumulation of any of them, but in dead cells, fatty acids are deposited. Peroxides formed during this process may destroy therapeutic constituents. Storage of Ergot causes rancidity and becomes inferior in quality. Therefore, powdered Ergot must be stored only in the defatted form.

Enzymatic Process : The enzymes of the fresh drugs are not destroyed completely during drying. However, when the water content of the tissues is reduced below 5%, enzymatic reactions are reduced. Hygroscopic materials absorb humidity from the atmosphere varying water content between 5 and 15 per cent. Therefore, crude drugs, such as Digitalis and Senna leaves, should be stored in closed containers over dehydrating agents such as lime or calcium chloride. This type of storage is costly and difficult.

Oxidative Processes : Drugs darken during storage due to oxidation reactions. Diffusion of oxygen into large pieces of a drug requires a longer time than diffusion into the interior of small particles. Therefore, drugs containing phenolic compounds lose activity more rapidly when stored in powder forms. Many essential oils on exposure to air develop typical odour and become viscous. Addition of oxygen to double bonds gradually forms peroxides, aldehydes, ketones, alcohols and acids. In bitter almond, benzaldehyde is partly converted to benzoic acid on storing the oil in air. Peroxides form many secondary products in the oil in the presence of oxygen. Anethole of Anise oil upon storage gives rise to ketone, aldehyde and acid. Therefore, the oils should be kept in completely filled bottles to eliminate the effect of oxygen. The bitter compound of Gentian root, gentiopicrin, is oxidized in air to gentiamarin and H_2O_2, and the aglycones of these two glycosides are further oxidized to a larger number of products.

Post-mortem oxidation is used for the improvement of some drugs. The fresh bark of Cascara sagrada contains the active constituents in the reduced form, anthranols, which have an irritating effect upon the mucous membranes and causes griping and nausea. During drying, a part of these compounds is oxidized to anthraquinones. Therefore, the drugs should be stored at least one year before used to destroy the griping property. The oxidation proceeds faster at elevated temperatures. Therefore, the drugs should also be heated for one hour at 100°. The colour of chrysarobin is changed from yellow to brown on storage in air and, hence, its antiseptic property is reduced.

Rancidification : Spoilage of fats during storage in called rancidification. New compounds are formed which may change the comsistency and therapeutic value of the fat. As inflamed areas of the skin are more sensitive to irritation, rancidified fats are undesirable for use in medicine.

The main types of rancidity are acid rancidity, carbonyl compound rancidity and peroxide rancidity. The fat splitting enzymes, lipases, produce free acids in the presence of water causing acid rancidity. Natural fats contain small amounts of water in disperse form. Therefore, natural fats should be stored under anhydrous conditions. The activity of lipases is inhibited by lowering the pH. The lipases are thermolabile, i.e., they are destroyed by heat. Many fats are exposed to steam for some time.

Oxidative rancidity is very important in the deterioration of fats. Microbes are developed when the fats contain water or proteins, e.g. lard and butter. By the action of microbes upon fat, methyl ketones having a strong and disagreeable odour are formed :

$$R-CH_2-CH_2-COOH \xrightarrow{-2H} R-CH = CH-COOH \xrightarrow{+H_2O}$$

$$R-CHOH-CH_2-COOH \xrightarrow{-2H} R-CO-CH_2COOH \xrightarrow{-CO_2}$$
$$R-CO-CH_3$$

Unsaturated fats absorb oxygen in the presence of light, increasing the weight, becoming more viscous and finally a solid material. The iodine value of the fat is decreased. At elevated temperatures, oxygen adds unsaturated acid to form peroxides which on rearrangement splits the molecule between the carbons forming aldehydes of disagreeable odour. The reaction is autocatalytic and started by UV light. Many substances, e.g. Fe, Cu, Co, Mn, hemin, and others accelerate the rate of oxidation. Such substances are called oxidants. Other substances retard the rate of oxidation and known as antioxidants. Carotenes, gallic and ascorbic acids, pomiferin, tocopherol (vitamin E) and nordihydroguaiaretic acid are used as antioxidants.

Racemization : In natural products, most physiologically active compounds occur in l-form. Racenization in dl-form has only half the activity. The racemic forms of atropine and ergot alkaloids lose half of their alkaloidal activity.

Light : Many substances are affected by light. Santonin of Levant wormseed turns yellow in the light. The carotenoids of Saffron is decolourized in the light. Essential oils turn gradually dark and viscous in the light. Vitamins A, B$_2$ and C are sensitive to light. The alkaloid content of Coca leaf, Stramonium leaf and of Veratrum root decreases faster when the drugs are dried in light.

Plant Growth Regulators

Plant growth regulators affect the morphological and physiological processes of plants in low concentrations. These are organic compounds which modify the plant growth. Some growth regulators occur naturally, e.g. plant hormones (auxins, gibberellins, zeatin); some of them are synthetic compounds, e.g. kinetin, adenine, 6-benzyl adenine, benzimidazole, N, N'-diphenyl urea and ethylene.

Five well known plant hormones are the auxins, gibberellins, cytokinins, abscisic acid and its derivatives and ethylene. They are specific in their action and show effects in very low concentration. They take part in cell division, organogenesis, senescence and dormancy. Their treatment influences the size of the plant, effects earlier growth and root development, improves the level of proteins and amino acids, and enhances the production of secondary metabolites.

Auxins : Auxins promote elongation of coleoptile tissues. Indoleacetic acid (IAA) is the principal natural auxin which occurs in actively growing tissues. Other similar natural compounds are indoleacetaldehyde, indoleacetonitrile and indolepyruvic acid. All these compounds are derived from tryptophan in plants. The synthetic auxins include indole-3-butyric acid, α-naphthyl acetic acid (NAA), naphthyl acetamide, 2,4-dichlorophenoxyacetic acid (2, 4-D), 5-carboxymethyl-N, N-dimethyl dithiocarbanate, etc.

Auxins elongate cells to increase the length of a stem; inhibit root growth and adventitious root production; and produce fruits in the absence of pollination. In low concentrations auxins accelerate the rooting of woody and herbaceous cuttings and in high concentrations they act as selective herbicides or weed-killers. They influence the physical and chemical properties in leaf abscission and inhibition of lateral buds.

In plants IAA oxidase controls the oxidative degradation of IAA. Orthodiphenols, e.g. caffeic and chlorogenic acids, inhibit the action of the enzyme and stimulate the growth.

Monophenols, e.g. p-coumaric acid, promote the action of IAA oxidase and inhibit the growth. α-Naphthyl acetic acid (NAA) is used for rooting of cuttings. IAA has been used for rooting of cuttings of *Cinchona, Carica, Coffea, Pinus* and other species. Auxins in specific concentration destroy some species of plants leaving other unaffected. 2, 4-Dichlorophenoxyacetic acid is toxic to dicotyledenous plants like dandelion and plantain. Treatment of seedlings and young plants of *Mentha piperita* with derivatives of NAA increases yield up to 40% of oil which contains 4.5 - 9% more menthol than the control. 2, 4-D produces abnormal and bizarre form of *D. stramonium;* an increase trichome production; and smooth fruits as distinct from those with spines.

Indole-3-acetic acid
(R = CH$_2$ COOH)

Indole-3-butyric acid
(R=CH$_2$CH$_2$CH$_2$COOH)

2, 4-Dichloro-
phenoxyacetic acid

α-Naphthyl acetic acid
(R = COOH)

α-Naphthylacetamide
(R = CONH$_2$)

Gibberellins : Gibberellins (GA) are the tetracyclic endrogenous plant hormones and were originally discovered as the phytotoxic metabolites of a rice pathogen, *Gibberella fugikuroi.* Many of their functional groups are attached on parent ring system. More than 40 gibberellins have been detected in plants and fungi. They are present in all plant organs. Commercially, they are used for promotion of vegetative and fruit growth, flower initiation, induction of parthenocarpy and breaking dormancy. Gibberellin A was found to be a mixture of about 6 components, e.g. GA$_1$, GA$_2$ GA$_3$ (Gibberellic acid), GA$_4$, GA$_7$ and GA$_9$. Gibberellins are synthesized in leaves and they usually accumulate in immature seeds and fruits.

Gibberellic acid (GA$_3$) : R = OH
GA$_7$: R = H

Gibberellins promote rapid expansion of plant cells, stimulate seed germination, breaking dormancy, induction of flowers, elongation of stem, increase in size of leaves and induction of parthenocarpic fruit leading to seedless fruit sets. The effects of gibberellins and auxins in cell division are almost similar. Gibberellins occur in plants in deactivated forms.

Application of GA shows various types of modifications in medicinal plants. Its spray on flowers of *Humulus lupulus* advances the maturity of the hops by 10 days. GA treatment on *Mentha piperita* has shown typical elongation of the internodes, changes in leaf shapes, loss of ribs on the stem, variation in chlorophyll content, fewer glandular hairs and decrease in the volatile oil yield up to 52.4 per cent. GA treatment on *Chenopodium ambrosioides* showed 33% increase in volatile oil. GA increases the volatile oil content of *Anethum graveolens* up to 50% and of *A. sowa* up to 30 per cent. The hormone increases yield of Digitalis glycosides per shoot. In *Hyoscyamus niger* the hormone elongates the stem having narrow leaves, shows more rapid onset of flowering and decreases of overall yield of alkaloids. Similar reduction of alkaloid contents of *Datura* species, Tobbaco, *Duboisia* species, *Catharanthus roseus*, *Rauwolfia serpentina* and *Thea sinensis* has been observed. Application of GA decreases sennosides in *Cassia angustifolia* and glycoside rutin in buckwheat plant.

Gluconeogenic enzymes effects the action of gibberellic acid. The hormone induces the synthesis of α-amylase and other hydrolytic enzymes and involves in mobilizing seed storage reserves during germination.

Cytokinins : Cytokinins have a specific effect on cell division. They regulate the pattern and frequency of organ production and have an inhibitory effect on senescence. These hormones are either natural (zeatin) or synthetic (kinetin) compounds. Zeatin is a 6-substituted adenine derivative. Cytokinin promotes cell division in the formation of adventitious buds and shoots; inhibits senescence; influences the expansion of cells in leaf discs and cotyledons; delays breakdown of chlorophyll; and degradates protein in ageing leaves. Kinetin treatment of *Datura meteloides* showed shorter and bushier plants, decreased growth and no change in alkaloid content. Cytokinin activity on *Duboisia* hybrids increased 18% in leaf yield and 16% increase in hyoscine. With *Cassia angustifolia*, there was a slight increase in sennoside content. Kinetins take part in nucleic acid metabolism and protein synthesis. In plants, some RNA shows cytokinin-type activity. They act on some enzymes which form amino acids.

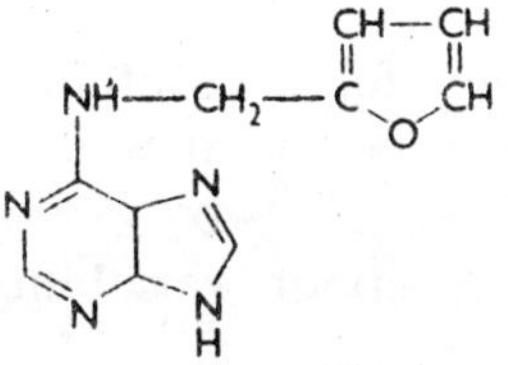

Kinetin

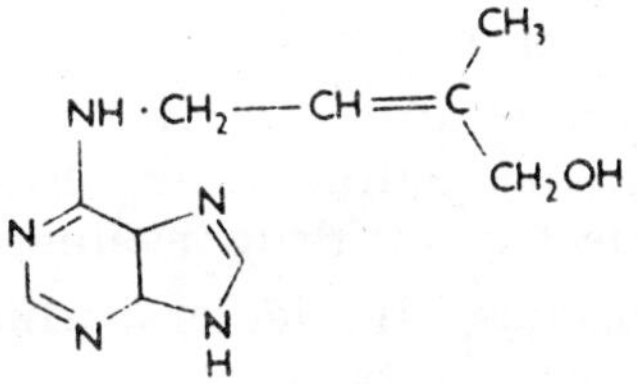

Zeatin

Growth Inhibitors : Natural growth inhibitors affect bud opening, seed germination and development of dormancy. Abscisic acid, a natural growth inhibitor, has been isolated from the fungus, *Cenospora rosicola*. The synthetic growth inhibitor, N-dimethylamino-succinamic acid, reduced the height of *Datura* species and there was up to 90% increase in the alkaloidal content. Phosphon produced the same effects on *D. ferox.*

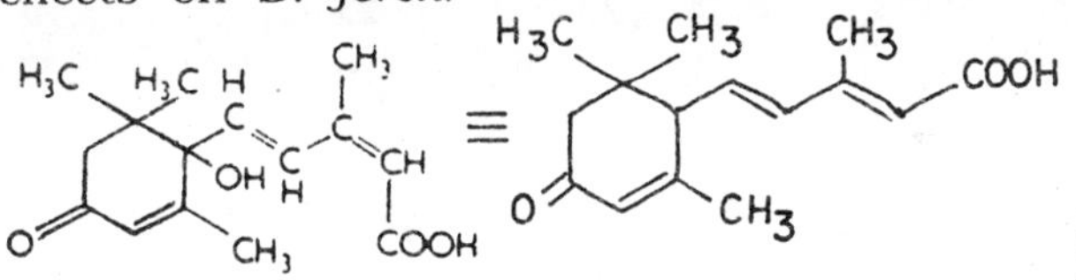

Abscisic acid (ABA)

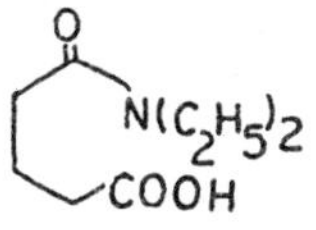

N-dimethylamino Succinamic

Ethylene : Ethylene, $CH_2 = CH_2$, is a colourless, flammable gas which induces growth responses in plants. It occurs in ripening fruits, flowers, and other plant organs. Commercially, it is used for induction of fruit abscission, breaking dormancy and stimulation of latex flow from 36 to 136% in rubber plants. At low concentrations it increases the sennoside concentration in *Cassia angustifolia.* It stimulates the production of phytuberin and phytuberol.

QUESTIONS

1. Enumerate the genetic factors that influence the quality of crude drugs. Give an account of chemical races.

2. What do you understand by ontogenetic variations of secondary plant metabolites ? Give suitable examples where such variations are of pharmaceutical significance.

3. Describe the genetic or exogenous factors which affect the plant constituents. Give suitable examples under each class.

4. Discuss genetic methods of improving drug yielding plants. Explain the terms selection, polyploidy and chemical races.

5. Enumerate factors responsible for variability of phytoconstituents in medicinal plants and how do they affect plant-drug evaluation.

6. Discuss the factors which bring about variability of constituents.

GLOSSARY

BOTANICAL TERMS

Accentric hilum : Hilum not present in the centre.

Acene : (1) A dry, one-seeded fruit with a firm, close fitting pericarp which does not split along regular lines, i.e., indehiscent. (2) The seed lies in the ovary except for its attachment by the funiculus.

Acicular : Having projections which are needle-like.

Acuminate : Having a small terminal point, with a very sharply tapering point; with an acute point.

Acute : Pointed, less than a right angle, sharp edged.

Adnate : Designating the union of unlike parts such as scales attached to stems, anthers attached along their entire length.

Adnation : (1) The fusion with or attachment to another plant structure by its whole length from the beginning of growth. (2) The union of vascular bundles.

Adventitious : Accidental; out of usual place; developing in an abnormal position, e.g. roots developing from stems.

Aerenchyma : Respiratory tissue formed by phallogen, cortical tissue containing airspaces in the parenchyma.

Albuminous cell : (1) Cells rich in nitrogenous contents (2) Parenchyma cells in gymnosperm phloem associated with sieve cells but not derived from the same source.

Aleurone : Protein granules of globulins and peptones found in ripe seeds; Crystalloid proteins in seeds.

Alluvial soil : Soil, deposited by water, a flood plain.

Anastomose : (1) United like the parts of a network. (2) Fused, as vascular bundles at nodes.

Annual : Yearly; living only one year; with a life cycle of one year's duration.

Annulate : Marked with rings; ring-shaped.

Annulations : Rings; belts, or circles.

Anther : (1) Upper part of the stamen in which pollen is produced; the pollen groups. (2) The microsporangium.

Apical : At the tip of apex.

Apicle : A small tooth or point at the apex.

Apicule : (1) Short, often sharp at one end of the spore. (2) A small acute projection.

Ascospore : A spore formed in an ascus and characteristic of ascomycetes.

Asexual : Not sexual; without male or female sex organs; sexless.

Axile : In the axis of any structure; situated in or belonging to an axis.

Axial placentation : Placentation in which the ovules are borne on a central axis in separate chambers of the fruit.

Axillary bud : A lateral bud borne in the axil of a leaf.

Bark : The outer covering of a trunk or branch; all tissues found outside the cambium; the cortical covering of a stem.

Berry : A fleshy fruit without a stone usually containing many seeds embedded in the pulp.

Bicarpellary : Having two carpels, i.e., modified floral leaves.

Bicollateral : Having two sides alike.

Biennial : A plant which completes its life history (cycle) in two growing seasons; usually fruiting during the second season.

Bifacial : Having two faces, as the distinct upper and lower surfaces of a leaf.

Bifurcate : Divided or forked into two branches; having two prongs.

Bilabiate : Two-lipped, as in the corolla of the mint.

Bilocular : With two cavities; having two chambers; two-celled.

Binate : (1) In pairs as of a simple leaf nearly divided into two parts. (2) A leaf composed of two leaflets at the ends of a common petiole.

Blossom : The flower, the corolla.

Bracteole : A small bract; a secondary bract particularly as borne on the pedicels.

Bulbous base : Swollen base.

Calex : A cup like part or organ.

Calyx : The outer floral envelope of the flowering plants usually green in colour and composed of sepals.

Cambium : A thin layer of formative tissues beneath the bark of dicotyledons and gymnosperms from which new wood and bark originate.

Capsule : (1) Dry dehiscent fruits formed from a compound ovary with various types of dehiscence to release the seeds. (2) The spore cases of mosses and ferns. (3) The perithecia or receptacles of fungi.

Cariaceous : Of a leathery texture.

Carpels : Modified floral leaves in the seed plants which form the simple or compound gynoecium of the flower in which seeds are formed.

Carpophore : Central stalk.

Caruncle : A small fleshy excrescence.

Caryophyllaceous : Resembling the pink family, *Caryophyllaceae;* having connate-perfoliate leaves and stems swollen at the nodes; having petals with long tapered bases or claws.

Cataphyll : A scale-like leaf as found in buds, rhizomes, etc.

Caulicle : (1) A small scale. (2) The initial stem as in embryo.

Chalaza : The point at which the nucleus and integuments of the ovule are united; the place where the seed coat unites with the rest of the ovule.

Channels : (1) Longitudinal grooves. (2) The interstices between the ribs on the fruits of Umbelliferous plants.

Coccus : (1) A one-seeded carpel (2) A mericarp. (3) A spherical bacterium.

Collateral : Being side by side, as in fibrovascular bundles.

Collenchyma : The first formed strengthening tissue of stems composed of elongated cells thickened only at the angles by material like cellulose.

Columella : A small column or central axis.

Commissural : The coherence of two carpels by their faces, as in Umbelliferae.

Conidiophore : A specialized hypha of a fungus mycelium which produces a conidiospore.

Connate : Joined into one organ as opposite leaves united at the base.

Conspicuous : Clearly seen.

Cordate : Heart shaped.

Corm : A solid, fleshy, underground base of a stem, usually spherical in shape, covered with thin membranes.

Corolla : The inner circle of petals which is usually the conspicuous part of a flower.

Cortex : A cylinder of parenchymatous cells lying between the epidermis and the vascular tissue in a young stem.

Cortical : Pertaining to the bark or cortex.

Cotyledon : The seed leaf, a leaf-like organ within a seed in which food for the new plant is stored.

Cremocarp : A dry, seed-like fruit which is composed of two one-seeded carpels which are invested by an epigynous calyx and separated into mericarps at maturity.

Crenate : Of leaf margins, with broad rounded teeth separated by narrow open spaces.

Crown : (1) A corona (2) The chaffy scales at the tip of an achene. (3) A part of a rhizome with a large bud suitable for propagation. (4) A short root stalk.

Cruciferous : Cross-shaped.

Crumple : To fall into small particles, becomes distintegrated.

Cuticle : (1) A continuous, non-cellular layer consisting of cutin and containing no cellulose. (2) A water repellent outer membrane of plant parts.

Cuticularized cells : Cells provided with a cuticle layer.

Debris : The mixture of leaves, twigs, wood, etc.

Deciduous : Falling off at certain season or stage of growth.

Decompound : Having divided leaflets compounded more than once, pinnate twice.

Decorticated : Destitute of bark, debarked.

Decortication : The act of stripping off the bark, rind or outer coat.

Decurrent : (1) Of a gill, descending or slopping down the stem. (2) Applied to an organ extending along the side of another. (3) Extending below the point of insertion.

Decussate : In pairs alternately crossing at right angles; applied to leaves and branches arranged in pairs and alternately crossing each other.

Dehisce : To open spontaneously for the exposure of seeds, spores, pollens, etc.

Dehiscence: The natural opening of fruit capsules; the act of splitting to open.

Dentate : Having teeth; having a toothed margin.

Dichasial : In two rows.

Dichotomous cyme : A cyme with two axes running in opposite direction.

Dioecious : Unisexual; having the staminate and pistillate flowers on separate individuals; producing male and female organs on diffrent individual.

Dissepiment : (1) A partition in capsule; the partition between the cells of seed vessels. (2) The trama in certain fungi.

Divergency : The fraction of a stem circumference; The separation of parts.

Dome : The growing point of the receptacle of a flower.

Dorsal : Referring to the back or outer surface of an organ.

Drip or drooping point : The acuminate apex of a leaf from which water drips.

Drupe : A one seeded, usually indehiscent fleshy fruit in which the endocarp is stony, the mesocarp fleshy, and the exocarp skin-like.

Drupaceous : Resembling or bearing drupes.

Ellipsoid : A solid body which is elliptic in section.

Endosperm : The multicellular food-storing tissue formed inside a seed.

Entire : Concerning leaf margins or gills without teeth; with a continuous, even margin.

Epicarp : The outer layer of the ovary wall.

Epidermis : The thin external layer of protective cells of a plant.

Epigynous : Having the calyx, corolla and stamens growing from the top of an inferior ovary.

Epipetalous : Having the stamens seated on the petals or corolla borne on the petals.

Exalbuminous : Without albumen, lacking endosperm and reserve food stored in the cotyledons.

Exserted : Projected as a stamen.

Exfoliation : The shedding of leaves or scales from a bud, peeling off.

Exudation : (1) Any discharge through an incision or pores (2) The loss of liquid through hydathodes.

Fibrous : Composed or covered with tough string-like tissues.

Fibrovascular : Composed of both fibres and ducts.

Filiform : Having shape of a thread or filament; Thread-like.

Fimbricate : Having the edge minutely fringed.

Foliaceae : The frondose vascular cryptogams leaf-like structures.

Follicle : A dry, one-celled, capsular fruit dehiscing longitudinally by a suture on one side.

Fracture : Act of breaking.

Fusiform : Spindle-shaped.

Gelatinization : The process in which a membrane breaks down into a jelly-like mass.

Glabrous : Without hairs, bristles, or scales; smooth.

Glandular : Consisting of a gland.

Glaucous : Covered with fine white or sea green bloom which is easily rubbed off; silvery.

Globulus : The fruit of *Hepaticae*. (2) The deciduous shield of some lichens.

Glossy : Having a smooth, shining surface.

Glutinous : Adhesive, glney.

Gritty : Sandy; containing fine, stony or hard particles.

Hemispherical : One half of a sphere or globe.

Herbaceous perennial : A plant having annual stems from a perennial root.

Hilum : (1) The scar at the point of attachment of the seed, The eye of a seed (2) The nucleus of a starch grain.

Horny : Any pointed projection or process in plants.

Hypanthium : The tube of the receptacle upon which the calyx, corolla, and stamens are borne.

Hypodermis : The tissue just beneath the epidermis.

Imbricate : Overlapping like the shingles on a roof.

Incise : To cut sharply and deeply on the margin.

Inconspicuous : Not easily perceived.

Indehiscent : Not opening naturally at maturity; not splitting regularly.

Inflate : To distend with air or gas; having a cavity within.

Inflorescence : (1) A reproductive shoot composed of or bearing a number of shoots of limited growth. (2) An arrangement of flowers on a stem (3) A cluster of reproductive organs in bryophytes.

Internodal : Below a node; Between to nodes

Involucre : A cluster of modified leaves or bracts at the base of a flower cluster.

Isobilateral symmetry : The condition of flowers and other parts of plants which can be divided into symmetrical halves by two distinct planes.

Kernel : The seed inside the stony endocarp of a drup; the seed within the coat.

Lactiferous : (1) Of trama, having a milky juice. (2) Producing latex.

Lamella : The membrane between any two cells.

Lamina : (1) A layer. (2) The blade or extended part of a leaf.

Lanceolate : Resembling a lance; much longer than broad, widest in the middle and tapering to a pointed apex.

Legume : A fruit formed from a single carpel opening by two sutures.

Lenticel : A small breathing pore in the bark of trees and shrubs.

Lenticular : Lens-shaped or resembling a lentil, orbicular and convex on both faces.

Lignification : The hardening or thickening of the cell wall by secondary deposits.

Lignified layer : The layer of cells immediately above the separation layer in leaf fall.

Lobe : A rounded division of a plant organ.

Longitudinal : Lengthwise; parallel with the axis from the base toward the summit or apex.

Lumen : A cell cavity.

Lustrous : Luminous, bright.

Matrix : (1) The body upon which lichens and fungi grow. (2) The ground substance of connective tissues.

Medullary layer : A thick subcortical layer of the thallus of some lichens.

Mericarp : A one-seeded portion of a fruit which splits at maturity.

Mesocarp : The middle layer of the pericarp which consists of three layers.

Mesophyll : The soft tissue between the upper and the lower epidermis of the leaf which is chiefly concerned in photosynthesis.

Micropyle : (1) A tiny opening in the integument at the apex of an ovule through which the pollen enters. (2) The tiny opening in the testa of seed through which water enters.

Molasses : Any of several dark coloured, thick syrups, produced during the refining of sugar or sorghum.

Monoecious : Having stamens and pistils in separate flowers on the same plant.

Mucilage : A gummy secretion; dissolved vegetable jelly.

Napiform : Turnip-shaped.

Nectary : The nectar-secreting organ.

Nematode : (1) Thread-like worms (2) The filamentous algae.

Node : (1) The joint of a culm (grass stem). (2) The place on the stem where leaves ordinarily arise.

Oblong : Rectangular and having the length greater than breadth.

Obtuse : Blunt-pointed, rounded.

Orbicular : Circular in outline, nearly rounded and flat, rotund, disk-shaped.

Ovary : The enlarged base part of the pistil or carpel in which the ovules appear.

Ovate : Shaped like the longitudinal section through a hen's egg.

Palea, Pale or palet : (1) The inner bracteole, thin and membraneous which encloses the grass flower.

Palisade cells : (1) A layer of elongated cells set at right angles to the surface of a leaf underlying the upper epidermis (2) Terminal.

Papilla : A soft superficial protuberance; a small, nipple-like elevation.

Papilionaceous : Butterfly-like, as the corollas of the pea flowers.

Papillate : Nipple-shaped.

Papillose : Having minute nipple-shaped projections.

Paripinnate : Having a pinnately compound leaf which has no terminal leaflet.

Patches : A clap on a piece.

Pedicel : (1) A slender stalk or stem. (2) The stalk of a single flower, a peduncle.

Peduncle : A primary flower stalk supporting an inflorescence or a solitary flower.

Perennial : A plant which lives for more than two years.

Perianth : The calyx and corolla collectively. (2) The outer envelope of a flower. (3) The cup-shaped or tubular sheath.

Pericarp : The ı mature ovary wall, the wall of the fruit or seed vessel developed from the wall of mature ovary.

Periderm : A protective outer cylinder of tissues formed in woody stems which consists of cork cambium and phellogen.

Perisperm : The albumen of the seed.

Persistent : Retaining its place, shape or structure; evergreen.

Petiolate : Having a petiole.

Petiole : The leaf stalk.

Phloem : Cortical tissue.

Pinnate : With leaflets or veins on each side of a common stem or vein in a feather-like arrangement.

Pinnate-pinnatifid : Once pinnate then pinnatified, feather-like.

Pinnatifid : Pinnately cleft to the middle or beyond, deeply cut into segments nearly to the midrib.

Pitch : The soft tissue in the interior which often disappears.

Pithy : Containing pith.

Placenta : The part of the ovary to which the ovules are attached. The ovule-bearing part of the ovary.

Placentation : The method of which ovules are atttached.

Plano-convex : Plane on one side and convex on the other.

Plasmodesmata : Fine protoplasmic strands between the different walls of endosperm cells.

Plumule : The embryonic shoot or bud in the seed located between cotyledons which develops into the stem and leaves of the plant.

Polygamous : Having unisexual and bisexual flowers on the same plant.

Polyploid : A cell, tissue or organism having three, four or more times the normal number of chromosome in its nuclei.

Procumbent : Prostrate but not taking root at the nodes, lying on the ground, trailing.

Propolis : A resinous material collected by the hive bees from the opening buds of various trees.

Protuberance : A rounded projection on surface.

Pseudoparenchyma: (1) False parenchyma, tissue which resembles parenchyma. (2) Hyphae of fungi which are divided into short cells and resemble in parenchyma.

Pubescent : Hairy or downy.

Pyriform : Pear-shaped.

Raceme : An inflorescence composed of pedicelled flowers arranged along the axis which elongates for an indefinite period. The lower flower blooms first.

Radial : Belonging to the ray as in the flowers of *Compositae*.

Radicle : The embryonic root, the portion of the embryo below the catyledons.

Ranunculaceous : (1) Buttercup yellow. (2) Allied to the genus *Ranunculus*.

Raphe : The continuation of the seed stalk along the side of an anatropous ovule or seed.

Receptacle : (1) In fungi, a spore-bearing structure, usually concave. (2) In algae, a swollen end of a branch containing reproductive organs (3) In mosses, a group of sexual organs surrounded by bracts. (4) In flowering plants, the elongated end of the flower stalk or the enlarged end of the peduncle which bears the flowers of a composite floweer.

Reniform : Kidney-shaped

Reticular : Net-like.

Reticulate cells : Cells having reticulate thickenings of the walls.

Rhizome : A thickish, prostrate, more or less subterranean stem producing roots and leafy shoots.

Rhomboid : Diamond-shaped.

Rhytidome : (1) A plate of cellular tissue within the liber (2) An external covering of a plant member made up of alternating sheets of cork and dead cortex or dead phloem.

Rosette : (1) A dense, flat, imbricated cluster of leaves growing from a short stem at the base of a plant. (2) A collection of leaves growing close together.

Rubiaceous : Belonging to or resembling to the family *Rubiceae*.

Scale : A small, thin, semitransparent bract or leaf-like structure.

Scaly : Scale-like.

Scar : The mark left by the natural separation of leaf or other organ.

Schizocarp : A dry compound fruit which splits apart into single-seeded segments at maturity.

Schizogenesis : Reproduction by fission.

Schizolysigenous cavity : An intercellular space formed in part by the separation of cells and in part by the dissolution of the cell wall.

Sclerenchyma : Cells with thick lignified-wall.

Sclerotium : (1) A resting body of small size composed of a hardened mass of hyphae from which fruit bodies may develop. (2) A hard, compact, tuber-like body containing stored food.

Segment : (1) A multinucleate portion of a hypha or filament delimited by transverse walls. (2) A portion of a blade of a leaf when deeply lobed but not divided into two leaflets.

Sepal : Each part of the calyx, a segment of the calyx.

Septate : Having septa.

Septicidal : Dehiscing along the partitions, dividing through the middle of the ovary septa.

Serrate : With teeth pointing toward the apex, saw-toothed.

Sessile : Without a stalk; sitting directly on the base.

Sheath : (1) A gelatinous envelop surrounding a plant (2) A tubular envelop (3) A cylindrical tube surrounding organs or cells.

Slender : Small in circumference in proportion to height or length.

Solitary : Alone; growing singly.

Speck : A tiny spot; a particle.

Sphacela : The apical cell metabolism.

Sphaeraphides : Spherocrystals.

Sphaero : Conical.

Spine : A thorn; a sharp process originating in the wood.

Splintery : A rough piece of wood, usually long thin and sharp.

Stalk : The lengthened above-ground support to which organs are attached, as the petiole of a leaf.

Stamen : The male organ of a flower.

Stellate : Relating to the centre.

Stipule : A leafy appendage at the base of the petiole, usually one on each side.

Stolon : A modified propagating stem above ground creeping and rooting at the tip.

Stoma : An opening surrounded by guard cells which opens into internal air cavities, the breathing apparatus in the epidermis of leaves.

Stratification : An arrangement in layers, the thickening of a wall by the depositing of successive layers of materials.

Striate : Having minute radiating furrows.

Striation : Markings due to the manner of formation in bands.

Strophiole : An excrecence or appendage at or about the hilum of a seed.

Style : The narrowed neck above the ovary which is surrounded by the stigma.

Stylopod : The enlarged bases of the styles in *Umbelliferae*.

Subarbicular : Nearly circular.

Subcaulescent : With a very short stem.

Suberin : A complex fatty or waxy substance found in cell wall

Suberization : Conversion into cork.

Subulate : Awl-shaped, tapering from a broad or thick base to a sharp point.

Succulents : The succulent plant, such as cacti and other xerophytes.

Syngenesious : In a ring, as the anthers in *Compositae*; having stamens united by their anthers.

Tear : A solid transparent drop.

Testa : The outer integument, the seed coat.

Tetradelphous : In four bundles.

Texture : Structure or constitution.

Tomentose : Woolly, hair.

Tortuous : Flashy.

Tracheids : The woody sieve-like conducting cells in secondary xylem.

Tracheidal vessels : A group of vessels composed of lignified cells without protoplasmic contents.

Traumatism : An abnormal growth resulting from an injury.

Trichome : A hair-like outgrowth of the epidermis.

Tubercle : (1) A wart-like or knob-like excrescence (2) A nodule. (3) The persistent base of the style.

Tubular : With sepals united except at the toothed margins.

Umbellate : Arrangement in an umbel.

Umbelliferous : Having umbellate flowers.

Unctuous : Having a greasy appearance.

Unifacial : With one face or principal surface.

Urceolate : Like a pitcher or contracted at the mouth, as the flowers of many heaths.

Vascular : Furnished with vessels or ducts through which fluid is conveyed.

Vascular strand : A strand of conducting tissue consisting of xylem and phloem sometimes separated by cambium.

Verticillate : Disposed in or forming verticles or whorles, as flowers, leaves, hairs etc.

Villous : Having long soft hairs

Viscid : Sticking or adhering, covered.

Vitta : An oil tube such as is found in Coriander (Umbelliferae fruits).

Wedge : A lip which broadens strongly outward.

Wiry : Wire-like

Wrinkle : A small ridge or furrow, formed by the folding; a small fold in the skin.

Xerophyte : A plant adapted to dry conditions of air and soil.

Xylem : The portion of vascular bundle which consists of tracheal tissue and wood parenchyma, woody tissue, the wood of the vascular bundle.

MEDICAL TERMS

Abortifacient : A drug that causes artifical abortion.

Abortion : Separation and expulsion of the contents of the pregnant uterus before the 28th week of pregnancy.

Abscess : A localized collections of pus.

Abstinance : A refraining from the use of or indulgence in food, stimulants or sexual intercourse.

Achyliagestrica : Absence of hydrochloric acid.

Acne : A chronic skin disease which affects practically all adolescents, eruption occurs on the face, back and chest.

Acrid : Sharp or biting to the taste.

Addiction : The state being strongly devoted; habitual; compulsive use of narcotics.

Addition's disease : consisting of a state of anaemia, extreme weakness, low blood pressure, dyspepsia, wasting, pigmentation of the skin and mucous membranes, and subnormal temperature.

Albuminuria : A condition in which albumin is present in the urine.

Alexipharmac : Antidotal, counter-poison.

Allergen : Any substance, usually protein, which is taken into the body, makes the body hypersensitive or allergic to it.

Allergy : Special sensitiveness of an individual to certain food, pollens or other animal products.

Alterative : Having a power to change.

Amoebia : A minute protozoan unicellular organism.

Amylolytic : Conversion of starch into sugar by an agent.

Anaemia : A condittion of inadequate red blood carpulses or haemoglobin in the blood.

Anaesthesia : Loss of power of feeling.

Anaesthetic : Drugs producing insensibility to external impressions.

Analgesia : Loss of power to feel pain without loss of consciounsess.

Analgesics : Drugs or other measures which cause temporary loss of the sense of pain without unconsciousness.

Anodynes : Curative measures which soothe pain.

Anthelmintics : Substances causing the death or expulsion of parasitic worms.

Anticholinergic : A substance that antagonizes acetylcholine.

Antidotes : Remedies which neutralize the effects of poisons.

Antigenic : A substance which causes the formation of antibodies.

Antihypertensive : Counteracting high blood pressure; an agent that reduces high blood pressure.

Anti-infective : Counteracting infection.

Anti-inflammatory : Counteracting or suppressing inflammation.

Anti-neoplastic : Inhibiting the development of neoplasms.

Antiperiodic : Preventing periodic recurrence of symptoms, as in malaria.

Antiprotozoal : Destroying protozoa.

Antipyretic : Drugs used to reduce temperature in fever.

Anti-rheumatism : Agent that prevents or relieves the pain of rheumatism.

Antiseptic : Substances which prevent putrefaction in dead animal or vegetable matter.

Antispasmodic : Any substance which lowers the tonus of pain muscle.

Antitussive : Agent that prevents or relieves cough.

Aperients : Medicines which produce a natural movement of the bowels as in constipation.

Aphrodisiac : Exacting sexual desire.

Aphthae : Small ulcers.

Appetite : Craving for food necessary to maintain the body.

Arrhythmia : Any variation from the normal regular rhythm of the heart-beat.

Arthritis : Inflammation of the joints; the gout.

Astringent : Contracting; styptic, contracting the organic tissues and canals of the body and thereby checking or diminishing bleeding or excessive discharge.

Atherosclerosis : A form of fatty degeneration of middle coat of the arterial walls.

Atony : Want of tone or vigour in muscles and other organs.

Bacteriocidal : Relating to killing of bacteria and part play in medicine, agriculture and industry.

Bacteriostatic : A process of bringing bacteria to a standstill by preventing their nourishment and growth.

Bilious : Concerned with disorder of the liver or bile.

Boil : A small areas of inflammation starting in the roots of hairs and due to the growth of a microorganism.

Bronchitis : Inflammation of mucous membrane of the bronchial tubes.

Bronchodilator : Agent that dilates the bronchi.

Bruccal : Check

Bruitis : A sound heard in auscultation.

Cachexia : Feeble state produced by serious disease, such as cancer.

Calculi : Concretion in the organs like bladder, kidney, gall bladder.

Cardiac : Relating to heart.

Carminative : Preparations to relieve flatulence.

Catarrh : A state of irritation of the mucous membranes associated with a copious secretion of mucus.

Cathartics : Substances which produce an evacuation of the bowels (purgative).

Celebral : Relating to brain.

Cerate : Thick ointment composed of oils, mixed with wax, resin, etc.

Cholagogues : Substances which increase the flow of bile by stimulating evacuation of the gall-bladder.

Cholera: An acute infectious disease characterized by severe intestinal disturbances.

Choleretic : Drug that stimulates the flow of bile.

Cholinergic : Relating to the basic compound choline which is essential to the function of liver.

Cinchonism : A disturbed condition of the body characteritized by dizziness, ear ringing, temporary deafness and headache due to overdose of quinine.

Coagulant : That which produces coagulation.

Colic : An attack of spasmodic pain in the abdomen.

Colitis : Inflammation of the colon.

Colostomy : The operation for the establishment of an artificial opening into the colon acting as anus.

Concentric : Having a common centre, as circle or spheres.

Condiment : A sauce, spice

Confections : Conserves and electuaries, form a method of prescribing bulky drugs mixed into a paste with sugar or honey.

Confectionary : Preparation of medicinal preparations with the aid of sugar, honey or sweet.

Congestion : Accumulation of blood in a part due to over-filling of its blood-vessels.

Congestion : An overcrowed condition; an unusual accumulation of blood in the vessels.

Constipation : A condition in which the bowels are opened to seldom or incompletely.

Convulsions : Rapidly alternating contractions and relaxations of the muscles, causing irregular movements of the limbs or body, and unusuallly accompanied by unconsciousness. Violent agitation or disturbance.

Cryptoichidism : A developmental defect characterized by failure of the testes to descend into the serotum.

Cyanosis : A condition of blueness seen particularly about the face and extremities and the blood is not properly oxygenated in the lungs.

Cytotoxic : Destructive to cells.

Dandruff : White scales cast off from the scalp.

Debility : A state of weakness.

Deliriant : A mental disturbance marked by illusions, hallucinations, etc.

Delirium : A state of preverted consciousness in which an irregular discharge of nervous energy goes on, causing incoherent talk, delusion, and ill-regulated muscular action.

Delivery : Final expulsion of the child in the act of birth.

Demulcent : A substance which exerts a soothing or protective influence upon the surface of the alimentary canal.

Dentifrice : A powder, paste, or liquid to use in cleaning the teeth.

Denture : False teeth.

Deobstruent : A substance that clears the natural passages of the body.

Depressant : Sedative, lowering the vital activities.

Depressor : A nerve by whose stimulation motion, secretion, or some other activity is restrained or prevented.

Dermatitis : Inflammation of the skin.

Diabetes insipidus : A disease characterized by excessive thirst and passing of large volumes of urine.

Diabetes mellitus : A constitutional disorder in which the power of muscles and other tissues to utilize sugar is diminished or lost.

Diaphoretics : Perspiration promoting remedies.

Diarrhoea : Looseness of bowels.

Diphtheria : Infectious disease caused by virulent strains of a bascillus.

Disinfection : The process of rendering harmless persons, articles, rooms, etc. which are liable to communicate disease.

Disinfestation : Destruction of insect pests.

Disintegrant : Separation of the component particles.

Diuretics : Substances which produce diuresis i.e., a copious excretion of urine by the kidneys.

Dropsy : An abnormal accumulation of fluid beneath the skin.

Drowsiness : Sleepy condition.

Dysentery : An infectious disease with a local lesion in the form of inflammation and ulceration of lower portion of the bowels.

Dysmenorrhoea : Painful menstruation.

Dyspepsia : A condition of pain or disorder of abdomen or chest which may be associated with other disturbances like nausea, flatulence, etc.

Dysuria : Difficulty or pain in urination.

Edema : A swelling due to excessive accumulation of fluid in a serous or connective tissues.

Emaciation : Pronounced wasting associated with repeated fever, tuberculosis, etc.

Embalming : Death involving burial, emblaming and cremation.

Embolism : Plugging of a small blood vessel by material carried through the larger vessels by the blood stream.

Emetic : Drugs or other means which produce vomiting.

Emission : The act of throwing or giving out.

Emmenagogues : Drugs which restore the flow at the menstrual periods when this is scanty or absent.

Emollients : Substances which have a softening and soothing effect upon the skin.

Emulsions : Mixtures containing oily substances in very fine division.

Emulsify : To form emulsion or milk-like substance.

Encapsulation : To enclose in a capsule.

Enema : An injection of fluid into the bowel.

Enuresis : Involuntary voiding of urine.

Epilepsy : Nervous disorder characterized by sudden loss of consciousness, attended with convulsions.

Episiotomy : The operation of cutting the outlet of the vagina in child hood to facilitate the birth of the child.

Erythrocytes : Red blood carpuscles.

Excipient : Inert substances added to a prescription.

Expectorants : Drugs assisting the removal of secretions from the air passages.

Febrifuges : Remedies employed to reduce the raised temperature of the body (antipyretics).

Febrile : Feverish.

Fibrillation : Rapid contraction of muscles especially abnormal action of the heart muscle.

Fibrositis : Non-articular rheumatism.

Fistula : An unnatural, narrow channel, leading from some natural cavity, such as a duct of a gland.

Fixative : Making fixed or permanent.

Flatulence : A collection of gas in the stomach or bowels.

Flocculation : Formation of clusters or masses of loosely united particles.

Flutter : A form of abnormal cardiac rhythm in which the atria contract at a rate of between 200-400 beats a minute.

Fungistatic : Inhibiting the growth of fungi.

Furunculosis : Relation to a boil or inflammatory sore.

Galactogogue : Drugs which increase the flow of milk in nursing women.

Gastroenteritis : Inflammation of the stomach and intestines.

Genito urinary tract : It consists of kindeys, ureters, bladder, and urethra or genital organs.

Germicide : A substance that destroys germs.

Gingivatis : Inflammation of the gingival margins around the teeth.

Glaucoma : A disease of eye after the age of 50 years.

Gonorrhoea : An inflammatory disease affecting the mucous membrane of urethra in the male and that of vagina in the female.

Gout : A constitutional disorder connected with excess of uric acid in the blood and inflammation of joints and morbid changes in organs.

Gravel : Any sediment which falls down in the urine, e.g., uric acid.

Haemolysis : Disintegration of elements in the blood.

Haemorrhage : Escape of blood from the vessels which naturally contain it.

Haemorrhoids : Pile; swelling at the anal region.

Haemostatics : Any means used to control bleeding.

Hallucinations : Errors in perception, affecting some sense organs.

Hay fever : As allergic condition of the mucous membranes of the eye, nose, and air passages.

Hemicrania : Headache limited to one side of the head.

Hepatitis : Inflammation of the liver.

Hoarseness : Husky, harsh, rough, or grating voice as when affected with a cold.

Hodgkin's disease : A condition in which the lymphatic glands undergo a progressive enlargement.

Hyaluronidase : An enzyme which hydrolyzes hyaluronic acid.

Hydragogue : A drug which produces a watery stool.

Hyperacidity : Excessive acidity.

Hypertension : High blood pressure.

Hypnotics : Measures including drugs, which produce sleep.

Hypotension : Unusual low blood pressure.

Hysteria : Overaction of some parts of the nervous system or failure of other parts to perform their necessary work.

Icterus : Jaundice.

Immunity : A principle by virtue of which the body is protected from the invasion of certain diseases or the action of certain poisons.

Immunization : A condition of being immunized.

Impotence : Inability to perform the sexual act.

Incense : Make angry.

Indolent : Causing little pain.

Infection : A process by which a disease is communicated from one person to another.

Infertility : The inability of a married couple to have children.

Inflammation : Reaction of tissues to any injury yielding redness, heat, pain and swelling.

Influenza : An acute infectious disease, characterized by a sudden onset, fever, aches and pains.

Infusions : Preparation of vegetable drugs made by steeping them for some time in water and straining.

Insanity : Mental illness.

Insecticides : Substances which are fatal to insects.

Insectifuge : A substance used for repelling insects.

Insomnia : Sleep; a periodic resting condition of the body and of the nervous system.

Intercellular : Situated between the cells.

Intoxication : State of poisoning.

Labour (Parturition) : The act of bringing forth young and ending of gestation or pregnancy.

Lactagogue : Galactagogue; promoting the flow of milk.

Lactation : The period during which an infant suckles on mother's breast.

Laparotomy : Operation in which the abdominal cavity is opened.

Laxative : Having the quality of loosening the intestines and relieving constipation.

Leprosy : A chronic disease which affects the skin, mucous membranes and nerves.

Leucoderma : A condition of the skin which becomes white as a result of various diseases.

Leucorrhoea : In women when the discharge is thick and white, consisting of pus or when the discharge is usually thinner and a clear mucous nature.

Ligature : A cord or thread used to tie round arteries in order to stop the circulation through them.

Linctus : Any thick syrupy medicine.

Liniments : Preparations intended for external application, generally with rubbing; mostly of oily nature.

Lotion : A fluid preparation intended for bringing in contact with, or for washing, the external surface of the body.

Lozenges : Small tablets containing drugs mixed with sugar, gum, glycerin-jelly or fruit-paste.

Lumbago : A painful ailment affecting the muscles of the lower part of the back.

Malaria : Periodic fever caused by the presence of certain parasites in the blood.

Mania : A mental disorder.

Mastication : Act of chewing.

Masticatory : Affecting the muscles of mastication.

Measles : An acute infectious disease in children causing disturbance of health, catarrh of the mucous membrane, sneezing, diarrhoea, fever and pulse rate.

Melanchoia : Mental illness.

Menorrhagia : An over-abundance of the menstrual discharge.

Menstrual : Pertaining to the menses of females.

Micturition : Act of passing water.

Migraine : A common condition of recurring intense headaches. accompanied by visual or gastro-intestinal disturbances, or both.

Miotic : An agent that causes the pupil to contract.

Miticide : A substance that kills mites.

Mucosa : A mucous membrane.

Mucus : Slimy secretion derived from mucous membranes.

Mumps : An infectious disease characterized by inflammatory swelling of the parotid and other salivary glands.

Muscular : Consisting or relating to muscles.

Muscularis : Relating to muscles.

Mydriasis : A state or unusual dilating of the pupil.

Mydriatics : Drugs causing unusual dilation of the pupil such as Belladonna and Cocaine.

Myeloid : Resembling marrow.

Narcotic : Drugs producing sleepness.

Nasal : Relating to the nose.

Nausea : Feeling that vomiting is about to take place; Vomiting sensation.

Nauseant : Causing upsetting of stomach often with an inclination to vomit.

Nephritic : Inflammation of the kidney.

Neuralgia : Nerve pain; untraceble origin of a pain..

Neurosis : Mental or emotional disturbance in which there is no serious disturbance of the personality.

Neuropsychiatric : Relating to neurology and psychiatry.

Neurosurgery : Surgery performed on some part of the nervous system.

Nocturia : Excess passing of urine during night.

Nostras : A disease endemic to a country.

Obese : Overweight.

Oedema : An abnormal accumulation of fluid beneath the skin or in cavities of the body (dropsy).

Oestrogen : Substance that induces oestrus or 'heat'.

Ointments : Semi-solid mixtures of medicinal substances with Lard, Benzoated Lard, Paraffin and Wool-fat, intended for external application.

Ophthalmia : Inflammation of the eye.

Ophthalmitic : Relating to eye.

Oxytocic : Promoting child birth.

Oxytocin : Extract isolated from the pituitary posterior lobe which stimulates the uterine muscle to contract.

Ozaena : A chronic disease of nose of an inflammatory nature, combined with atrophy of the mucous membrane.

Palpitation : A condition in which the heart beats forcibly or irregularly and the person becomes conscious of its action.

Pancreatitis : Inflammation of pancreas.

Paralysis : Loss of mascular power due to interference with the nervous system.

Paraplegia : Paralysis of the lower limbs accompanied by paralysis of bladder and rectum.

Parasympathetic nervous system : Part of the autonomic nervous system which is connected with the brain and spinal cord through certain nerve centres.

Parasiticide : A parasites destroying agent of preparation.

Parkinsonism : Neurological disorders characterized by hypokinesia, tremor and muscular rigidity.

Paroxysm : Spasm or seizure; symptoms that suddenly intensify or recur.

Pathogenic : Disease-producing bacteria.

Pediculicide : Destroying lice.

Perspiration : An excretion from the skin produced by the sweat glands.

Pertussis : Whooping cough.

Pestilles : A sweetened lozenge.

Pharyngitis : Inflammation of pharynx.

Phlogistic : Inflammatory.

Phthisis : Any wasting disease of whole body; pulmonary tuberculosis.

Piles : Consists of a varicose and inflamed condition of veins about the lower end of the bowel.

Pimples : Pustule of small size usually of face or neck.

Postpartum : After childbirth.

Poultice : Soft moist applications to the surface of the body.

Presor : Anything that increases the activity of a function, e.g., pressor nerve or pressor drug.

Prophylactic : Preventive, defending from or warding of disese.

Prophylaxis : Treatment for warding off disease.

Psoriasis : A chronic inflammatory disease of the skin.

Psychotomimetic : Producing manifestations resembling those of a psychosis, e.g., visual hallucination.

Pungent : Warm biting sensation.

Purgative : Drugs producing evacuation of the bowels.

Pyaemia : A form of blood-poisoning.

Pyorrhoea alveolaris : A suppurative process occurring in the suppressing tissues of the teeth.

Pyramidal : Like a triangular pyramid.

Pyrogen : A toxin that causes fever.

Refrigerants : Substances which relieve thirst and give a feeling of cooling.

Relaxant : A drug that relaxes tension, espicially of muscles.

Rennet : A substance prepared from the stomach of the calf to digest milk.

Repellant : Having the effect of driving back.

Resuscitation : Recovering from drowning.

Rheumatism : A group of diseases concerning inflammatory affections of the fibrous textures of joints, muscles and other parts.

Rhinitis : Inflammation of the mucous membrane of the nose.

Rickettsiae : A group of micro-organisms, which are intermediate between bacteria and viruses.

Rubefacient : Irritation of the skin causes congestion of the parts immediately below the skin.

Scarlatina : Relative to a contagious streptococcal disease characterized by fever, inflammation of throat and scarlet rash.

Sedative : Drugs which soothe over-excitement of the nervous system.

Septic : A substance which causes putrefaction.

Serosal : Serous membrane that covers most of the viscera of the intestine.

Sommolence : Sleepiness, drowsiness.

Somniferous : Causing or inducing sleep, as narcotic.

Soporifics : Measures which induce sleep.

Spasm : An involuntary and painful contracction of a muscle of a hollow organ with a muscular wall.

Spasmodic : Characterized by spasms; sudden and violent, but brief.

Spasmolytic : Remedies which diminish spasm.

Spermatorrhoea : Passage of semen without erection of the penis or organs.

Stiffness : A condition due to a change in the joints, ligaments, tendons, or muscles.

Stomachic : Exciting the action of stomach.

Stringent : Producing a contraction of the tissues of mouth.

Stupor : Disorder of the brain (unconsciousness)

Suppository : A small conical mass made of oil of theobroma, to which white beeswax and drugs are present and intended for introduction into the rectum.

Suppressant : An agent that stops secretion.

Suture : Closing of a wound.

Sympathomimetic : Drugs which produce on effect comparable to those produced by stimulation of the sympathetic nervous system.

Syndrome : A group of symptoms occurring together regularly and thus constituting a disease.

Syphilis : A contagious venereal disease.

Taeniacide : A remedy that destroys tapeworm.

Tetanus : A disorder of the nervous system consisting of increased excitability of the spinal cord.

Thrombosis : A universal harmless habit in infancy.

Tinnitus : A noise heard in the ear without any external cause.

Tonics : Substances given for strength and vigour to the body.

Tonsillitis : Inflammation of the tonsils.

Toxoid : A toxin whose toxic property has been eliminated.

Tranquillizer : Drug which induces a mental state free from agitation and anxiety, and renders the patient calm, serene and peaceful.

Trichuriasis : A world wide infection caused by whipworm in the tropics.

Tuberculosis : A disease of lungs or other organs due to the presence of *Mycobecterium tuberculosis.*

Typhus fever : An infective disease caused by microorganisms of the genus Rickettsia.

Ulcer : A breach on the surface of the skin or on the surface of the membrane lining any cavity within the body, which does not tend to heal quickly.

Ulceration : The action or progress or ulcerating; an ulcer or a group of ulcer.

Urethane : Ethyl carbamate.

Urethra : The tube which leads from the bladder to the exterior, and by which the urine is voided.

Urticaria : Nettle rash, chronic affection of the skin.

Uterine : Pertaining to the uterus or womb.

Vaccine : A substance of the nature of dead or attenuated living infectious material introduced into the body for increasing its power to resist or to get rid of a disease.

Vascoconstrictor : Serving to constrict blood vessels on stimulation; a drug, nerve or other agent causing constriction of blood vessels.

Venereal disease : Sexually transmitted diseases.

Vermifuge : Any substance causing expulsion of parasitic worms.

Vermine : Relating to an external animal parasite.

Vertigo : A condition in which the affected person loses the power of balancing himself.

Vesicants : Blistering agents.

Vomiting : The expulsion of the stomach contents through the mouth.

Vulnerary : Used in healing or curing wounds.

Warts : Small, solid growth, arising from the surface of the skin.

INDEX